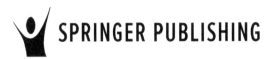 **SPRINGER PUBLISHING**

MW01029035

GET THE MOST FROM YOUR BOOK

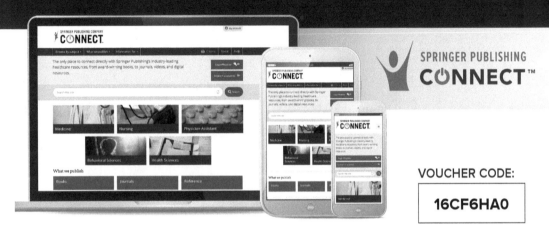

SPRINGER PUBLISHING
C⊙NNECT™

Online Access

Your print purchase of *Nurse Leadership and Management* includes **online access via Springer Publishing Connect**™ to increase accessibility, portability, and searchability.

Insert the code at https://connect.springerpub.com/content/book/978-0-8261-7795-7 today!

Having trouble? Contact our customer service department at cs@springerpub.com

Instructor Resource Access for Adopters

Let us do some of the heavy lifting to create an engaging classroom experience with a variety of instructor resources included in most textbooks SUCH AS:

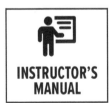

**INSTRUCTOR'S
MANUAL**

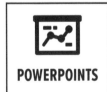

POWERPOINTS

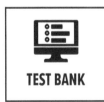

TEST BANK

Visit **https://connect.springerpub.com/** and look for the **"Show Supplementary"** button on your **book homepage** to see what is available to instructors! First time using Springer Publishing Connect?

Email **textbook@springerpub.com** to create an account and start unlocking valuable resources.

NURSE LEADERSHIP AND MANAGEMENT

Joyce J. Fitzpatrick, PhD, MBA, RN, FAAN, FNAP, FAANP(H), is director, Marian K. Shaughnessy Nurse Leadership Academy and Elizabeth Brooks Ford Professor of Nursing, Frances Payne Bolton School of Nursing, Case Western Reserve University (CWRU) in Cleveland, Ohio, where she was dean from 1982 through 1997. In 2020, she was named distinguished university professor at CWRU. She earned a BSN (Georgetown University), an MS in psychiatric-mental health nursing (The Ohio State University), a PhD in nursing (New York University), and an MBA from CWRU. Dr. Fitzpatrick has received numerous honors and awards; she was elected a fellow in the American Academy of Nursing in 1981, a fellow in the National Academies of Practice in 1996, and an honorary fellow of the American Association of Nurse Practitioners in 2019. She has received the *American Journal of Nursing* Book of the Year Award 22 times. In 2016, she was named a Living Legend by the American Academy of Nursing. In 2019, she received the Florence Nightingale International Foundation International Achievement Award in recognition of her significant achievement in influencing nursing internationally. Dr. Fitzpatrick is widely published in nursing and healthcare literature. She served as coeditor of the *Annual Review of Nursing Research* series, volumes 1 to 26. She has published several books with Springer Publishing Company, including four editions of the classic *Encyclopedia of Nursing Research (ENR)*.

Celeste M. Alfes, DNP, MSN, MBA, RN, CNE, CHSE-A, FAAN, is professor and assistant dean of academic affairs at the Frances Payne Bolton School of Nursing, Case Western Reserve University (CWRU) in Cleveland, Ohio. She earned a BSN (University of Akron), an MSN (University of Akron), a DNP (CWRU), and an MBA from CWRU. Dr. Alfes has 33 years of experience as a nurse educator and has made significant contributions pioneering simulation training including the development of North America's first high-fidelity helicopter simulator adapted for flight nurse training. Dr. Alfes is a fellow in the American Academy of Nursing; a Fulbright Specialist at the University of Rome Tor Vergata, Italy; an Inaugural Coldiron Fellow, Marian K. Shaughnessy Nurse Leadership Academy (MKSNLA), American Organization for Nursing Leadership, American Nurses Association, and Healthcare Financial Management Association; a member of the MKSNLA Founder's Circle; a recent visiting professor at the University of L'Aquila, Italy, and Aichi Medical University, Japan; and a National League for Nursing simulation leader and consultant. Dr. Alfes is a reviewer for the National Science Foundation and a regular contributor to the journals *Nurse Leader, Nursing Education Perspectives,* and *Clinical Simulation in Nursing*. Dr. Alfes has published several books with Springer Publishing Company including *Clinical Simulations for the Advanced Practice Nurse* (2020), *Innovative Strategies in Teaching Nursing* (2020), and the *Guide to Mastery in Clinical Nursing* (2019) series.

NURSE LEADERSHIP AND MANAGEMENT
Foundations for Effective Administration

Joyce J. Fitzpatrick,
PhD, MBA, RN, FAAN, FNAP, FAANP(H)

Celeste M. Alfes,
DNP, MSN, MBA, RN, CNE, CHSE-A, FAAN

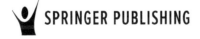

SPRINGER PUBLISHING

Springer Publishing Company, LLC
11 West 42nd Street, New York, NY 10036
www.springerpub.com
connect.springerpub.com

Executive Acquisitions Editor: Joseph Morita
Director, Content Development: Taylor Ball
Production Editor: Rachel Haines
Compositor: S4Carlisle Publishing Services

ISBN: 978-0-8261-7794-0
ebook ISBN: 978-0-8261-7795-7
DOI: 10.1891/9780826177957

SUPPLEMENTS:
Instructor Materials:

 A robust set of instructor resources designed to supplement this text is located at http://connect.springerpub.com/content/book/978-0-8261-7795-7. Qualifying instructors may request access by emailing textbook@springerpub.com.

Qualified instructors may request supplements by emailing textbook@springerpub.com
Instructor's Manual: 978-0-8261-7796-4
Instructor's PowerPoints: 978-0-8261-7797-1

22 23 24 25 26 / 5 4 3 2 1

The author and the publisher of this Work have made every effort to use sources believed to be reliable to provide information that is accurate and compatible with the standards generally accepted at the time of publication. The author and publisher shall not be liable for any special, consequential, or exemplary damages resulting, in whole or in part, from the readers' use of, or reliance on, the information contained in this book. The publisher has no responsibility for the persistence or accuracy of URLs for external or third-party internet websites referred to in this publication and does not guarantee that any content on such websites is, or will remain, accurate or appropriate.

Library of Congress Cataloging-in-Publication Data

Names: Fitzpatrick, Joyce J., 1944- author. | Alfes, Celeste M., author.
Title: Nurse leadership and management : foundations for effective
  administration / Joyce J. Fitzpatrick, PhD, MBA, RN, FAAN, FNAP,
  FAANP(H), Director, Marian K. Shaughnessy Nurse Leadership Academy,
  Elizabeth Brookes Ford Professor of Nursing, Frances Payne Bolton School
  of Nursing, Distinguished University Professor, Case Western Reserve
  University, Cleveland, Ohio, Celeste M. Alfes, DNP, MSN, MBA, RN, CNE,
  CHSE-A, FAAN, Professor, Assistant Dean for Academic Affairs, Inaugural
  Coldiron Fellow, Marian K. Shaughnessy Nurse Leadership Academy,
  American Organization for Nursing Leadership, American Nurses
  Association, Healthcare Financial Management Association, Frances Payne
  Bolton School of Nursing, Case Western Reserve University, Cleveland,
Identifiers: LCCN 2022022587 (print) | LCCN 2022022588 (ebook) | ISBN
  9780826177940 (cloth) | ISBN 9780826177957 (ebook)
Subjects: LCSH: Nursing services--Administration. | Leadership.
Classification: LCC RT89 .F537 2023 (print) | LCC RT89 (ebook) | DDC
  362.17/3068--dc23/eng/20220713
LC record available at https://lccn.loc.gov/2022022587
LC ebook record available at https://lccn.loc.gov/2022022588

Contact sales@springerpub.com to receive discount rates on bulk purchases.

Publisher's Note: New and used products purchased from third-party sellers are not guaranteed for quality, authenticity, or access to any included digital components.

Printed in the United States of America by Gasch Printing.

CONTENTS

Competencies Grid *viii*
Contributors *xiii*
Foreword Deborah Zimmermann, Erik Martin *xix*
Preface *xxi*
Acknowledgments *xxiii*
Instructor Resources *xxv*

SECTION I: INTRODUCTION

1. **Leading in Challenging Times** **3**
   Angela S. Prestia

2. **Professionalism** **31**
   Germaine C. Nelson

3. **Nurse Manager and Leader Competencies** **55**
   Linda Q. Everett and Benjamin J. Farber

SECTION II: RELATIONAL LEADERSHIP IN PRACTICE

4. **The Importance of Relationships** **73**
   Mary Beth Modic and Amy Windover

5. **Emotional Intelligence** **99**
   Mary T. Quinn Griffin and Lauraine Spano-Szekely

6. **Relationship-Based Leadership Theories** **119**
   Rosanne Raso and Rae Jean Hemway

7. **The Coaching and Mentoring Process** **147**
   M. Lisa Hedenstrom and Susan M. Dyess

SECTION III: INNOVATIVE AND EXPANDING MODELS OF CARE DELIVERY

8. **Value-Based Contracting** 171
   Kristine Adams and Nicholas Engelhardt

9. **Population and Community Health: Leveraging Leadership and Empowering Nurses to Understand and Positively Impact Social Determinants of Health** 199
   Natalia Cineas and Donna Boyle Schwartz

10. **Telehealth** 243
    Noreen B. Brennan

11. **Innovation** 259
    Cole Edmonson and Tim Raderstorf

SECTION IV: ORGANIZATIONAL ANALYSIS

12. **Structures, Processes, and Organizational Goals** 285
    Deirdre O'Flaherty and Mary Joy Garcia-Dia

13. **Strategic Development and Planning** 307
    Moreen Donahue

14. **System Perspectives for Organizations** 331
    Michele P. Holskey and Reynaldo R. Rivera

SECTION V: ESSENTIAL MANAGEMENT ISSUES

15. **Quality and Safety** 353
    Mary Cathryn Sitterding and Amy Dee Wilson

16. **Information Management and Big Data** 381
    Andrew P. Reimer

17. **Human Resource Management** 411
    MariLou Prado-Inzerillo and Bertha Ku

SECTION VI: HEALTHCARE FINANCE AND BUDGETING

18. **Macro Components of Healthcare Financing** 435
    Nathanial Schreiner and Todd Nelson

19. **Developing Financial Acumen for Nurse Leaders** 451
    Deborah J. Stilgenbauer

SECTION VII: GOVERNANCE

20. Board Leadership and Responsibilities   477
Kimberly J. Harper and Laurie S. Benson

21. Relationships Between Board and Management   503
Pamela Austin Thompson

SECTION VIII: SPECIAL TOPICS

22. Unanticipated Transitions   521
Theresa L. Champagne and Ashley M. Carlucci

23. The Nurse Leader's Role in Philanthropy   539
Kate Judge

SECTION IX: CASE STUDIES FOR NURSE MANAGERS AND EXECUTIVES

24. Comprehensive Case Studies   551
   Comprehensive Case Study 1: Human-Centered Leadership   552
      Kay Kennedy, Lucy Leclerc, and Susan Campis

   Comprehensive Case Study 2: Effective Mentoring Through Relational Leadership   555
      K. David Bailey and Joseph P. De Santis

   Comprehensive Case Study 3: Telehealth   561
      Mary Joy Garcia-Dia

   Comprehensive Case Study 4: Nurse-Led Innovation to Reduce Occupational Heat Stress of Operating Room Personnel   569
      Jill Byrne

   Comprehensive Case Study 5: Leadership to Drive Quality Through Direct-Care Nurse Feedback Using an Electronic Health Record Dashboard   575
      Anne Pohnert and Mary A. Dolansky

   Comprehensive Case Study 6: Resiliency   579
      Deirdre O'Flaherty and Mary Joy Garcia-Dia

   Comprehensive Case Study 7: Main Hospital: Perioperative Transition Unit   585
      Garry Brydges

   Comprehensive Case Study 8: Competition Within Healthcare Industry   589
      Nathanial Schreiner and Stuart D. Downs

Index   595

COMPETENCIES GRID

	Chapter	AONL Nurse Executive Competencies					AONL System CNE Competencies		
		Communication	Knowledge	Leadership	Professionalism	Business Skills	Communication	Knowledge	Leadership
1	Leading in Challenging Times	X	X	X	X	X	X	X	X
2	Professionalism	X	X	X	X		X	X	X
3	Nurse Manager and Leader Competencies	X	X	X	X	X	X	X	X
4	The Importance of Relationships	X	X	X	X		X	X	X
5	Emotional Intelligence	X	X	X			X	X	X
6	Relationship-Based Leadership Theories	X		X	X		X		X
7	The Coaching and Mentoring Process	X	X	X	X		X	X	X
8	Value-Based Contracting	X	X	X	X	X		X	X
9	Population and Community Health	X	X					X	X
10	Telehealth	X	X	X	X	X	X	X	X
11	Innovation	X	X	X	X	X	X	X	X
12	Structure, Processes, and Organizational Goals	X	X	X	X	X			
13	Strategic Development and Planning	X	X	X	X	X	X	X	X
14	System Perspectives for Organizations	X	X	X	X	X	X	X	X
15	Quality and Safety	X	X	X	X	X	X	X	X
16	Information Management and Big Data			X					X
17	Human Resource Management	X	X	X	X				
18	Macro Components of Healthcare Financing	X	X	X	X	X	X	X	X
19	Developing Financial Acumen for Nurse Leaders	X	X	X	X	X	X	X	X
20	Board Leadership and Responsibilities	X	X	X	X	X	X	X	X
21	Relationships Between Board and Management	X	X	X	X	X			
22	Unanticipated Transitions	X		X		X	X		X
23	The Nurse Leader's Role in Philanthropy	X	X	X		X	X	X	X

(continued)

		AONL Post-Acute Care Competencies					AONL Nurse Manager Competencies			AONL Nurse Executive Population Health				
Professionalism	Business Skills	Communication	Knowledge	Leadership	Professionalism	Business Skills	Science/Managing the Business	Leader Within/Creating Leader in Self	Art/Leading the People	Communication	Knowledge	Leadership	Professionalism	Business Skills
X	X	X	X	X	X	X	X	X	X	X	X	X	X	X
X		X	X	X	X			X		X	X	X	X	
X	X	X	X	X	X	X	X	X	X	X	X	X	X	X
X		X	X	X	X			X		X	X	X	X	
		X	X	X				X	X	X	X	X		
X		X		X	X			X	X	X		X	X	
X		X	X	X	X			X	X	X	X	X	X	
X	X		X	X	X	X	X				X	X	X	X
							X		X	X	X	X	X	X
X	X	X	X	X	X	X	X			X	X	X	X	X
X	X							X	X					
							X	X	X					
X	X	X	X	X	X	X	X	X	X	X	X	X	X	X
X	X	X	X	X	X	X	X	X	X	X	X	X	X	X
X	X	X	X	X	X	X	X	X	X					
							X							
							X	X	X					
X	X						X	X	X					
X	X						X	X	X					
X	X	X	X	X	X	X	X	X	X	X	X	X	X	X
							X	X	X					
X	X						X	X	X					
X	X	X	X	X	X	X		X	X	X	X	X	X	X

(Additional competencies on next spread)

	Chapter (*repeated for convenience*)	AACN Essentials: Domains for Nursing Education							
		Knowledge for Nursing Practice	Person-Centered Care	Population Health	Scholarship for Nursing Practice	Quality and Safety	Interprofessional Partnerships	Systems-Based Practice	Information and Healthcare Technologies
1	Leading in Challenging Times								
2	Professionalism	X	X			X	X		
3	Nurse Manager and Leader Competencies	X					X		
4	The Importance of Relationships	X	X				X		
5	Emotional Intelligence								
6	Relationship Based Leadership Theories						X		
7	The Coaching and Mentoring Process	X	X				X		
8	Value-Based Contracting	X		X			X	X	
9	Population and Community Health	X	X	X		X	X	X	
10	Telehealth	X	X	X	X	X	X	X	X
11	Innovation								
12	Structure, Processes, and Organizational Goals	X				X	X	X	X
13	Strategic Development and Planning								
14	System Perspectives for Organizations	X	X	X	X	X	X	X	
15	Quality and Safety	X	X	X	X	X	X	X	
16	Information Management and Big Data					X			X
17	Human Resource Management								
18	Macro Components of Healthcare Financing	X				X	X		
19	Developing Financial Acumen for Nurse Leaders	X				X	X		
20	Board Leadership and Responsibilities	X	X	X	X	X	X	X	X
21	Relationships Between Board and Management	X	X			X	X	X	
22	Unanticipated Transitions								
23	The Nurse Leader's Role in Philanthropy						X		

(continued)

Professionalism	Personal, Professional, and Leadership Development	AACN Concepts Woven through the AACN Domains									QSEN Graduate Level Competencies					
		Clinical Judgement	Communication	Compassionate Care	Determinants of Health	Diversity, Equity, and Inclusion	Ethics	Evidence-Based Practice	Health Policy	Social Determinants of Health	Patient-Centered Care	Teamwork and Collaboration	Evidence-Based Practice	Quality Improvement	Safety	Informatics
X	X	X	X			X	X	X		X		X	X			
X	X		X									X	X	X		
X	X		X	X		X					X	X				
X			X										X			
X	X		X			X	X						X			
X	X	X	X	X			X	X					X	X	X	X
					X		X		X			X	X	X		X
	X	X		X	X	X		X	X	X	X	X	X	X	X	
X	X	X	X	X	X	X	X	X	X	X	X	X	X	X	X	X
X	X		X			X	X	X	X			X	X	X	X	X
X	X	X	X	X	X	X	X	X			X	X	X	X	X	
X	X	X	X	X			X	X	X		X	X	X	X	X	X
								X			X	X		X		X
X	X	X	X					X								
X	X	X	X					X	X		X	X	X		X	X
X	X	X	X					X	X		X	X	X		X	X
X	X	X	X	X	X	X	X	X	X	X		X	X	X	X	X
X	X		X				X						X		X	X
X	X			X	X								X		X	

CONTRIBUTORS

Kristine Adams, MSN, CNP   Associate Chief Nursing Officer, Care Management & Ambulatory Services, Cleveland Clinic, Cleveland, Ohio

K. David Bailey, PhD, MBA, MSN, RN, CCRN-K, NEA-BC, FACHE   Chief Nursing Officer, UCLA Health – Santa Monica Medical Center, Santa Monica, California, President, Association for Leadership Science in Nursing, Birmingham, Alabama

Laurie S. Benson, BSN   Nurse Entrepreneur, Executive Director, Nurses on Boards Coalition, Monona, Wisconsin

Noreen B. Brennan, PhD, RN-BC, NEA-BC   Chief Nurse Executive, James J. Peters VA Medical Center, Bronx, New York, Inaugural Coldiron Fellow, Marian K. Shaughnessy Nurse Leadership Academy, Frances Payne Bolton School of Nursing, Case Western Reserve University, American Organization for Nursing Leadership, American Nurses Association, Healthcare Financial Management Association, Cleveland, Ohio

Garry Brydges, PhD, DNP, MBA, CRNA, ACNP-BC, FAANA, FAAN   Chief Nurse Anesthetist, Department of Anesthesia, Critical Care, and Pain Medicine, University of Texas MD Anderson Cancer Center, Houston, Texas, Inaugural Coldiron Fellow, Marian K. Shaughnessy Nurse Leadership Academy, Frances Payne Bolton School of Nursing, Case Western Reserve University, American Organization for Nursing Leadership, American Nurses Association, Healthcare Financial Management Association, Cleveland, Ohio

Jill Byrne, PhD, RN, CNOR   Assistant Professor, Frances Payne Bolton School of Nursing, Case Western Reserve University, Visiting Nurse Researcher, Anesthesia Outcomes Research, Cleveland Clinic, Cleveland, Ohio

Susan Campis, MSN, RN, NE-BC   Senior Principal, Chief Wellness Officer, uLeadership, Atlanta, Georgia

Ashley M. Carlucci, MSN, MHA, RN, CEN   Chief Nursing Officer, University Hospitals East & West Market, Cleveland, Ohio, Miller Fellow, Marian K. Shaughnessy Nurse Leadership Academy, Frances Payne Bolton School of Nursing, Case Western Reserve University, Cleveland, Ohio

Theresa L. Champagne, DNP, MSN, RN, CNOR   Former Chief Nursing Officer, LRG Healthcare, Laconia, New Hampshire, Miller Fellow, Marian K. Shaughnessy Nurse Leadership Academy, Frances Payne Bolton School of Nursing, Case Western Reserve University, American Organization for Nursing Leadership, American Nurses Association, Cleveland, Ohio

Natalia Cineas, DNP, RN, NEA-BC, FAAN Senior Vice President, Chief Nursing Executive, Co-Chair, Equity and Access Council, New York City Health + Hospitals, New York, New York, Inaugural Samuel H. and Maria Miller Foundation Fellow, Marian K. Shaughnessy Nurse Leadership Academy, Frances Payne Bolton School of Nursing, Case Western Reserve University, Coldiron Fellow, Marian K. Shaughnessy Nurse Leadership Academy, Frances Payne Bolton School of Nursing, Case Western Reserve University, American Organization for Nursing Leadership, American Nurses Association, Healthcare Financial Management Association, Cleveland, Ohio

Joseph P. De Santis, PhD, APRN, ACRN, FAAN Associate Professor, University of Miami School of Nursing and Health Studies, Coral Gables, Florida

Mary A. Dolansky, PhD, RN, FAAN Sarah C. Hirsh Endowed Professorship in Nursing, Director, Sarah Cole Hirsh Institute for Best Nursing Practices Based on Evidence, Member, Founder's Circle, Marian K. Shaughnessy Nurse Leadership Academy, Frances Payne Bolton School of Nursing, Case Western Reserve University, Coldiron Fellow, Marian K. Shaughnessy Nurse Leadership Academy, American Organization for Nursing Leadership, American Nurses Association, Healthcare Financial Management Association, Cleveland, Ohio

Moreen Donahue, DNP, RN, FAAN, NEA-BC Former System CNE, Western Connecticut Health Network, Danbury, Connecticut, Member, Founder's Circle, Adjunct Faculty, Marian K. Shaughnessy Nurse Leadership Academy, Frances Payne Bolton School of Nursing, Case Western Reserve University, Cleveland, Ohio

Stuart D. Downs, DNP, RN, NEA-BC, CENP, CPHQ, FACHE, FAONL Nursing Administrator, Northside Hospital Gwinnett, Lawrenceville, Georgia, Inaugural Coldiron Fellow, Marian K. Shaughnessy Nurse Leadership Academy, Frances Payne Bolton School of Nursing, Case Western Reserve University, American Organization for Nursing Leadership, American Nurses Association, Healthcare Financial Management Association, Cleveland, Ohio

Susan M. Dyess, PhD, RN, NE-BC, AHN-BC Professor of Nursing and Associate Dean, Wellstar College of Health and Human Services, Kennesaw State University, Kennesaw, Georgia

Cole Edmonson, DNP, RN, NEA-BC, FACHE, FAONL, FNAP, FAAN Chief Clinical Officer, AMN Healthcare Inc., Coppell, Texas

Nicholas Engelhardt, MBA Senior Product Owner, Interoperability Solutions, MCG Health, Part of Hearst Health Network, Cleveland, Ohio

Linda Q. Everett, PhD, RN, NEA-BC, FAAN, FAONL Professor, Member, Founder's Circle, Marian K. Shaughnessy Nurse Leadership Academy, Frances Payne Bolton School of Nursing, Case Western Reserve University, Cleveland, Ohio

Benjamin J. Farber, DNP, RN, CNL, NEA-BC, CENP Vice President Patient Care Services and Chief Nursing Officer, Eisenhower Health, Rancho Mirage, California, Miller Fellow, Inaugural Coldiron Fellow, Marian K. Shaughnessy Nurse Leadership Academy, Frances Payne Bolton School of Nursing, Case Western Reserve University, American Organization for Nursing Leadership, American Nurses Association, Healthcare Financial Management Association, Cleveland, Ohio

Mary Joy Garcia-Dia, DNP, RN, FAAN Program Director, Nursing Informatics, Information Technology Department, New York-Presbyterian Hospital, New York, New York, Member, Founder's Circle, Inaugural Coldiron Fellow, Marian K. Shaughnessy Nurse Leadership Academy, Frances Payne Bolton School of Nursing, Case Western Reserve University, American Organization for Nursing Leadership, American Nurses Association, Healthcare Financial Management Association, Cleveland, Ohio

Mary T. Quinn Griffin, PhD, RN, FAAN, ANEF The May L. Wykle Endowed Professor and Associate Dean for Global Affairs, Frances Payne Bolton School of Nursing, Case Western Reserve University, Cleveland, Ohio

Kimberly J. Harper, MS, RN, FAAN CEO, Indiana Center for Nursing and Indiana Action Coalition, Board Chair Emeritus, Nurses on Boards Coalition, Indianapolis, Indiana

M. Lisa Hedenstrom, PhD, RN, MBA, NEA-BC Assistant Professor of Nursing, Wellstar School of Nursing, Wellstar College of Health and Human Services, Kennesaw State University, Kennesaw, Georgia

Rae Jean Hemway, MPA, BSN, RN, RNC-NIC Director of Nursing-Department of Pediatrics, Komansky Children's Hospital/Alexandra Cohen Hospital for Women & Newborns, New York-Presbyterian/Weill Cornell Medical Center, New York, New York

Michele P. Holskey, DNP, RN, NEA-BC Magnet Program Director, NewYork-Presbyterian Westchester Behavioral Health Center, NewYork-Presbyterian Weill Cornell Medical Center Psychiatry Program, Gracie Square Hospital, New York, New York

Kate Judge, BA Executive Director, American Nurses Foundation, Silver Spring, Maryland

Kay Kennedy, DNP, RN, NEA-BC, CPHQ Senior Clinical Instructor, Nell Hodgson Woodruff School of Nursing, Emory University, Chief Executive Officer, uLeadership, Atlanta, Georgia

Bertha Ku, DNP, MPH, RN, NEA-BC Director of Nursing, NewYork–Presbyterian/The Allen Hospital, New York, New York

Lucy Leclerc, PhD, RN, NPD-BC Assistant Professor, Massachusetts General Hospital, Institute of Health Professions, Boston, Massachusetts, Chief Learning Officer, uLeadership, Atlanta, Georgia

Mary Beth Modic, DNP, APRN-CNS, CDCES, FAAN Clinical Nurse Specialist, Office of Advanced Practice, Cleveland Clinic, Member, Founder's Circle, Coldiron Fellow, Marian K. Shaughnessy Nurse Leadership Academy, Frances Payne Bolton School of Nursing, Case Western Reserve University, American Organization for Nursing Leadership, American Nurses Association, Healthcare Financial Management Association, Cleveland, Ohio

Germaine C. Nelson, DNP, MBA, RN, NEA-BC, CPXP, CEN Director of Nursing, Icahn School of Medicine at Mount Sinai, New York, New York, Member, Founder's Circle, Coldiron Fellow, Marian K. Shaughnessy Nurse Leadership Academy, Frances Payne Bolton School of Nursing, Case Western Reserve University, American Organization for Nursing Leadership, American Nurses Association, Healthcare Financial Management Association, Cleveland, Ohio

Todd Nelson, MBA, FHFMA   Chief Partnership Executive, Healthcare Financial Management Association, Westchester, Illinois, Collaborative Partner, Coldiron Fellowship Program, Marian K. Shaughnessy Nurse Leadership Academy, Frances Payne Bolton School of Nursing, Case Western Reserve University, American Organization for Nursing Leadership, American Nurses Association, Healthcare Financial Management Association, Cleveland, Ohio

Deirdre O'Flaherty, DNP, MSN, APN-BC, NEA-BC, ONC, FFNMRCSI   Senior Director Patient Care, Lenox Hill Hospital, Northwell Health, New York, New York, Member, Founder's Circle, Marian K. Shaughnessy Nurse Leadership Academy, Frances Payne Bolton School of Nursing, Case Western Reserve University, Cleveland, Ohio

Anne Pohnert, MSN, RN, FNP-BC   Lead Director of Clinical Quality, MinuteClinic, Woonsocket, Rhode Island

MariLou Prado-Inzerillo, DNP, RN, NEA-BC   Vice President, Nursing Operations, NewYork–Presbyterian, New York, New York, Member, Founder's Circle, Marian K. Shaughnessy Nurse Leadership Academy, Frances Payne Bolton School of Nursing, Case Western Reserve University, Cleveland, Ohio

Angela S. Prestia, PhD, RN, NE-BC   Director of Patient Care, Trustbridge Hospice and Palliative Care, West Palm Beach, Florida, Adjunct Professor of Nursing, Christine E. Lynn College of Nursing, Florida Atlantic University, Consultant, Marian K. Shaughnessy Nurse Leadership Academy, Adjunct Professor of Nursing, Frances Payne Bolton School of Nursing, Case Western Reserve University, Cleveland, Ohio, President-Elect, Association for Leadership Science in Nursing (ALSN), Boca Raton, Florida

Tim Raderstorf, DNP, RN, FAAN   College of Nursing, The Ohio State University, Columbus, Ohio

Rosanne Raso, DNP, RN, NEA-BC, FAAN, FAONL   Chief Nursing Officer and Vice President, New York-Presbyterian/Weill Cornell Medical Center, New York, New York, Editor-in-Chief, *Nursing Management*, Member, Founder's Circle, Marian K. Shaughnessy Nurse Leadership Academy, Frances Payne Bolton School of Nursing, Case Western Reserve University, Cleveland, Ohio

Andrew P. Reimer, PhD, RN, CFRN   Assistant Professor, Frances Payne Bolton School of Nursing, Case Western Reserve University, Research Coordinator, Transport Nurse, Critical Care Transport, Cleveland Clinic, Cleveland, Ohio

Reynaldo R. Rivera, DNP, RN, NEA-BC, FAAN   Director of Nursing Research and Innovation, Center for Professional Nursing Practice, Department of Nursing, New York-Presbyterian, New York, New York, Member, Founder's Circle, Marian K. Shaughnessy Nurse Leadership Academy, Frances Payne Bolton School of Nursing, Case Western Reserve University, Cleveland, Ohio

Nathanial Schreiner, PhD, MBA, RN   Assistant Professor, Faculty, Marian K. Shaughnessy Nurse Leadership Academy, Frances Payne Bolton School of Nursing, Case Western Reserve University, Cleveland, Ohio

Donna Boyle Schwartz, MSJ, BSJ   Assistant Director—Marketing, Office of Patient Centered Care, Nursing Administration New York City Health + Hospitals, New York, New York

Mary Cathryn Sitterding, PhD, RN, CNS, FAAN Vice President, Nursing Quality and Regulatory Affairs, Ascension, St. Louis, Missouri

Lauraine Spano-Szekely, DNP, MBA, BSN, RN, NEA-BC Vice President Nursing and Patient Care Services, NYU Langone Health, New York, New York, Member, Founder's Circle, Marian K. Shaughnessy Nurse Leadership Academy, Frances Payne Bolton School of Nursing, Case Western Reserve University, Cleveland, Ohio

Deborah J. Stilgenbauer, DNP, MA, RN, NEA-BC Sigma Theta Tau, Trusted Health Care Advisory Council, Consultant, Greater New York Hospital Association (GNYHA), 1199SEIU League Training and Upgrading Fund, Member, Founder's Circle, Marian K. Shaughnessy Nurse Leadership Academy, Frances Payne Bolton School of Nursing, Case Western Reserve University, Cleveland, Ohio

Pamela Austin Thompson, MS, RN, FAAN Chair, System Value/Quality Committee, Member, Dartmouth Health Board of Trustees, Manassas, Virginia

Amy Dee Wilson, DNP, RN, CPHQ Senior Vice President, Nursing Center of Excellence, Ascension, St. Louis, Missouri

Amy Windover, PhD Clinical Psychologist, Home Based Primary Care, VA Northeast Ohio Healthcare System, Cleveland, Ohio

FOREWORD

Around the world, nurses confront the unknown with grace and grit. In the face of uncertainty, we lean in with a spirit of inquiry, fueling innovation, research, and exponential changes in practice across the care continuum. As the most trusted profession, we convene key stakeholders and collaborate to identify solutions supporting seamless care for our patients.

Now is the time to recognize nurses as full partners in national healthcare policy making and redesign. The COVID-19 pandemic exposed disparities in the United States and required swift action to eliminate barriers to care. Without skipping a beat, nurses pivoted and were at the forefront of reshaping care delivery and leading innovations that demonstrated significant outcomes and positive impact. Nurses are change agents and expanding our influence will facilitate the expansion of these advances and promote programs providing effective, efficient, equitable, and accessible care.

As a profession, we are at a tipping point. We are in a position to successfully influence and lead the redesign of healthcare. Nurses must be experts in organizational analysis, leadership theory, the changing dynamics of healthcare, healthcare finance, governance, and the use of data. Elevating the health of our communities requires us to build relationships and to be adept at leading innovation.

The authors of these chapters—and editors Joyce J. Fitzpatrick and Celeste M. Alfes— are the thought leaders of the largest profession on Earth. They are innovators, strategists, provocateurs, transformational leaders, and compassionate clinicians. Their advice is based on evidence and years of experience and serves as a guide for leaders to overcome constraints and lead the nation to better health. While the content is foundational for new leaders and executives, the advice from these leaders is an inspiration to all.

Deborah Zimmermann, DNP, RN, NEA-BC, FAAN
Chief Executive Officer, DAISY Foundation
President-Elect, American Organization for Nursing Leadership
Anacortes, Washington
Global Advisory Board Member
Marian K. Shaughnessy Nurse Leadership Academy
Cleveland, Ohio

Erik Martin, DNP, RN, CENP
VP, Patient Care Services, and Chief Nursing Officer
Norton Children's Hospital
President, American Organization for Nursing Leadership
Louisville, Kentucky
Inaugural Coldiron Fellow, Marian K. Shaughnessy Nurse Leadership Academy
Frances Payne Bolton School of Nursing
Case Western Reserve University
American Organization for Nursing Leadership
American Nurses Association, Healthcare Financial Management Association
Cleveland, Ohio

PREFACE

We have been teaching leadership for years, both formally and informally, modeling the way for new nurse leaders at all levels. We have been encouraged by the leadership roles that graduates have assumed, charting new territory in healthcare delivery, in academic leadership, and in policy changes within society. We firmly believe that management and leadership skills can be taught. This conviction, and the fact that there was no comprehensive leadership and management book that met our teaching needs, led us to prepare this book. Graduate nursing students in management and leadership courses will benefit from the wisdom imparted in each chapter by distinguished nurse leaders. We know that this book will lead to substantial changes in how nurses view themselves and the leadership roles they can embrace in the future.

There are some unique features of the book that we believe are noteworthy. While we have embedded the content within the American Organization for Nursing Leadership core competencies for nurse managers and leaders, we have gone beyond these competencies. Each chapter also includes attention to the American Association of Colleges of Nursing Essentials for master's and doctoral education. We have included nine sections; each chapter within the section follows a structured format, a feature that is especially useful to beginning graduate students. The sections are Introduction (leading in challenging times, professionalism, and descriptions of the core competencies); Relational Leadership in Practice (relational leadership theories, emotional intelligence, coaching and mentoring); Innovative and Expanding Models of Care Delivery (social determinants of health, telehealth, value-based contracting, and innovation and entrepreneurship); Organizational Analysis (goals and strategic planning); Essential Management Issues (quality and safety, information management, and human resource management); Healthcare Finance and Budgeting (macro and micro financial planning); Governance (board leadership and management); Special Topics (unexpected transitions and the nurse's role in philanthropy); and Case Studies for Nurse Managers and Executives (extensive case studies on selected topics).

We are convinced that this work will make a significant contribution to the preparation of future leaders in nursing and healthcare. We look forward to significant outcomes in the years to come.

Joyce J. Fitzpatrick
Celeste M. Alfes

ACKNOWLEDGMENTS

We are indebted to the chapter authors who have shared their expertise, often within a compressed schedule. They have shared their knowledge, much of which was gained through extensive clinical leadership careers. All of the authors were cognizant of the need for graduate students and aspiring leaders to benefit from experienced leaders in the field. Thus, each chapter includes real-life management and leadership scenarios, constructed to guide the students' learning.

We also wish to acknowledge the many graduate students who participated through comprehensive reviews of the literature for selected topics and assistance in preparing materials for use in the accompanying materials. We hope that in doing so they enriched their own knowledge of the state of the science and the practice of leadership and management in nursing.

Also, special thanks to the publishing team at Springer Publishing, to Joe Morita, Taylor Ball, and Hannah Hicks. Each contributed their expertise to enhance the quality of this book and, along the way, provided the encouragement to move toward a high-quality book.

Thank you, all.

INSTRUCTOR RESOURCES

A robust set of resources designed to supplement this text is located at http://connect
.springerpub.com. Qualifying instructors may request access by emailing textbook@
springerpub.com.

Available resources include:

- **Instructor Manual:**
  - Teaching strategies
  - Discussion questions
  - Learning exercises
- **Chapter-Based PowerPoint Presentations**

SECTION I
INTRODUCTION

CHAPTER 1

LEADING IN CHALLENGING TIMES

Angela S. Prestia

"The only thing to fear is fear itself!"

President Franklin Delano Roosevelt

LEARNING OBJECTIVES

- Summarize the importance of perpetual readiness.
- Demonstrate understanding of the concept and complexities of courageous caring.
- Experiment with strategies to approach failed predictions and daily challenges.
- Create a mission critical checklist for daily use.

INTRODUCTION

Leadership takes courage; the courage that is steeped in caring so much, there is a primal "call to action." The desire to care is an essential component of nursing leadership. Boykin and Schoenhofer (2001) discuss the importance of caring leadership as the foundation for the actualization of those nursed. Courageous caring is the framework guiding the art of leading in challenging times.

In his seminal work, *On Caring*, Mayeroff (1971) identifies courage as the main ingredient for leading into the unknown. "The greater the sense of going into the unknown, the more courage is called for in caring" (p. 35). Consider if you will what has been identified as the "Moses effect" (Porter-O'Grady, 2011). Moses led the Israelites into the wilderness in search of freedom and the Promised Land. We may remember the miraculous manner with which he parted the Red Sea. This was not a leadership moment. The true leadership moments occurred when he quelled their grumbling and complaints (Rev. A. Lacy, personal communication, December 9, 2020). His courage was exemplified when he gave them strength to forge ahead, despite their hunger, weariness, and desire to return to Egypt. He negotiated a second chance for them after they had broken the Covenant by worshipping a false idol. These examples of courageous leadership are steeped in caring. He places his people first.

George Washington exemplified the perfect combination of courageous and caring leadership. "In his own day he was seen as the indispensable man, the American Moses" (Stazesky, 2000, p. 1). His desire to forge a new nation caused him to leave his very comfortable life. Washington led and his men followed in conditions incompatible with human existence: frigid cold, exhaustion, and hunger. His reputation as an ethical, caring, steadfast leader was reciprocated with their belief in him. He showed immense courage.

Lillian Wald was a nurse activist who lived at the turn of the 20th century. This time period was no less challenging than the present time. Scientific discoveries and technical advances flooded the country (Miami Dade College, n.d.). The invention of electricity, the automobile, and radio radicalized daily living. Social reform, however, did not keep pace. Lillian Wald's response was to courageously care. She cast aside her comfort and privilege (Rothberg, n.d.).

Recognizing that the densely populated, poorly lit, and unventilated "tenement" houses on Manhattan's Lower East Side were vectors for the proliferation of disease, Lilian Wald's focus became singular. The Spanish flu pandemic served to magnify the need for improving substandard living conditions. Her name is synonymous with public health. She garnered social and financial support creating the Visiting Nurses Association of New York City, as well as the Henry Street Settlement house. This urban development, criticized by many, became a place of refuge, healthcare, education, and dreams fulfilled. This incredibly courageous and caring nurse continued her advocacy for women, children, and nursing until her death.

Courage is described by Enright and White (2012) as unwavering commitment, necessary for positive change and forward progress. Leadership requires a boldness that is exemplified through advocacy in spite of contrary conditions or opinions. Nurse leaders require courage to enter the healthcare wilderness. The current milieu is fraught with the unknown. Daily events can bring challenges never imagined. Pandemics, artificial intelligence, gene-mapping, ethical dilemmas, psychological strain, human and material resource shortages, and illicit designer drug use all contribute to this unchartered and dangerous landscape. The courageous nurse leader readies themself as a warrior but not for battle. Their quest is one of knowledge: how better to lead. The warrior has significant resolve, which drives determination (Prestia, 2020a). The warrior is courageous; "guardian of society, of the people served" (p. 163). The reason for this is simple: they care about people.

This chapter discusses the dynamics of courageous caring as an essential element for leading in challenging times. It is not a chapter solely focused on leading during a crisis. There is a distinct difference. Although crises may cause challenges, they may be singular events (e.g., a hurricane, a bus casualty, or an overcrowded obstetrical department). Challenging times are more enduring, a prolonged time of existing and living, with the tumultuous nature of healthcare fueled by societal issues. Examples of this may be governmental regulations, unconscious bias, the increasing numbers of Alzheimer's disease diagnoses, human trafficking, artificial intelligence, or a new variant strain of virus (Pennic, 2019; Prestia, 2020a). This chapter includes the exploration of character, preparation, and the importance of leadership self-care required to sustain staff, patients, and person, into perpetuity. It provides useful tools that can be operationalized daily to guide leadership decisions during challenging times. Most importantly, it examines leadership purpose, prioritizing the precious responsibility of serving all people with courageous care.

LEADERSHIP CHARACTER

Good leaders are relatively easy to identify. They exhibit certain behaviors that encourage the heart of their followers to envision forward progress and eventual goal attainment. It is not difficult to be a good leader when times are plentiful, and routines are predictable. Challenging times require phenomenal leaders, courageous caring leaders—those who are not brave for a solitary, defined moment, but those who exhibit "guts and nerve" along with the mental and moral fortitude to "venture, persevere, and withstand danger, fear, or difficulty" (Enright & White, 2012, p. 807).

It is difficult to comprehend the essence of courageous caring leadership. What ethereal forces combine to create such character? There is a palpable difference, an indelible mark per se, a *"je ne sais quoi,"* an aura of unrelentless commitment to those served, despite the recognition of potential self-consequences. The desire to place oneself in a precarious position to make a difference is an amalgamation of familial values, early influences, and life experiences. Love, empathy, compassion, and an understanding of the human connection to be responsible for others forms the essence of a courageous leader. This understanding was evidenced by the Chief of the World Health Organization (WHO), Tedros Adhanom Ghebreyesus, when discussing lessons learned from the COVID-19 pandemic: ". . . attempts to improve human health are 'doomed' without tackling climate change and animal welfare . . . The pandemic has highlighted the intimate links between the health of humans, animals, and planet" (France24, 2020, pp. 1–2). Not only does this statement demonstrate an understanding of connection, it exemplifies leadership that is courageously caring.

A hallmark of nursing leadership character is the foundational importance of courageous caring. Caring nursing theorists establish a unique dimension to the profession. Their theories have been affirmed through research and positively impact patient outcomes (Dyess et al., 2010). The nurse leader understands the importance of this evidence and works to synthesize its essence into practice. The nature of the courageous nurse leader compels them to intentionally connect with staff. Each encounter is valuable and meaningful, facilitating the co-creation of caring relationships (Boykin & Schoenhofer, 2001; Watson, 2006). The collective intra-disciplinary staff longs for leadership that understands their basic human needs: food, shelter, safety, and socialization (McLeod, 2020; Figure 1.1). They work because they have a plethora of responsibilities, including families to feed, homes to maintain, and tuition to pay. They expect leadership behaviors that preserve their livelihood.

MORAL CHARACTER

In the previous scenarios, the nurse leader potentially risks livelihood to ensure evidence-based processes are not compromised. The willingness to take risk-laden action is described as moral courage (Corley, 2002). This is an essential leadership characteristic required for challenging times. The American Nurses Association's (ANA's) Code of Ethics includes a provision requiring the articulation of nursing values. Courageously caring nurse leaders are obligated to preserve the integrity of the profession (ANA, 2015). They are held to a higher level of ethical standards.

Through the exhibition of moral actions, nurse leaders help to reduce staff confliction (Edmonson, 2010). This encourages behaviors of courageous advocacy for patients. When staff recognize moral action by their leaders it becomes a cultural norm. A climate where truth can be spoken without fear can benefit the leaders in the face of uncertainty. The leader needs to hear the truth from staff, "The emperor has no clothes" (Christian-Andersen, 1998)! This candidness can potentially reduce negative consequences (Edmonson, 2010). It is reciprocal in nature and a true reflection of leadership moral courage.

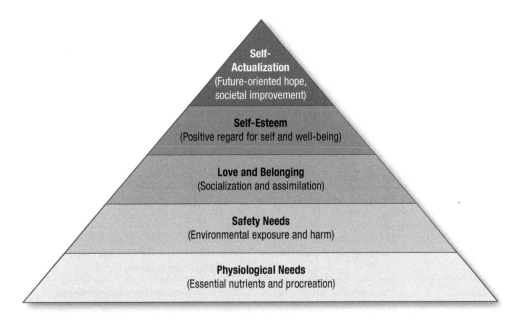

FIGURE 1.1: Maslow's hierarchy of needs.

Source: Adapted from Maslow, A. H. (1969). *Psychology of science: A reconnaissance.* Maurice Bassett Publishing.

Although the discussion scenarios are specific examples of morally courageous actions, "leadership character is not just seen in leaders' behaviors related to crisis, in the presence of stress, or in situations involving an ethical dilemma; it shows up in all behaviors and in *everything they do or fail to do*" (Klann, 2007, p. 7).

AUTHENTIC PRESENCE/CARING COMPORTMENT

"Showing up" is literally what courageous caring leaders do to connect with staff. Being available and responsive to the needs of the staff is paramount to leading at any time, not just during times of particular challenge. This means that leaders are fully and authentically present. They are committed, fully engaged, and connected to staff. Staff cannot be expected to follow an absent leader (Prestia & Dyess, 2020).

There are several strategies for living leadership presence. Prestia (2016a, 2016b) melds the work of nurse theorist Marilyn Ray (1997) and economist Sylvia Hewlett (2014) to examine three important elements of caring leadership comportment. In basic language, these three elements are: how you act, how you speak, and how you look.

How You Act

How a leader acts is a reflection on the leader's integrity. It contributes to 67% of living leadership presence. It includes the courageous behavior of decisiveness and the caring behavior of gracefulness. Purposefully rounding is an example of caring action. During rounds, the leader has an opportunity to engage with staff, giving of self by listening to staff frustrations or actually visualizing issues of concern. How powerful the message of care if the nurse leader solves the problem immediately. If the issue is unable to be resolved during rounds, accountable, timely follow-up is essential to building trust.

How You Speak

The second element of authentic presence is how a leader speaks. This element accounts for 28% of leadership comportment (Hewlett, 2014). Oral communication is mindful of tone, body language, and the critical element of holding the audience's attention. Conveying important information affecting the entire staff should not be left to assistants or subordinates. Crucial conversation must be messaged by the leader. Staff expect and deserve truthful, mindful, relevant, and trustworthy messaging (Prestia, 2016a, 2016b; see Table 1.1). The effective leader portrays courageous caring through the mindful understanding of the audience's needs, especially at times of challenge.

How You Look

Speaking in front of an anxious audience requires self-respect. When all eyes are on the leader, appearance must be dignified and confident. Although, the third element of authentic

TABLE 1.1: Impactful Messaging

Messaging Type	Definition	Example
Truthful	Verify the facts knowing that they can be fluid	"As of the end of quarter 1, HCAHPS scores for *Nurse Listened* exceeded the target!"
Mindful	Consideration for the composition of the audience	"I realize the majority of the ICU staff in attendance have over 10 years' experience in the critical care specialty."
Relevant	Messages that speak directly to the individual or audience	"I want to publicly thank the emergency department staff for their performance during the recent *Code Black*."

HCAHPS, Hospital Consumer Assessment of Healthcare Providers and Systems.

presence—how you look—only contributes 5% to total comportment, its impact is major (Prestia, 2016a, 2016b). It is the first filter from which intent is determined. If the leader appears disheveled or casually attired, the subconscious impression may damage credibility. Appearance does require context. If the leader has been at the helm of the hurricane command center for 24 hours, then staff will be more forgiving of appearance. However, if the leader is addressing a prescheduled quarterly "all-staff town hall" slovenly in appearance, staff may be less than inspired. Appearance is "a sign of legitimacy and identity" (Roach, 2002, p. 65).

SELF-CARE

The elements of authentically present leadership require caring for self as a prerequisite to caring for others. Self-care was found to be an intentional practice for nurse leaders (Dyess et al., 2015). This means it is not something a leader thinks about doing if and when there is time. It is an engrained way of being. It is proactive attention to the health cues of mind, body, and spirit. In its basic form, it is the intentional practice of proper nutrition, hydration, physical and mental rest, exercise, and the expression of gratitude. Self-care provides comfort, nourishes resiliency, and sustains a leader's well-being. It is discussed in further detail later in the chapter.

Leading in challenging times requires foundational character work. Successful leaders consciously prepare to ensure the harmonious alignment of behaviors necessary to ensure ethical decision-making. Detailed awareness of authentic leadership presence is required to connect with staff. When pressures mount, there can be no vacillation as to the correct path to follow.

◼ WHAT EVERY NURSE EXECUTIVE NEEDS TO KNOW

Courageous caring leadership requires the authentic presence of an engaged nurse executive. Existing in chaos, staff expect their leader to be available and ready to honestly message the situation. The leader is self-aware and models behaviors they expect their staff to reciprocate.

◼ WHAT EVERY NURSE MANAGER NEEDS TO KNOW

The nurse manager balances the needs of the patient with the needs of the staff. There will be times of uncertainty; however, when in doubt, keep the patient central to the decision. Remember that leadership is a journey requiring life-long learning.

PREPARING FOR CHALLENGES

The daunting reality is that healthcare challenges are endless. They are ever evolving and often unimaginable. Over the last 40 years, rapid growth of technology has created profound ethical issues. An unprecedented global pandemic has forced changes in treatment and care modalities. The cumulative forces of economic volatility, climate change, terrorism on American soil, social unrest, and political division continue to erode the already vulnerable mind, body, and spirit that is human health.

Being prepared for the unthinkable may seem impossible. There are, however, strategies that courageous caring leaders can employ, as Moses and Washington did, to position their teams to face the unknown.

PREPAREDNESS REQUIRES LEADERSHIP INVESTMENT

Preparedness requires a state of readiness, of being proactive and not reactive. Vulnerabilities need to be identified and planned for by leaders and staff (DiSciullo et al., 2021). The confluence of challenges does not allow the leader to select and tackle one problem at a time.

This may be a key difference between leading during a singular crisis versus leading in challenging times. Although crises have moving parts, there is one over-arching problem. Chaos may be time limited. Alternately, challenging times create diverse complexities that disallow leadership the luxury of a singular focus.

Leaders need to invest in being prepared. There is a myriad of investments that need to be considered. The leader invests in themselves, in human and material resources, in relationships, and in capacity and contingency planning (Arnold et al., 2006; Lee et al., 2019). There is precedent and context that can be provided to initiate and sustain an investment plan for leading in complex challenging times.

INVESTING IN SELF

Advanced education is required to understand the enormity of complex issues defining healthcare. Accessing existing frameworks and resources for venturing into the unknown requires knowledge and skill. The American Organization for Nursing Leadership (AONL) is a nursing association dedicated to the preparation and advancement of nurse leaders at all levels (2021). Their position statement on education endorses nurse leaders to be minimally prepared with a bachelor's degree or master's degree in nursing (American Organization of Nurse Executives, 2015). It further recommends that those seeking the nurse executive roles be prepared at the doctoral level.

Certification adds another dimension to the nurse leader's educational preparation. Achieving certification validates a leader's knowledge and skills against a rigorous set of national standards (American Association of Critical-Care Nurses [AACN], 2021a). Research supports a feeling of empowerment and increased confidence in decision-making when certification is achieved. The power of education cannot be underestimated. It can be the difference between being unsuspecting or prepared, being stagnant or innovative (Lee et al., 2019).

ROAD MAPS AND RESOURCES

It is not possible for the leader to predict the future of healthcare. However, the leader is required to create a cache of resources from which to depend on. The advanced practice nurse utilizes the nursing literature, but understands the need to expand beyond, courageously exploring trends, predictions, and priorities of other professions to determine their impact on healthcare. Consideration is given to this information. It is used as a guide in anticipation of future needs. Here are just a few to consider.

POLITICAL AGENDAS

Healthcare organizations are truly just microcosms reflective of societal issues. For example, 2021 brought a new president with a new agenda. Acknowledging the issues of the economic downturn, tackling COVID-19, and addressing climate change and racial injustice provide insight into the president's administrative priorities (Jaffee, 2021). Consider, then, how these issues may impact your organization. Planning for their impact will help in preparing for challenges yet to be experienced.

THE INSTITUTE FOR HEALTHCARE IMPROVEMENT

The Institute for Healthcare Improvement (IHI), a think tank of healthcare leaders, developed a useful tool from which to prioritize preparedness. The Triple Aim of Healthcare, now the Quadruple Aim, was developed to optimize organizational performance (Berwick et al., 2008; Bodenheimer & Sinsky, 2014). Attention to the four aims is required of the nurse leader, and they are: improving population health; improving the patient experience to include safe, quality care; improving the clinicians' experience; and reducing costs (Figure 1.2). The courageous caring leader consciously assimilates these aims and carefully considers a plan to invest in them all.

Reducing Costs

- Productivity
- Sustainability
- Cost effective
- Comparatively effective

Population Health

- Risk management through pooling
- Preventive care
- Socio-economically impactful

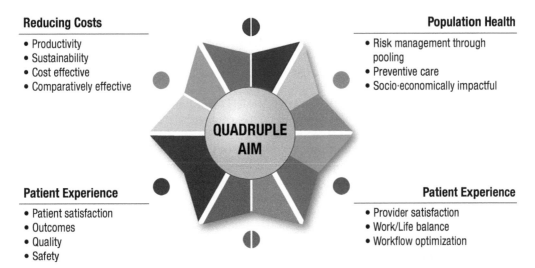

QUADRUPLE AIM

Patient Experience

- Patient satisfaction
- Outcomes
- Quality
- Safety

Patient Experience

- Provider satisfaction
- Work/Life balance
- Workflow optimization

FIGURE 1.2: The Quadruple Aim.

Source: Reproduced with permission from the University of Arkansas for Medical Sciences.

THE FUTURE OF NURSING 2020–2030

The Robert Wood Johnson Foundation supported a 2010 initiative to examine the future of nursing. The new decade creates an opportunity to re-assess, revise, and reformulate those initiatives (National Academies of Sciences, Engineering, Medicine, 2021). An interdisciplinary committee was appointed and tasked with reducing health disparities and improve well-being for all U.S. citizens. They will examine contributing factors to current health and societal demands. There are nine imperatives for this committee to consider (Box 1.1). Careful consideration of this list of action items helps inform the nurse leader of challenges they may experience and prepare for in their organizations.

BOX 1.1: FUTURE OF NURSING 2020–2030 IMPERATIVES

The role of nurses in improving the health of individuals, families, and communities by addressing social determinants of health and providing effective, efficient, equitable, and accessible care for all.

The current and future deployment of all levels of nurses across the continuum, including collaborative practice models to address the challenges of building a culture of health.

System facilitators and barriers to achieving a workforce that is diverse, including gender, race, and ethnicity across all levels of nursing education.

The role of the nursing profession in assuring that the voice of individuals, families, and communities are incorporated into design and operations of clinical and community health systems.

The training and competency-development skills needed to prepare nurses, including advanced practice nurses, to work outside of acute care settings and to lead efforts to build a culture of health and health equity and the extent to which current curricula meets these needs.

The ability of nurses to serve as change agents in creating systems that bridge the delivery of healthcare and social needs care in the community.

The research needed to identify or develop effective nursing practices for eliminating gaps and disparities in healthcare.

The importance of nurse well-being and resilience in ensuring the delivery of high-quality care and improving community health.

The role of nurses in response to emergencies that arise due to natural and man-made disasters and the impact on health equity.

Source: Reproduced with permission from National Academies of Sciences, Engineering, & Medicine. (2021). *The future of nursing 2020–2030.* Author.

TECHNOLOGICAL ADVANCES

Proactively planning for the complexities of healthcare requires constant vigilance regarding the advances in information technology (IT). Annual reports, participation at conferences, and weekly/daily updates from the chief clinical officer (CCO) and/or nurse informaticist help inform nurse leaders of the cutting-edge innovations that may be suitable for implementation. At the height of the COVID-19 pandemic, IT solutions helped connect patients to their healthcare teams as well as their families (Drees & Dyrda, 2020).

The Healthcare Information Management Systems Society (HIMSS) is a not-for-profit organization dedicated to transforming healthcare through research, education, and fundraising (HIMSS, n.d.). Some examples of current trends include the internet of things (IoT), ambient voice technology, the use of artificial intelligence (AI) developing predictive models, and the seamless transferability of patient records between providers. Following information released by HIMSS can help anticipate investments and conserve human and material resources when unknown challenges present themselves.

INVESTING IN HUMAN AND MATERIAL RESOURCES

Think back on the previous discussion regarding human needs as identified by Maslow. If food, water, warmth, and rest are foundational, then the courageous caring leader understands that assuring their employees have work is priority number one. This requires the leader to be a fiscal steward and organizational advocate grounded in prudent decision-making. If the need for security and safety is next, then the leader, for example, works to acquire the proper amount of equipment, maintained in proper working order. The nurse leader, as an important member of the facilities plant and operations team, endorses the development and adherence to preventive maintenance schedules. In another example, the nurse leader convinces colleagues of the need for appropriate quantities of supplies to meet staff and patient usage.

RECOGNIZING SHIFTING PARADIGMS

Addressing the remainder of needs outlined by Maslow's hierarchy requires further understanding of the way humans think, and an "awareness of social context" (Tideman et al., 2013, p. 21). These needs are belonging, esteem, and self-actualization. It is important to understand that human beings are emotional creatures, interdependent on others for survival. Despite the well-intentioned preparation of a leader, other factors may influence the success of any plan.

RELATIONSHIPS

In its basic form, context is created through the understanding of society influences and human needs. Leaders are significantly aware of these issues and hone proficiencies, becoming competent in various healthcare leadership skills. However, patients and staff are not cared for in a vacuum. The courageous nurse leader steps out of the silo and carefully develops relationships that support the interdependent nature of quality patient-centric healthcare.

Mastering all types of relationships is essential in preparation for successfully tackling the tumultuous state of healthcare. The first relationship any nurse leader needs to cultivate is that with the chief executive officer (CEO). It may be systems nurse leader and systems CEO, CEO–chief nursing officer (CNO), medical director of orthopedics and patient care director of orthopedics, and so on, whatever that dyad may look like. Transparent, authentic communication between both parties nurtures trust (Prestia, 2014). Building on foundational trust requires evidence of the value a nurse leader contributes to the organization. Examples of this are excellent metrics related to nurse-sensitive data, patient falls and/or central line infections, Hospital Consumer Assessment of Healthcare Providers and Systems (HCAHPS) scores, Leapfrog scores, and the maintenance of accreditations. Be forthcoming and celebrate successes. If the data is not trending positively, the courageous leader is authentic in recognizing the deficiency, following up with a solid action plan to improve.

When the CEO–nurse leader dyad is based on trust, the CEO can confidently align other key stakeholders in support of organizational preparedness efforts. These key stakeholders may be governing board members (BOG), foundation board members, and key physician leaders. The nurse leader seeks every opportunity to formally or informally present information to the BOG or medical executive committee members. Nursing's professional voice is a valuable and meaningful contributor.

Additional Relationships

The importance of relationship building was supported in a qualitative research study designed to understand how chief nursing officers were sustained in their work. The support of fellow administrative staff, subordinates, and other nurse leader colleagues was deemed vital to sustainment (Prestia, 2015). The ability to call on colleagues with whom you have fostered strong relationships facilitates problem-solving. Networking allows for the leaning-on and learning from others. It can save precious time when challenges present themselves.

FAILED PREDICTIONS

Predictions are just that: educated guesses. They can be fallible. Consider if you will discussion of the ever-present nursing shortage. Demographic statistics predicted the mass retirement of the baby boomer generation, born between 1946 and 1964. This foreshadowing was worrisome, as it projected an enormous loss of professional knowledge and clinical experience (Lee et al., 2019). What transpired instead was the 2009 economic downturn due to a crash of the housing market (Stichler, 2013). Nurses could no longer afford to retire as liquidity of assets was no longer an option. Leaders were then faced with a new set of challenges. One in particular was how to create work environments to accommodate aging personnel. The creation of more conducive work environments benefitted all the generations of working nurses. The prepared nurse leader finds a solution to an alternate problem.

Fast forward now to 2020, the year annihilated by the COVID-19 pandemic. Nurses came out of retirement to assist their fatigued colleagues. Deploying these clinical although rusty experts was essential to existing with the pandemic. They successfully practiced as buddies with current employees to provide activities of daily living (ADLs), dressing changes, functional assistance, and administration of medications. They assisted with inoculations when the vaccines became available.

Both examples support the unpredictability of the future and the human emotional response. Courageous caring leaders learn the art of pivoting. The term "pivot" is one used in basketball (Prestia, 2021a, 2021b, 2021c). In order to move the ball down court, players are required to bounce the ball with every step. When they are heavily guarded, their forward motion is halted. The pivot allows the player to keep one foot on the ground and move right or left. This move buys the player time to decide on the best course of action. When unexpected changes thwart preparation, pivoting allows the courageous caring leader to evaluate options, develop a new plan, and perhaps find a better direction. It may also increase awareness of the resiliency of self.

Nurse leaders are extremely knowledgeable and can be a tremendous resource to all stakeholders. They will come to be recognized as healthcare experts. This status places the nurse leader in a favorable position of serious consideration; when necessary, resources are requested to meet challenges.

◼ WHAT EVERY NURSE EXECUTIVE NEEDS TO KNOW

The nurse executive reaches beyond the scope of the nursing literature in anticipation and preparation of future trends. The information is shared at all levels of the organization. Careful consideration is given to the feedback/ideas received from staff. It may just help light the way.

◨ WHAT EVERY NURSE MANAGER NEEDS TO KNOW

The nurse manager understands societal trends and develops contingency plans to ensure the continued smooth operation of their unit. Best practices are shared with the executive team, peers, and staff.

THE NECESSITY OF SELF-CARE

The energy required to be prepared for leading in complex times begins with self-care. Staff deserve a leader who is sustained and resilient. Self-care begins with genuine self-love (Dyess et al., 2015; Prestia, 2020b). The courageous caring leader believes their personhood is worthy of love. Permission to love self, despite flaws and shortcomings, helps with the realization that others—staff and colleagues—are deserving of loving care. Appreciation for self and others is expressed through caring behaviors that value, preserve, refresh, and renew personhood.

Protecting physical, mental, and emotional reserves requires a daily commitment to self-care. How is this commitment lived? Research conducted to identify how CNOs were sustained supported the conscious effort of maintaining work/life balance (Prestia, 2015). Self-preservation behaviors were described as setting boundaries, managing the daily calendar, and participating in diversionary activities. Participants articulated the need to be energized to be their best self for their staff.

A secondary analysis of the previously discussed study further identified self-care behaviors (Dyess et al., 2015). An important finding was attentiveness to self-cues. Knowing self and acknowledging fatigue, emotional and nutritional imbalances, and hydration needs were critical to role sustainability. Awareness of the need for time away to regroup was paramount to self-preservation.

In times of great challenge and constant pressure, however, routine self-care behaviors may not be enough. Normal practices of yoga, meditation, immersion in fiction, or travel may no longer yield expected results. Schedules may no longer allow for even a working lunch. It is at these times that next-level self-care should be employed. Next-level self-care is one of change so engaging that it prohibits the mind from wandering and worry (Prestia, 2021a, 2021b, 2021c). It is not increased intensity or duration of any one activity. The science behind next-level self-care recognizes that change in routine creates new neural pathways, causing the brain to take notice, providing nourishment instead of comfort. Activities of next-level care are personally defined by the leader. For example, if adult coloring books have been a diversion, reach out of the comfort zone and try painting with watercolors. If relaxation is found in cooking, change course. Challenge your mind and create desserts worthy of "bake-off" challenges. Sharing these creations with older neighbors can provide emotional nurturance. Find activities that challenge the mind, body, and spirit. It takes courageous caring to disengage from the routine and nurture the soul, which are both essential elements for leading in challenging times.

◨ WHAT EVERY NURSE EXECUTIVE NEEDS TO KNOW

Self-care is not a luxury. It is an essential requirement to remain energized and lead in challenging times. Alter the routine of self-care if it no longer provides comfort. Share the importance of experiences with staff. Approve their requests for time away to re-charge.

◨ WHAT EVERY NURSE MANAGER NEEDS TO KNOW

Be a self-care role model by utilizing your vacation time for diversionary activities. Create schedules conducive for staff to do the same. During the workday, encourage staff to take their breaks and go outside (if safety allows) to walk, stretch, or simply feel the sun on their face.

TACKLING THE CHALLENGE OF THE DAY

Chaotic challenges can present themselves, individually, subsequently, in random order, or all at once. As stated previously, the challenge of the day reflects the challenges of society. Today, the leader may be dealing with a union strike, developing gender-neutral nomenclature, and/or an influx of homeless individuals on a hot summer's day. If due diligence is adhered to, trends monitored, and contingency plans developed, tackling the issues may be less daunting; however, they will still be formidable. A glimpse of courage and his solid methodological approach can be found when reviewing the first 100 days of Franklin Delano Roosevelt's presidency.

When FDR, the 32nd president of the United States, assumed office, he faced a financial crisis of monumental proportion (Goodwin, 2018). Banks were closing, Americans had no access to their hard-earned savings, and the New York Stock Exchange had shut down with no inkling of when trade would resume. Assuming an undaunted comportment, and with conviction, FDR set into motion a time-defined, concrete plan to tackle the crisis. An extrapolation of his ideas is identified, and they lend themselves to a formalized methodology for adaptation by nursing leadership (Box 1.2).

BOX 1.2: TACKLING CHALLENGES: THE 10-STEP METHODOLOGY OF FRANKLIN DELANO ROOSEVELT

Create unity of purpose and communicate a clear vision
Approach the problem with optimistic realism
Follow the law
Acknowledge your fear and courageously continue
Assemble a team to tackle the issue
Develop a timeline and work toward a deadline
Hold yourself and your staff accountable
Align key stakeholders
Have patience—there will be slow adapters
Recognize momentum and celebrate successes

Source: Reproduced with permission from Kearns, D. K. (2018). *Leadership in turbulent times.* Simon and Schuster.

CREATE UNITY OF PURPOSE COMMUNICATED THROUGH A CLEAR VISION

From the outset of his term, FDR provided a clear vision steeped in hope (Goodwin, 2018). This practice provided clarity of communication, which is essential to conveying a precise understanding of intention (Prestia, 2017). Wheatley states that leaders should "fill all of space with messages we care about," to combat chaos and shape it into a common goal that staff can understand and align behind (Wheatley, 2006, p. 57). Conviction and transparency of messaging helps minimize the formation of individual agendas and subsequent conflict. It is the instrument from which the melodic harmony of purpose is created.

APPROACH THE PROBLEM WITH OPTIMISTIC REALISM

Optimistic realism requires the leader to publicly acknowledge the gravity or importance of a situation. The leader authentically communicates the weaknesses, barriers, and difficulties anticipated in achieving a particular goal. This is done while still fostering a sense of positivity and a "can-do" spirit. It is a fine balance. The message becomes one of confidence in the abilities of reporting staff and the current mission.

FOLLOW THE LAW

The leader ensures that the mission's journey occurs with the utmost transparency. Abiding by all laws is essential. These "laws" may be governmental regulations, accreditation standards, workmen's compensation procedures, or the principles of biomedical ethics (i.e., autonomy, nonmaleficence, beneficence, and justice [Beauchamp & Childress, 2009]). The nurse leader is not expected to know every nuance of the laws; however, the prudent leader consults with content experts to fully understand guidelines and restrictions. The courageously caring nurse leader, by virtue of the compassionate nature of the profession, engages in "principle-guided" decisions (Beauchamp & Childress, 2009, p. 38).

ACKNOWLEDGE YOUR FEAR AND COURAGEOUSLY CONTINUE

As mentioned earlier in this chapter, following one's moral compass to conduct business in an ethical fashion requires courage. Depending on the environmental culture, this may at times cause conflicts with other members of the administrative team. In her account of reversing a medical center fraught with public and private scrutiny, Yancer (2012) called upon her "internal well of courage" (p. 67), one she says that all nurses draw upon by virtue of their clinical compassion. She contemplates decisions made that could have been career altering. However, she followed the advice of trusted mentors, and often forged out of her comfort zone to build trust and accomplish her mission.

ASSEMBLE A TEAM TO TACKLE THE ISSUE

The courageous caring leader possesses a firm belief that collective intelligence is the life force from which innovative solutions spring (Mayo & Woolley, 2016). The engaged guidance of diplomatic leadership astutely assimilates talent to solve the challenge of the day (Prestia, 2017). Multidisciplinary, multicultural, multigender, and multigenerational teams are better equipped to develop solutions due to the variety of experience, expertise, ideas, and values they possess (Mayo & Woolley, 2016; Morley & Cashell, 2017). However, teams need to be encouraged to share ideas and evidence without the fear of censorship, boundary issues, or humiliation. The very nature of composite teams can create participant fear and untoward conflict based on the formal ranking of positions.

It is essential for the nurse leader to extract the best from every team member. They do not need to participate as a member themselves to accomplish this. Instead, through the establishment of carefully laid ground rules, alignment of key players, and periodic updates on team progress, barriers can be minimized. Successful teams have leaders that create an environment where goals are clear, team members are all equal, ideas and opinions are respected, and everyone is treated with dignity. Meetings are considered "judgment-free zones" (Duhigg, 2016).

In their quest to identify why certain teams were successful and others were not, the researchers at Google discovered that psychological safety was a key factor (Duhigg, 2016). Psychologically safe teams exhibited care and concern for one another. They participated in two important behaviors, "conversational turn-taking" and "average social sensitivity" (Duhigg, 2016). These terms support the importance of fully listening, non-interruption, and an astute awareness of team member feelings. The team identifies the importance of their work, the integral nature of their role, and the value of the collective whole. These teams excel at coordination, cooperation, and shared decision-making. They become true partners in solving the task at hand (Morley & Cashell, 2017). The courageous caring leader sets the expectation for this type of conduct in facilitating peak team performance in solving complex challenges.

Courageous caring leadership is instrumental in aligning the organization behind strategies to tackle the complex challenges of healthcare. The role is multifaceted, requiring an unrelentless commitment to ultimately achieve the goal of quality patient outcomes. This is not easy. The courageous caring nurse leader must find their internal grit; their passion to persevere in even the most trying of times (Lee & Duckworth, 2018). The next section will present a daily-use checklist to assist leaders through the complexity.

DEVELOP A TIMELINE AND WORK TOWARD A DEADLINE

Every project has a planning phase, a build-up phase, an implementation phase, and a close-out (Harvard Business Review [HBR] Editors, 2016). Hiring/contracting with an experienced project manager to assist in assuring these four phases are accomplished and deadlines are met may be worth investing in. The leader works in tandem with the project manager, providing direction at key junctures.

Timelines are best developed by working backwards from significant dates (HBR Editors, 2016). For example, if the medical executive committee needs to approve an aspect of the project, then a deadline may be the third Tuesday of the month. Review the calendar and determine when the impactful dates arise, and work to provide enough flexibility in the plan for revision. Continuous forward motion is an important aspect of project management.

HOLD YOURSELF AND YOUR STAFF ACCOUNTABLE

Courageous caring leadership requires delegation of certain tasks. This requires a skillful approach to maintaining just enough responsibility—but not too much—and avoiding overcommitment, diminishing time to plan and contemplate other priorities (Prestia & Platas, 2019). The leader holds self-accountable for the aspects of team selection, guidance, surveillance, supervision, evaluation, and feedback (Joint Statement on Delegation, ANA & National Council of State Boards of Nursing [NCSBN], 2019). The leader holds staff accountable for project, attendance, engagement, deliverables, and the respectful comradery necessary for goal attainment. Although the leader's time can be limited, interaction with staff must always be a priority.

ALIGN KEY STAKEHOLDERS

Working through challenging times is not done in isolation. The courageous caring nurse leader must leave the office to connect with all stakeholders. These are the people most affected by the project (HBR Editors, 2016). They are integral in providing the human and material resources necessary to ensure a beneficial outcome. Connecting is accomplished by rounding on units and/or scheduling nursing/staff "town halls" to discuss the initiative and build consensus. This is a time to test the plans with the actual audience. Some will be supportive, and others will have trepidations or simply not agree. A critical competency at this juncture is listening. This is a time to solicit support from even the staunchest of naysayers. The nurse leader must understand the stakeholder concerns, fears, and reservations regarding the challenge. These must be addressed, or the project will be doomed from the onset.

HAVE PATIENCE—THERE WILL BE SLOW ADAPTERS

As time consuming as this may seem, exhibiting patience is a key leadership competency. Patience is the "intermediate state between the two extremes of . . . recklessness and sloth" (Schnitker, 2012, p. 264). Patient leaders who calmly communicate their vision, as many times as required, positively influence staff. There is a sense of value when leadership takes the time to provide further explanation. A recent study supported that leadership patience improved staff productivity, creativity, and collaboration (Strauss, 2020). These are three very important attributes to goal achievement. The benefits of the reward are still achievable if the leader exhibits patience.

RECOGNIZE MOMENTUM AND CELEBRATE SUCCESSES

Rewarding even the smallest of successes is important for motivating self and team. Caring leadership requires presence. At these times, the leader enthusiastically recognizes team performance and shares how their initiative impacts the overall goal. This is not a time for leadership ego. It is a time to praise and give gratitude to all those contributors. Personal experience supports leader recognition of staff and generosity as a great moral booster. Investing in kind gestures (e.g., handwritten notes, scratch off tickets, gift cards in small sums, buying lunch, or distributing full size candy bars) has been well received. Remember, as St. Francis of Assisi said, "It is in the giving that we receive" (Pass It On, 2021).

◼ WHAT EVERY NURSE MANAGER NEEDS TO KNOW

Delegation does not relieve you from project oversight. If time prohibits meeting participation, consider being more of a sponsor and less of a facilitator. You are still responsible for assuring project completion, so hold staff and yourself accountable for deliverables. Remember to be generous with your staff, rewarding them with gratitude.

◼ WHAT EVERY NURSE EXECUTIVE NEEDS TO KNOW

Overcommunicate your expectations using multimedia: written comments, verbal comments, email, flyers, Zoom, or Webex. Have a trusted associate read and re-read your communication for understanding. Use aesthetically pleasing graphics and fonts. Change up your selection process for assigning participants to teams. Give others a chance to be a part of an award-winning team. Never miss an opportunity to praise staff for their contributions to the success of a project. Remember, no matter how much you personally contributed to the success of an initiative, give the team the credit.

⬡ CASE SCENARIO
REVEALING UNQUALIFIED CANDIDATES
SITUATION

The CNO of a not-for-profit medical center is approached by the CEO and told the CNO must seriously consider the hiring of the friend of the chairman of the foundation for the open position of director of perioperative services. The chairman of the foundation has a seat at the governing board and is quite influential in all organizational decisions. The CNO understands the importance of the foundation board in raising funds to support the medical center. They currently fund a nursing scholarship program for those staff members pursuing registered nurse and advanced nursing degrees.

The CNO receives the potential candidate's resume and determines that their experience is not commensurate with the position requirements. The position requires progressive leadership experience, plus a master's degree in nursing, with a certification from the Association of periOperative Registered Nurses (AORN). The candidate requires a Monday to Friday schedule, 8-hour shifts. Additionally, the CNO has been grooming the assistant director of perioperative services for this role.

APPROACH

The CNO is in a precarious position. The first course of action is to discuss the situation with the chief human resources officer (CHRO). The CNO's relationship with the CHRO is strong, as they have worked together on numerous employee concerns. The CNO is advised and agrees to have an authentically transparent discussion with the CEO, sharing the position description and the candidate's resume. Additionally, the CNO will suggest an alternative position to hire the potential candidate into (e.g., a quality analyst role for surgical services). The CNO believes this is a good compromise, as it requires no weekends and no holidays.

OUTCOME

When the CNO discusses the situation and the compromise with the CEO, the CEO is unmoved and directs the CNO to hire the candidate into the director of peri-op role. The CEO will accept no compromise.

DISCUSSION QUESTIONS

1. What elements of the Nursing Leadership Mission Critical Checklist would apply to this scenario?
2. What should the CNO do? If they do not hire the candidate, are they at risk of losing their job?
3. What are the ethical implications of this scenario?

● CASE SCENARIO

REVEALING METRIC FALSIFICATION

SITUATION

FR is a systems chief nurse at a large regional hospital. They have been in this role for approximately 16 months. It has come to FR's attention that the flagship medical center in one of their regions has falsified the reports of their quality metric results for hospital-acquired infections.

APPROACH

The systems chief nurse has a responsibility to ensure the safety of all patients. FR also has a responsibility to role model transparency, setting the expectation for all those CNOs who report to them. Falsification of any records or reports is unacceptable. There are several approaches that must occur simultaneously to tackle this issue. The first order of business is to share this finding with the corporate administrative team. The corporate compliance officer will be tasked with completing a thorough independent investigation. This must be done with the complete assistance of the facility infection control practitioner, director of clinical quality, the chief nursing officer, and any staff responsible for collection and ultimate reporting of this data.

Simultaneously, FR will travel to the facility and speak with the CNO to ascertain the CNO's knowledge of the validity of the report. There needs to be some sense of transparency of reporting.

OUTCOME

The investigation reveals that the data has been falsified for the last two quarters. The explanation is that it is the result of pressure placed on the quality abstractors from the director of clinical quality to meet the company goals. Staff report bullying behaviors, specifically related to the application of definitions for any "gray area" metrics. The quality staff require emotional support due to the incivility they experienced. They knew the director of clinical quality's behavior in applying the definitions was questionable. However, they all need their jobs and were fearful that if they utilized the chain of command, they would be the recipients of retaliation.

DISCUSSION QUESTIONS

1. What elements of the Nursing Leadership Mission Critical Checklist would apply to this scenario?
2. Would you consider the systems chief nurse as courageously caring in this situation? If so, why?
3. Should the CNO be held accountable, and perhaps lose their job, due to the false reporting?

THE NURSING LEADERSHIP MISSION CRITICAL CHECKLIST©

The literature is replete with evidence to support how to "stay the course" and accomplish quality patient outcomes. As complexity presents copious daily challenges, it is difficult, however, to know which "course" to take. As stated previously, the nurse leader does not have the luxury to work on one challenge at a time. When complex challenges diverge, the nurse leader needs a tool to help center and ground their daily work. This author developed a comprehensive nursing leadership checklist of evidence-based tactics for just this purpose. Entitled The Nursing Leadership Mission Critical Checklist©, it can be referred to and effectively operationalized on a daily basis to help "stay the course" (Exhibit 1.1).

EXHIBIT 1.1: THE NURSING LEADERSHIP MISSION CRITICAL CHECKLIST

Are my leadership decisions evidence-based and supported by reliable data?	
NOTES:	
Caring	
Decisions are optimized to preserve the patients' individual human dignity.	
Decisions are optimized to preserve the staffs' individual human dignity.	
NOTES:	
Improving the patient experience—quality and safety	
Communication invites truthful dialogue.	
Communication is responsiveness, reciprocal, and drives accountability.	
NOTES:	
Improving the staff experience	
Practice environment is conducive to creating joyous and meaningful work.	
NOTES:	

(continued)

EXHIBIT 1.1: THE NURSING LEADERSHIP MISSION CRITICAL CHECKLIST (continued)

Reducing healthcare costs	
Resource management is balanced.	
Information technology is leveraged.	
Talent is engaged in continuous learning.	
NOTES:	
Relationships	
How have I nurtured self?	
Am I self-aware?	
Have I reflected on situations?	
Have I networked internally and externally?	
Have I provided emotional support to team members?	
NOTES:	

Source: © Angela Prestia (2021).

CHECKLISTS

Checklists have been touted by the aviation industry as a significant tool to reduce "human performance deviation" (Staff Writers, 2018, p. 5). When used properly, they are meant to ensure minimum standards are met and quality is maintained. Effective checklists categorize information in a sequential practical fashion. Each critical element reminds flight leadership of an essential process that must be performed to reduce vulnerability. Checklists are designed for both routine and abnormal/emergency situations (Captain David Becker, American Airlines—Retired, personal communication, October 2020). "Routine checklists can be completed by an individual," states Captain Becker. "Emergency checklists can also be completed by one individual, i.e., single pilot airplanes, or by challenge, response, and verification," thus requiring two people.

Humans are fallible. Their imperfections may be due to "memory, vigilance, attention, concentration . . ." and be exacerbated by "fatigue, sleep-deprivation, excessive task demands, stress, and anxiety" (Suresh et al., 2011, p. 97). Checklists can assist in maintaining focus on mission critical elements. When used daily, the nurse leader can decrease the possibilities of missed opportunities.

The aviation checklist was eloquently extrapolated for use in the healthcare arena by Dr. Atul Gawande in his book entitled *The Checklist Manifesto* (2009). The book details his quest with WHO to decrease overall complications during surgery. His research resulted in understanding the importance and applicability of checklists to healthcare. Checklists had been successfully used in the skyscraper construction industry. They were also integral for the safe set-up of musical sound stages for grandiose rock concert performances. "Under conditions of complexity, not only are checklists a help, they are *required* for success" (Gawande, 2009, p. 79).

Over the last 10 years, checklists have become a staple in the pre-procedural arena. Their implementation has prevented catastrophic errors, decreased infection rates, and improved the overall safety and quality of care provided to patients (Gawande, 2009). If the disciplined use of a checklist is this impactful, it most assuredly can assist the nurse executive in navigating daily chaos and complexity.

Checklists are not developed to address every possible scenario requiring attention. Instead, they are developed to assist with "memory recall" (Gawande, 2009, p. 39). They are meant to remind us of the least number of steps; "5–9 at the most" to ensure achievement (Gawande, 2009, p. 123). The leanness of elements helps expedite thought processes and assists the leader to focus on what is truly crucial for success.

COMPONENTS OF THE NURSING LEADERSHIP MISSION CRITICAL CHECKLIST

The development of The Nursing Leadership Mission Critical Checklist began with a literature review related to the prioritization of nurse leadership responsibilities. There is not a plethora of articles on this topic. However, several articles were key to understanding what elements were important and why they should be included in the checklist. The Quadruple Aim framework was also used as a foundation.

COMMITTING TO EVIDENCE

Each day, the checklist begins with the overarching commitment to make decisions steeped in evidence and supported by reliable data. No matter how impassioned a nurse leader feels about a situation, decisions made in an emotional state may be detrimental to patients, staff, and self. "Decisions made in haste may yield unsustainable and erroneous compromises" (Prestia & Platas, 2019, p. 155). Staff disillusionment with leadership can result from improperly contemplated decisions. Leaders need to allow themselves the time to collect and/or examine the literature or organizationally acquired data. It is imperative for evidence to ground all practice (Arnold et al., 2006).

The leader competently utilizes evidence-based practice (EBP) when problem-solving. This approach integrates the conscientious use of evidence in combination with professional expertise and consumer/customer preferences and values (Melnyk et al., 2012). The use of EBP in decision-making can ensure the nurse leader is "fixing" the correct problem. Dissecting and therefore refining the evidence helps accurately understand and solve the right issue.

There are several tools available to ensure data is used to discern the correct issue at hand. The plan-do-check/study-act (PDCA) methodology is one of them (The Deming Institute, n.d.). Additionally, the use of Lean Six Sigma and the define-measure-analyze-improve-control (DMAIC) methodology can also assist (American Society for Quality, n.d.). Both of these methodologies use data to improve processes. Again, the nurse leader should have knowledge regarding these data analyzing techniques, but does not have to be expert at them. Preparing educators in the use of these methodologies is a sound investment. It empowers employees with the tools to improve quality at the grass-roots level. Credentialed facilitators exist and can also be contracted with to help provide services.

CARING—THE PRESERVATION OF HUMAN DIGNITY

Nurse leaders champion healthy work environments, creating an optimal culture from which to care. The benefits of this impact both the patient and the staff.

PRESERVING PATIENT INDIVIDUALITY

The myriad of conflicting priorities often causes the nurse leader to lose sight of their core responsibility, which is quality patient care. Nurse leaders define "caring" as alleviating suffering by maintaining clinical presence, listening, respecting, facilitating dialogue, balancing limited resources, and affirming relationships (Prestia & Dyess, 2020, p. 330). The effort a nurse leader exerts in being visually present to staff solidifies the importance of their daily work in caring for the patients. Part of rounding includes visiting patients, greeting families, telephoning, or videoconferencing to connect. Even with this limited engagement, nurse leaders are assessing the environment, evaluating staffing, and gaining an understanding of barriers that may affect patient care.

Additionally, a key to supporting patient individuality is to ensure processes exist to secure living wills and, for example, "Do Not Resuscitate" (DNR) orders. The patient's wishes must be honored. "Nurse leaders strive to prioritize their duty to know patients, protect them from harm, and influence the development of procedures supporting the best possible care" (Solbakken et al., 2018, p. E13).

PRESERVING STAFF INDIVIDUALITY

Living caring leadership creates hope in staff that they are "known and supported" in their personhood (Boykin & Schoenhofer, 2001, p. 34). The nurse leader works to cultivate the best in people (Kennedy et al., 2020). When staff feel they are respected and cared for, they are more efficient and productive (Robbins, 2007). They trust that their contributions are meaningful, and their value is recognized. As discussed earlier, the courageous caring leader recognizes staff uniqueness, and honors their individuality through a commitment to prioritizing their needs (Prestia & Dyess, 2020). They make mindful decisions.

IMPROVING THE PATIENT EXPERIENCE—QUALITY AND SAFETY

"No matter the practice setting, the collective purpose is to provide a transformative patient experience, rich in artfully skilled holistic caring" (Dyess et al., 2019).

Improving the patient experience does not mean offering chai lattes to every patient and family member on admission to the organization. Patient experience is a comprehensive approach to assuring safe, effective, quality care that is individualized and in alignment with the patient's goals.

The nurse leaders' role in assuring safe, quality patient care is an imperative. At first glance, this may seem difficult to control, as the leader is not responsible for the actual provision of direct patient care. However, the nurse leader is responsible for the creation and sustainment of a healthy work environment, which is fundamental to the delivery of safe quality of care. Research designed to understand the role of the nurse leader in advancing such work environments supports the importance of nurse leader; influence, advocacy, and innovation, in both the recognition and removal of barriers to safe, quality care (Bowles et al., 2019). The researchers identified the barriers of workplace incivility, generational differences, lack of utilizing best practices, and forgetting the centrality of the patient, as deterrents to safe quality patient care. Additionally, if nurse leaders did not have access to data, their power to effect change was limited.

Data requires reporting transparency. This translates to courageous acceptance of information from a staff that trusts they will not be retaliated against for reporting the truth. If the leader holds self-accountable for role modeling this behavior, clinicians providing direct patient care recognize this as an organizational expectation.

COMMUNICATION: INVITING TRUTHFUL DIALOGUE THAT IS ACCOUNTABLE AND RECIPROCATED

The importance of mindful, relevant, and trustworthy messaging was discussed earlier. There are several important points to reinforce at this juncture. Relevance describes the topic at hand, not a tangential dialogue, with little connectiveness. It also describes the timeliness of the subject matter. Entertaining discourse about a situation that occurred a month ago may no longer be pertinent. Additionally, relevance requires examples. The mindful leader has data to support the discussion, not inference or interpretation.

The courageous caring leader invites this dialogue, unencumbered by negative personal emotions. Listening carefully as staff extol the underperformance of the leadership team does not mean that the nurse leader is a failure. Consider the reciprocity of truthful dialogue as a gift, something to be explored, with an opportunity to be rectified. This reciprocity requires approachability, action, and feedback. The nurse leader utilizes the mission critical checklist as a reminder to continuously create an environment that appreciates honest, nonjudgmental communication that is lovingly shared. When this is accomplished, patient care can only benefit.

IMPROVING THE STAFF EXPERIENCE

The importance of a well-cared for workforce, pulsating with meaning-driven purpose, is critical to surviving and thriving in complex challenging times. The courageously caring nurse leader must understand the criticality of this. Fortunately, both the IHI, along with the AACN (2021b), have shed light on the importance of staff experience. Different though symbiotic, the AACN's standards focus on creating healthy work environments, while the IHI identifies the contributory nature of "joy in work" for sustaining satisfaction (Perlo et al., 2017).

In the committee-developed white paper, the IHI identifies four steps for leaders to help discover and sustain joy and meaning in work. These four steps are:

- Ask staff, "What matters to you?"
- Identify unique impediments to joy in work in the local context.
- Commit to a systems approach to making joy in work a shared responsibility at all levels of the organization.
- Use improvement science to test approaches to improving joy in work in your organization.

Courageous caring leaders ask "What matters?" without fearing the answers. They are committed to understanding the barriers and using data to focus on removing the correct ones. Interestingly, the document encourages progress to be measured by using the AACN's Healthy Work Assessment tool. This can be found at www.aacn.org/hwe.

The six standards for creating and sustaining healthy work environments identified by the AACN are: skilled communication, true collaboration, effective decision-making, appropriate staffing, meaningful recognition, and authentic leadership (AACN, 2021b). Although these six standards are enmeshed to create healthy work environments, there is again a focus on meaningful recognition to improve staff experience.

The workforce requires timely, individualized appreciation and recognition. This appreciation should be given at many junctures, not just when goals are accomplished. An example of this would be extolling appreciation for the contributory nature of everyone's work on a daily basis. "All team members need to be valued for their human worth regardless of outcomes" (Prestia, 2017, p. 243). When given freely, appreciation is the catalyst for continued effort. Contributory effort is the catalyst for continued appreciation.

Individualized appreciation is as important as the act of bestowing appreciation. Some staff may find public praise embarrassing. Others may lavish in it. Chapman and White (2010) identified five languages of appreciation: words of affirmation, quality time, acts of service, tangible gifts, and physical touch. A word about the latter: Physical touch requires situational consideration. During this time of pandemic, it may require a virtual application (Table 1.2). Imagine the staff's surprise when the leader recognizes them in their preferred manner.

TABLE 1.2: The Five Languages of Appreciation in the Workplace

Language of Appreciation	Workplace Example
Words of affirmation Specific/individualized	"I could not do my job without you!" "Thank you for following up with that family."
Quality time Giving of self	"Let me answer the phones while you take a break." "I'm happy to take your week of call for you."
Acts of service Random expressions of kindness	"Let me help complete the job requisition, so you can focus on staffing." "Getting your car washed was the least I could do!"
Tangible gifts Small tokens of gratitude	"Enjoy the fruit basket!' "I'm so lucky you work for me. Good luck with the scratch off ticket."
Physical touch*	Elbow bumps Gloved-handed high 5's Socially distant virtual hugs

*Always with permission/may be virtual.

Source: Adapted from Chapman, G., & White, P. (2010). The 5 languages of appreciation in the workplace. Northfield Publishing.

REDUCING HEALTHCARE COSTS

One of the main tenets of the IHI's Quadruple Aim for improving healthcare is reducing healthcare costs. Organizational finances are not the siloed responsibility of the chief financial officer (CFO). The nurse leader takes a significant interest in "the bottom line." An earlier discussion identifies that nurse leaders understand this and embrace it as an expression of caring leadership (i.e., balancing limited resources). Nurse leaders have a fiscal responsibility to ensure organizational solvency, to continue to have monies available to provide care to the community they serve and meaningful work for all those employed.

Daily, the nurse leader is faced with making decisions related to cost. Examples of this are identifying census trends in the development of staffing plans, careful scrutiny of agency personnel use, supporting antibiotic stewardship, prioritizing capital expenditures, phasing in minor equipment purchases, leveraging technology and automation, and developing a robust retention plan.

RELATIONSHIP BUILDING

The last section of the mission critical checklist reminds the nurse leader to participate in behaviors that build relationships. This begins with the relationship the leader has with self.

Nurturing and Self-Care

Leaders can be caught "off-guard" and respond emotionally or hastily in certain situations. The Nurse Leadership Mission Critical Checklist reminds the leader to invest in self to yield positive returns. The importance of self-care and the nourishment that next-level self-care provides has been previously discussed. These practices perpetuate a balanced state from which perspective can be gained. Perspective allows the nurse leader an opportunity to take a step back, ask questions, review the data, gain insight, make rational decisions, and provide space for reflection.

Creating the Space to Reflect

Intentional use of reflection is an important leadership skill attributed to several U.S. presidents (Kearns, 2018; Scipioni, 2020). It has been linked to understanding event outcomes, as well as reducing stress and improving resiliency (Prestia, 2019). President Barack Obama touted the benefits of his 1-minute walk to and from the Oval Office to reflect on his day's agenda. "It was along this walkway that I'd gather my thoughts for the day, preparing for conversations with members of Congress and constituents, reviewing plans and proposals to move the country forward" (Scipioni, 2020). At the end of the day, the president welcomed his sojourn back to the White House, as it aided in decompression. This time helped provide perspective prior to being with family.

The practice of reflection allows for an honest evaluation of major events, minor conversations, accomplishments, and remaining opportunities, the outcome of which assists the nurse leader to develop tangible approaches to problem-solving. It can further strengthen their resolve (Prestia, 2019). Its power lies in shaping personal and professional conduct. If done in the spirit of self-improvement, reflection can help identify "unconscious bias, core beliefs and facilitate learning" (Prestia, 2019, p. 466).

Different sources outline specific methodology in the practice of reflection. One prescribes a four-step approach including a conscious understanding of the experience, the reflection, lessons learned, and the implementation of those lessons (EDShare, n.d.). Another methodology is discussed in the book *The Practice* (Schmidt, 2014). Here, the author identifies reflective activities to aide in the release of negativity and the recognition of opportunities. Her overarching framework of waking up, living present, and letting go has subcategories, saturated with mediative and reflective approaches to understanding the construct of events. It was found that this pensive approach decreased perceived stress in nurse leaders (Dyess et al., 2018). The methodology is less important than creating the space in which to reflect.

Networking

The power of connectedness both external to and within the work environment emerged as a vital force to CNO sustainment (Prestia, 2015). The nurse leader must work to cultivate these relationships on a daily basis. As discussed earlier, staff content experts can assist the nurse leader to problem-solve. Daily diligence to strengthen these relationships will improve responsiveness to challenges. Additionally, when conscious effort is made to come to know other nurse leaders, a network of experts is only a phone call away. The scope of the network should be broad, not just limited to those within your company's system. Build relationships with nurse leaders working for "the competition," with academicians, with experts outside of the nursing profession. "Ask to meet with professionals you admire" (Prestia, 2016a, 2016b). Invite them to coffee, lunch, or a Zoom call. Send a follow-up note, thanking them for the idea, or their time. A reciprocal relationship is important to foster. One cannot just take. One also has to freely provide innovations, best practices, listening, and emotional support when needed.

Emotional Support

The nurse leaders' responsibility to provide emotional support links back to the previous discussion regarding Maslow's Hierarchy of Needs. Staff and colleagues must experience the caring side of the nurse leader in the most fundamental way. Offering support to every individual staff member may seem impossible. The courageously caring nurse leader recognizes this and develops the infrastructure necessary to provide robust support inclusive of reward, education, programs, and technological networking (Prestia, 2021a, 2021b, 2021c). An example of this may be an educational program regarding the signs and symptoms of posttraumatic stress disorder (PTSD) and related support via the employee assistance program (EAP). Investing in an advanced practice employee health nurse versed in various mental health websites can provide emotional support to all staff members. The nurse leader can promote positive supportive health agendas on a daily basis.

SUMMARY

In general, the power of checklists supports a decrease in missed opportunities. The use of The Nurse Leader Mission Critical Checklist requires further evaluation to understand its true value. However, without a sequential reference of imperatives, even the most organized nurse leader can be overwhelmed by complexity and succumb to chaos. Forward motion may be thwarted, and setbacks can occur.

SETBACKS

"In any moment of decision, the best thing you can do is the right thing. The worst thing you can do is nothing."

Theodore Roosevelt

The courage and care required to lead during challenging times may be magnified when anticipated outcomes are not achieved. Despite understanding the importance of vision, relationships, execution, and the daily use of The Nurse Leader Mission Critical Checklist, success may be elusive (Bellack & Dickow, 2019). This does not mean failure. Reimagine this as a setback, requiring the fortitude to continue nuancing the plan.

Often there exists underlying issues that nurse leaders are not consciously aware of. Uncompromising superiors who may offer no alternative options, staff noncompliance, or sheer jealousy may create "no-win" situations (Prestia, 2020c). Timing may also be a consideration. A successful plan may now be unsuccessful due to a change in personnel, unexpected life events, or both. For example, remote work for supporting staff was unheard of prior to the COVID-19 pandemic. It is now the "new normal."

When visions fall short of implementation, the courageous caring leader, committed to self-improvement, listens more intently, networks more fully, and reflects more deeply. Remove failure from leadership vocabulary to avoid the emotional consequences that can disrupt the importance of the nurse leader's work (Prestia, 2020c).

◼ WHAT EVERY NURSE MANAGER NEEDS TO KNOW

The Nurse Leader Mission Critical Checklist provides a solid foundation on which to ground professional practice. Research and understand the importance of every element within the checklist. Start off small, focusing on one of the elements each day, until such time that the checklist in its entirety becomes an effortless tool to assist in goal attainment. Begin with grounding every decision in evidence-based data.

◼ WHAT EVERY NURSE EXECUTIVE NEEDS TO KNOW

It is difficult to remember to infuse the daily practice of nursing leadership with identified critical elements without a framework. The Nurse Leader Mission Critical Checklist provides a sequential reference of essential elements for leading in challenging times. Its use can help decrease unintentional missteps. Even with consistent use, there will be times that setbacks occur. Reference the checklist again to reflect and help identify those areas that could have been strengthened to ensure successful outcomes.

KEY POINTS

- Courageous caring leadership requires authentic presence and constant mindful consideration.
- Nurse leaders must exist in a state of proactive preparation.
- Nurse leaders must create and nurture trusting relationships.
- Self-care is not an option. It must be lived and modeled.
- Inclusive composite teams are essential for innovation.
- Nurse leaders hold themselves and their staffs accountable.

SUMMARY—MAINTAINING AND SUSTAINING DURING CHALLENGING TIMES

In this chapter, concepts, tools, and research are offered to support the nurse leaders' journey through challenging times. The information provides a solid foundation for daily progress toward quality patient-centered care, provided by a supported workforce. It reminds the leader to prepare through education, relationship building, data analysis, and comes full circle to committing to a foundation of continual learning.

In a recent article, now-President Joseph Biden coined the phrase, "the art of the possible" (Viser & Linskey, 2021). This is so apropos to leading in challenging times. Success is possible. Keep patients central. Remember your staff's needs. Be brave. Stay true to your ethics and morals. Ask questions of your network. Be still enough to listen for the answers. Work the checklist every day. Align key stakeholders, develop action plans, and wait for the right time. Remember, challenges are impermanent; they come into being and then disappear.

The professional practice of nursing leadership requires courageous caring: courage to envision beneficial outcomes, and caring comportment to evoke sincerity among staff to operationalize the dream. Lead with the soul of a warrior (Prestia, 2020a). Have the fortitude to journey to enlightenment, despite the challenges of chaos and complexity.

END-OF-CHAPTER RESOURCES

◧ DISCUSSION QUESTIONS

1. How could the leader of a community-based public health department best utilize AI to predict the impact of a viral pandemic?
2. How might ambient voice technology assist a certified RN midwife during an obstetrical emergency?
3. A nonverbal hospice patient is transferred from a skilled nursing facility in the middle of the night due to a fall. What technology might an ED nurse leader use to determine if aggressive treatment is the correct plan of action?

◧ LEARNING EXERCISES FOR STUDENTS

1. Consider the following scenarios which truly test the commitment of nurse leaders to stay true to assuring positive long-term outcomes for staff and patients despite potential consequences:

   - The CHRO reports that merit increases will be capped at 1% due to a poor financial margin during the recent pandemic. Additionally, those employees furloughed at any time during the year are ineligible for an increase as they did not work the whole year.
   - The director of orthopedics complains to you that the pre-op protocol meeting lasted for 2 hours and no progress was made.
   - A request from a staff RN for a 10-day vacation was denied by her manager. Six days were approved. The requesting employee met with a human resources representative for an explanation. When asked why the employee did not resolve the issue by following the chain of command, she stated, "Our director is unapproachable."

- On December 15, six agency nurses were hired for the Intensive Care Unit (ICU) to supplement the staffing for the next 13 weeks. At the end of February, the ICU director determined that the critical needs had subsided and cancelled two of the nurses at week 10.

- A town hall meeting turned tearful during which time a staff RN accused the CNO of breaking his promise to ensure safe staffing levels. When pressed for specifics, no details were provided, just a collective sentiment of being overworked.

A robust set of instructor resources designed to supplement this text is located at http://connect.springerpub.com/content/book/978-0-8261-7795-7. Qualifying instructors may request access by emailing textbook@springerpub.com.

REFERENCES

American Association of Critical-Care Nurses. (2021a). *Certification benefits patients, employers and nurses.* https://www.aacn.org/certification/value-of-certification-resource-center/nurse-certification-benefits-patients-employers-and-nurses

American Association of Critical-Care Nurses. (2021b, March). *AACN standards for establishing and sustaining healthy work environments.* https://www.aacn.org/WD/HWE/Docs/ExecSum.pdf

American Nurses Association. (2015). *Code of ethics for nurses: With interpretive statements.* https://www.nursingworld.org/practice-policy/nursing-excellence/ethics/code-of-ethics-for-nurses/coe-view-only

American Organization for Nursing Leadership. (2021, February). *American Organization for Nursing Leadership homepage.* https://www.aonl.org

American Organization of Nurse Executives. (2015). *AONE position statement on educational preparation of nurse leaders.* https://www.aonl.org/sites/default/files/aone/educational-preparation-nurse-leaders.pdf

American Society for Quality. (n.d.) *The define, measure, analyze, improve, control (DMAIC) process.* https://asq.org/quality-resources/dmaic

Arnold, L., Drenkard, K., Ela, S., Goedken, J., Hamilton, C., Harris, C., Holecek, N., & White, M. (2006). Strategic positioning for nursing excellence in health systems: Insights from chief nursing executives. *Nursing Administration Quarterly, 30*(1), 11–20. https://doi.org/10.1097/00006216-200601000-00004

Beauchamp, T. L., & Childress, J. F. (2009). *Principles of biomedical ethics.* Oxford Press.

Bellack, J. P., & Dickow, M. (2019). Why nurse leaders derail: Preventing and rebounding from leadership failure. *Nursing Administration Quarterly, 43*(2), 113–122. https://doi.org/10.1097/NAQ.0000000000000345

Berwick, D. M., Nolan, T. W., & Whittington, J. (2008). The Triple Aim: Care, health, and cost. *Health Affairs, 27*(3), 759–769. https://doi.org/10.1377/hlthaff.27.3.759

Bodenheimer, T., & Sinsky, C. (2014). From Triple to Quadruple Aim: Care of the patient requires care of the provider. *Annals of Family Medicine, 12*(6), 573–576. https://doi.org/10.1370/afm.1713

Bowles, J. R., Batcheller, J., Adams, J. M., Zimmermann, D., & Pappas, S. (2019). Nursing's leadership role in advancing professional practice/work environments as part of the Quadruple Aim. *Nursing Administration Quarterly, 43*(2), 157–163. https://doi.org/10.1097/NAQ.0000000000000342

Boykin, A., & Schoenhofer, S. O. (2001). *Nursing as caring.* Jones & Bartlett.

Chapman, G., & White, P. (2010). *The 5 languages of appreciation in the workplace.* Northfield Publishing.

Christian-Andersen, H. (1998). *The emperor's new clothes: An all-star retelling of the classic fairy tale.* Harcourt Brace.

Corley, M. C. (2002). Nurse moral distress: A proposed theory and research agenda. *Nurse Ethics, 9*(6), 636–650. https://doi.org/10.1191/0969733002ne557oa

The Deming Institute. (n.d.). *PDSA cycle.* https://deming.org/explore/pdsa

DiSciullo, B., Clafin, D., Hickerson, K. A., Kubis, S. E., Patton, A. M., Simpson, C. J., & Figuero-Altmann, A. (2021). Strategies for success in regulatory readiness. *The Journal of Nursing Administration, 51*(2), 6–8. https://doi.org/10.1097/NNA.0000000000000958

Drees, J., & Dyrda, L. (2020). *10 emerging trends in health IT for 2021*. https://www.beckershospital review.com/healthcare-information-technology/10-emerging-trends-in-health-it-for-2021.html

Duhigg, C. (2016). *What Google learned from its quest to build the perfect team*. https://www.nytimes. com/2016/02/28/magazine/what-google-learned-from-its-quest-to-build-the-perfect-team.html

Dyess, S., Boykin, A., & Rigg, C. (2010). Integrating caring theory with nursing practice and education: Connecting with what matters. *The Journal of Nursing Administration, 40*(11), 498–503. https://doi .org/10.1097/NNA.0b013e3181f88b96

Dyess, S. M., Prestia, A. S., Marquit, D. E., & Newman, D. (2018). Self-care for nurse leaders in acute care environment reduces perceived stress: A mixed-methods pilot study merits further investigation. *Journal of Holistic Nursing, 36*(1), 79–90. https://doi.org/10.1177/0898010116685655

Dyess, S. M., Prestia, A. S., Marquit, D. E., & Newman, D. (2019). Self-care for nurse leaders in acute care environments reduces perceived stress: A pilot study merits further investigation. *Journal of Holistic Nursing*. https://doi.org/10.1177/089801016685655

Dyess, S. M., Prestia, A. S., & Smith, M. (2015). Support for caring and resiliency. *Nursing Administration Quarterly, 39*(2), 104–116. https://doi.org/10.1097/NAQ.0000000000000101

Edmonson, C. (2010). Moral courage and the nurse leader. *OJIN: The Online Journal of Issues in Nursing, 15*(3), Manuscript 5. https://doi.org/10.3912/OJIN.Vol15no03Man05

EDShare. (n.d.). *Reflective learning theory*. University of South Hampton. http://edshare.soton.ac .uk/11124/1/index.htm

Enright, S. M., & White, S. J. (2012). Leadership courage. *Hospital Pharmacy, 47*(1), 807–810. https:// doi.org/10.1310/hpj4710-807

France24. (2020, December 26). Covid-19 pandemic will not be the last: WHO chief. *France24*. https:// www.france24.com/en/live-news/20201226-covid-19-pandemic-will-not-be-the-last-who-chief

Gawande, A. (2009). *The checklist manifesto: How to get things right*. Henry Holt.

Goodwin, D. K. (2018). *Leadership in turbulent times*. Simon & Schuster.

Harvard Business Review Editors. (2016). The four phases of project management. *Harvard Business Review*. https://hbr.org/2016/11/the-four-phases-of-project-management

Healthcare Information Management Systems Society. (n.d.). Who we are. https://www.himss.org/ who-we-are

Hewlett, S. (2014). *Executive presence*. Harper Collins.

Jaffee, A. (2021, January). *Harris prepares for central role in Biden's White House*. https://apnews.com/ article/joe-biden-race-and-ethnicity-symone-sanders-south-asia-coronavirus-pandemic-d11545d0 9f132366909d492822df692d

Joint Statement on Delegation, American Nurses Association & the National Council of State Boards of Nursing. (2019). *National guidelines for nursing delegation*. https://www.ncsbn.org/NGND -PosPaper_06.pdf

Kearns, D. K. (2018). *Leadership in turbulent times*. Simon & Schuster.

Kennedy, K., Campis, S., & Leclerc, L. (2020). Human-centered leadership: Creating change from the inside out. *Nurse Leader, 18*(4), 227–231. https://doi.org/10.1016/j.mnl.2020.03.009

Klann, G. (2007). *Building character: Strengthening the heart of good leadership*. John Wiley and Sons.

Lee, E., Daugherty, J., & Hamelin, T. (2019). Reimage health care leadership, challenges and opportunities in the 21st century. *Journal of PeriAnesthesia Nursing, 34*(1), 27–38. https://doi.org/10.1016/j .jopan.2017.11.007

Lee, T. H., & Duckworth, A. L. (2018). Organizational grit. *Harvard Business Review*. https://hbr. org/2018/09/organizational-grit

Maslow, A. H. (1969). *Psychology of science: A reconnaissance*. Maurice Bassett Publishing.

Mayeroff, M. (1971). *On caring*. HarperPerennial.

Mayo, A. T., & Woolley, A. W. (2016). Teamwork in health care: Maximizing collective intelligence via inclusive collaboration and open communication. *AMA Journal of Ethics, 18*(9), 933–940. https:// doi.org/10.1001/journalofethics.2016.18.9.stas2-1609

McLeod, S. (2020). *Maslow's hierarchy of needs*. https://www.simplypsychology.org/maslow.html

Melnyk, B. M., Fineout-Overholt, E., Gallagher-Ford, L., & Kaplan, L. (2012). The state of evidenced based practice in US nurses: Critical implications for nurse leaders and educators. *The Journal of Nursing Administration, 42*(9), 410–417. https://doi.org/10.1097/NNA.0b013e3182664e0a

Miami Dade College. (n.d.). *History of Modernism*. https://www.mdc.edu/wolfson/academic/ artsletters/art_philosophy/humanities/history_of_modernism.htm

Morley, L., & Cashell, A. (2017). Collaboration in health care. *Journal of Medical Imaging and Radiation Sciences, 48*, 207–216. https://doi.org/10.1016/j.jmir.2017.02.071

National Academies of Sciences, Engineering, and Medicine. (2021). *The future of nursing 2020-2030*. https://www.nationalacademies.org/our-work/the-future-of-nursing-2020-2030

Pass It On. (2021). *For it is in giving that we receive*. https://www.passiton.com/inspirational-quotes/ 7241-for-it-is-in-giving-that-we-receive#:~:text=%E2%80%9CFor%20it%20is%20in%20giving, Francis%20of%20Assisi%20%7C%20PassItOn.com

Pennic, J. (2019). *Top 10 challenges, issues and opportunities for healthcare executives in 2019*. https://hitconsultantnet/2018/09/28/challenges-issues-opportunities-healthcare-executives/ #XZ5GvmZ7mUk

Perlo, J., Balik, B., Swensen, S., Kabcenell, A., Landsman, J., & Feeley, D. (2017). *IHI: Framework for improving joy in work*. IHI White Paper. Institute for Healthcare Improvement.

Porter-O'Grady T. (2011). *Presentation at Florida Atlantic University*, September 27, Boca Raton, Florida.

Prestia, A. S. (2014). Strengthening the CNO/CEO relationship: A model of collaboration. *Nurse Leader, 12*(6), 79–83. https://doi.org/10.1016/j.mnl.2014.04.004

Prestia, A. S. (2015). Chief nursing officer sustainment: A phenomenological inquiry. *The Journal of Nursing Administration, 45*(11), 575–581. https://doi.org/10.1097/NNA.0000000000000266

Prestia, A. S. (2016a). A fresh approach to impactful messaging. *Nurse Leader, 16*(3), 163–166. http:// doi.org/10.1016/j.mnl.2018.03.004

Prestia, A. S. (2016b). Transformational resiliency. *Nurse Leader, 14*(5), 354–357. https://doi.org/ 10.1016/j.mnl.2016.05.001

Prestia, A. S. (2017). The art of leadership diplomacy. *Nursing Management, 48*(4), 52–55. https://doi .org/10.1097/01.NUMA.0000514068.76314.4d

Prestia, A. S. (2019). Reflection: A powerful leadership tool. *Nurse Leader, 17*(5), 465–467. https://doi .org/10.1016/j.mnl.2019.01.004

Prestia, A. S. (2020a). Leading with the soul of a warrior. *Nurse Leader, 18*(2), 163–166. https://doi .org/10.1016/j.mnl.2019.09.015

Prestia, A. S. (2020b, August). The moral obligation of nurse leaders: COVID-19. *Nurse Leader, 18*(4), 326–328. https://doi.org/j.mnl.2020.04.008

Prestia, A. S. (2020c, December). Failure: Is it personal? *Nurse Leader, 18*(6), 616–619. https://doi .org/10.1016/j.mnl.2019.11.015

Prestia, A. S. (2021a). Next level self-care for nurse leaders. *Nurse Leader, 19*(3), 305–307. https://doi .org/10.1016/j.mnl.2021.02.006

Prestia, A. S. (2021b). Nurse executive mental health. *Nurse Leader, 19*(4), 378–382. https://doi. org/10.1016/j.mnl.2020.03.016

Prestia, A. S. (2021c). The remote influence of nursing leadership. *Nurse Leader, 19*(2), 184–187. https://doi.org/10.1016/j.mnl.2020.06.005

Prestia, A. S., & Platas, C. N. (2019). The over-committed nurse executive. *Nurse Leader, 17*(2), 155–158. http://doi.org/10.1016/j.mnl.2018.09.011

Prestia, A. S., & Dyess, S. M. (2020). Losing site: The importance of nurse executive's balancing caring essentials. *Nurse Leader, 18*(4), 329–332. https://doi.org/10.1016/j.mnl.2020.04.005

Ray, M. (1997). The ethical theory of existential authenticity: The lived experience of the art of caring in nursing administration. *Canadian Journal of Nursing Research, 29*(1), 111–126. http://hdl.handle .net/10822/902039

Roach, M. S. (2002). *Caring, the human mode of being*. CHA Press.

Robbins, M. (2007). *Focus on the good stuff: The power of appreciation*. Jossey-Bass.

Rothberg, E. (n.d.). *Biography: Lillian Wald*. https://www.womenshistory.org/education-resources/ biographies/lillian-wald

Schmidt, B. (2014). *The practice: Simple tools for managing stress, finding inner peace and uncovering happiness*. Health Communications.

Schnitker, S. A. (2012). An examination of patience and well-being. *The Journal of Positive Psychology, 7*(4), 263–280. http://doi/10.1080/17439760.2012.697185

Scipioni, J. (2020, November). The 1-minute destresser Barack Obama used during his presidency to 'clear his mind'. *CNBC Make It*. https://www.cnbc.com/2020/11/11/trick-barack-obama-used -during-his-presidency-to-clear-his-mind.html

Solbakken, R., Bergdahl, E., Rudolfsson, G., & Bondas, T. (2018). International nursing: Caring in nursing leadership—A meta-ethnography from the nurse leader's perspective. *Nursing Administrative Quarterly, 42*(4), E1–E19. https://doi.org/10.1097/NAQ.0000000000000314

Staff Writers. (2018). *One thing at a time: A brief history of the checklist.*https://www.flightsafetyaustralia.com/2018/11/one-thing-at-a-time-a-brief-history-of-the-checklist

Stazesky, R. C. (2000, January). *George Washington, genius in leadership.* https://washington papers.org/resources/articles/George-washington-genius-in-leadership

Stichler, J. F. (2013). Healthy work environments for the aging workforce. *Journal of Nursing Management, 21*, 956–963. https://doi.org/10.1111/jonm.12174

Strauss, T. (2020, November). *Organizational factors underlying the adoption of a patient-centered approach in physician-patient interaction* (Publication No. 28745417) [Master's dissertation, University of Haifa (Israel)]. ProQuest Dissertations Publishing. https://www.proquest.com/dissertations-theses/organizational-factors-underlying-adoption/docview/2593014088/se-2

Suresh, G. K., Godfrey, M. M., Nelson, E. C., & Batalden, P. B. (2011). Improving safety and anticipating hazards in clinical microsystems. In E. C. Nelson, P. B. Batalden, M. M. Godfrey, & J. S. Lazar (Eds.), *Value by design* (pp. 87–130). Jossey-Bass.

Tideman, S. G., Arts, M. C., & Zandee, D. P. (2013). Sustainable leadership: Towards a workable definition. *The Journal of Corporate Citizenship*, (49), 17–33. https://go.gale.com/ps/i.do?p=AONE&u=anon~a0bcf113&id=GALE|A347968416&v=2.1&it=r&sid=googleScholar&asid=31a589cb

Viser, M., & Linskey, A. (2021). 'The art of the possible': Biden lays out pragmatic vision for his presidency. https://www.washingtonpost.com/politics/biden-pragmatic-agenda/2021/03/25/d8fec310-8da2-11eb-a730-1b4ed9656258_story.html

Watson, J. (2006). Caring theory as an ethical guide to administrative and clinical practice. *Nursing Administrative Quarterly, 30*(1), 48–55. https://doi.org/10.1097/00006216-200601000-00008

Wheatley, M. J. (2006). *Leadership and the new science.* Berrett-Koehler.

Yancer, D. A. (2012). Betrayed trust: Healing a broken hospital through servant leadership. *Nursing Administration Quarterly, 36*(1), 63–80. https://doi.org/10.1097/NAQ.ObO13e31823B458b

CHAPTER | 2

PROFESSIONALISM

Germaine C. Nelson

"Professionalism demonstrates the hallmark of one's character."
S. Moore (personal communication, February 14, 2021)

LEARNING OBJECTIVES

- Define professionalism, self-care, and mindfulness.
- Differentiate leadership and management behaviors that build professionalism within individuals, teams, mentees, and organizations.
- Apply the elements of advocacy and support with individuals and groups with information to build advocacy involvement and foundational precepts.
- Formulate individual and team strategies to engage in wellness, self-care, and mindfulness practices.

INTRODUCTION

Professionalism is demonstrated through the adherence to or development of standards, practice guidelines, and behaviors that are supported by licensing agencies, professional organizations, organizational structures, and thought leaders in the profession. The American Nurses Association's (ANA's) *Nursing Scope and Standards of Practice* provides the professional framework for nursing standards and practice. Professionalism is demonstrated through a commitment to ethical standards; a commitment to quality and patient safety; the commitment to skills acquisition and competency development; the commitment to behaviors that foster mindfulness and self-care; the commitment to behaviors that foster a culture of respect, as well as support diversity, equity, and inclusion; and the commitment to lifelong learning. Currently there are an estimated 28 million nurses worldwide, and in the 2020 calendar year nurses received additional exposure as the COVID-19 pandemic brought media attention to the work they perform daily. Their roles included exposure to organisms and diseases that could equal potentially fatal exposures and negative sequela as nurses provided life-saving care to others. With images of nurses' faces structurally impacted by lines and often skin breakdown from prolonged periods of wearing masks, coupled with the physically exhaustive work requirements experienced daily, nursing became a point of interest on nightly news programs. The public viewed a barrage of images of nurses, witnessed real-time patient care innovation, and became acutely aware of the professional role that nurses have within the complex worldwide and U.S. healthcare delivery systems. This all displayed the essential nature of the work done by a highly skilled healthcare worker—the professional nurse.

Professionalism demonstrated while managing emergencies, and in the mitigation of COVID-19–related risks, was credited to the professional nurse as part of a dynamic healthcare team, which included the professional nurse leader and professional nursing organizations as advocates. All this occurred during 2020, the "Year of the Nurse and Midwife," so named in honor of the 200th birth anniversary of Florence Nightingale. While historically significant, only one year—2020—was devoted to recognizing the professionalism of nurses. "The values and ethics of the profession should be affirmed in all professional and organizational relationships whether local, inter-organizational, or international" (ANA, 2015, p. 35).

Widening the lens and extending the "Year of the Nurse and Midwife" into 2021, one asks, what is professionalism in nursing? Professionalism has many components. It is understanding and upholding the mission, vision, and values of one's practice and the organizations to which one belongs when employed or working within collaborative relationships. Professionalism is maintaining the standards of practice, ethics, integrity, and accountability. Professionalism is practicing advocacy at the local, national, and global level to assist in building better health-related outcomes for patients and communities. It is understanding and engaging in social justice and championing equity. It is building one's knowledge of the financial issues within the healthcare delivery system and committing to resource stewardship. It is innovating. It is demonstrating executive presence and engaging in self-care and mindfulness. Professionalism is not a singular process but the weaving of multiple elements and moving to the mastery of the stated capabilities and competencies. "All registered nurses are expected to engage in professional role activities, including leadership, appropriate to their education and position" (ANA, 2021, p. 5). Professionalism is codified as one of the common core competencies for health leadership by the American Organization for Nursing Leadership (AONL). Table 2.1 reviews significant milestones within the profession of nursing.

TABLE 2.1: Historical Milestones in Nursing

Year(s)	Historical Milestones in Nursing
1820	Florence Nightingale was born May 12
1853 through 1856	The Crimean War military conflict was fought October 1853 to February 1856; in 1854, Florence Nightingale brought 38 volunteer nurses to provide care to British soldiers
1860	Florence Nightingale credited for the professionalization of nursing in healthcare
1879	Mary Eliza Mahoney was the first African American to graduate from an American school of nursing
1881	Clarissa Harlowe Barton founded the American Red Cross
1893	National League for Nursing (NLN) founded the first professional organization within the body of nursing
1896	The Nurses' Associated Alumnae of the United States and Canada was founded
1899	International Council of Nurses (ICN) was founded
1911	The Nurses' Associated Alumnae of the United States and Canada became the American Nurses Association (ANA)
1922	Sigma Theta Tau International Honor Society of Nursing was founded
1948	The World Health Organization (WHO) was founded April 7
1950	The ANA Code of Ethics for Nurses was adopted
1953	The ICN Code of Ethics for Nurses was adopted
1954	National Nurses Week was initially established in October
1964–1966	The American Academy of Nursing (AAN) was first approved

(continued)

TABLE 2.1: Historical Milestones in Nursing *(continued)*

Year(s)	Historical Milestones in Nursing
1965	Dr. Loretta Ford and Dr. Henry Silver develop the first nurse practitioner (NP) program at the University of Colorado
1967	The American Hospital Association (AHA) Council of Nursing was organized, a membership group of the AHA; today, it is known as the American Organization for Nursing Leadership (AONL), previously known as the American Organization for Nurse Executives (AONE)
1971	The National Black Nurses Association (NBNA) was organized
1975	The National Association of Hispanic Nurses (NAHN) was founded
1978	The National Council of State Boards of Nursing (NCSBN) is founded
1979	The Philippine Nurses Association of America, Inc. (PNAA) is established
1985	Public Health law 99-158 authorizes the National Center for Nursing Research (NCNR) at the National Institutes of Health (NIH)
1992	The Asian American/Pacific Islander Nurses Association, Inc. (AAPINA) was formed
1993	The National Institute of Nursing Research (NINR) was established
1993	The Delegate Assembly adopted the Model Legislation Language and Model Administrative Rules for Advanced Nursing Practice
1998	The National Coalition of Ethnic Minority Nurse Associations (NCEMNA) was incorporated
2020	WHO declares "The Year of the Nurse and Midwife" in recognition of the 200th birth anniversary of Florence Nightingale
2020	Sandra Lindsay, a nurse, was the first person to receive the COVID-19 vaccine in the United States on December 14
2021	WHO extends "The Year of the Nurse and Midwife" in recognition of the 200th birth anniversary of Florence Nightingale

PROFESSIONALISM AND STANDARDS OF PRACTICE

Foundational to nursing professionalism are the nursing scope and standards of practice. "Nursing occurs when there is a need for nursing knowledge, wisdom, caring, leadership, practice, or education, anytime, anywhere" (ANA, 2021, p. 3). The National Council of State Boards of Nursing states "[s]afe, competent nursing practice is grounded in the law as written in the state nurse practice act (NPA) and the state rules/regulations" (National Council of State Boards of Nursing, n.d., para. 1). "To be accountable, nurses follow a code of ethical conduct that includes moral principles such as fidelity, loyalty, veracity, beneficence, and respect for the dignity, worth, and self-determination of patients as well as adhering to the scope and standards of nursing practice" (ANA, 2015, p. 15). Globally as stated by the International Council of Nurses (ICN) Code of Ethics, "[n]urses have four fundamental responsibilities: to promote health, to prevent illness, to restore health and to alleviate suffering" (2012, p. 1).

Health promotion can occur with each patient contact, and by engaging with communities to raise awareness of specific disease-related concerns. Professional nurses can also engage patients and communities through social media to highlight priority areas for wellness integration. Restoration of health can occur at the stretcher-side, bedside, or through critical decisions made in the boardroom. Clinical competency demonstrated by providing the best technical care and leadership skills allows for patients to experience improvement or health maintenance in their current level of illness. The alleviation of suffering occurs with the compassionate and empathetic caring that is the cornerstone of nursing professionalism.

It is through ongoing education, involvement in research, designing quality improvement structures, and the development of evidence-based practices that professional nurses impact care. "Research-focused nurses engage in the science of nursing and spirit of inquiry by designing, implementing, and evaluating research studies directed to the generation of new knowledge to improve and reform nursing practice and the systems in which nursing practice occurs" (ANA, 2021, p. 31). Great care should be taken to uphold the scope and standards of practice.

Nurse managers and nurse executives enhance the maintenance in professional standards of practice by maintaining the competencies of leadership, professionalism, business skills and principles, knowledge of healthcare and the environment, and communication and relationship management, a framework developed by the Healthcare Leadership Alliance.

PROFESSIONALISM REQUIRES ETHICS AND INTEGRITY

Professionalism requires integrity, ethics, and accountability. In 2020 and for the 19th consecutive year, nurses were ranked by Gallup as the most trusted professionals in the United States. The most trusted ranking carries with it a significant level of professional responsibility and vigilant protection of the public's trust. In 1990, the ANA established the Center for Ethics and Human Rights to assist nurses in obtaining a thorough understanding of the ethical issues encountered in a rapidly changing practice landscape (ANA, 2020). Currently, the Center for Ethics and Human Rights inbox is ethics@ana.org, and connects leaders to 12 nurse ethicists. By reviewing the standards for the professions, various practice organizations, and by reviewing interpretative and evidence-based guidelines, nurses are positioned to uphold the maintenance of acceptable standards. Nursing-executive leadership is key to the maintenance of ethics and integrity. "Healthcare organizations must be led and managed with integrity and consistent adherence to organizational values, professional and ethical standards" (American College of Healthcare Executives, 2020, para. 1).

Ethical standards and a commitment to professionalism are enhanced through skillful decision-making that demonstrates integrity, ethics, and accountability. "Decision making is defined by the following attributes: information gathering, critical thinking, and use of a defined process" (Quinn Griffin et al., 2016, p. 178). Evaluating situations and considering decision points as shown in Box 2.1 may aid in decision-making that meets the standards of ethics and integrity.

BOX 2.1: POINTS TO CONSIDER WHEN MAKING DECISIONS BASED ON STANDARDS, ETHICS, AND INTEGRITY

- Analyze what is guiding the decision. Through the gathering of information, determine if there are any clinical decision support tools, research, quality data, predictive analytics, professional organization white papers or position statements, regulatory mandates, or metrics that can assist in the decision-making process.

- Are all team members in alignment with the decision, and have dissenting views been considered? Critically analyze opposing views and ideas.

- Is there diversity of clinical expertise, skill, gender, age, and backgrounds within the decision-making team?

- Would a professional weighing the specifics of ethics and integrity make the same decisions, or draw the same conclusions?

(continued)

BOX 2.1: POINTS TO CONSIDER WHEN MAKING DECISIONS BASED ON STANDARDS, ETHICS, AND INTEGRITY *(continued)*

- Is the decision in alignment with the ANA's *Code of Ethics for Nurses With Interpretive Statements* or the *Nursing Scope and Standards of Practice?*

- Has there been a review or usage of ethical analysis models? The MORAL Model or the DECIDE Model can be considered.

- Has a culture been created where concerns related to ethical standards or decisions are raised without fear of reprisal or career compromise?

- Is there a clear and readily identifiable process for the report of ethics-related concerns?

- Does this decision require additional discussion with the corporate compliance department, the ethics committee, peers with content expertise, or legal counsel?

- Does the decision make sense when considering ethics, integrity, or accountability guideposts?

To create an ethical culture, healthcare executives should support the development and implementation of ethical standards of behavior, including ethical, clinical, leadership, management, research, and quality improvement practices; ensure effective and comprehensive ethics resources, including an ethics committee, exist and are available to develop; propagate and clarify such standards of behavior when there is ethical uncertainty; support and implement a systemic and organization-wide approach to ethics training (including the consequences of social disparities in healthcare) and corporate compliance; and exemplify diversity, inclusion, and equity as core organizational values in creating an ethical culture (American College of Healthcare Executives, 2020).

There is no gradation for ethical standards.

THE ORGANIZATIONAL ROLE IN ETHICAL STANDARDS IN PROFESSIONALISM

Organizations address ethical standards by developing mission and vision statements as part of their core business strategy. The corporate board's governance structure and executive leadership teams work to ensure that compliance processes support the mission and vision. "Mission is the central purpose of an organization; its reason for existence" (White & Griffith, 2019, p. 4). "The vision statement continues the expression of the desired service and the level of achievement necessary to achieve the mission" (Porter-O'Grady & Malloch, 2015, p. 180). Employee handbooks outline the behaviors that are expected to guide practice and assimilation of the corporate mission and vision statements. Effective handbooks point employees to daily performance and ethical standards, the organization's "true north" and direction of excellence, and provide structure to support metric-related goals. At the organizational level, a continued analysis of the ethical standards conveyed by the mission and vision statements, ethical alignment with professional standards, quality structures, ethics committee protocols, and clinical practice guidelines must be critically appraised on an ongoing basis. Nurse executives' competencies dictate that the leader: "uphold ethical principles and corporate compliance standards; hold self and staff accountable to comply with ethical standards of practice; and discuss, resolve and learn from ethical dilemmas" (American Organization of Nurse Executives [AONE] & AONL, 2015a, p. 9). Figure 2.1 provides an overview of the flow of organizational ethical standards responsibility, development, and refinement.

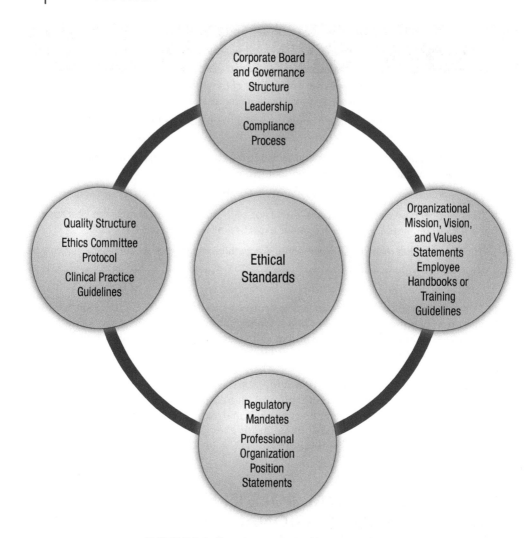

FIGURE 2.1: Organizational ethical standards flow.

PROFESSIONALISM AND ETHICS AT THE INDIVIDUAL LEVEL

At the individual level, professionalism dictates the continual process of self-reflection and an analysis of competency-related ethics knowledge. Continually assessing one's strengths, weaknesses, opportunities, and threats (SWOT analysis) and developing an individual development plan (IDP) to build in identified strategic areas for ethics knowledge improvement is essential. "People learn and develop when what they want to change matters deeply and will affect them both personally and professionally" (McKee et al., 2008, p. 7). Figure 2.2 highlights the flow for individual development of ethics knowledge and competency.

SOCIAL MEDIA PRESENCE AND PROFESSIONALISM

Social media includes applications, tools, and technologies that facilitate communication among individuals and groups; these are used to share information (Society for Human Resource Management, 2016). Social media has influenced the way both individuals and organizations communicate, and social media presents a public relations opportunity for

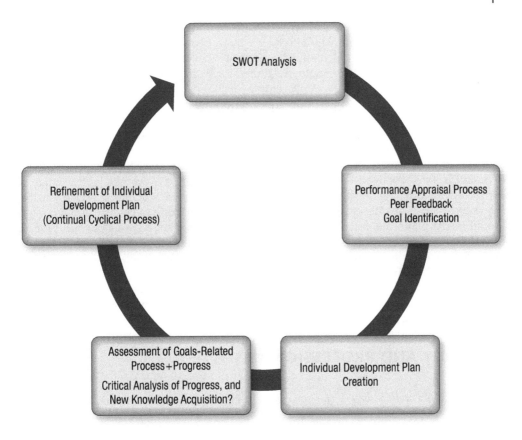

FIGURE 2.2: Flow for individual development of ethics knowledge and competency.

SWOT, strengths, weaknesses, opportunities, and threats.

organizations to communicate with staff and the public, to recruit talent, and to facilitate partnership and collaboration (Society for Human Resource Management, 2016). Social media includes, but is not limited to, text messages, media message services (MMS), Twitter, Facebook, Instagram, Clubhouse, LinkedIn, YouTube, TikTok, and organizational internal and external websites. Nursing professionals must remain critically aware that there are codes of conduct directly linked to the usage of social media, publications, and verbal dialogue (e.g., podcasts). These codes involve upholding the values of respect, courtesy, and thoughtfulness, as well as the parameters for copyrighted material. A purposeful and deliberate pause before posting is beneficial and allows for an additional layer of analysis of social media content.

The ANA has developed guiding principles for social networking (ANA, n.d.-b):

1. Nurses must not transmit or place online individually identifiable information.

2. Nurses must observe ethically prescribed professional patient–nurse boundaries.

3. Nurses should understand that patients, colleagues, organizations, and employers may view postings.

4. Nurses should take advantage of privacy settings and seek to separate personal and professional information online.

5. Nurses should bring content that could harm a patient's privacy, rights, or welfare to the attention of appropriate authorities.

6. Nurses should participate in developing organizational policies governing online conduct.

The governing board and leaders of organizations continually assess threats to their brand and language that is not in alignment with their values. In the rapid-fire social media world, professionalism requires that a calculation be made of whether social media post sviolate established organizational values if employed. Professionalism dictates an understanding that every post is readily available to the public, employers, licensing agencies, and regulators. Information technology departments within organizations monitor every computer keystroke. Consistent review of policies allows for the understanding of allowed communication and expectations for appropriate social media behaviors. Reviewing the competency of personal and professional accountability draws the leader's attention to "role model standards of professional practice (clinical, educational, and leadership) for colleagues and constituents" (AONE & AONL, 2015a, p. 9). Analysis of strategic management highlights "promote[s] the image of nursing and the organization through effective media relations" (AONE & AONL, 2015a, p. 10) and demonstrates the expectation for nurse leaders. Narratives created through posts on social media platforms, publications, or opinion pieces matter and are a powerful forum for the dissemination of information. Information, whether texted, posted, tweeted, or published, does not have an expiration date. The tone and tenor of published content matter and should be in alignment with the standards of professionalism.

The maintenance of one's professional image and reputation must be curated daily. Consider consulting with the marketing and communications department when available or branding experts (e.g., BRANDPRENUER, http://nickfnelson.com).

ADVOCACY AND PROFESSIONALISM

"Change will not come if we wait for some other person or some other time. We are the ones we've been waiting for. We are the change that we seek."

President Barack Obama

In 2020, nurses raised their voices to advocate for uniformity with the requirements for availability and usage of personal protective equipment (PPE) when providing care to patients with COVID-19, and the need for an integrated national logistics plan for the distribution of PPE. Professional nurses advocated for the dissemination of updates regarding masking requirements and provided their voice to "stay home" campaigns during 2020. Nurses used advocacy to activate their political power and call-to-action protocols and practices that were directly impacting life and health. Through electronic petitions, providing expert testimony, and having a presence within the news media, nurses used a collective voice to challenge politicians and world leaders to emergently address the PPE safety needs of their colleagues at the bedside. The ANA political action committee (PAC) provides an avenue for political engagement and support for candidates who support ANA's legislative agendas. Nurses Day at the Capitol provides a chance for elected officials to hear from nurses engaged in the political process and hear position statements on legislative items impacting healthcare. Utilizing their advocacy to address healthcare economics and policy is a competency for the nurse executive.

Nurses can become involved at the local level by attending community board meetings, attending local town hall events, or drafting letters to the editor at the community and national level. To learn more and have a formalized structure for advocacy review, the ANA Advocacy Toolkit (ANA–toolkit [aristotle.com]). "Nurses instinctively advocate for their patients, in their workplaces, and in their communities: but legislative and political advocacy is no less important to advancing the profession and patient care" (ANA, n.d.-a, para. 1). Committing to evaluating constructive change that can be formulated through strong advocacy-related work is essential and is paramount to public health. Vulnerable populations can only be impacted when professionals, professional organizations, communities, and political systems form collaborative relationships that are goal-directed to improving health. "Implementing change to address SDOH (social determinants of health) and advance health equity will require the contributions of nurses in all roles and all settings, and recognition that no one nurse can successfully implement change without the collaboration of others" (Wakefield et al., 2021, p. 277).

PROFESSIONALISM AND ADVOCACY THROUGH MEMBERSHIP

Professional memberships allow for nurses, including executives, to engage with peers with common interests, common clinical expertise, and interest in the development of and dissemination of research; draft position statements and policy/programmatic guidelines; and provide a forum for continued education, specialty certification, and advocacy. It has been reported that there are more than 130 nursing organizations across an array of practice areas, ethnic groups, and national affiliations. Professional organization membership and board-related responsibilities can enhance the development of professionalism through committee involvement, offer opportunities to author advocacy-related publications, develop policy, and foster opportunities to serve in roles that build one's ability in advocacy-based development. Through professional organization social media campaigns and media-related activities, professional organizations provide additional streams of information to their membership and the public. A comprehensive list of professional nursing organizations can be found on the worldwide web, or by visiting the Sigma Theta Tau International Honor Society of Nursing website: Professional Nursing Organizations (sigmanursing.org).

 CASE SCENARIO

ADVOCACY

SITUATION

Nurse Manager JS is familiar with the role of advocacy as it pertains to their individual patients' responsibilities. Over the last year, they attended several rallies for very public social justice movements. They would like to utilize their professional voice on an ongoing basis to champion causes that raise awareness and address concerns related to equity in housing, equity-related research in women, and the lack of diversity within executive leadership in healthcare, including their present organization. Their organization's senior leadership team has posted several position statements on equity-related gaps on the employee intranet and has stated that there will be a plan to address equity at the organizational level.

APPROACH

Nurse Manager JS has reviewed an analysis of housing in the community where they reside, as well as within the community where the hospital Nurse Manager JS works at is located (the poverty rate in these areas was 23.3% in 2019 compared to 16% citywide and the life expectancy rate was 11 years shorter than in the more affluent areas of the city). Nurse Manager JS has met with several hospital-based nurse researchers to gain more information and insight on the research process and inclusion of women in government-funded studies, and they have read all the materials on the intranet from the hospital's Office for Diversity and Inclusion. Nurse Manager JS also began reading position statements from the two professional organizations they belong to and the PAC information available on the ANA website at https://ana.aristotle.com/SitePages/pac.aspx.

OUTCOME

Nurse Manager JS will do the following:

- They will begin to attend the hospital-based community advisory committee meetings that are held monthly so Nurse Manager JS can become more informed about the community needs and participate in an organized effort to rally for low- and middle-income housing in the community. They will sign up for notifications from the mayors' and governors' offices on housing lotteries, as well as community zoning and planning meetings.

- They will begin to attend the hospital-based research council meetings. They will also become active in Sigma Theta Tau and will attend virtual events to build research-based knowledge.
- They will join the employee resource group within the hospital to participate in discussions and activities that will facilitate discussions related to leadership diversity that are both ongoing and solutions oriented. They have volunteered to mentor one student in a community-based mentoring program supported by the hospital's executive leadership team.
- They have also sent an email to their immediate manager and the chief nurse executive to determine workgroup and volunteer activities that are specific to advocacy.

DISCUSSION QUESTION

1. Draft an advocacy-based project that could be implemented for National Nurses Week that would involve a cross-section of units and job functions.

EXEMPLARY PROFESSIONAL PRACTICE AND PROFESSIONALISM

When evaluating exemplary professional practice, the American Nurses Credentialing Center (ANCC) Magnet® criteria for nursing excellence is the framework for discussion. "The true essence of a Magnet organization stems from exemplary professional practice within nursing" (ANCC, n.d., "III. Exemplary Professional Practice"). This occurs through evaluating both the professional practice model (PPM) and the care delivery system (CDS). Exemplary professional practice incorporates patients, patient-centered care, interprofessional collaboration practice, standards, and professional organization standards of practice, patient safety, and autonomy into the organizational nursing practice. Nurses consistently engage with the healthcare system to ensure that the design of the CDSs are in alignment with the improvement of the patient's outcomes and the patient and family experience. Advocacy is key to evaluating those systems designed to consider inclusion. Another key is providing a tangible mechanism to assess professionalism based on metrics that can be trended. Global issues in nursing and healthcare are also reviewed utilizing both the PPM and CDS. The role of the nurse leader is to build an environment that hardwires the components of the PPM and supports advocacy-related projects that positively impact clinical outcomes validated by metrics.

THE ROLE OF THE NURSE RESEARCHER WITHIN ADVOCACY

The knowledge and learning that occurs within a profession should be guided by evidence-based research. Understanding communities through research, including but not limited to ethnographic studies, can impact the quality of lives and can improve the patient care experience. Rivera and Fitzpatrick noted, "It is important that as clinical leaders, nurses have the most accurate, most up-to-date, and evidence-based information available so that they can always do the right thing" (2021, p. xxiv). Conducting studies, participating in research, or participating in professional organizations that further research-based knowledge is a competency and goal when building professional advocacy. The nurse executive is charged with the "use [of] data and other sources of evidence to inform decision making" (AONL, 2015a, p. 7). The nurse leader as advocate should be committed to an environment that fosters research to ensure that all patient populations receive care tailored to their individual needs and that the evidence and PPM are in alignment.

EQUITY, SOCIAL JUSTICE, AND ALLYSHIP

"Professionalism is the confidence to be one's authentic, amazing self, knowing that— despite what structural '-ism' and '-phobias' suggest—individuality alone does not subvert a

team's shared mission and vision. In tandem, professionalism is the competence to motivate, appreciate, and navigate others doing the same."

O. Byers (personal communication, February 14, 2021)

"Equity is defined as the process by which we achieve fairness, equality, and inclusion that includes the reallocation of resources and implementation of policies and structures that work to eliminate historical, systemic advantage" (Winters, 2020, p. 161). In 2020, there were two historic events that galvanized many to have greater discussions regarding equity, social justice, and allyship. On May 25, 2020, George Floyd was placed under arrest as part of an investigation into the use of an alleged $20 counterfeit bill. What was witnessed by millions was a 9 minute and 29 second video of an arrest and what has now been ruled after a jury trial to be a murder. Simultaneously the COVID-19 pandemic highlighted the disparities in health experienced by communities of color. On April 8, 2021, the Centers for Disease Control and Prevention (CDC) and the administrator of the Agency for Toxic Substances and Disease Registry (ATSDR) declared racism a serious public health threat. "Racism is a system—consisting of structures, policies, practices, and norms—that assigns value and determines opportunity based on the way people look or the color of their skin" (CDC, n.d., para. 1). "There are many moments in history that are an inflection point, where it illuminates all the dark corners of our experience, and that is what these last two years have done: they've forced us to confront so many things etched by racism" (Lonnie G. Bunch as cited in Mount Sinai, 2021, para. 4). These things and disparities impacted who lived and died.

Healthcare and, more importantly, the profession of nursing are uniquely positioned to address equity, social justice, and allyship within healthcare leadership including healthcare organizations, equity where care delivery occurs, equity in the community, and equality and social justice within the healthcare industry. Nurses are change agents and innovators. "The current unrest worldwide in response to unjust killings of Black and Brown people as well as higher rates of COVID-19 within these communities, has emphasized more clearly the need for social justice reform that address[es] racism and realigns structures to enable the attainment of better health regardless of race, ethnicity, gender, social group, or geography" (ANA, 2020, para. 2).

Professionalism dictates that nurses committed to equity, equality, allyship, and change consider the following points:

- Do I understand the equity, equality, and power dynamic of this situation?
- Has the clinical impact of decisions made or proposed been evaluated from a lens of equity, equality, diversity, and inclusion?
- Am I contributing daily to an environment that fosters equity, equality, diversity, inclusivity, and allyship?
- When attending meetings or organized events, is there diversity within the meeting group, and can I request the addition of representative attendees?
- Have I reviewed position statements of professional organizations or community groups related to the specific discussion or decisions? Have the SDOH been considered or been impacted by this decision or project?
- "Commit to do your part to eradicate injustices as part of our collective responsibility" (Winters, 2020, p. 157).

PROFESSIONALISM AND CULTURAL HUMILITY, INCLUSIVITY, AND ACCESS

Nurses must provide care that is equitable and culturally competent, while understanding the tenets of cultural humility. Cultural competency in healthcare describes the ability of systems to provide care to patients with diverse values, beliefs, and behaviors, including the tailoring of healthcare delivery to meet the patient's social, cultural, and linguistic needs

(American Hospital Association [AHA], 2021). Cultural humility involves understanding the complexity of identities—that even in sameness there is difference—and that a clinician will never be fully competent about the evolving and dynamic nature of a patient's experiences (Khan, 2021). Understanding that people are not a monolith allows the healthcare professional to expand one's view of culture by asking key questions and listening to cultural norms from patients, caregivers, and colleagues. Nurse leaders should not make care-related determinations based on appearance or presumed ethnic group affinity, as this speaks to bias. Before a healthcare organization becomes culturally competent, leaders must understand the local community and the role the organization plays within the community (AHA, 2021). Cultural competence, healthcare equity, and access-related equity occur when patients are seen as individuals and are treated based on their life experiences at the time they engage with the healthcare delivery system. Healthcare professionals embracing their role on increasing professionalism within practice must continue to educate themselves regarding biases occurring within healthcare and partner to disrupt cultures that do not address unequal access to care. It is through ongoing education that the human experience for peers, patients, and communities that have been marginalized will be positively impacted.

HEALTHCARE TEAMS

Professionalism is found in high functioning executive triad (executive nursing, executive physician, and financial operations leadership) and dyad (nursing and physician leadership) teams. "The purpose of a dyad leadership approach is to help organizations meet strategic goals, enhance the leadership skills of new clinical leaders, promote shared accountability across divisions, and model partnering throughout the organization as a means of collectively improving clinical outcomes" (AHA, 2018, p. 3). Additionally, triad and dyad teams are committed to collaboration and coalition building, designing structures that allow for pivoting to address emerging, emergent (e.g., pandemics), and urgent concerns, while simultaneously building and navigating the patient and family experience. "The shift of health care delivery toward value-based care requires the blending of clinical and administrative expertise to ensure alignment of incentives between physicians and hospitals" (AHA, 2018, p. 2). While it is true that no one structure works for all organizations, a shift is needed to ensure that organizations remain nimble, innovative, and financially stable. Nurse leaders within these frameworks "create the operational objectives, goals and specific strategies required to achieve the strategic outcome" (AONL, 2015a, p. 10).

Optimizing strategy allows for a positive patient, family, and community engagement experience. In 2020, it was clear that health and wellness in the community directly impacted the ability for healthcare organizations to manage both capacity and flow. For example, a few healthcare organizations became vaccination distribution hubs for entire communities and regions. It is through community engagement and reviewing current structures for care and making changes to care delivery structures that healthcare can be impacted. In the greater New York area in calendar year 2020, several healthcare organizations such as Northwell Health and the New York Presbyterian Healthcare System partnered with community groups and religious organizations to provide vaccinations and offer webinars to address vaccine hesitancy. The Mount Sinai Health System deployed a van that engaged with the Long Island community to provide vaccines. These are just a few examples of how redeploying resources, building community coalitions, and modifying care delivery models address emerging trends.

Engaging the community also allows for the voice of the patient and family to be heard, allows for organizations to continue with investments into population health, and allows for the navigation of the patient and family experience in a patient-centered manner. Press Ganey (www.pressganey.com) and The Beryl Institute (www.theberylinstitute.org) are two organizations that provide a number of patient solutions, tools, and educational materials that emphasize the patient and family experience. Nurse leaders can reference these sites to acquire additional knowledge and build programs specific to patient experience.

PROFESSIONALISM AND EXECUTIVE PRESENCE

In the simplest terms, executive presence is your ability to inspire confidence—inspiring confidence in your subordinates that you are the leader they want to follow, inspiring confidence among peers that you are capable and reliable, and, most importantly, inspiring confidence among senior leaders that you have the potential for great achievements (Valentine, 2018). Hewlett et al. (2012) found: "Pillars of executive presence are gravitas, communication, and appearance."

Gravitas is a leadership quality that conveys knowledge, confidence, and decisiveness (Sherman, 2019). Gravitas is indeed a reflection of one's natural character and personality but is also a set of skills—interpersonal and communication—that a leader can develop (Bavister, 2017). Authority is not only one's corporate or positional title. "Holistic leaders with executive presence are relational beings—they magnetize people with ideas, effective meeting management, and inclusive engagement" (Bleich, 2020, p. 152). There are leaders who command attention merely by entering a room. One can encounter an individual without a formal title, and they are the "go to" person. What is it about them that commands a high level of respect? What is it about them that draws both internal and external customers to them? It is executive presence.

Competency building and working toward mastery of one's professionalism instills confidence. Learning and leaning into the acquisition of knowledge allows a nurse leader to become a key content authority. This occurs through ongoing education and assuming responsibilities that provide additional learning opportunities. AONL (2015) highlights, as part of clinical practice knowledge competency, that the chief nurse executive "partner with academic colleagues to create life[long] learning opportunities for self, nursing leaders and staff" (AONE & AONL, 2015b, p. 5). The nurse executive will "learn from setbacks and failures as well [as] successes" (AONE & AONL, 2015b, p. 8). The leader, through building competencies, opportunity management, and networking, continues to build executive presence. The additional layers of presence, appearance, and communication are linked. It is expected that one's appearance signals a professional tone; if a leader is not appropriately dressed, few will listen to the information that needs to be conveyed.

Communication in today's environment occurs in several forums. Message boards, emails, electronic feeds, and person–person offer the ability for nurse leaders to share information. Preparation should occur whenever possible. Talking points, or an executive summary, offer leaders the ability to develop a strategy for the information that needs to be highlighted. Town halls are another communication strategy that can be utilized, and web-based meetings with question-and-answer periods have also become popular. Commercially available web applications (e.g., Microsoft Teams) allow for internal communication within teams and service lines. High-level and consistent communication is always evolving and a foundational component of executive presence.

⬡ CASE SCENARIO

TRANSFORMATIONAL LEADERSHIP

SITUATION

A nurse manager was an external hire to lead a unit that has seen the turnover of assistant nurse managers and frontline staff, including registered nurses, medical assistants, EKG technicians, and the unit registration and clerical staff. The unit had been discussed at the last patient family advisory council committee meeting as a place where "no healing could ever occur." The patient services department has asked the executive leadership team to make this unit a priority focus area, after a review of the last patient experience data. It has been said that this unit requires transformational leadership to make an emergent turnaround.

APPROACH

The nurse manager has reviewed the organizational strategic plan, the unit's practice council minutes, and clinical quality data for the last 12 months. They have also reviewed the notes from the patient family advisory council and met with the patient services department. The nurse manager has met with the unit leadership from two nursing units that have excellent quality metrics (exceeding all benchmarks), high levels of staff engagement, and staff that were the recipients of internal and external awards over the last 24 months. There are three themes based on information gathering: culture of respect, teamwork, and responsiveness to patient and family needs.

OUTCOME

The nurse manager has engaged with the talent development and nursing education departments within the organization. There are three existing courses for the staff that can be scheduled on demand. This course work framework is culture of respect, team building, and responsiveness to patient and family needs. There is the commitment for a talent development specialist to facilitate culture of respect and teamwork discussions at unit practice council meetings for the next 6 months. Information related to quality metrics and patient experience data has been posted strategically throughout the unit and has been emailed to all staff that work in or float into this specific unit. A weekly email has also been developed that provides an overview of unit-based operations and opportunities for improvements. The nurse manager has also worked to have real-time patient experience data operationalized at the time of discharge using a portable tablet.

The chief nurse executive has rounded on the unit to highlight the involvement and commitment to work with the interprofessional team and monitor clinical outcomes in alignment with patient safety and AONL competencies.

DISCUSSION QUESTION

1. Draft a unit-specific mission and vision statement. What are the key behaviors included?

Healthcare systems and leaders that are identified as transformational will be able to remain viable and viewed by at-risk communities as safe places for care and information, as well as places where work is done to address the impact of SDOH. Economic stability, education access and quality, healthcare access and quality, neighborhood and built environment, and social and community context can all be impacted through transformational leadership. "Leaders must learn to shift from the 'individual expert' model so common in today's healthcare systems and move toward a model that leverages cross boundary groups and teams and spans disciplines, levels, functions, generations, and professions" (Browning et al., 2016, p. 1).

"The transformational leadership component of the Magnet model comprised three categories: (1) strategic planning; (2) advocacy and influence; and (3) visibility, accessibility, and communication" (Burke & Erickson, 2020, p. 7). "The defining attributes of transformational leadership are inspiration, influence, and motivation" (Khan, 2016, p. 284). Khan (2016) further states "the transformational leader is able to inspire staff to become actively engaged in their environment" (p. 284).

"To achieve and sustain a high-performing nursing organization, the nurse manager must be specifically trained in transformational leadership: how to encourage associates, respond to recurring questions, implement process and protocol changes, and celebrate gains" (White & Griffith, 2019, p. 220). The transformational nurse leader utilizes and builds leadership experiences to support teams within a shared governance structure to drive outcomes tied to operational excellence and goal setting, data management and logistics, innovation and problem-solving, and business acumen. "Nurse Executives must embody the principles of transformational leadership to meet the leadership imperative of achieving high-quality outcomes in this ever-changing healthcare environment" (Pearson, 2020, p. 142). This is done by building trust while simultaneously, leveraging quality decision-making.

PROFESSIONALISM REQUIRES MENTORSHIP, ALLYSHIP, AND SPONSORSHIP

The healthcare delivery process is challenging and simultaneously ever changing. With many organizations and hospitals merging and becoming systems, the ability to move seamlessly from one individual free-standing hospital or company to the next is more difficult. Mentoring nurse leaders to develop competencies and confidence in creating a shared vision, educating interprofessional and executive stakeholders on the financial implications of patient care decisions, and constructing and presenting a business case for adequate nursing resources are all critical in today's healthcare landscape (Ducharme, 2018). Building, maintaining, and actively managing your professional career portfolio is a critically important process embedded in professionalism.

Identifying mentors, allies, and sponsors are key in professional development. Mentors often guide us through some of our toughest challenges and help us achieve advancement in sometimes complex environments (Beltran, n.d.). While some debate the merit of mentorship within its traditional parameters, when it is expanded to include sponsorship and advocacy, it is proven to be a critical element of success by providing protégés with the opportunity to broaden their perspective, build social capital, navigate organizational politics more strategically, and muster up the confidence to "lean in" and speak up when it matters most (Warrell, 2017).

Recognize that each day you can pursue relationships that expand professional development and mentorship. Care should be taken to ensure that, as part of professional development, curating mentorship experiences that are not homogeneous is a priority.

The mentoring process is not unidirectional. A mentoring relationship must be managed and nurtured (Abbajay, 2019). Mentored employees advance faster, are more productive, and are better accustomed to navigating the company's culture (Beltran, n.d.). Abbajay (2019) states the chances of creating and sustaining a successful mentoring relationship are enhanced by adopting a few simple practices: designing the alliance, getting to know each other, and setting the agenda. In setting the agenda, you can utilize specific, measurable, achievable, realistic, and time-bound (SMART) goals.

SPONSORS IN THE PROFESSIONAL WORLD

The critical difference in a sponsorship relationship versus mentorship is the dynamic of a position of influence or authority (Brine, 2020). Sponsors help you to navigate your career advancement in a different way by strategizing stretch assignments, key introductions, and vertical moves (Brine, 2020). This involves having a key sponsor assist the individual and organization with succession planning for key positions and identifying individuals who are potentially ready now for positions. Through detailed discussions and, at times, facilitating an individual's acquisition of specific job skills, the sponsor has a specific role in a candidate's role attainment. Sponsors, by definition, use their position and power to achieve business objectives by advancing a protégé's career (Anderson & Smith, 2019). They are influential leaders who intentionally invest in, and rely on, the skills and contributions of their protégé's highest potential (Anderson & Smith, 2019).

The role that a nurse leader plays in the career development of professionals through mentorship and sponsorship is significant. Coaching others in developing their own career paths (AONL, 2015a) is a competency of the nurse executive. The identification of talent by nurse leaders, as well as the development of professional attributes and competency-related skills through sponsorship and allyship, allows for the healthcare industry to thrive. Great sponsors purposefully look for people who bring different experiences and perspectives from their own and have the results, potential, and ambition to make a larger contribution (Anderson & Smith, 2019).

"Succession planning is a strategy for identifying and developing future leaders at your company—not just the top but for major roles at all levels" (Half, 2020, "What Is Succession Planning?"). "Leaders of healthcare systems will need to hire and develop talented individuals who can see the next wave of plausible solutions and innovations and lead transformational change" (Browning et al., 2016, p. 6). Organizations have both formal and informal processes to identify personnel across functional job descriptions, which are often linked to the performance appraisal process. Professionalism dictates that clinicians and leaders function at the top licenses and position requirements, and that they position organizations, clinical units, and companies to thrive through succession planning. Assessment of practices for identifying top talent and developing team members is performed with succession planning as a goal. Succession planning is a key element of employee engagement and an essential element for the sustainability of any organization. Several specific questions and statements related to succession planning are found in Box 2.2.

BOX 2.2: QUESTIONS FOR ORGANIZATIONAL SUCCESSION PLANNING

- Is there a process in place that identifies team members for current and future positions? Who is at risk of leaving the organization or transitioning into alternative positions?

- Is there a process in place to identify top-level talent team members and determine their interest in movement as part of the succession plan (e.g., timing, ready now, or not interested)?

- Is there a process in place that facilitates ongoing development for key positions, and personnel identified as part of the organizational succession plan?

- Is there a process in place for skills and ongoing competency review for all team members? This allows for leadership to analyze all available information regarding the organization's employees' abilities.

- Have all the facts regarding your teams' positions and managerial abilities been identified? Does the annual performance appraisal process address employee career goals?

- Is there a process in place that evaluates the commitment to diversity, equity, and inclusion as part of succession planning? Is the process transparent? Are metrics associated with the delineated process?

- Is there a process in place that allows for identified team members to have exposure to additional projects, or an expanded scope of responsibility, across departments? This allows for better preparation for potential positions, a shortened transition period for new areas of responsibility, and proactive succession management.

⬡ | CASE SCENARIO

SELF-CARE AND MINDFULNESS

SITUATION

Nurse Manager AB has become aware that a few nurses on their unit have highlighted an inability to engage in self-care and have stated that they are feeling increased levels of work-related stress. They have stated that the last year increased their work-related hours and a summary of verbatim statements reveals "this has pushed the limits of what we are able to physically do."

APPROACH

The spiritual services, employee assistant consultant, and employee resilience team were activated. A list of resources for immediate use by the staff was sent to all teams by email and posted on the unit as a reminder to all levels of staff. An analysis of available days off were reviewed and posted on the electronic message board to allow staff to apply for additional paid time off. Time was scheduled for each staff member to utilize several resilience building resources being offered within the organization over the next 30 days. Offerings included classes on mindfulness moments, nutrition for commuters, sleep hygiene, chair yoga, and managing children's academic needs in the remote world.

OUTCOME

Nurse Manager AB created a formalized plan for the next 18 months of events and support-related activities available to staff. Nurse Manager AB created a resilience channel in Microsoft Teams for staff to share activities and ideas. Nurse Manager AB has increased wellness rounding with specific questions provided by the employee assistance department and has partnered with the mental health department to offer monthly sessions on requested topics. The chief nurse executive has also begun a review of resilience-based programs after hearing of the concerns raised by the staff on Nurse Manager AB's unit and in line with the competency to "formulate programs to enhance work–life balance" (AONE & AONL, 2015a, p. 10).

DISCUSSION QUESTIONS

1. Are there any additional ideas or tools recommended to build self-care and mindfulness practices into unit-based or organizational programs?
2. Are there specific programs that have worked for you or members of your team? Please discuss.

The healthcare industry is engaging in dialogue that analyzes and evaluates the impact the work environment is having on the ability for workers to engage in self-care and mindfulness practices. In August of 2021, the U.S. Senate passed the Dr. Lorna Breen Health Care Provider Protection Act (S. 610). This legislation, named after an emergency department physician, would provide funding to develop programs that address the mental health needs of frontline healthcare workers, and also validates the urgency to address well-being. The focus is building and developing programs that address the mental, physical, and spiritual health and optimize the professional caregiver's ability to provide quality care. The AONL addresses the promotion of healthful work environments and the formulation of programs that enhance work–life balance as components of the nurse executive and system chief nurse executive competencies. Healthcare burnout is well documented in the literature. Burnout continues to be reported by registered nurses across a variety of practice settings nationwide (Shah et al., 2021). Additionally, COVID-19–related work has modified and often called for increases in work-related responsibilities. With the advent of telecommuting and hybrid models of work (in-person and remote work), there is no longer a fixed end to the workday pattern. When do professional nurses disengage? When do professional nurses or any member of the healthcare team engage in self-thought time?

Leaders who have positioned themselves to consistently engage in self-care practices and encourage their teams to do the same will be the model. This involves committing to, and embodying, self-care and mindfulness practices. Leaders through modeling can demonstrate that professional nurses have tools (i.e., commitment to daily self-care and mindfulness practices) at their disposal that can create better individual health. Mandatory behaviors should be operationalized by the professional nurse each day. The World Health Organization (WHO) defines "self-care" as "the ability of individuals, families and communities to promote health, prevent disease, maintain health, and to cope with illness and disability with or without the support of a healthcare provider" (WHO, 2018, para. 1). Journaling, heart-centered breathing, meditation, massage, enjoying nature, and all forms of artistic expression—singing, movement, and dance—can contribute to self-love and self-compassion (Watson, 2018). To have time for self-care you'll need to advocate for yourself and your needs to make it happen (Saunders, 2021).

"Mindfulness is the ability to notice one's thoughts and feelings, to have an awareness of the present moment and react nonjudgmentally with self-acceptance" (Matthes, 2016, p. 209).

Present is the art of being in the moment, the luxury of pausing, the virtue of stillness (Zalani, n.d.). Mindfulness has roots in Buddhist traditions dating back more than 2,500 years (Matthes, 2016). Jon Kabat-Zinn states, "mindfulness is a whole repertoire of formal meditative practices aimed at cultivating moment-to-moment nonjudgmental awareness" (Kabat-Zinn, as cited in Mindful, n.d., "Jon Kabat-Zinn MasterClass"). "Research suggests that mindfulness meditation training not only reduces stress and anxiety following a stressful episode, but that practicing it can mitigate stress in the moment" (Mascarelli, 2020, p. 8). Mindfulness meditation may help boost immune function (Mascarelli, 2020). Certainly, more research is needed to evaluate the connection between mindfulness and health; in the meantime, these practices remain a viable option within the workplace and life. Sustaining mindfulness in the midst of constant career and life pressures is not easy (McKee et al., 2008). "Setting aside time to practice mindfulness builds a reservoir of the ability to focus on what is important in the real world" (Pipe, 2018, p. 258).

There are several technology applications that can be used to engage in self-care and mindfulness practices. There are websites; web-based applications that can be downloaded to your mobile phone or personal wearable technology devices; blogs, newsletters, and magazines; and podcasts that offer ideas and strategies to build the framework for individual self-care and mindfulness practices. Many of these web-based applications that offer guided meditation and instructions can be found on any number of popular websites and are free. Sources can be found in Box 2.3.

BOX 2.3: SELF-CARE AND MINDFULNESS IDEAS AND RESOURCES

SELF-CARE

- Complete a self-care assessment inventory.
- Define individual self-care goals.
- Self-care does not mean take a vacation, although that could be one element. Identify what is being done daily to fill your cup of intentional self-care.
- Evaluate sleep hygiene practices, including your individual sleep pattern. Are you getting enough sleep?
- Remember that sleep hygiene matters!
- Did you take time for eating, hydration, and toileting?
- Hydration applications:
  - Hydro Coach (https://hydrocoach.com)
  - Drink Water Reminder (www.healthline.com/health/hydration-top-iphone-android-apps-drinking-water#my-water)
  - My Water: Daily Water Tracker (https://apps.apple.com/us/app/my-water-daily-drink-tracker/id964748094)

MINDFULNESS

- Meditate for at least 5 minutes in your day. There are several 5-minute guided meditation videos available.
- Did you take time to conduct breathing exercises?
- Inhale deeply, hold 3 to 5 seconds, and exhale deeply (complete 5 cycles and check in with yourself after the breathing exercise). When you inhale deeply, think of pulling in air as if you are sipping a cup of water. This allows you to breathe deeply and intentionally.
- Did you notice the tension in your body?

(continued)

BOX 2.3: SELF-CARE AND MINDFULNESS IDEAS AND RESOURCES *(continued)*

- Did the tension dissipate?
- Are you avoiding multitasking? The literature is clear there are no real good multitaskers!
- Meditation applications:
  - HEADSPACE (www.headspace.com/)
  - INSIGHT TIMER (https://insighttimer.com)

Self-care + Mindfulness = Building an intentional roadmap to wellness

---

Healthcare organizations have also developed internal websites and web-based applications that facilitate the ability for employees and internal stakeholders to engage in health-promoting practices during their daily work schedules. A mindfulness moment or pause is available at any time. Professional nurse leaders can initiate the development or serve as executive sponsors of programmatic development if their organizations do not currently offer programs that foster self-care and mindfulness practices. In celebration of Nurses Month 2021, the ANA identified week 1 as self-care, a demonstration of the importance and commitment to these practices. The role and existence of employee assistance programs (EAP) must also be highlighted. The idea that professional nurses possess endless stores of energy and health without requiring self-care and mindfulness practices must be retired.

WHAT EVERY NURSE MANAGER NEEDS TO KNOW ABOUT PROFESSIONALISM

- The nurse manager is committed to lifelong learning.
- Nursing management is a daily lesson in competency management and competency development.
- Continually assessing ongoing SWOT analysis allows for refinement of the many components of professionalism.
- Media management is critical in leveraging communication that is impactful; it expands the individual as well as the brand of the nursing profession.
- Appropriate media management has licensure implications for the leader, as well as the team members being managed, mentored, coached, or sponsored. The nurse manager is a role model and brand.
- The usage of professional organizations to acquire more knowledge and information related to professionalism builds expertise.
- At the broadest levels of nursing leadership and management are knowledge of the healthcare environment, communication and relationship management, financial acumen, business skills, and business principles.
- Keeping abreast of evidence-based practices, nursing research, and professional standards and protocols are key to the maintenance of professional standards.
- It is critical to understand the importance of leading on issues of diversity, equity, equality, and inclusion. This process is ongoing.
- Cultural competence and cultural humility build a better understanding of staff, patients, and the community.
- Self-care and mindfulness = wellness as a journey.
- Ethical standards must be maintained at all times.

WHAT EVERY NURSE EXECUTIVE NEEDS TO KNOW ABOUT PROFESSIONALISM

- The nurse executive is a strategist.
- The nurse executive is visionary and is integral in the establishment of professionalism-related guideposts for individuals and teams.
- The nurse executive may be the only nurse in the room, and it is imperative that they advocate for nursing practice at the highest levels of licensure, quality, safety, and ethics.
- Partnership with physician colleagues and collaborative teams is the exemplar.
- A transformational nurse executive is required for healthcare delivery for today and in the future.
- The nurse executive understands that a commitment to diversity, equity, equality, and inclusion matters, and develops projects that foster environments of change.
- The nurse executive evaluates decision-making that impacts the SDOH.
- The nurse executive utilizes communication to share the mission and values of the organization while advocating for essential causes within the profession and community.
- The nurse executive is the creator of brand strategy, and mentors managers at all levels through robust succession planning.
- The nurse executive is committed to learning and building healthcare delivery models.
- The support of practice innovation is required.
- Systems can only thrive through a commitment to professionalism.
- The strategy for maintaining ethical standards of professionalism are developed by the nurse executive.
- Collaboration across disciplines, and at the senior level, occurs through triad and dyad structures, and is essential in today's healthcare arena.
- The commitment to diversity, equity, equality, and inclusion across systems is facilitated by the transformational leadership of the nurse executive.
- Branding for the profession, professional organizations, and the leader occur through executive presence.
- Communication is a priority area for employees and communities.
- Ethical standards must be maintained at all times.

KEY POINTS

- Professionalism is demonstrated through the adherence to or development of standards, practice guidelines, and behaviors that are supported by licensing agencies, professional organizations, and organizational structures and standards, or thought leaders within the profession.
- The professional nurse is committed to lifelong learning and building of competencies.
- The nurse manager is a role model and brand.
- Building mentoring relationships and identifying sponsors are key in continued professional development.
- The commitment to membership and involvement in professional organizations is integral to professional growth.
- Self-care and mindfulness = wellness as a journey.

- The commitment to diversity, equity, equality, and inclusion across systems is facilitated by the transformational leadership of the nurse executive.
- Collaboration across disciplines and structures is essential in today's healthcare arena.
- Ethical standards must be maintained at all times.

SUMMARY

Professionalism is foundational to nursing. Within the body of nursing, evolution of practice continues. On May 16, 2021, Dr. Anthony Fauci, director of the National Institute of Allergy and Infectious Diseases, told graduates of the Emory College of Arts and Sciences to expect the unexpected (Steig, 2021). The disease processes witnessed in the 2020 calendar year were certainly unexpected. Nurses in action embracing their individual professionalism have been, can, and should continue to be at the forefront of revolutionary and essential change related to pandemic preparedness. Emerging pathogen preparedness directly impacts local, regional, national, and global health. The additional public health concerns of gun violence, Black infant-maternal mortality, vaccine hesitancy, equity within healthcare delivery and research, the lack of diversity within the highest levels of the nursing profession including academia, and creating a different and inclusive future can all be addressed through the tenets of professionalism.

How we continue to ignite and innovate change will impact the shift that needs to occur within the operational and administrative levels of nursing as we continue to build the culture of excellence, while managing fiscal responsibility. "The nurse, in all roles and settings, advances the profession through research and scholarly inquiry, professionalism standards development and the generation of both nursing and health policy" (ANA, 2015, p. 27). Nurses utilize their voices within the advocacy framework and work within professional organizations to make essential improvements in practice and care delivery. Professionalism is what nurses embody, always considering knowledge of nursing practice, person-centered care, population health, interpersonal partnerships, system-based practice, informational and healthcare technologies, and personal, professional, and leadership development. Nurse managers, nurse academicians, and nurse executives are equipped to drive processes in organizations that are the model for health and wellness for the future. As stated by Marian K. Shaughnessy, "nurse leaders will be the agents of change responsible for providing others with a path for positive changes in the health care field and in society" (Warshawsky & Fitzpatrick, 2020, p. 212).

END-OF-CHAPTER RESOURCES

◆ DISCUSSION QUESTIONS

1. You have had time to reflect on professionalism. Are there content areas for which you would consider drafting an IDP to address nursing leadership and management-related professional behaviors?
2. Ethics are foundational to nursing professionalism, and there is no gradation for ethical standards. How will you assist professionals that you mentor in building ethical decision-making processes?
3. Are you a member of a professional organization? If not, how can you engage with members to find out more information? If yes, how will you increase your organizational involvement including the recruitment of peers who are not currently members?

4. Advocacy is foundational to nursing. What advocacy related causes can you lend your professional voice to?

5. The pillars of executive presence have been identified as gravitas, communication, and appearance. Is there a specific area you would like to develop in the next calendar year? Can you draft a goal-directed plan?

6. What self-care and mindfulness practices can you hardwire into your professional practice today?

◼ ADDITIONAL RESOURCES

Coyle, D. (2018). *The culture code: The secrets of highly successful groups.* Bantam Books.

Dang, D., & Dearholt, S. L. (2018). *Johns Hopkins evidence-based practice: Model and guidelines.* Sigma Theta Tau International.

Diangelo, R. (2018). *White fragility: Why it's so hard for White people to talk about racism.* Beacon Press.

Dufu, T. (2017). *Drop the ball: Achieving more by doing less.* Flatiron Book.

Kabat-Zinn, J. (2005). *Wherever you go there you are: Mindfulness meditation in everyday life.* Hachette Books.

Love, R. (2019, January 21). *How nurses can help drive healthcare innovation.* TEDxBeaconStreet: https://www.ted.com/talks/rebecca_love_how_nurses_can_help_drive_healthcare_innovation/up-next

Newport, C. (2016). *Deep work: Rules for focused success in a distracted world.* Hachette Books.

Southwick, S. S., & Charney, D. S. (2018). *Resilience: The science of masterings life's greatest challenges* (2nd ed.). Cambridge University Press.

Thich, N. H. (1987). *The miracles of mindfulness.* Beacon Press.

Wider, M. A. (2020). *The worthy wardrobe: Your guide to style, shopping & soul.* New Degree Press.

 SPRINGER PUBLISHING CONNECT™ A robust set of instructor resources designed to supplement this text is located at http://connect.springerpub.com/content/book/978-0-8261-7795-7. Qualifying instructors may request access by emailing textbook@springerpub.com.

REFERENCES

Abbajay, M. (2019, January 20). *Mentoring matters: Three essential elements of success.* https://www.forbes.com/sites/maryabbajay/2019/01/20/mentoring-matters-three-essential-element-of-success/?sh=7623c39045a9

The American Association of Colleges. (2021, April 6). *The essentials: Core competencies for professional nursing education.* https://www.aacnnursing.org/Education-Resources/AACN-Essentials

American College of Healthcare Executives. (2020). *Creating an ethical culture within the healthcare organization.* https://www.ache.org/about-ache/our-story/our-commitments/ethics/ache-code-of-ethics/creating-an-ethical-culture-within-the-healthcare-organization

American Hospital Association. (2018, August). *A model for clinical partnering how nurse and physician executives use synergy as strategy.* https://www.aha.org/system/files/2018-08/plf-issue-brief-clinical-partnering.pdf

American Hospital Association. (2021, May 30). *Becoming a culturally competent health care organization.* https://www.aha.org/ahahret-guides/2013-06-08-becoming-culturally-competent-health-care-organization

American Nurses Association. (n.d.-a). *Advocacy.* https://www.nursingworld.org/practice-policy/advocacy/

American Nurses Association. (n.d.-b). *Social.* https://nursingworld.org/social

American Nurses Association. (2015). *Code of ethics for nurses with interpretive statements.* American Nurses Association.

American Nurses Association. (2020). *The American Academy of Nursing and the American Nurses Association call for social justice to address racism and health equity in communities of color.* https://www.nursingworld.org/news/news-releases/2020/the-american-academy-of-nursing-and-the-american-nurses-association-call-for-social-justice-to-address-racism-and-health-equity-in-communities-of-color

American Nurses Association. (2021). *Nursing scope and standards of practice* (4th ed.). Author.

American Nurses Credentialing Center. (n.d.). *Magnet-model: Creating a Magnet culture*. https://nursingworld.org/organizational-programs/magnet/magnet-model

American Organization for Nurse Executives & American Organization for Nursing Leadership. (2015a). *Nurse executive competencies*. https://www.aonl.org/system/files/media/file/2019/06/nec.pdf

American Organization for Nurse Executives & American Organization for Nursing Leadership. (2015b). *Nurse executive competencies: System CNE*. https://www.aonl.org/system/files/media/file/2019/06/nec-system-cne.pdf

Anderson, R. H., & Smith, D. G. (2019, August 7). What men can do to be better mentors and sponsors to women. *Harvard Business Review*. https://hbr.org/2019/08/what-men-can-do-to-be-better-mentors-and-sponsors-to-women

Bavister, S. (2017, October 18). *Gravitas: What it is and how it can help you to be more successful, influential and charismatic*. https://blog.speak-first.com/gravitas-what-it-is-and-having-it

Beltran, W. (n.d.). *Mentoring works: Mentoring women for leadership*. https://chronus.com/blog/mentoring-women-for-leadership

Bleich, M. R. (2020). Exploring executive presence: Leadership traits or skills? *The Journal of Continuing in Nursing, 51*, 152–154. https://doi.org/10.3928/00220124-20200317-03

Brine, C. (2020, March 13). *Mentorship & sponsorship: Why you need both*. https://www.linkedin.com/pulse/mentorship-sponsorship-why-you-need-both-chantal-brine

Browning, H. W., Torain, D. J., & Patterson, T. E. (2016). *A six-part model for adapting and thriving during a time of transformative change*. Collaborative Healthcare Leadership. http://www.ccl.org/wp-content/uploads/2015/04/CollaborativeHealthcareLeadership.pdf

Burke, D., & Erickson, J. I. (2020). Passing the chief nursing officer baton: The importance of succession planning and transformational leadership. *The Journal of Nursing Administration, 50*(7-8), 369–371. https://doi.org/10.1097/NNA.0000000000000901

Centers for Disease Control and Prevention. (n.d.). *Racism and health*. https://www.cdc.gov/healthequity/racism-disparities

Ducharme, M. (2018). Professional practice environment. In J. Adams, J. Mensik, R. P. Ponte, & J. Somerville (Eds.), *Lead like a nurse: Leadership in every healthcare setting* (pp. 23–29). The American Nurses Association.

Half, R. (2020, March 20). *What is succession planning? 7 Steps to success*. https://www.roberthalf.com/blog/management-tips/7-steps-to-building-a-succession-plan-for-success

Hewlett, S. A., Leader-Chivée, L., Sherbin, L., Gordon, J., & Dieudonné, F. (2012). *Executive presence: Key findings*. Coqual. https://coqual.org/wp-content/uploads/2020/09/26_executivepresence_keyfindings-1.pdf

International Council of Nurses. (2012). *The ICN code of ethics for nurses*. https://www.icn.ch/sites/default/files/inline-files/2012_ICN_Codeofethicsfornurses_%20eng.pdf

Khan, B. (2016). Transformational leadership. In J. J. Fitzpatrick, & G. McCarthy (Eds.), *Nursing concepts analysis: Applications to research and practice* (pp. 283–288). Springer Publishing Company.

Khan, S. (2021, March 9). Cultural humility vs. cultural competence—and why providers need both. *Boston Medical Center HealthCity Newsletter*. https://www.bmc.org/healthcity/policy-and-industry/cultural-humility-vs-cultural-competence-providers-need-both

Mascarelli, A. (2020). Feel better starting today. *Yoga Journal*, 6–15.

Matthes, J. (2016). Mindfulness. In J. J. Fitzpatrick & G. McCarthy (Eds.), *Nursing concept analysis: Applications to research and practice* (pp. 209–214). Springer Publishing Company.

McKee, A., Boyatzis, R., & Johnston, F. (2008). *Becoming a resonant leader*. Harvard Business School Publishing.

Mindful. (n.d.). *Everyday mindfulness with Jon Kabat-Zinn*. https://www.mindful.org/everyday-mindfulness-with-jon-kabat-zinn

Mount Sinai. (2021, May 26). *Noted historian Lonnie G. Bunch, III, PhD, discusses COVID-19, the death of George Floyd, and combating racism in health care*. https://health.mountsinai.org/blog/noted-historian-lonnie-g-bunch-iii-phd-discusses-covid-19-the-death-of-george-floyd-and-combating-racism-in-health-care

National Council of State Boards of Nursing. (n.d.). *Find your nurse practice act*. https://www.ncsbn.org/npa.htm

Pearson, M. M. (2020, March). Transformation leadership principles and tactics for the nurse executive to shift nursing culture. *The Journal of Nursing Administration, 50*, 142–151. https://doi.org/10.1097/NNA.0000000000000858

Pipe, T. (2018). Mindfulness and leadership. In J. Adams, J. Mensik, P. R. Ponte, & J. Somerville (Eds.), *Lead like a nurse: Leadership in every healthcare setting* (pp. 253–276). The American Nurses Association.

Porter-O'Grady, T., & Malloch, K. (2015). *Quantum leadership: Building better partnerships for sustainable health* (4th ed.). Jones & Bartlett Learning.

Quinn Griffin, M. T., Stilgenbauer, D. J., & Nelson, G. (2016). Decision making by nurse managers. In J. J. Fitzpatrick & G. McCarthy (Eds.), Nursing concept analysis: Applications to research and practice (pp. 177–185). Springer Publishing Company.

Rivera, R. R, & Fitzpatrick, J. J. (2021). *The peace model: Evidence-based practice guide for clinical nurses.* Sigma Theta Tau International Honor Society of Nursing.

Saunders, E. G. (2021, April 1). Make time for "Me Time." *Harvard Business Review.* https://hbr.org/2021/04/make-time-for-me-time

Shah, M. K., Gandrakota, N., Cimiotti, J., Ghose, N., Moore, M., & Ali, M. K. (2021). Prevalence of and factors associated with nurse burnout in the US. *JAMA Network Open, 4*(2), e2036469. https://doi.org/10.1001/jamanetworkopen.2020.36469

Sherman, R. O. (2019, September 5). *Honing your executive presence.* Emerging RN Leader. https://www.emergingrnleader.com/honing-your-executive-presence

Society for Human Resource Management. (2016, January 19). *Managing and leveraging workplace use of social media.* Society for Human Resource Management. https://www.shrm.org/Resources-AndTools/tools-and-samples/toolkits/Pages/managingsocialmedia.aspx

Steig, C. (2021, May 16). Dr. Anthony Fauci to Emory University graduates: Embrace change and 'expect the unexpected.' *CNBC Make It.* https://www.cnbc.com/2021/05/16/watch-live-dr-anthony-fauci-speaks-at-emory-university-graduation.html

Valentine, G. (2018, July 31). Executive presence: What is it, why you need it, and how to get it. *Forbes.* https://www.forbes.com/sites/forbescoachescouncil/2018/07/31/executive-presence-what-is-it-why-you-need-it-and-how-to-get-it/

Wakefield, M. K., Williams, D. R., Le Menestrel, S., & Flaubert, J. L. (Eds.). (2021). *The future of nursing 2020–2030: Charting a path to achieve health equity.* National Academies Press. https://nap.nationalacademies.org/catalog/25982/the-future-of-nursing-2020-2030-charting-a-path-to

Warrell, M. (2017, June 24). Mentoring matters: How more women can get the right people in their corner. *Forbes.* https://www.forbes.com/sites/margiewarrell/2017/06/24/women-mentoring/?sh=7d07844c22db

Warshawsky, N. E., & Fitzpatrick, J. J. (2020). Leader to honor: Marian K. Shaughnessy, DNP, RN. *Nurse Leader, 18*(3), 211–215. https://doi.org/10.1016/j.mnl.2020.03.001

Watson, J. (2018, June 11). *Caring science starts with self-care for nurses.* Nurse.com. https://www.nurse.com/blog/2018/06/11/caring-science-starts-with-self-care

White, K. R., & Griffith, J. R. (2019). *The well-managed healthcare organization* (9th ed.). Health Administration Press.

Winters, M.-F. (2020). *Inclusive conversations.* Berrett-Koehler Publishers.

World Health Organization. (2018, June 15). *What do we mean by self-care?* https://www.who.int/news-room/feature-stories/detail/what-do-we-mean-by-self-care

Zalani, R. (n.d.). *Why we need to be present to enjoy our lives, not just productive.* Tiny Buddha: https://tinybuddha.com/blog/why-productivity-without-presence-is-a-recipe-for-burnout-and-misery

CHAPTER 3

NURSE MANAGER AND LEADER COMPETENCIES

Linda Q. Everett and Benjamin J. Farber

"If your actions inspire others to dream more, learn more, do more, you are a leader."

John Adams

LEARNING OBJECTIVES

- Describe the meaning and relevance of nurse leader competency.
- Understand nurse leader competency within the broader context of healthcare leadership competencies.
- Differentiate frameworks for nurse leader competencies.
- Critique the similarities and differences among frameworks for nurse leader competencies.
- Investigate emerging competencies that will be required in the future.

INTRODUCTION

In the nursing literature there is much written on the topic of "competency," what it is and what it is not. These discussions largely center on knowledge, skills, and abilities (KSA) to perform assessments and technical skills. In other words, and rightly so, the focus has been on point-of-care providers. There is little documented literature on competency as it relates to nurse management and leadership. In a dynamic, complex, and uncertain healthcare environment, the concept of "leader competency" takes on greater significance. The nurse leader at any level and in any care setting must be competent in a myriad of domains including, but not limited to, quality and safety, finance, regulatory, legal, human resources, staff engagement, and patient/family satisfaction.

Nursing as a profession is a service to society with social responsibilities and expectations. These responsibilities and expectations are discussed in Fowler's *Guide to Nursing's Social Policy Statement* (2015). It is about the relationship—the social contract—between the nursing profession and society and their reciprocal expectations. Knowledge, skill, and competence are among these expectations, as "the profession will ensure the knowledge, skills and competence of those newly entering the practice and those in practice, at every level and in every role" (Fowler, 2015, p. 20).

The International Council of Nursing's (ICN's) *Code of Ethics* (2012) maintains that nurses have personal responsibility for nursing practice and for maintaining competency through lifelong learning. To ensure that these responsibilities and expectations are fulfilled, the nursing profession is regulated and monitored by the concept of competency. Hager and Gonzezi (1996) view competence as "a possession of a series of desirable attribute including knowledge of appropriate sorts, skills and abilities such as problem solving, analysis, communication, pattern recognition and attitudes of appropriate kind" (p. 15).

Competencies can be conceptualized as a shared language across application in the context of an organization's business and talent management system (Griffiths & Washington, 2015).

Nurses are hired, evaluated, promoted, and dismissed based on a defined level of competency based on KSA. In this chapter the meaning and relevancy of nurse leader competency from nurse manager to executive level across the continuum of care is discussed.

LITERATURE REVIEW

The literature on competencies for healthcare executives is limited in scope and recent in publication, with most of the studies being published in the last 20 years. While this chapter addresses competencies from non-nursing organizations, the focus is on competencies for nurse managers and nurse executives, and as such, the literature review is focused on nursing competency. A total of 23 articles were reviewed for content; seven of those articles were written by international authors and published in international journals. The current standard for nurse leader competencies in the United States is the American Organization for Nursing Leadership (AONL) Nurse Executive Competencies (NEC) and Nurse Manager Competencies (NMC). Aside from the AONL standards, the American Nurses Association (ANA) published a revised Nursing Administration Scope and Standards of Practice in 2016 aimed at providing standards for the entire spectrum of nursing leadership. While the ANA Scope and Standards of Practice are noteworthy, it is not a competency document, and defers to both the Healthcare Leadership Alliance (HLA) and AONL competencies, so discussion in this chapter will be limited (ANA, 2016).

NURSE EXECUTIVE COMPETENCIES

Initially published in 2005, the AONL NEC has been used to inform education, certification standards, and job postings (Waxman et al., 2017). As noted in the competency crosswalk at the beginning of this book, the AONL NEC are grouped into five domains: communication and relationship management, professionalism, leadership, knowledge of the healthcare environment, and business skills and knowledge. These domains are shared with the other five organizations within the HLA (HLA, 2017) as common requirements for healthcare leaders across the continuum. The HLA includes the American College of Healthcare Executives (ACHE), American College of Physician Executives (ACPE), the AONL, the Healthcare Financial Management Association (HFMA), and the Healthcare Information and Management Systems Society (HIMSS; Stefl, 2008). A crosswalk detailing the consistency among nursing and non-nursing frameworks as described in the HLA Directory 2021 are shown in the comopetency grid at the beginning of this book.

A review of 17 articles was completed by Crawford et al. (2017). According to the review, a successful chief nursing officer (CNO) must have four characteristics and nine categories with 11 subcategories of competencies. The four traits the CNO must possess include one overarching trait, being a super integrator, and three traits to support super integration: being dynamic, driven, and determined; being realistic; and being well-educated and experienced. The nine competency categories are:

Communication and relationship-building, knowledge of healthcare and technical environments, leadership skills, healthcare economics and business acumen skills, clinical practice knowledge, foundational thinking skills, shared decision-making, professionalism, personal journey disciplines. (Crawford et al., 2017, p. 303)

The AONL NEC includes all nine categories. Further discussion in the review included the rapid change of the role, with increased complexities requiring additional "responsibilities, traits, and competencies" (Crawford et al., 2017, p. 306). Finally, the review identified a lack of clarity in CNO responsibilities, due to a lack of defined responsibilities and traits. Two other nursing leadership frameworks to validate competency are the Quality and Safety Education for Nurses (QSEN) and the American Academy of Colleges of Nursing (AACN).

The Institute of Medicine's (IOM's; 2011) *The Future of Nursing: Leading Change, Advancing Health* report made it clear that the role of the nursing executive was changing. Enhanced identified skills included an increased understanding of data, financial acumen, collaboration, innovation, and change management (Prestia, 2015). These competencies are all embedded in the AONL NEC; however, very little is included about sustainment/resilience of the nurse executive.

The National Academies of Sciences, Engineering, and Medicine's (NASEM's) *The Future of Nursing 2020–2030: Charting a Path to Achieve Health Equity* (Wakefield et al., 2021) provides a comprehensive list of recommendations for educators, practicing nurses, researchers, policy makers, healthcare system leaders, and payors to support nurses in creating a culture of health. Reductions in health disparities and improvement in health and well-being for the population is a worthy and commendable goal. Moving forward, nurses and nurse leaders will need to learn and adapt to new and emerging competencies to meet these recommendations and the challenges they impose.

Calhoun and colleagues (2008) described an evidence-based interprofessional competency model for healthcare leadership. The framework addresses three overarching domains including behavioral and technical competencies. Each competency is composed of prescriptive behavioral indicators, or levels, for the development and assessment as leaders progress through their careers from the entry-level to advanced stages of lifelong professional development. The model supports identification of opportunities for leadership improvement in both academic and practice settings.

The previously noted professional nursing leadership associations, AONL, QSEN, and AACN, have adopted this competency-based framework to guide nursing leaders in practice and education (Morse & Warshawsky, 2021). The Association for Leadership in Nursing Science (ALSN) is discussed in the text that follows. Examining nursing leadership from a competency-based perspective allows educators and practitioners to understand different dimensions of leader qualities and capacities (Morse & Warshawsky, 2021). The education-based QSEN competencies and The Essentials: Core Competencies for Professional Nursing Education are not listed in the HLA Directory and are also discussed in the text that follows.

NURSE MANAGER COMPETENCIES

Published in 2015, the AONL NMC are not based upon the HLA model. They include three domains: the science, the art, and the leader within. Each of those domains contains four to seven categories with individual competencies listed under each category. These will be discussed in more detail in the "What Every Nurse Manager Needs to Know" section of this chapter. Orchard et al. (2017) recommend shifting from the traditionally recommended leadership styles—transactional, servant, transformative, and authentic—to a collaborative model. Clausen et al. (2019) recommend a competency-building program that encourages and builds resilience, a necessary competency that has been left out of formal models.

Overwhelmingly, the basic recommended competencies for nurse managers cited in the literature mirror those listed in the AONL NMC. The competencies necessary to function at the nurse manager and nurse executive level are discussed in greater detailed later in this chapter. While the research and literature are limited, the competencies identified remain consistent, not only within the realm of nursing leadership, but across the healthcare continuum.

QUALITY AND SAFETY EDUCATION FOR NURSES COMPETENCIES

The QSEN project was originally funded by the Robert Wood Johnson Foundation at the University of North Carolina-Chapel Hill in 2005. In 2012 QSEN was transitioned to the QSEN Institute at the Frances Payne Bolton School of Nursing, Case Western Reserve University (QSEN Institute, n.d.-b).

> The Quality and Safety Education for Nurses (QSEN) addresses the challenge of preparing future nurses with the knowledge, skills, and attitudes (KSAs) necessary to continuously improve the quality and safety of the healthcare systems within which they work. (QSEN Institute, n.d.-a, para. 1)

QSEN used the IOM competencies to define quality and safety competencies for nursing and identified specific content for the KSAs to be developed in nursing pre-licensure and graduate programs for each competency (Cronenwett et al., 2007, 2009).

Six domains are defined: patient-centered care; teamwork and collaboration; evidenced-based practice; quality improvement; safety; and informatics. Subcompetencies in each of these domains have relevance for nursing leadership in education and in practice in any care setting and are consistent with the AONL competencies.

ASSOCIATION FOR LEADERSHIP IN NURSING SCIENCE PERSPECTIVE ON LEADERSHIP COMPETENCIES

The ALSN, formerly the Council for Graduate Education for Administrative Nursing (CGEAN), was established in 1970 (ALSN, 2021). The 2019 name change reflects the association's "mission to unite nursing leadership, practice, education, and research. We advance the science that informs nursing leadership education and practice" (Morse & Warshawsky, 2021, pp. 65–66). ALSN does not have a defined set of competencies. In the spirit of academic-practice partnerships, ALSN aligns their mission and goals with respect to leadership with AONL and HLA and is consistent with the ANA Scope and Standards of Practice (ALSN, 2021).

AMERICAN ASSOCIATION OF COLLEGES OF NURSING: THE ESSENTIALS—CORE COMPETENCIES FOR PROFESSIONAL EDUCATION

The AACN was established in 1969 and represents over 840 member schools of nursing. It is recognized as the national voice for academic nursing:

> The American Association for Colleges of Nursing (AACN) works to establish quality standards for nursing education; assists schools in implementing those standards; influences the nursing profession to improve healthcare; and promotes public support for professional nursing education, research, and practice. (AACN, n.d., para. 1)

AACN has published The Essentials series that provides the educational framework for the preparation of nurses at 4-year colleges and universities since 1986. Given changes in higher education and the rapidly evolving and uncertain healthcare environment, in 2019 AACN created a new Vision for Academics with creative thinking and innovative approaches to nursing education. In 2021, to prepare the nursing workforce of the future, The Essentials: Core Competencies for Professional Nursing Education was published. This document combines the three previously published versions of The Essentials that detailed separate specific guidelines for baccalaureate, master's, and doctoral education for advanced nursing practice. The new Essentials provides a framework for preparing individuals as members of

TABLE 3.1: American Association of Colleges of Nursing Professional Practice Domains

Domain 1	Knowledge for Nursing Practice
Domain 2	Person-Centered Care
Domain 3	Population Health
Domain 4	Scholarship for the Nursing Discipline
Domain 5	Quality and Safety
Domain 6	Interprofessional Partnerships
Domain 7	Systems-Based Practice
Domain 8	Informatics and Healthcare Technologies
Domain 9	Professionalism
Domain 10	Personal, Professional, and Leadership Development

the discipline of nursing across the trajectory of nursing education and applied experience from entry-level through advanced practice. The Essentials are designed to bridge the gap between education and practice (AACN, 2021).

In this current document, competencies for professional nursing practice are made explicit. These Essentials introduce 10 domains that represent the essence of professional nursing practice and the expected competencies for each domain. The domains are shown in Table 3.1.

All domains and their specific competencies and subcompetencies are salient for nursing leadership, especially at the advanced level. The Personal, Professional, and Leadership Development domain clearly demonstrates the alignment of education and practice with respect to nursing leadership. The descriptor for this domain states:

> Participation in activities and self-reflection that fosters personal health, resilience, and well-being; contributes to lifelong learning; and supports the acquisition of nursing expertise and the assertion of leadership. (AACN, 2021, p. 60)

The focus for this domain for the first time clearly highlights the significance of the well-being of the nurse, resiliency, lifelong learning, assertion of control, influence, and power, which includes advocacy for patients and the nursing profession. These competencies are consistent with the mission goals of the AONL, QSEN, and ALSN reviewed earlier.

⬛ WHAT EVERY NURSE MANAGER NEEDS TO KNOW

The nurse manager is a pivotal role for smooth operations and strategy implementation at a unit or clinic level. In contrast to the five domains in the executive framework, the AONL NMC (AONL, 2015) are based on the three domains of the Nurse Manager Learning Domain Framework: The Science: Managing the Business; The Art: Leading the People; and The Leader Within: Creating the Leader in Yourself. This section introduces the basic skills for a novice nurse manager to perform the job, the necessary competency building blocks to transition to an executive role, and opportunities for attaining competency.

FORMAL NURSE MANAGER COMPETENCIES

When one considers competencies necessary to function in the nurse manager role, start with the formal structure discussed in the AONL NMC (AONL, 2015). There are three domains: The Science; The Art; and The Leader Within. The Science includes financial and human resource management, performance improvement, foundational thinking skills, technology, strategic management, and appropriate clinical practice knowledge. These are the hard skills you can study to learn through formal education programs, certification review courses, conference attendance, and other forms. The Art includes human resource leadership skills, relationship management and influencing behaviors, diversity, and shared decision-making. These are the soft skills, learned over time, through life and job experience. The Leader Within includes personal and professional accountability, career planning, personal journey disciplines, and optimizing the leader within. These are the competencies that will help the new nurse manager to build, expand, and sustain a professional career.

FROM BEDSIDE TO MANAGER

When transitioning into the first manager role, it is important to approach it from a lens of learning. The new manager may have completed nursing leadership education, an AONL fellowship, or an internal leadership program, but the first position will help expand and develop the tools offered in those programs. In the past, the prerequisite to becoming a nurse manager was being a strong clinical nurse. That belief is no longer reliable. Schlaak (2019) found a positive correlation between advanced nursing education and nursing professionalism, and it has a correlated direct impact on caregiver experience and retention.

INCREASING RESPONSIBILITY

The nurse manager position provides excellent opportunities for growth and learning. Ensure you have completed a self-assessment of your current competency understanding (i.e., AONL online competency self-assessment), and have written, and tracked, a self-guided development plan to continue your growth. Consider taking advantage of every learning opportunity offered to you: stretch assignments, fellowships, additional education, and certification. As you feel more confident in your role, review the AONL NEC competencies and use them to add to your development plan to ensure consistent movement toward your next leadership goal.

 CASE SCENARIO

CONFLICT RESOLUTION

SITUATION

You are the nurse manager over two units with experienced charge nurses on both units. In the morning, you triage which unit needs your most immediate presence and choose the unit with severe, unanticipated staffing issues due to no call, no shows. As you are working through possible options to find additional staff, you get a call from a caregiver on your other unit, which is on a different floor of the hospital.

This caregiver is calling to let you know a traveling bedside RN, JP, and the charge nurse, ST, are loudly arguing in the nurse's station and that the argument is rapidly escalating. The caregiver requests you come to the unit immediately. By the time you arrive on the unit, the argument has escalated to ST and JP shouting at each other in front of the rest of the unit staff in the middle of the nursing station. Aside from the shouting, accusations are being made about competency, derogatory language use, and hospital risk. There are no patients or family present to witness the argument. *What would you prioritize as your immediate action, and what formal leadership competencies would you rely on?*

APPROACH

After separating JP and ST into separate spaces on the unit and dispersing the unit team, you start interviewing the two nurses. You learn that ST was making their morning rounds and heard a conversation they felt may lead to future and professional risk to JP, due to the amount of personal information being shared. ST initially pulled JP away from the bedside and reminded them of unit policies and the importance of guarding all information. During that conversation, JP escalated the situation and felt that ST was questioning their nursing judgment. JP's escalation caused ST to start escalating, and what started as a conversation with positive intent turned into an argument. While speaking with ST, ST owns that they escalated inappropriately, but they reiterate their perception of future risk for JP, describing the information given.

OUTCOME

While speaking with JP, they do admit to sharing the information, but they make excuses as to why the policy should not have applied in this situation. JP goes on to state that it is not ST's job to counsel them or question their nursing judgment, and they share that they were triggered by that questioning. JP does not take responsibility or any ownership for the escalation of the argument, nor does JP state understanding and agreement with the policies in place. JP then goes on to question others' behaviors and begins loudly exclaiming that they have never had a manager question them the way you are.

DISCUSSION QUESTIONS

1. From a competency-based approach, what are your next steps?
2. What do you do to ensure a situation like this doesn't occur in the future?
3. What competencies have we discussed in this chapter that you will rely on to arrive at a final outcome for this situation?

◼ WHAT EVERY NURSE EXECUTIVE NEEDS TO KNOW

The role of the nurse executive has evolved over the past decade to include much more than the responsibility and accountability for provision of safe and quality care to patients. As a member of the senior leadership team, the nurse executive must be competent in a myriad of subjects. These include the need for continuous education, the role of professional associations, the imperative of interprofessional teams, the value of mentoring, and the sustainment of lifelong learning. These competencies are discussed in the text that follows.

FORMAL NURSE EXECUTIVE COMPETENCIES

CONTINUOUS EDUCATION

The leadership competencies reviewed in this section serve as a framework to guide the professional development of nurses in executive positions or those preparing for that role. There are several strategies to cultivate and develop leader competencies. Formal academic courses are the most structured method. Most of the entry-level leadership courses begin with a self-assessment tool. More advanced courses use a 360-degree feedback process that includes not only the supervisor but peers, direct reports, and other colleagues to evaluate an employee's performance. The analysis includes how the employee perceives themself and how others perceive them (Economic Times, 2021). Webinars, podcast, blogs, TED Talks and other digital video platforms often bring a different perspective to leadership development education. Textbooks, professional journals, newsletters, and self-help books on leadership are also great resources.

MEMBERSHIP IN PROFESSIONAL ASSOCIATIONS

Membership and engagement in professional nursing organizations and decision-making boards offer value-added resources (Cherry et al., 2019). Networking with peers and colleagues is one of the most valued benefits of these memberships. For example, AONL and Sigma, The International Honor Society for Nursing, frequently host leadership programs with continuing education units with no or nominal cost to members. AONL offers a myriad of programs from early careerist to nurse executive. Certificate programs in finance at the manager and executive levels are offered. Certification at the manager and executive levels are also offered. A fellowship designation at the executive level is available (AONL, n.d.).

Sigma (n.d.) offers products and services to advance learning and professional development. These programs focus on education, leadership, career development, evidence-based nursing, research, and scholarship in practice and academia. The goal is to improve the health of "the world's people" (Sigma, n.d., para. 6).

INTERPROFESSIONAL HEALTHCARE TEAMS

The healthcare system is rapidly moving in nontraditional care delivery models that extend beyond organizational role boundaries. Advances in medical and nursing science, information systems, and telehealth applications demonstrate a need for nursing leaders to form collaborative partnerships with other members of the healthcare team. To meet the Institute for Healthcare Improvement (IHI) Quadruple Aim to provide high quality, positive patient experience, cost effectiveness, and healthy work environments, collegial partnerships must be forged (Bodenheimer & Sinsky, 2014). These relationships not only include physicians but other members of the senior executive team. Departmental leaders representing pharmacy, respiratory therapy, social work, finance, information technology, human resources, and legal and supply chain management must also be included. Engagement with associations such as ACHE, HFMA, and HIMSS provides an excellent way to develop effective interprofessional relationships.

The global pandemic of 2020 catapulted the need for interprofessional collaborations to a new level. In the wake of this catastrophic contagion, the healthcare industry was rocked to the core. In acute care, command centers were established overnight, isolation units were created in obscure areas, the search for personal protective equipment (PPE) became a scavenger hunt, and nurse staffing became a nightmare. To manage this collection of challenges required a team effort, a healthcare team effort. Other sectors such as ambulatory centers, primary care clinics, and home care services also felt the weight of the pandemic. It became clear that, in times of crisis, working in interprofessional teams to meet the needs of the population was critical (Tannenbaum et al., 2021). The AONL NEC (AONL, 2015) domain of Communication and Relationship Management provides the tools to develop effective interprofessional healthcare teams.

MENTORING

Mentorship and coaching can be some of the most powerful tools in directing a nurse leader's career. Leaders that have relationships with a mentor frequently attribute their success as a leader, as well as attainment of roles, to their mentor (McCloughen et al., 2013). Coaching can take place in one-on-one or small group settings, with different benefits being attained from each setting (Steinberg & Watkins, 2021). While coaching can be helpful, this chapter is dedicated to nurse leader competencies and, as such, will focus on the formal competency of mentoring.

Mentoring is considered a competency of nursing leadership and credited with growth for both the mentor and mentee. It is widely believed that the importance of the mentor role can be formally taught, but the skills associated with being a mentor and leader often start informally in childhood. The mentor/mentee relationship may be formal or informal and is more effective the longer it lasts, but may be fluid in terms of formality of discussion, with various phases of growth and separation. Most nurse leaders recognize that they are in a mentor/mentee relationship without formally structuring the relationship (McCloughen et al., 2013). Mentoring resources and connections are available on the AONL Leader2Leader Member Community. The coaching and mentoring process is discussed in Chapter 7, "The Coaching and Mentoring Process."

LIFELONG LEARNING

In partnership with the Robert Wood Johnson Foundation/AARP Future of Nursing Campaign for Action, the IOM (now known as the National Academy of Medicine [NAM]) has published two reports on the future of nursing. The first report, *The Future of Nursing: Leading Change, Advancing Health* (2011), identified five key messages and eight recommendations to assist the nursing workforce in meeting the objectives set forth in the 2010 Affordable Care Act. The second nursing report, released in 2016, *Assessing Progress on the IOM Report The Future of Nursing* (Altman et al., 2016), highlighted progress made since the 2011 report while recognizing that much more needed to be accomplished.

The NASEM and the Robert Wood Johnson Foundation released a third report, *The Future of Nursing 2020–2030: Charting a Path to Achieve Health Equity* (Wakefield et al., 2021), in May 2021. The partners continued their resolute collaboration toward promoting a culture of health for all. Major themes from the 2021 report include social determinants of health (SDOH) and health equity, the role of nursing in improving healthcare access and quality, paying for equity in health and healthcare, disaster preparedness, public health emergency response, nurses leading change, and supporting the health and professional well-being of nurses. The report includes eight recommendations and a health sciences research agenda to achieve health equity in the United States built on strengthened nursing capacity and expertise.

The first IOM report, *The Future of Nursing: Leading Change, Advancing Health* (2011), recommended: "Ensure that nurses engage in lifelong learning" (IOM, 2011, p. 282). This report underscores the necessity to engage in lifelong learning to gain and sustain competencies needed to provide for diverse populations across the continuum of care and life span. At no other time in recent history is lifelong learning more vital than in the aftermath of the global pandemic in 2020. The need for new leadership skills emerged in areas including but not limited to crisis management, telehealth, informatics, and disaster preparedness. The need to recognize and address the impact of health disparities and inequities on communities became a focal point. New skills mandate new competencies. Achieving and sustaining competencies in leadership in a dynamic, complex, and uncertain healthcare environment requires active engagement in the learning process.

◼ WHAT EVERY NURSE EXECUTIVE NEEDS TO KNOW ABOUT THE SYSTEM CHIEF NURSE EXECUTIVE

The system level CNO, frequently referred to as the chief nurse executive (CNE) or system CNE (SCNE), is primarily accountable for systemwide or corporate leadership. The role is considered a subspecialty of nursing leadership and, given the complex and dynamic healthcare environment in the United States, requires its own set of competencies. The American Organization of Nurse Executives (AONE) system level competencies developed in 2015 are an expansion of the competencies AONE developed for the nurse executive in 2004.

FORMAL NURSE EXECUTIVE COMPETENCIES

In the Crawford et al. (2017) integrative review referred to earlier in this chapter, the authors conclude that the SCNE has additional roles and responsibilities. As a strategic member of the senior leadership team, this role reports to the system president, chief executive officer (CEO), and/or chief operating officer (COO). The SCNE serves as a boundary spanner across various facilities and care settings involving multiple obligations (AONE, 2015; Bradley, 2014; Burkman et al., 2012; Clark, 2012). Salient to the SCNE role is to represent corporate authority as well as the voice of nursing in multiple and diverse healthcare settings across the system (Burkman et al., 2012) by creating and communicating a vision for nursing and coordinating the work of entity nurse executive groups (Clark, 2012; Kerfoot & Luquire, 2012).

In recent years, new competencies have emerged; for example, partnering within and coordinating interprofessional healthcare teams, focusing on employee engagement and healthy work environments, and enhancing knowledge of information systems and telehealth technology. Recommendations for 2020 post-pandemic implications are discussed in the next section.

⬡ CASE SCENARIO

EVALUATING COMPETENCY FOR NURSE EXECUTIVES

SITUATION

A large Magnet®-designated academic health system in the Midwest has begun the search for a new role, an associate chief nurse executive (ACNE). This position is critical to the nursing enterprise. The chosen candidate will be mentored to succeed GB, the current CNE, when they plan to retire in 18 months.

APPROACH

A job description was developed for the new role. In addition to the position summary, information included reporting relationships and responsibilities. Personal data included candidate qualifications: education/certifications, knowledge and work experience, and leadership competencies.

A search committee was convened and led by GB. Influential system leaders and the dean of the school of nursing were members of the committee. There were no viable internal candidates, so a talent firm was hired to conduct the search.

OUTCOME

The firm presented four external applicants for the position. All four participated in the first round of interviews via videoconferencing with the committee. The search committee eliminated two candidates at this phase of the process. These decisions were based on the depth of their experiences and their responses to competency-based interview questions.

The remaining two candidates, JS and RJ, were invited to campus to meet the search committee. On paper, these nurse leaders appeared to be comparable in education and experience. JS earned a doctor of nursing practice (DNP) from a private university and was the CNO of a small teaching hospital in New England. They were a former board member of the AONL and are certified in nursing administration. All of their references highlighted remarkable accomplishments in performance and professionalism.

RJ earned a DNP from a state university. They were an executive director in a large academic health system in the South. RJ was actively engaged in regional leadership associations and served as president of the AONL affiliate in their state. They too submitted glowing references.

Both interviews were scheduled over a 2-day period for each candidate. The committee was impressed with both candidates. It was decided to invite both back to meet other senior leaders and influential members of the health system and school of nursing.

On the second visit, the candidates were asked to respond to what were considered competency-based interview questions. The questions included topics such as describe your leadership style, what are your strengths and weaknesses, and so forth. Experiences with finance, human resources, change management, and other related topics were explored. JS and RJ responded well to these questions. No discernible difference between the candidates was identified by the committee.

These questions can help evaluate soft skills, such as communication, leadership, teamwork, and more. Hiring leaders can also gain insight into the ability to multitask, solve problems, and think critically. That said, do they really evaluate nurse leader competency?

GB convinced the committee to take a deeper dive into the issue of competency. GB's approach was scenario-based. Each candidate was asked to describe their responses to real-life leader situations in storytelling or narrative style (Fitzpatrick et al., 2019).

These narratives not only provided insight into relationship management, communication skills, systems thinking, and financial management, but other competencies as well. These included personal and professional accountability competencies such as culture, ethics, patient and family centeredness, mentoring, and self-awareness (AONL, 2015).

After thoughtful deliberation, the committee recommended RJ for the ACNE position. GB supported the decision and offered the ACNE position to RJ.

DISCUSSION QUESTIONS

1. How do you evaluate leader competency?
2. If you were the hiring CNE, would you place more weight on finance and human resources competencies or culture, ethics, patient and family centeredness, mentoring, and self-awareness?
3. Narrative nursing is becoming popular as a teaching modality. Do you use this technique in your leadership practice?

IMPLICATIONS FOR ORGANIZATIONS

Evidence-based professional competencies discussed in this chapter serve to guide organizations in talent management; for example, position descriptions, hiring, firing, role expectations, evaluation criteria, compensation, promotions, succession planning, and professional development of the nursing workforce.

During the recovery from the global pandemic, it became clear that leadership roles across the spectrum looked different. Nurse managers functioned as crisis managers, figuring out how to accept excessive numbers of patients and handle difficult staffing situations moment to moment, often while providing direct care themselves. CNOs moved outside of their typical roles to assist with day-to-day operations and ensure patient safety was met while functioning outside of typical healthcare practice.

After the first three waves of the pandemic passed, the recovery was characterized by a need to rapidly return to more traditional operations. This meant that nursing leaders with strong competence in quality, caregiver and patient engagement, and bias toward action thrived. There was, and is, a need to take all that has been learned in 2020 to 2021 and apply it to the healthcare organization of tomorrow, instead of reverting to pre-pandemic thinking, practices, and operations. The release of the latest *Future of Nursing* report (2021) and the new AACN Core Essentials (2021) have emphasized emerging competencies with respect to nurse well-being and healthy work environments.

AONL is in the process of revising their competencies that will also address the need for these new competencies. While it is likely that the core elements of the AONL competency structure will be similar, there will likely be changes that build upon the learning from the pandemic and take advantage of the rapidity of change made to continue high-quality and safe care for our communities and to ensure continued functioning of our healthcare organizations. These emerging competencies should include disaster management, identification and mitigation of contagious microbes, and enhanced technological knowledge and skills.

FUTURE IMPLICATIONS FOR NURSE LEADERS

The global pandemic in 2020 and the subsequent release of the NASEM's *The Future of Nursing 2020–2030: Charting a Path to Achieve Health Equity* (Wakefield et al., 2021) emphasize the evolving human competencies in an ever dynamic, complex, evolving, and digitalized healthcare environment that will be required. These include diversity equity and inclusion, health inequities, and health disparities and social inequities.

DIVERSITY, EQUITY, AND INCLUSION

Diversity, equity, and inclusion (DEI) has long been an issue in the U.S. nursing system, starting from the colonization of America and the slave trade (Iheduru-Anderson, 2020). While there has been conversation around DEI for several decades, 2020 brought renewed conversation and calls to action. While this chapter does not focus on DEI, it would be incomplete without speaking to development of, and/or participation in, a DEI program as a vital competency for nurse managers and nurse executives.

HEALTHCARE INEQUITY

Long-term structural racism in the nursing profession has created an environment that precludes the nursing workforce from matching the patient population treated and created a lack of Black, Indigenous, and people of color (BIPOC) nurses in leadership positions. The lack of racial equity in nursing seeps into other segments of the healthcare environment and contributes to racial healthcare inequities. In order to dismantle centuries of structural racism, nursing leaders must commit to building a culture that supports racial equity. They will need to create partnerships and programs that address racism at all levels, from personal to structural. In order to be successful, they must learn the history and understand the context of American structural racism, and commit to understanding how it affects all persons, but especially BIPOC nurses (Nardi et al., 2020).

HEALTH DISPARITIES AND SOCIAL INEQUITIES

A patient's zip code is the greatest indicator of their overall health (Haggerty et al., 2018). Structural racism, food and housing insecurity, lack of transportation, and lack of healthcare coverage all play a role in a patient's ability to manage their health (Gollust et al., 2018). As with DEI programs, it is an absolute necessity for nurse leaders of the future to develop competency in identifying and eliminating barriers that contribute to healthcare disparities and inequity (Wakefield et al., 2021).

The good news is that there has been a change in healthcare provider attitudes over the last decade that shift blame for inability to manage from the patient to their circumstances (Gollust et al., 2018). With the good news, however, comes the bad: The continued shift toward pay for performance (PFP) punishes providers who care for patients that have difficulty with management of their care, as the quality outcomes may suffer (Haggerty et al., 2018). In order to start making progress toward equity, leaders need the ability to identify and speak to necessary changes to provide access to healthcare, policy and practice changes to allow equitable access, and the ability to speak to legislators about changes necessary in PFP programs to ensure addressing social disparities are accounted for when payments are calculated (Haggerty et al., 2018).

The future state of healthcare must address the needs of the entire community. While the competencies around healthcare equity are evolving, it is clear that nurse leaders will have a major role in shaping a healthcare system that cares for the entire community. *The Future of Nursing 2020–2030: Charting a Path to Achieve Health Equity* (Wakefield et al., 2021) connects suboptimal health outcomes and inequities in health and healthcare:

> If the nation is to achieve better population health, it will have to meet the challenge of mitigating these inequities. Herein lies the greatest contribution of the nursing workforce in the decade ahead. (Wakefield et al., 2021, p. 3)

KEY POINTS

- Competency attainment takes time; plan your growth but allow yourself time to get there.
- Lifelong learning and engagement in professional associations will provide knowledge and resources to develop evolving competencies.

- Identify a mentor(s) to provide coaching and guidance on your professional journey.
- Great bedside skills do not translate to great leadership skills.
- Knowledge and competency in evolving domains of diversity equity and inclusion, health inequities, and health disparities and social inequities are critical.
- Creativity and innovation are essential competencies in a post-pandemic healthcare environment.

SUMMARY

To successfully meet the challenges of a post-pandemic healthcare environment, nurse leaders must employ new knowledge and competencies to navigate the dynamic complexities of an uncertain future. These evidence-based competencies have been discussed in this chapter.

Sanford and Janney in a pre-pandemic article outlined five future healthcare leadership scenarios in the year 2025 (Sanford & Janney, 2019, p. 76):

- inpatient-centric care replaced with center of care in the home
- dissolution of traditional organizational boundaries
- new technologies disrupting old work practices
- leaders communicating across multiple channels
- staff meeting evolving to daily messages delivered through social platforms

In a post-pandemic healthcare environment, these scenarios become even more challenging. Demonstrating existing and emerging leadership competencies discussed in this chapter will create an empowering environment that inspires creativity and innovation to meet these challenges (Snow, 2019). Creativity and innovation have become an essential competency for nurse leaders at all levels in all care settings in the 21st century.

END-OF-CHAPTER RESOURCES

DISCUSSION QUESTIONS

1. Identify a recent situation you encountered. Which competencies do you believe you incorporated in the solution? After reading this chapter, do you believe this knowledge would have changed the outcome? If so, which additional competencies would you have utilized?
2. The COVID-19 pandemic required all of us to think outside the box, showcase leadership skills, and learn to do things differently. Are there any competencies you believe exist post-pandemic that were not identified in this chapter?
3. How do you plan to use these competency structures to build your own career? Along those lines, how will you review situations and outcomes to look for your own personal strengths and opportunities with regard to current competency knowledge and use?

ADDITIONAL RESOURCES

- TEDx Talks (2013, January 2). *Dr. Lorelei Lingard collective competence, TEDxBayfield* [Video]. https://youtu.be/vI-hifp4u40 (19.34 minutes)
- Consider the following questions:
  - How does your healthcare team communicate?

- How does your healthcare team's communication influence patient care?
- How does your organization educate healthcare professionals to improve patient care?
  - Is your organization adapting to collective competence?

- TEDx Talks. (2019, Septermber 10). *The human skills we need in an unpredictable world | Margaret Heffernan* [Video]. https://www.youtube.com/watch?v=w4OPtFCs_fw (15.30 minutes)
- Consider the following questions:
  - Have you made a "just in time management decision" when a "just in case decision" would have been better?
  - What skills will you need to build resiliency and strength in an unpredictable future?
  - Does your organization have the capacity to adapt to variation in an unpredictable future?
    - Does your organization use imagination and the art of invention to deal with uncertainty?

 A robust set of instructor resources designed to supplement this text is located at http://connect.springerpub.com/content/book/978-0-8261-7795-7. Qualifying instructors may request access by emailing textbook@springerpub.com.

REFERENCES

Altman, S. H., Butler, A. S., & Shern, L. (Eds.). (2016). *Assessing progress on the Institute of Medicine Report* The Future of Nursing. National Academies Press. https://www.ncbi.nlm.nih.gov/books/NBK350166

American Association of Colleges of Nursing. (n.d.). *Who we are.* https://www.aacnnursing.org/About-AACN

American Association of Colleges of Nursing. (2021). *The essentials: Core competencies for professional nursing education.* https://www.aacnnursing.org/About-AACN

American Nurses Association. (2016). *ANA scope and standards of practice* (3rd ed.). https://www.nursingworld.org/practice-policy/scope-of-practice

American Organization for Nursing Leadership. (n.d.). *AONL education programs.* https://www.aonl.org/education/overview

American Organization for Nursing Leadership. (2015). *AONL nurse leader competencies.* https://www.aonl.org/resources/nurse-leader-competencies

Association for Leadership Science in Nursing. (2021). *About ALSN.* https://www.nursingleadershipscience.org/about

Bodenheimer, T., & Sinsky, C. (2014). From Triple to Quadruple Aim: Care of the patient requires care of the provider. *Annuals of Family Medicine, 12*(6), 573–576. https://doi.org/10.1370/afm.1713

Bradley, C. (2014). Leading nursing through influence and structure: The system nurse executive role. *Journal of Nursing Administration, 44*(12), 619–621. https://doi.org/10.1097/NNA.0000000000000136

Burkman, K., Sellers, D., Rowders, C., & Batcheller, J. (2012). An integrated system's nursing governance model: A system chief nursing officer's synergistic vehicle for leading a complex health care system. *Nursing Administration Quarterly, 36*(4), 353–361. https://doi.org/10.1097/NAQ.0b013e31826692ea

Calhoun, J. G., Dollett, D., Sinioris, M. E. Wainio, J. A., Butler, P. W, Griffith, J. R., Pattullo, A., & Warden, G. L. (2008). Development of an interprofessional competency model for healthcare leadership. *Journal of Healthcare Management, 53*(6), 375–388.

Cherry, B., Caramonica, L., Everett, L. Q., Fennimore, L., & Scott, E. (2019). Leveraging the power of board leadership in professional nursing organizations. *Journal of Nursing Administration, 49*(11), 517–519. https://doi.org/10.1097/NNA.0000000000000805

Clark, J. S. (2012). The chief nurse executive role: Sign of the changing times? *Nursing Administration Quarterly, 36*(4), 299–305. https://doi.org/10.1097/NAQ.0b013e3182669440

Clausen, C., Emed, J., Frunchak, V., Purden, M., & Bruno, F. (2019). Toward resilient nurse leaders: The leadership-in-action program in nursing (LEAP-IN). *Nursing Leadership, 32*(3), 40–56. https://doi.org/10.12927/cjnl.2019.25973

Crawford, C., Omery, A., & Spicer, J. (2017). An integrative review of 21st-century roles, responsibilities, characteristics, and competencies of chief nurse executives: A blueprint for the next generation. *Nursing Administration Quarterly, 41*(4), 297–309. https://doi.org/10.1097/NAQ.0000000000000245

Cronenwett, L., Sherwood, G., Barnsteiner, J., Disch, J., Johnson, J., Mitchell, P., Sullivan, D., & Warren, J. (2007). Quality and safety education for nurses. *Nursing Outlook, 55*(3), 122–131. https://doi.org/10.1016/j.outlook.2007.02.006

Cronenwett, L., Sherwood, G., Pohl, J., Barnsteiner, J., Moore, S., Sullivan, D., Ward, D., & Warren, J. (2009). Quality and safety education for advanced nursing practice. *Nursing Outlook, 57*(6), 338–348. https://doi.org/10.1016/j.outlook.2009.07.009

Economic Times. (2021). Definition of '360-degree feedback.' https://economictimes.indiatimes.com/definition/360-degree-feedback

Fitzpatrick, J. J., Rivera, R. R., Walsh, L., & Byers, O. M. (2019). Narrative nursing inspiring a shared vision among clinical nurses. *Nurse Leader, 17*(2), 131–134. https://doi.org/10.1016/j.mnl.2018.12.002

Fowler, M. D. (2015). *Guide to nursing's social policy statement: Understanding the profession from social contact to social covenant*. American Nurses Association.

Gollust, S. E., Cunningham, B. A., Bokhour, B. G., Gordon, H. S., Pope, C., Saha, S. S., Jones, D, M., Do, T., & Burgess, D. J. (2018). What causes racial health care disparities? A mixed-methods study reveals variability in how health care providers perceive causal attributions. *The Journal of Health Care Organization, Provision, and Financing, 55*, 1–11. https://doi.org/10.1177/0046958018762840

Griffiths, B., & Washington, E. (2015). Competencies at work providing a common language for talent management. *Business Expert Press*. https://www.businessexpertpress.com/books/competencies-work-providing-common-language-talent-management

Haggerty, J., Chin, M. H., Katz, A., Young, K., Foley, J., Grolux, A., Perez-Stable, E. J., Turnbull, J., DeVoe, J. E., & Uchendu, U. S. (2018). Proactive strategies to address health equity and disparities: Recommendations from a bi-national symposium. *Journal of the American Board of Family Medicine, 31*(3), 479–483. https://doi.org/10.3122/jabfm.2018.03.170299

Healthcare Leadership Alliance. (2017). *About the HLA compentency directory*. http://www.healthcare leadershipalliance.org/directory.htm

Iheduru-Anderson, K. (2020). The White/Black hierarchy institutionalizes White supremacy in nursing and nursing leadership in the United States. *Journal of Professional Nursing, 37*(2021), 411–421. https://doi.org/10.1016/j.profnurs.2020.05.005

Institute of Medicine. (2011). *The future of nursing: Leading change, advancing health*. National Academies Press. https://www.ncbi.nlm.nih.gov/books/NBK209880

International Council of Nursing. (2012). *Code of ethics*. https://www.icn.ch/news/international-council-nurses-launches-consultation-revise-code-ethics-nurses

Kerfoot, K. M., & Luquire, R. (2012). Alignment of the system's chief nursing officer: Staff or direct line structure? *Nursing Administration Quarterly, 36*(4), 325–331. https://doi.org/10.1097/NAQ.0b013e3182669333

McCloughen, A., O'Brien, L., & Jackson, D. (2013). Journey to become a nurse leader mentor: Past, present, and future influences. *Nursing Inquiry, 21*(4), 301–310. https://doi.org/10.1111/nin.12053

Morse, V., & Warshawsky, N. E. (2021). Nurse leader competencies today and tomorrow. *Nursing Administration Quarterly, 45*(1), 65–70. https://doi.org/10.1097/NAQ.0000000000000453

Nardi, D., Waite, R., Nowak, M., Hatcher, B., Hines-Martin, V., & Stacciarini, J. (2020). Achieving health equity through eradicating structural racism in the United States: A call to action for nursing leadership. *Journal of Nursing Scholarship, 52*(6), 696–704. https://doi.org/10.1111/jnu.12602

Orchard, C., Olubukola, S., Morse, A., Collins, J., & Al-Hamad, A. (2017). Collaborative leadership, part 1: The nurse leader's role within interprofessional teams. *Nursing Leadership, 30*(2), 14–25. https://doi.org/10.12927/cjnl.2017.25258

Prestia, A. (2015). Chief nursing officer sustainment: A phenomenological inquiry. *The Journal of Nursing Administration, 45*(11), 575–581. http://doi.org/10.1097/NNA.0000000000000266

QSEN Institute. (n.d.-a). *About*. https://qsen.org/about-qsen

QSEN Institute. (n.d.-b). *Project overview.* https://qsen.org/about-qsen/project-overview

Sanford, K., & Janney, M. (2019). Preparing the nurse executive of the future. *Journal of Nursing Administration, 49*(4), 171–173. https://doi.org/10.1097/NNA.0000000000000732

Schlaak, M. (2019). From nurse to nurse manager. *Viewpoint: The Official Publication of the American Academy of Ambulatory Care Nursing, 41*(2), 1, 13–14.

Sigma. (n.d.). *Sigma organizational fact sheet.* https://www.sigmanursing.org/why-sigma/about-sigma/sigma-organizational-fact-sheet

Snow, F. (2019). Creativity and innovation: An essential competency for the nurse leader. *Nursing Administration Quarterly, 43*(4), 306–312. https://doi.org/10.1097/NAQ.0000000000000367

Stefl, M. (2008). Common competencies for all healthcare managers: The Healthcare Leadership Alliance model. *Journal of Healthcare Management/American College of Healthcare Executives, 53*(6), 360–374. https://doi.org/10.1097/00115514-200811000-00004

Steinberg, B., & Watkins, M. (2021). The surprising power of coaching. *Harvard Business Review.* https://hbr.org/2021/04/the-surprising-power-of-peer-coaching

Tannenbaum, S. I., Traylor, A. M., Thomas, E. S., & Salas, E. S. (2021). Managing teamwork in the face of pandemic: Evidence-based tips. *BMJ Quality & Safety, 30*, 59–63. https://qualitysafety.bmj.com/content/30/1/59.abstract

Wakefield, M. K., Williams, D. R., Le Menestrel, S., & Flaubert, J. L. (Eds.). (2021). *The future of nursing 2020–2030: Charting a path to achieve health equity.* National Academies Press. https://doi.org/10.17226/25982

Waxman, K., Roussel, L., Herrin-Griffith, D., & D'Alfonso, J. (2017). The AONE nurse executive competencies: 12 years later. *Nurse Leader, 15*, 120–126. https://doi.org/10.1016/j.mnl.2016.11.012

SECTION II

RELATIONAL LEADERSHIP IN PRACTICE

CHAPTER 4

THE IMPORTANCE OF RELATIONSHIPS

Mary Beth Modic and Amy Windover

"We believe that a person is a person through other persons, that my humanity is caught up, bound up, inextricably, with yours."

Archbishop Desmond Tutu

LEARNING OBJECTIVES

- Summarize the relationship between "sense of belonging" and the development of flourishing relationships.
- Assess the impact of person-centered, strength-based, empathic language on relationships.
- Evaluate behaviors that nurture relationships.
- Plan rituals that foster communities of caregivers.

INTRODUCTION

Since the beginning of time, human beings have sought out companionship. We have a need for human connection and social interaction. We are social by nature. It is well known that babies who are deprived of human contact fail to thrive. Agrawal (2018) suggests that "we were literally born in community attached to someone else" (p. 16). Individuals who are made to feel welcome, acknowledged for their contributions, and invited to participate in decisions that affect them feel a sense of belonging. Clarke tenders that respect, community, and connectedness are all essential for a sense of belonging to exist (Clarke, 2019). Cultivating a sense of belonging allows individuals to feel like their authentic selves without fear of alienation or rejection. Individuals who enjoy their work believe they work closely with someone who cares about them as a person (Mann, 2018). Nurses recognize the importance of belonging and work diligently to foster relationships that are affirming, nurturing, and supportive with patients, colleagues, and the communities in which they live.

In healthcare, individuals are asked to come together and align around a common mission and vision and embrace a set of values aimed at caring for others. We are often asked to set our personal needs aside to focus on meeting the needs of those for whom we serve. Yet, there are as many ways of interpreting how best to carry out the mission and values as there are people. Leaders are often challenged to create communities. This chapter offers behaviors, strategies, and novel techniques that nurse leaders can use to foster collegial relationships and promote a feeling of genuine belonging and community.

BELONGING

Leaders are in the unique position to create vibrant, inclusive, and collaborative communities and to ensure a sense of belonging. A definition of belonging proposed by Finnish researchers states that belonging is "an experience of personal involvement in a system or environment so that persons feel themselves to be an integral part of that system or environment" (Hagerty, 1996, p. 238). Radha Agrawal (2018), a social influencer, defines belonging as "a feeling of deep relatedness and acceptance: a feeling of I would rather be here than anywhere else" (p. 17). Community can best be described as both a feeling and a set of relationships among people (Vogl, 2016). Communities differ from groups because members feel a sense of connection and are committed to the welfare and success of one another. To nurture a flourishing community, it is essential that the community's core values be clearly articulated and embraced by the members. Shared values are what attracts people to an organization in the first place. Creating a community so that each individual can flourish is an effective retention strategy (Manion & Bartholomew, 2004).

One critical behavior that indicates a sense of belonging is the exchange of help, not only offering help, but the comfort in asking for it. Ninety percent of helping in the workplace is in response to requests for help (Murthy, 2020). Often, there is a fear that asking for help may be perceived as being lazy, weak, or incompetent. When asking and offering help is incorporated into an organization as a core value, people feel it promotes an atmosphere of solidarity and connection.

Findings from a qualitative study in which nurse and social managers were queried about their perceptions of factors that influence the sense of belonging revealed six elements that contributed to a sense of belonging and five that impeded it (see Tables 4.1 and 4.2). Many of the fostering behaviors reported—listening, collaborating, and strong work ethic—can be

TABLE 4.1: Factors That Foster a Sense of Belonging Among Social and Healthcare Managers

Open Interaction	Effective Communication Culture	Support and Encouragement	Common Values	Shared Vision of the Work	Structure of Leadership
Listening to one another	Joint meetings Regular meetings Joint conversations Time together	Helping each other Encouraging each other Collegiality Sharing work experiences Open flow of information Professional guidance Personal relationships and networks	Humor Trust Respect Appreciation Honesty Sharing of same values	Mutual goals and modes of operation at work Common rules of agreement and the commitment to them Collaboration	Functional practices Good superior/ subordinate relationships

Source: Data from Lampinen, M. S., Konu, A. I., Kettunen, T., & Suutala, E. A. (2018). Factors that foster or prevent sense of belonging among social and healthcare managers. *Leadership in Health Service, 31*(4), 468–480. https://doi.org/10.1108/LHS-09-2017-0054.

TABLE 4.2: Factors That Prevent a Sense of Belonging Among Social and Healthcare Managers

Negative Work Atmosphere	Lack of Common Time	Structural Components of the Organization	Problems That Occur at Organizational Level	Problems Related to Leadership and Management
Distrust	Urgency	Organizational structure	Financial situation	Poor flow of information
Competition	Lack of common time	Distance between fundamental units	Lack of shared vision	Bypassing of organizational lines of leadership
Envy	Workload	Organizational changes	Lack of common goals	
Underestimating another person			Lack of communication	
Talking behind someone's back			Lack of cooperation	
Self-interest				
Lack of appreciation				
Inappropriate interactions				

Source: Data from Lampinen, M. S., Konu, A. I., Kettunen, T., & Suutala, E. A. (2018). Factors that foster or prevent sense of belonging among social and healthcare managers. *Leadership in Health Service, 31*(4), 468–480. https://doi.org/10.1108/LHS-09-2017-0054.

attributed to what is often referred to as "soft skills." Soft skills are behaviors, personality traits, and work habits that help individuals flourish at work (Dziados, 2019; Kroning, 2015). Soft skills are often underappreciated but essential in forming and sustaining relationships, generating trust, and contributing to a successful career as a leader. The impeding elements that were identified—organizational change, lack of cooperation, and lack of communication—can be overcome by the wise use of soft skills.

MASLOW'S HIERARCHY OF NEEDS

In 1943, the psychologist Abraham Maslow proposed a hierarchy of needs. Maslow's theory, while never empirically validated, rank ordered needs according to necessity for survival. Maslow believed that all behaviors are predicated on needs. The needs are housed in one of the most recognized pyramids in the management literature with the most basic needs located at the bottom. The needs in ascending order are:

- **Physiological Needs:** Air, food, water, shelter, clothing, sleep
- **Safety and Security:** Health, employment, property, family, and social stability
- **Love and Belonging:** Friendship, family, intimacy, sense of connection
- **Self-Esteem:** Confidence, achievement, respect of others, the need to be a unique individual
- **Self-Actualization:** Morality, creativity, spontaneity, acceptance, experience purpose, meaning and inner purpose

Maslow averred that healthy individuals seek to become fully formed persons by optimizing their talents, capabilities, and sense of purpose. Maslow placed love and belonging in the third tier. He espoused that human beings need to feel a sense of belonging and community, whether it comes from large organizations or small networks of family and friends. Researchers have continued to study the impact of love and belonging needs on well-being and have found that social connections impact a sense of physical health and well-being (Waldinger, 2015).

Radha Agrawal (2018) suggests that Maslow's hierarchy needs some updating. Agrawal believes that the need for belonging is as fundamental as air, food, and water. She reconstructs Maslow's work and proposes four major needs: basic human needs, physical and mental well-being, purpose, and joy. She contends that a sense of purpose is integral to self-actualization and that the culmination of a well-lived life is joy, brought about by a sense of wonder, curiosity, and playfulness throughout one's life.

INTERPERSONAL RELATIONSHIPS

Hildegard Peplau, the founder of psychiatric nursing, proposed the theory of interpersonal relations which emphasized the significance of the nurse–patient relationship. Her research identified that patients and nurses pass through three phases to experience a therapeutic relationship. In the first phase, which Peplau named the orientation phase, the nurse enters as a stranger skillfully gathering important information about the patient and prioritizing worries, fears, and anxieties all the while conveying respect and attention. The working phase is the second phase and encompasses the majority of time that nurses care for patients. It is during this phase that the patient experiences the myriad of interventions the nurse provides—comfort, education, and physiological, emotional, and environmental safety. The nurse uses a myriad of communication skills to reflect on the patient's understanding of illness and hopes for recovery. The final phase is known as the termination phase and is most often associated with discharge planning and the validation of learning. The nurse and patient relationship comes to an end.

Peplau's theory has relevance for clinical leaders. Nurses who are new to the clinical unit or leadership team go through an enculturation. Individuals enter the group as a stranger to the norms, values, and practices. They are welcomed enthusiastically, introduced to others with respect, and reassured that their presence has been expected with great anticipation and excitement. The working phase is associated with the knowledge and skill acquisition required for the position. During this phase, the new member to the group undergoes a transformation as information and affirmation are provided. Relationships that evolve during the working phase confirm a new professional identity, foster a sense of belonging, and provide social support (Peplau, 1994). The termination phase would be represented by the relinquishment of a position and change in relationships. Hildegard Peplau's revolutionary work continues to provide guidance on the nuances of developing and sustaining relationships. She propagated the ethos "that a team nourishes its own member so that their interrelated functions become more meaningful" (Peplau, 1991, p. 7).

MULTIGENERATIONAL WORKFORCE

Today's workforce is multigenerational. Generational diversity provides opportunities for nurse leaders to harness different communication patterns, work practices, and career expectations. Multigenerational organizations committed to diversity can employ as many as five distinct generations: Traditionalists, Baby Boomers, Generation X, Millennials, and Gen Z. Baby Boomers who were born from 1946 to 1964 are currently the largest generation in the workforce, although it is predicted that more than 500,000 nurses will retire by 2022, including 75% of nurse leaders (ANA, n.d.). This loss of strategic thinkers will impact how nursing care is delivered without their stewardship (Stichler, 2013).

Millennials born between 1981 and 1996 will represent 75% of the U.S. workforce by 2025 (Louis, 2017). Given the number of leadership vacancies because of retirements, Millennials may be promoted into positions for which they are not prepared (Stichler, 2013). However,

Millennials may be the generation most interested in community building and fostering a sense of belonging as compared to any previous generation. They have been connected through digital technology since infancy (Martin, 2020).

Leaders need to appreciate the generational preferences for job searches, marketing strategies, learning and career advancement opportunities and the perks or benefits that will entice different generations to remain in their jobs. The use of technology and communication preferences account for the greatest difference among the generations. As a result, this generational divide necessitates that leaders be multilingual in their communication strategies using texting, email, social media platforms, or hosting in person conversations to ensure that each team member, regardless of generational affiliation, feels a sense of belonging and being valued.

BELONGING FOR EVERYONE: DIVERSITY, EQUITY, AND INCLUSION

Forming relationships and fostering a sense of belonging begins with knowing everyone's name on the healthcare team and calling them by their preferred name. Atul Gwande (2010), a surgeon and patient safety advocate, stresses the importance of relationships, collegiality, and cooperation in providing safe and quality care. He calls attention to the need to know the names of colleagues because "people who don't know one another's names, don't work together nearly as well as those who do" (p. 108). Manion and Bartholomew (2004) describe the experience of a new nurse manager who learned that the physicians who routinely admitted patients to her unit were unable to identify any of the nurses by name, many who had worked on the unit for 15 years.

Fostering a sense of belonging in the workplace necessitates the need for leaders to appreciate that many individuals are entering the workplace with gender identities and expressions that are different from the way gender has been identified in the past. Gender expansive individuals may choose to use pronouns "they, them, and theirs."

Diversity, equity, and inclusion (DEI) are essential elements of workplace culture. The workforce should reflect the composition of society at large. The workplace needs to be a place where all individuals feel welcomed, respected, and have opportunities for success. Creating a DEI workplace where all individuals can flourish means that all team members have an obligation to imagine how others might experience daily life and encourage full participation. The National Academy of Medicine (NAM) released a report entitled *The Future of Nursing 2020–2030: Charting a Path to Achieve Health Equity*, which describes the activities the profession of nursing must embrace to create an inclusive and diverse workforce. Additionally, the report calls on nursing to be integral leaders in the eradication of socioeconomic and environmental factors that impede access to equitable healthcare and the promotion of healthy communities (NAM, 2021).

PROFESSIONAL CITIZENSHIP

Encouraging team members to expand their professional relationships and current networks by joining professional nursing organizations can impact patient outcomes and promote collegiality with nurses outside of their organization. As a member of a professional nursing organization, members can expand their knowledge and become familiar with healthcare policies that affect their clinical specialty as well as the nursing profession. Fulton (2019) posits that membership in a nursing organization is a professional citizenship responsibility which allows nurses to participate in the creation of nursing's desired future. Hildegard Peplau (1952) called for nurses to be active participants in a democratic society.

A strong professional alliance allows nurses to examine issues with like-minded individuals. In the United States, there are over 180 professional nursing organizations in which nurses can avail themselves (Nurse Organization, n.d.). In addition to exploring clinical and healthcare policy issues, members can serve in leadership positions which afford them skills in public speaking, facilitating meetings, organizing events, and managing budgets. Clinical leaders should encourage relationship building beyond the confines of their organizations. Sharing journal articles, news of conferences, and dates for submission of podium presentations at local, regional, and national conferences may provide the incentive for a team member to join and enjoy the innumerable benefits of membership.

UBUNTU

"Ubuntu" is a South African word that originates from the Zulu tribe. Ubuntu means "I am because you are." It offers a person a way of interacting with other human beings so that they can welcome the gifts that only others bring to relationships. People are not viewed as competitors or adversaries, but human beings who are respected and valued for their unique talents, experiences, and wisdom. Ubuntu was popularized by South African President Nelson Mandela and Archbishop Desmond Tutu in the 1990s to educate the world about the dangers of apartheid. Ubuntu personifies the importance of relationship in its purest form. At its core, Ubuntu provides the genesis for all relationships, as that is how communities are formed (Nolte & Downing, 2019). Two other South African words are frequently used to convey community: "saubona," which means "I see you," and "sikona," which means "I am here to be seen." Clarke, in her 2019 TED Talk, implies that the use of the two words together translate to *Until I see you, I do not exist.* She suggests that each of us is dependent on one another for our humanity. This richness of recognition is dependent on the quality of human relationships (Peplau, 1994).

Ubuntu serves as the underpinning for this chapter on relationships as its principles promote the concepts of caring and belonging. The philosophical intentions of Ubuntu suggest that

- the organization be recognized as a community filled with deep relationships,
- the good of all its members should be encouraged, and
- all members of the community thrive (Lutz, 2009).

Cross et al. (2021) proffer that a rich network of relationships can help us bounce back from difficulties by

- helping us *shift work or manage surges,*
- helping us to *make sense of people or politics in a given situation,*
- helping us find the confidence to *push back* and *self-advocate,*
- helping us see *a path forward,*
- providing *empathic support so we can release negative emotions,*
- helping us to *laugh at ourselves and the situation,*
- reminding us of the *purpose or meaning* in our work, and
- broadening us as individuals so that we maintain *perspective* when setbacks happen.

LANGUAGE

Language is our most powerful form of communication. It reflects the way we think about others as well as ourselves. Words matter. They can heal, inspire, and teach or they can hurt, demean, or incite. Words reveal what we think, believe, and value. Every day, nurses care for patients as compassionate strangers and offer words of hope, encouragement, and comfort to attenuate suffering. We can also use judgment-laden labels to describe the individuals entrusted to our care when communicating with other caregivers. Nurses have been enculturated into a world that uses disease- and deficit-based language: "The patient is hypertensive, obese, and noncompliant. The patient can't swallow, walk, or speak." The medical model of disease and disability pathologizes illness and chronic conditions. What leaders model by the words they use can be deeply impactful and demonstrate an inclusive environment for both patients and caregivers (McMaster, 2014), It demonstrates a commitment to the best possible care and promotes relational excellence (Koloroutis, 2020).

PERSON-CENTERED, STRENGTH-BASED LANGUAGE

Until recently, most nurses have been unaware of the negative consequences of deficit-based language. A "language movement" has been embraced by other fields of research for years. The literature is now replete with language recommendations for establishing, developing, and engaging relationships with patients, their families, and other caregivers. There is compelling evidence that a strength-based vocabulary heals and empowers (Crocker & Smith, 2019; Dickinson et al., 2017; Granello & Gibbs, 2016; Kapitan, 2017).

Patient-first language has been in the literature for decades. Yet there remains a delay in implementation of this evidence-based practice. On acute and critical care units, caregivers can be observed discussing patients based on their disease. "The diabetic in bed 3"; "he's autistic"; "she's an alcoholic"; and "the patient is nonverbal" are all labels unconsciously used by nurses to hand off care from one nurse to another or communicate care needs in what is thought to be an effective use of language. While the intention in nurse handoffs is not to be deliberately disrespectful, disease-first language diminishes patients, promotes the idea that the disease is a characteristic of the person, and fosters negative stereotypes. Opportunities for a linguistic upgrade also encompass the phasing out of pejorative words including "nonadherent," "noncompliant," "difficult," "demanding," and "frequent flyer" (see Table 4.3).

As leaders, person-centered, strength-based, empathic language extends beyond the patient care arena to daily conversations with other caregivers and colleagues (see Table 4.4). A leader's vocabulary that is egalitarian and strength-based can highlight the unique work of the nurse and may be significant in elevating the profession's status and identity.

EMPATHIC LANGUAGE

Empathy is the ability to imagine what another person is thinking and feeling. While nonverbal cues like the tilt of one's head or furrowing of one's brow convey care and concern, verbal statements of empathy can be powerful in connecting with others. S.A.V.E. is a mnemonic that outlines four different types of empathic statements (support, acknowledgment, validation, and emotion naming). Statements of support convey partnership and let others know that they are not alone. For instance, "I'm here for you. Let's work together." Statements of acknowledgment convey respect for what someone has gone through or accomplished, such as, "This has been hard for you," or "I wish there were better options." Validation statements are often mistaken for agreement with another person. Instead, these statements legitimize the emotion experienced by another person. For example, "Anyone in your position would feel upset," or "Most people would feel the way you do." Validation is most effective when someone is feeling embarrassed or ashamed, such as apologizing profusely for crying at work. Last, emotion naming are statements that identify the emotion the other person is experiencing. Examples include, "You seem sad," or "You sound worried." The more accurate we can be in identifying the person's emotion, the more effective the empathy and connection. However, if we don't name the emotion accurately, most people are happy to correct us and still appreciate our intent (Windover et al., 2014).

TABLE 4.3: Person-Centered, Strength-Based Language Examples in Care of Patients

Current Language	Recommended Language
Adherence	Engagement
Control	Manage
Alcoholic, autistic, bipolar, diabetic, druggie	A person with alcoholism, autism, bipolar disorder, diabetes, or has a substance abuse disorder
Noncompliant	Struggling
Suffering	Living with/being treated for
Value-laden labels assigned to stereotypical behavior	
Angry	Intense emotion
Complained of	Expressed concern/reported
Demanding/difficult	Made repeated requests
Entitled	Aware of one's rights
"Frequent flyer"	Utilizes services and supports when needed
Helpless/hopeless	Unaware of opportunities
Nasty, rude, mean	Used offensive language
Needy	Sought reassurance
Refused	Declined
Resistant	Chooses not to/is not ready
Unmotivated	Preferred options unavailable
Unrealistic	High expectations

Source: Adapted from Counseling at Northwestern. (n.d.). *Inclusive language guide.* https://counseling.northwestern.edu/blog/inclusive-language-guide; Dickinson, J. K., Guzman, S. S., Maryniuk, M.-D., O'Brien, C. A., Kadohiro, J. K., Jackson, R. A., D'Hondt, N., Montgomery, B., Close, K. L, & Funnell, M. M. (2017). The use of language in diabetes care and education. *Diabetes Care, 40*(12), 1790–1799. https://doi.org/10.2337/dci17-0041.

TABLE 4.4: Relationship-Promoting Language

Current Language	Recommended Language
Ask the doctor	Consult with physician/healthcare team
Confront	Reconcile
Coworker	Colleague
Doctor	Professional role—physician, pharmacist, physical therapist, audiologist, nurse, psychologist
Feedback	Feedforward
Floor, frontline, staff nurse	Clinical nurse

(continued)

TABLE 4.4: Relationship-Promoting Language (*continued*)

Current Language	Recommended Language
He, she	Preferred pronoun
Legal name	Preferred name
Just a staff nurse	Clinical nurse, essential caregiver, integrator of care
Midlevel, nonphysician provider	APRN, PA
Newbie	Newly licensed RN
Nursing floor (RNF)	Med–surg, step down, or other as appropriate
Older nurse	Clinical expert
Works on the floor	Practices on the unit
Write-up/disciplinary action	Corrective conversations—"I believe in you"

APRN, advanced practice registered nurse; PA, physician assistant; RN, registered nurse; RNF, regular nursing floor.

FEEDFORWARD

Feedforward is a novel idea that is attributed to author and leadership innovator Marshall Goldsmith (2012). It originated out of his observation that, while feedback is essential to performance improvement, it may not be well presented or well received. Feedforward is predicated on the idea that one cannot change the past but can influence the future. Rather than debriefing about a performance or decision that was ineffective, feedforward concentrates on solutions for the future. Hirsch (2017) posits that feedforward unleashes performance possibilities. By using feedforward concepts and language, leaders can explore growth opportunities for the future. Hirsch suggests the use of the mnemonic REPAIR to remember the benefits of feedforward:

- Regenerates talent
- Expands possibilities
- Is Particular
- Is Authentic
- Has Impact
- Refines group dynamics (Hirsch, 2017, p. 17)

Feedforward requires a mindset change because it is not an analysis of past performance but an opportunity to rehearse and plan for the future. It encourages team members not to perseverate on past mistakes, but plan for behaving differently moving forward. It promotes feelings of self-confidence and reinforces views of what is possible.

THE LANGUAGE OF APOLOGY

Being responsible for the well-being of others is simultaneously gratifying and demanding. At times, it can prove overwhelming when there are competing time demands or workload exceeds one's capacity. On occasion, tempers may flair and words are uttered that are hurtful, disrespectful, and regrettable. An apology is necessary to repair and preserve a collegial relationship.

Aaron Lazare was a psychiatrist who dedicated much of his career to studying the act of apology. He was curious about characteristics that made apologies successful or fail and contributed to reconciliation. His research revealed that the most prevalent misstep was the lack of acknowledgment of the offense by the offending individual. Most often, vague or incomplete apologies were offered. Statements such as "if I offended you," "a mistake was made," or "sorry for whatever I did" were expressed in his study. Lazare's research revealed that an effective apology consists of four components, although not every apology requires all four (Box 4.1).

BOX 4.1: COMPONENTS OF AN EFFECTIVE APOLOGY

1. A valid acknowledgment of the offense that makes clear who is the offender and who is the offended

2. An effective explanation, which shows an offense was neither intentional nor personal and is unlikely to recur

3. Expressions of remorse, shame, and humility, which show that the offender recognizes the suffering of the offended

4. A reparation of some kind, in the form of a real or symbolic compensation for the offender's transgressions

Source: Adapted from Lazare, A. (2004). *On apology.* Oxford Press.

Effective apologies are an essential tool for leaders to use in assuaging feelings of humiliation, reconciling misunderstandings, and restoring peace to a tumultuous work environment. Without heartfelt apologies, grudges can fester, relationships are tarnished, and the work environment is negatively impacted.

In sum, the sense of belonging is reduced to the most basic of questions: "Do I know you as a person?" "Do I have a relationship with you that enriches my life?" "Do I contribute to your self-worth in a meaningful way?" Knowing the essence of another person brings that individual into our consciousness. We miss people with whom we have relationships when they are not present. Their absence creates a void (McMaster, 2014).

RITUALS

In healthcare, we do not have significant time to invest in establishing and maintaining relationships. Rituals are an efficient and effective way to foster a sense of belonging and community. Rituals can be defined as a set of actions that occur in a particular order and may be positioned into a daily work schedule at the beginning or end of a shift or as a transition between two activities. Rituals allow for sharing of values, perspectives, and personal histories. There are many different types of rituals that can be used to foster a sense of belonging and create communities.

CHECK-INS AND SETTLING PRACTICES

Check-ins meet people where they are by first acknowledging and validating their thoughts and feelings before orienting everyone to a shared goal or activity. They consist of requesting a word or phrase from each team member to convey how they are showing up or feeling in the moment. Check-ins provide a safe space to briefly connect with people on a personal or emotional level. They also remind us of our humanity and lives outside of work, while helping the individuals doing the check-in to say what is on their mind and more readily transition to the work at hand. It's a deliberate process meant to elicit meaningful, as opposed to perfunctory, responses (Box 4.2). Examples include:

- *How are you showing up today?*
- *What is especially present for you in this moment?*
- *What three adjectives would you use to describe how you are feeling right now?*

BOX 4.2: CHECK-INS AND SETTLING PRACTICES

Traditional check-ins

- How are you showing up today?
- What is especially present for you in this moment?
- What three adjectives would you use to describe how you are feeling right now?

Check-in variations

To infuse fun and creativity:

- If your mood is a weather forecast, what would it be?
- What song best reflects how you're showing up today?
- What movie or television show best reflects how you're feeling as a result of our work today?

To promote appreciation and gratitude:

- What is one thing you appreciate in this moment?
- What is one thing you are proud of today?
- What is one thing you appreciate about our team or a specific team member?

To elicit feedback or assess the impact of an activity:

- What is something you are taking away from today, and how will you incorporate it into your work?
- What did you appreciate most about today's meeting? What's one thing we might consider doing to make meetings even better?
- What surprised you about our time together?

Many variations exist on the traditional check-in that can serve different relational objectives. For example, some check-ins can infuse fun and creativity:

- *If your mood is a weather forecast, what would it be?*
- *What song best reflects how you're showing up today?*
- *What movie or television show best reflects how you're feeling as a result of our work today?*

Other check-ins promote a spirit of appreciation and gratitude:

- *What is one thing you appreciate in this moment?*
- *What is one thing you are proud of today?*
- *What is one thing you appreciate about our team or a specific team member?*

Still others serve to elicit feedback or assess the impact of an activity:

- *What is something you are taking away from today, and how will you incorporate it into your work?*
- *What did you appreciate most about today's meeting? What's one thing we might consider doing to make meetings even better?*
- *What surprised you about our time together?*

In addition to check-ins, there are a myriad of settling rituals that focus attention and create a sense of interconnectedness. Mindfulness meditation is one of the most common and consists of purposeful observation of one's thoughts and feelings in the present moment without judgment. Before starting, minimize any distractions and direct attention to the breath. Invite people to accept each new thought or feeling, whether good or bad, as just one of many clouds gently moving across the sky. Practicing collectively, even a few minutes a day, is helpful in realizing the benefits of this ritual. In addition to improved personal well-being, mindfulness meditation has been shown to improve a nurse's capacity to manage stress and communicate effectively with patients and one another (Guillaumie et al., 2017). Several online resources (such as Headspace, Calm, and Buddhify) exist to provide guided mindfulness meditation.

Grounding is another technique that focuses attention on the present moment by bringing awareness to the five senses. After finding a comfortable seated position with feet flat on the floor, invite people to take a few diaphragmatic breaths in through their nose for a count of three and out through their mouth for a count of four. Then, invite them to take a few moments to identify five things they see, followed by four things they feel, three things they hear, two things they smell, and one thing they taste.

WARM-UP ACTIVITIES

Warm-up activities are one of three elements in sociodrama, a therapeutic technique developed by Jacob Moreno to examine deep emotional conflict. Not to be mistaken with icebreakers, warm-up activities are characterized by learning through action. For example, people are invited to respond to a series of prompts by positioning themselves on different sides of a room, standing on an imaginary continuum, or stepping into a circle based on their thoughts, feelings, or attitudes in that moment. Prompts are chosen based on the individual characteristics and needs of a group (e.g., group size, familiarity with one another). Warm-ups serve many community-building functions including gradual familiarity with others in a group, the promotion of creativity, openness and collaboration, and validation of private attitudes and emotions that are often shared among group members (Modic, 2016a, 2016b).

There are four different types of warm-up activities: polarities, spectragrams, locograms, and step-in circles. Polarities consist of asking people to move to one of three different spaces depending on their preference for two criteria posed. For example, you might say, "Do you prefer cake or ice cream? If you prefer cake, move to the right side of the room. If you prefer ice cream, move to the left side of the room. For those that may like or dislike both equally, stand in the middle of the room."

Spectragrams entail asking people to position themselves along an imaginary continuum, standing shoulder to shoulder in a straight line facing forward according to a specific criterion. For example, while walking the imaginary line, the meeting facilitator might say, "Stand shoulder to shoulder in a straight line and face me according to the time it took you to get here today, from the least amount of time to the greatest amount of time."

Locograms consist of asking people to stand in designated areas, often quadrants, based on their preference. For instance, while moving to the four different quadrants of the room you might say, "Now I'd like you to go stand in the group that resonates most with you. If you could have any superpower, would you prefer to have super strength, the ability to read minds, the ability to be invisible, or the ability to fly? If you prefer something I didn't mention, please feel free to stand in the middle." Other examples of light or neutral criterion include the four seasons, favorite footwear, and favorite types of music or movie genres, whereas more serious criterion might include topics like knowledge or experience with a given subject, factors causing the most stress, or implicit norms impacting the group.

Step-in circles are the last warm-up activity. Group members stand in a circle facing forward and are invited to take one step forward if a particular statement resonates with them. Step-in circles allow people to choose more than one option, all the options, or none of the options. It allows team members to efficiently acknowledge significant elephants in the room and move forward without the need to enter into a debate or difficult conversation.

There are several considerations in planning warm-up activities. One consideration involves choosing criterion that won't embarrass or humiliate anyone. What could be considered an innocent warm-up may contribute to a person feeling alienated. For example, using dogs and cats as a polarity may prove isolating if a single woman stands alone in her preference for cats, resulting in jokes about the stereotypic "cat lady." Another consideration in developing criterion and warm-ups is to go in order of least threatening or personal to more personal. This allows people to become more comfortable and familiar with one another. After establishing a sense of safety and trust, the group can move to more sensitive criterion and topics such as validating shared challenges or acknowledging thoughts and feelings that may be creating discord and impeding performance within the group. A third consideration is in when and how to solicit additional reflection. For less personal criterion, a comment or two about what led people to place themselves in a particular criterion may be solicited. However, for more personal or serious questions, it's important to hear from everyone that wants to contribute a reflection. Finally, when facilitating warm-ups, it's important to provide clear, concise instructions using action to demonstrate where people should stand for each criterion and how.

MINUTE MATRIX

Teams are most productive and resilient when strong connections are formed among all members. Minute matrix is a group formation activity, much like speed dating, that facilitates initial connections with every member of a group. Individuals are asked to form two lines facing one another to form pairs. A facilitator then asks a question and provides 30 to 60 seconds to answer in their pairs. When the time is up, one line remains stationary while the other line shifts one person forward and the first person moves to the back so that everyone has a new partner. Since the connection times are brief, the exercise generates a lot of playful energy and openness. Incorporate a range of questions that are personal, yet safe from contention, such as those involving politics or religion. Examples of prompts include a favorite childhood memory, your favorite book, your favorite home remedy when you are sick, a motto you live your life by, your biggest accomplishment, and your ideal day off.

STEPPING STONES

Ira Progroff offered a technique to promote self-reflection via an activity he called "Stepping Stones." This activity can also be used as a community-building exercise. Participants are broken into small groups consisting of three to four individuals. The participants are instructed to write down on a sheet of paper events, milestones, or names of individuals (not exceeding six) who have influenced them as nurses, leaders, or activists and two to three sentences about what or who they have written. (Not all people or events that are identified are positive.) Stones of different sizes, shapes, colors, and textures are needed for this activity. Each participant is asked to select stones that represent the events or people they have written down. After selecting the stones, each participant presents the stone and the story that accompanies it to members of the small group. The stories that are shared are compelling and illuminating. Participants can learn about influential people or life-altering events of colleagues with whom they work (Modic, 2016a, 2016b).

INSIDE SCOOP

Vivek Murthy, the 19th and 21st U.S. surgeon general, describes how his staff developed "Inside Scoop" as a way of getting to know and appreciate the rich life experience within his expanding team. The activity became a standing 5-minute agenda item during weekly meetings. Team members take turns sharing pictures via a PowerPoint presentation that reveals personal aspects of their lives they wish their colleagues to learn about them while the rest of the team listens actively. Murthy reported that the team members expressed delight in having the opportunity to get to know their colleagues from a different vantage point. They have indicated that this is one of the highlights of the weekly meetings (2020). Personal stories dismantle hierarchies; allow for a deeper insight into another's perspectives, values, and motivation; and foster esprit de corps (Smith, 2012).

IF YOU KNOW ME

Since organizations across the globe have committed to ensuring a diverse workforce, it is imperative that relationship-building opportunities be incorporated into regular meetings to promote understanding among diverse groups (Jacob et al., 2020).

An activity that promotes dialogue is called "If You Knew Me." Some sample statements include:

- *"At work, I add value by. . ."*
- *"When I am having a bad day, I need. . ."*
- *"When I am under pressure, my colleagues can help me by. . ."*
- *"I think email is a good way to communicate for. . ."*
- *"A meeting should never be. . ."*
- *"Three words that describe how I expect to be treated at work are. . ."*

TEAM CHARTERS

Team charters serve to involve and align everyone in dialogue about what success would look like if the team worked optimally (Exhibit 4.1). From there, the group explores how the

EXHIBIT 4.1: TEAM CHARTER

Team Name: Date:	Team Members:	What Does Success of Our Team Working Together Look Like? Optional: Vision/Mission:	
Team Member Strengths	**Roles and Responsibilities**	**Trust**	**Decision-Making**
■ What strengths does each member bring to this team? ■ How can those strengths contribute to team success? ■ How can we structure our work to ensure everyone can play to their strengths?	■ What are each individual's roles and responsibilities on this team? ■ Is there any overlap in roles/responsibilities? If so, do we need to clarify or make changes? ■ How will each of the roles interact with each other?	■ How will we build trust?	■ How will decisions be made on this team? ■ Who will make decisions, and who will provide input? ■ When there is disagreement about a decision, do we agree that the lead makes the final call?
Accountability	**Conflict**	**Other Team Norms**	
■ How will we hold each other accountable? ■ Examples: deadlines, clear assignments, reiterate action items at meetings, standups	■ How will we handle conflict?	■ What other norms/expected behaviors do we want to establish as a team?	

group will function, first identifying individual strengths of each member and clarifying roles and responsibilities, and then discussing how the team will build trust, make decisions, hold one another accountable, and manage conflict. Such charters can be established for an overarching team (e.g., nurses working on an inpatient unit) or for smaller teams committed to working on a particular time-limited goal (e.g., a safety and quality committee).

THE FAILURE BOW

Mistakes or failures are inevitable in life. Despite this, failure often results in a sense of shame that can make acknowledging the mistake hard. This, in turn, reduces our ability to learn from it and move forward. The failure bow is an important ritual to encourage public acknowledgment of failure followed by validation and support from the rest of the team. In so doing, it allows everyone to remain in the present moment and move forward. To establish this ritual, invite your team to assume an exaggerated posture of someone who has made an error, and ask them to look at one another. Are they inspired by what they see? When a trapezist falls from the air into a safety net, they immediately roll out and take a large sweeping circus bow. In response, the audience thunders its applause, and the trapezist climbs right back up to go again. Imagine what the entertainment value would be if trapezist artists instead slunk off in shame? Finally, ask everyone to practice taking a dramatic circus bow with arms held straight up in the air and saying, "I failed." Allow them to practice several times until people become comfortable with the grand gestures. Finally, offer a professional bow as an alternative and demonstrate by rolling shoulders back, lifting hands up from the elbows, and saying, "Thank you." Explore how it felt to take a failure bow and how it might benefit you and your team. Invite team members to take a professional failure bow whenever they make an error as a way of normalizing mistakes and promoting acceptance and moving forward.

SUMMARY

Several rituals that foster a sense of belonging and community have been offered. To the uninitiated, such rituals can feel awkward and uncomfortable. Some may even question the value of spending time practicing circus bows and standing in quadrants representing their favorite superpower. At these times, it can be helpful to trust the process. Acknowledge any discomfort and allow those who are disengaged to experience not only the rituals but also the benefits that occur over time.

Rituals serve many functions in establishing and maintaining a community. One function is identifying commonalities among a group. Affinity bias is the human tendency to feel more connected to, and interact more with, others who are similar to us. For instance, during a check-in, if someone shares the birth of a baby, other parents in the room may resonate with the feelings of joy and exhaustion often associated with welcoming a new baby. Identifying others who prefer summer or the beach during warm-ups can lead to further conversation and bonding over their love of summer. Not only do these moments increase job satisfaction and engagement, but they also create regular opportunities to develop cohesion, shown to drive effectiveness and interprofessional collaboration (Appelbaum et al., 2020).

A second function is one of normalizing and appreciating differences in others. Diversity has been associated with effective team processes and outcomes (Lemieux-Charles & McGuire, 2006). While inclusive hiring practices can expand the diversity of a team, they cannot ensure that such differences will be valued and respected. However, by providing a safe, supportive space to share and learn about one another and varying points of view, rituals can create space for leaders to model curiosity and validation of different worldviews. This is essential for minimizing groupthink and improving team performance and innovation.

Rituals function in other ways to optimize performance, such as helping to establish and reinforce norms, expectations, and team culture. For example, use of a team charter outlines a team's mission and values while also clarifying roles and responsibilities. Introducing the failure bow and encouraging its use sends the message that mistakes are to be expected, accepted, and acknowledged as an opportunity to learn.

Moreover, rituals provide regular boosters of resiliency and burnout prevention that are much needed in times of stress (Box 4.3). When challenges or adversities arise, the structure and regularity of rituals that provide a spirit of fun and/or foster cohesion and connectedness serve as the oxygen mask donned by the team prior to assisting others. For example, Montross-Thomas et al. (2016) found that hospice workers who engage in rituals to cope with the death of their patients, such as attending memorials, reported significantly higher levels of compassion and lower levels of burnout compared to counterparts who did not engage in such rituals.

BOX 4.3: RELATIONAL FUNCTIONS OF RITUALS

- Identify commonalities among a group.
- Normalize and appreciate differences in others.
- Help establish and reinforce norms, expectations, and team culture.
- Provide regular boosters of resiliency and burnout prevention.

NURTURING BEHAVIORS

The future of healthcare is dependent on its ability to transform how it is delivered. Healthcare must be accessible and affordable to all, predicated on science, and delivered by an ensemble of educated, skilled, and empathic individuals. For this to occur, all caregivers—nurses, physicians, social workers, pharmacists, aides, and housekeepers, to mention just a few—will need to embrace radical thinking.

Beverly Malone, former president of the American Nurses Association (ANA) and current chief executive officer (CEO) of the National League for Nursing, in her assessment of the State of the World Nursing Report, challenged governments, academic institutions, healthcare organizations, and public and private agencies to collaborate in designing an "equitable and sustainable access to outstanding, inclusive, culturally sensitive universal healthcare" (Malone, 2021, p. 6). Nurse leaders will need to be the translators and integrators of these changes across the healthcare continuum. Forming and sustaining relationships will be central to the ability to carry out this work.

Nurturing behaviors which challenge thinking, encourage curiosity, and promote the social role and privilege of the nurse as healer, teacher, and advocate are dependent upon meaningful relationships with others. Nurse leaders' ability to foster a sense of belonging has been the genesis for this chapter. There is an array of nurturing behaviors nurse leaders can employ with staff to create an inclusive and affirming work environment. Several are offered for special consideration:

- **Be present:** Being physically and emotionally attentive. Being present conveys a sense of value and respect, that every person is worthy of unadulterated attention. Presence entails more "being" than "doing." It necessitates leaders disengaging from technology while participating in meetings and conversing with staff. Being fully present sends the message that "You are important to me. Your worry is worthy of my full attention. Thank you for bringing your concern to my attention." Being present also means being visible so that staff can engage and dialogue with their leaders in person.

- **Listen:** Thoughtful attention is being given to the words being used. Listening is an underrated skill that requires taking in as much information as possible and filtering the essential facts, feelings, and intention with which information is shared. Effective listeners create an atmosphere of unhurried conversations. Skilled listeners allow for silence and interject only to seek more information. "I'd like to hear more about that if you are willing to share. Tell me more?"

- **Express empathy:** Empathy is a gift of generosity. It is the ability to recognize and relate to another. It is one of the most coveted human qualities that attenuates suffering. Empathy fosters connections. "It sounds like you are having a tough time." "I hear worry in your voice." "You must feel so proud of yourself!"

- **Apologize:** Heartfelt apologies help to acknowledge humiliation and suffering. Offering an apology is not a sign of weakness but of strength. It signifies that the relationship is important and worthy of mending. "I am sorry that I embarrassed you. It was insensitive and I apologize." "I kept you waiting. I am sorry. I know that your time is valuable, and I appreciate it." "I was rude to you the other day and I diminished you as a person. For that I am deeply sorry."

- **Forgive:** Forgiveness is an act of kindness and compassion. It is about offering mercy to individuals who have disappointed or hurt us or have caused harm to another. Forgiveness does not require that we minimize or overlook the significance of the action. Leader behavior has a tremendous impact on organizational culture. Leaders who model forgiveness demonstrate authenticity, humility, and wisdom, and promote healthy relationships.

- **Break bread together:** The phrase "break bread together" means to share a meaningful connection with another person. Food is central to celebrations. Each culture uses food to honor events: birth or adoption of a child, birthdays and anniversaries, graduations, marriage, or to recognize transitions, promotions, relocation, retirement, and funerals. Sharing a meal or a snack provides an opportunity for relationship building. Team members value the opportunity to connect and build deeper relationships. Dedicating time to gather is a way of conveying respect and appreciation, as well as acknowledging success.

- **Express gratitude:** There are a variety of ways that gratitude can be conveyed. It can be as simple as saying "thank you" to another person, either publicly or in private. An individual can be recognized at a department meeting or at the beginning of the shift huddle. A "gratitude wall" can be created, so that team members can be acknowledged publicly by their colleagues. A handwritten note acknowledging the action and placed in the mail shows a deeper investment in effort as it requires more time than texting appreciation or sending an email. The importance of expressing gratitude cannot be overstated. Expressing gratitude authentically and regularly to members of your team will improve well-being, create a high-performing team, and help your team flourish.

- **Give gifts:** Giving gifts is a way to contribute to a flourishing work environment. It is another way to recognize or celebrate contributions. Gifts do not need to be elaborate or require an expense report. Gifts can be a collection of affirmations from colleagues printed in different fonts and placed in a decorated brown lunch bag with the title "Nourishment for the Soul." Playlists of favorite songs from team members can be sent to a new colleague before beginning work. A favorite poem can be printed, rolled into a scroll, wrapped in a ribbon, and placed at every seat before a meeting. Noting graduations or work anniversaries with a few packages of seeds to acknowledge "growth" can be a novel way to recognize accomplishments. Leaders find a way to celebrate everyone because creating a sense of community ensures that no one is made to feel left out.

◎ WHAT EVERY CHIEF EXECUTIVE OFFICER NEEDS TO KNOW

Nurses are well positioned to assume leadership of healthcare organizations because of their ability to view other people as a whole. Nurses are educated to care for others, work with others, and act on behalf of others. A relationship-centered orientation provides the moral compass for which all decisions are based. This requires asking for and honoring the contributions of others.

CASE SCENARIO

HONORING THE WORK OF OTHERS

SITUATION

MB is in the midst of their fourth day as CEO of a specialty hospital. MB is new to the organization, the position, and the city. Throughout their career, MB has held a myriad of progressive leadership positions including nurse manager, clinical director, assistant director of nursing, senior vice president, and chief operating officer (COO).

MB is invited into one of their first meetings as CEO with physician and administrative leaders to discuss the recommendation to cancel all pediatric surgeries for the next day due to both physician and nurse staffing issues. The decision to cancel pediatric surgeries had always resided with the staff of the Pediatric Intensive Care Unit (PICU) in this organization who had issued the decision earlier in the day.

MB began exploring the issue by asking the team to review the surgery schedule for the next day. MB inquired about each patient on the schedule and asked members of the team to share the patient's medical and personal history. The team was able to speak about each patient with great clarity and knowledge. Of significance was the patient story of a 12-year-old who was to undergo their fourth surgery for a brain tumor. The child and their parents lived 200 miles away. MB placed a star by the child's name on the notes they were taking.

MB then began to query the group about the decision-making process that led to the cancellation of surgeries. MB asked the group to reflect on what the work was like when the resources were available. MB asked them to envision a process which maintained patient safety and quality of care. MB asked them to imagine their 12-year-old patient and the child's parents traveling 200 miles in anticipation of another surgery. What would be the myriad of emotions they would experience learning that the surgery had been cancelled? MB asked them to generate several alternatives to cancelling the surgeries for the next day. MB requested that these recommendations be implemented immediately and that the surgeries be performed as scheduled. Lastly, MB asked that the group reconvene to explore contingency plans to prevent this issue from reoccurring and that they meet as a group by the end of the month to reformat the standard operating procedure.

DISCUSSION QUESTIONS

1. What were the relational-based approaches that MB used to explore the ramifications of cancelling surgeries?
2. How did MB, being new to the organization, introduce their approach to problem resolution?
3. What are your thoughts on how MB was received by their new executive team?

WHAT EVERY NURSE EXECUTIVE NEEDS TO KNOW

The chief nurse executive (CNE) promotes the contributions of nurses and the impact they have on patient outcomes. They establish the vision for all nursing staff. They are central to the creation of safe work environments and promoting interprofessional collaboration. CNEs also play an integral role in strategic decision-making and the creation or adoption of equitable healthcare policies.

CASE SCENARIO

ALIGNING VALUES FOR A SHARED PURPOSE

SITUATION

TR is the CNE of a large healthcare system in the Southwest. Prior to their selection as CNE, TR held every nursing position available in the organization: patient care nursing assistant, clinical nurse, charge nurse, assistant nurse manager, clinical coordinator, nurse manager, and clinical director. TR was chosen for the CNE position by the CEO and chief medical officer (CMO), both of whom were physicians. TR was recognized for their ability to bring disparate groups of people together to achieve important outcomes, to celebrate individuals at all levels of the organization, and to be an astute thinker who places the patient at the center of every decision.

The previous 18 months had been chaotic for the organization as it had acquired several hospitals. The executive leadership team was struggling with merging the new hospitals, welcoming thousands of new caregivers, and integrating all service lines to become one healthcare system. The previous CNE had been unsuccessful in fostering a sense of unity and belonging among the nursing staff, honoring the past traditions of the newly acquired hospitals, and validating the nurses' worries, fears, and anxieties that their contributions would become diminished and unrecognized.

APPROACH

Prior to accepting the CNE position, TR sought out unwavering support and commitment from the CEO and CMO, acknowledging that TR would make mistakes along the way. TR wanted to be assured that they could seek the CEO's and CMO's counsel and advice yet be the individual responsible for making the ultimate decisions affecting nursing practice for the healthcare system. Their assurances were freely given, and TR's authority was conveyed to all key stakeholders in the organization.

OUTCOME

TR committed themself to having a visible presence at each hospital. Working with nursing clinical leaders throughout the healthcare system, TR began to uncover similarities in workflow processes, inconsistencies in hospital policies and procedures, and inequitable allocation of resources. Resolute with the goal of integrating all the hospital nursing departments, TR began by reassuring the CNOs of TR's commitment to their success. TR reduced turnover in the CNO position, dedicated meeting time to relationship-building activities, and celebrated personal and professional successes among their executive leadership team.

The integration of nursing as one entity was not without its missteps. However, 10 years later, critical processes have been adopted in welcoming new hospitals into the healthcare system and TR remains the CNE.

DISCUSSION QUESTIONS

1. What was inherent in TR's success as the CNE?
2. What activities did TR use to solicit support in integrating the nursing department?

◘ WHAT EVERY NURSE MANAGER NEEDS TO KNOW

Nurse managers create the environment that allows nurses to flourish. They must establish expectations and hold colleagues accountable while, at the same time, acknowledging the competing demands of the clinical nurse. The nurse manager is integral to the acceptance of change, nurse engagement, and fostering a sense of community.

◆ CASE SCENARIO

NURTURING THE CAREER ASPIRATIONS OF COLLEAGUES

SITUATION

JH has been the nurse manager of a 36-bed mixed neuroscience unit for 3 years. Prior to their promotion, JH had been an associate nurse manager for 2 years and a clinical nurse for 17 years, working 2 years as a travel nurse. JH felt extremely prepared to assume the role of nurse manager as the former nurse manager had announced their retirement 3 months prior to their departure and worked with JH to ensure a seamless transition.

The unit is highly regarded for its specialized evidence-based practice nursing care. The patient population is comprised of people with a variety of brain and spinal cord diseases and/or injuries. Nurses on the unit care for a myriad of neurosurgical patients as well as general neurology conditions. The unit is a designated comprehensive stroke center specializing in the care of people who have experienced a complex stroke. The unit also has nine hard-wired rooms to perform epilepsy monitoring to care for people with unrelenting seizures. The unit participates in a post-baccalaureate nurse residency program in which two new clinical nurses, on average, are hired per year to fill vacancies.

Prior to the COVID-19 pandemic that began overwhelming hospitals across the globe in March of 2020, turnover was low on the unit. JH was considered an exemplary manager because of their visible presence on the unit, their ability to create an environment where nurses felt empowered, and their intentionality to learn about their staff's real selves. JH enjoyed leading a unit comprised of clinical experts who had been providing care on the unit, many as long as 10 years. JH promoted membership in professional organizations and obtaining specialty certification. Several of JH's senior staff nurses had been the recipients of national nursing awards. Most held the certification of certified neuroscience registered nurse (CNRN), awarded by the American Association of Neuroscience Nurses. The nurses embodied the concept of teamwork. The unit was a model for collaboration, inclusion, and innovation.

The COVID pandemic took its toll on the nursing staff. The unit quickly converted to a "COVID unit" because all non-emergent neurosurgery cases were cancelled. After several months of caring for people with COVID, some members of the nursing staff experienced moral distress and compassion fatigue. Several decided that it was time to walk away from nursing and took early retirement, while others left to join the workforce as travel nurses. For the first time in their nurse manager role, JH was confronted with many vacancies. In the span of 3 months, JH hired nine new graduate nurses.

APPROACH

JH immersed themself in getting to know their new staff. They worked tirelessly at rebuilding a "community of caregivers." JH held virtual meetings on their off time with groups of new staff when they were not working and compensated them for their time. JH wanted to learn more about what brought each of them into nursing, their families, their hobbies and outside interests, and what they enjoyed about being a nurse. JH learned about their concerns and worries as well as their aspirations.

OUTCOME

JH became aware that the Neuro Intensive Care Unit (ICU) would be offering an additional orientation and two of JH's staff, who had just completed their 1-year anniversary on the unit, had expressed interest in working in the Neuro ICU. Knowing that these two nurses did not meet the application criteria for clinical experience but aspired for critical care experience, JH met with the nurse manager of the Neuro ICU to advocate for them. An exception was made, and the two nurses were accepted into the Neuro ICU. Their departure was bittersweet for JH and the rest of the staff as these two young staff members had thrived on the unit and demonstrated great leadership potential. Although the transfer required recruiting additional staff, one of JH's leadership principles is that "people should be where they want to be," and JH saw it as their responsibility to facilitate the transfer.

DISCUSSION QUESTIONS

1. Considering strategies on optimizing a sense of inclusion, what practices influenced JH's leadership decisions?
2. How was JH able to reconcile their staffing issues with the professional growth and development of the two nurses?

◻ WHAT EVERY PRESIDENT OF A PROFESSIONAL ORGANIZATION NEEDS TO KNOW

Presidents of professional organizations advocate for one or more disciplines. This position draws heavily on the ability to connect with others from a multitude of different interests and practice environments. Inherent in this role must be the ability to energize, inspire, and capture the imagination of others.

⬡ CASE SCENARIO

PROMOTING PROFESSIONAL CITIZENSHIP

SITUATION

GR is the president of a national nursing organization that relies heavily on volunteer participation. GR's entry into the leadership world began when they joined their professional organization. GR was encouraged to become more active in the organization by a colleague and after 3 years of active membership ran for a position on the board. GR's contributions were so exceptional that after 2 years GR was selected as president elect of the organization.

GR brought exuberance, optimism, and a strong financial background to the helm. The organization had experienced some recent turmoil, with a significant number of members not renewing their membership. GR set out to reverse this trend.

APPROACH

GR began by soliciting the vision for the organization from each board member. After agreeing on a shared vision for the next year, GR began to energize the committees by reassigning responsibilities and fostering autonomy. GR collaborated on reorganizing the committee leadership structure so that each committee was led by two co-chairs rather than one individual, allowing for smooth transitions of authority. GR instituted quarterly calls with each of the committees so that committee members could raise concerns, solicit advice, and build connections and speak directly with the president of the organization. GR used every opportunity to communicate their vision for the organization and reiterate the value of membership. The president's message, published bimonthly in the organization's professional journal, described opportunities in which members could become more engaged, capture their financial contributions, and mentor others. GR promoted the concept of "professional citizenship" and the impact the organization had on healthcare reform initiatives.

OUTCOME

By the end of their tenure as president, GR had reawakened the membership. Student membership in the organization had increased by 15%, new membership was up 8%, and renewed membership of those who had their membership lapse was 23%. Applications to serve on committees had tripled. Attendance at the national meeting during GR's presidency had exceeded previous attendance records by 39%. In GR's final act as president, each board member and committee co-chair received a handwritten note of gratitude highlighting their unique contribution to the organization.

DISCUSSION QUESTIONS

1. What did GR do to awaken the membership of the organization?
2. What are the benefits of cultivating a sense of "professional citizenship" among nurses?

KEY POINTS

- A sense of belonging is essential to a person's personal and professional sense of well-being.

- Words matter. The use of person-centered, strength-based, empathic language conveys value and respect while promoting inclusion.

- Rituals are an efficient and effective way to foster a sense of belonging and community. They allow for sharing of values, perspectives, and personal histories.

- There is an array of nurturing behaviors nurse leaders can employ with staff to create an inclusive and affirming work environment.

SUMMARY

Investing in relationship building will require a time commitment. Effective leaders know their staff, not just their names or where they went to school. They know about their colleagues' families, outside interests, preferences, strengths, and aspirations. Impactful leaders care about the people they lead and foster a sense of belonging and community using rituals, strength-based language, and appreciative practices. When people feel that they belong and are cared for, they are more collaborative, resilient, and productive.

The practice of ubuntu provides the foundation for which all nurturing and affirming behaviors emanate. The behaviors espoused in this chapter will take practice and fine tuning. Take delight in the success of others and dedicate your leadership practices to promoting the well-being of others while preserving your own. The desired outcome of inclusive, egalitarian, and respectful relationships is that each person in the caregiving community led by you will flourish and believe that they are making a difference in the lives of their patients, their colleagues and society as a whole.

END-OF-CHAPTER RESOURCES

◆ DISCUSSION QUESTIONS

1. How does a "sense of belonging" contribute to flourishing relationships?
2. What is the impact of person-centered, strength-based empathic language on relationships?
3. What rituals foster communities of caregivers?
4. What behaviors nurture relationships?

◆ ADDITIONAL RESOURCES

TED TALKS

- Perel, E. (2021, March). *The routines, rituals, and boundaries we need in stressful times* [Video]. TEDSalon: DWEN. https://www.ted.com/talks/esther_perel_the_routines_rituals_and_boundaries_we_need_in_stressful_times#t-75562
- Clarke, C. (2019, August). *The essential power of belonging* [Video]. TEDxBeacon Street. https://www.ted.com/talks/caroline_clarke_the_essential_power_of_belonging
- Levy, J. (2019, November 8). *Driving change: The power of ubuntu* [Video]. TEDx. https://www.ted.com/talks/jordan_levy_driving_change_the_power_of_ubuntu

- Richards, S. (2019, October 5). *Ubuntu: The one word to change how you love, live, and learn* [Video]. TEDx, South Lake Tahoe. https://www.ted.com/talks/shola_richards _ubuntu_the_one_word_to_change_how_you_work_live_and_lead
- Hirsch, J. (2019, August 25). *The joy in getting feedback* [Video]. TEDx, Tarrytown. https://www.ted.com/talks/joe_hirsch_the_joy_of_getting_feedback
- TEDx Talks. (2019, Setember 20). *The ART of relational leadership | Rowan Kevin van Dyk | TEDxSwakopmund* [Video]. YouTube. https://www.youtube.com/ watch?v=MjqkqNUHS0g
- TEDx Talks. (2018, April 22). *The one thing all great teachers do | Nick Fuhrman | TEDx-UGA* [Video]. YouTube. https://www.youtube.com/watch?v=WwTpfVQgkU0
- TEDx Talks. (2016, January 25). *Lessons from nursing to the world | Kathleen Bartholomew | TEDxSanJuanIsland* [Video]. YouTube. https://www.youtube.com/ watch?v=Qh4HW3yx00w
- Waldinger, R. (2015, November 15). *What makes a good life? Lessons from the longest study on happiness* [Video]. TED. https://www.ted.com/talks/robert_waldinger_what _makes_a_good_life_lessons_from_the_longest_study_on_happiness?language=en
- TEDx Talks. (2016, October 7). *The simple cure for loneliness | Baya Voice | TEDxSaltLake-City* [Video]. YouTube. https://www.youtube.com/watch?v=KSXh1YfNyVA&t=797s
- McGonigal, K. (2013, June). *How to make stress your friend* [Video]. TEDGlobal. https:// www.ted.com/talks/kelly_mcgonigal_how_to_make_stress_your_friend
- Brown, B. (2010, June). *The power of vulnerability* [Video]. TEDx Houston. https://www .ted.com/talks/brene_brown_the_power_of_vulnerability
- Adichie, C. (2009, July). *The danger of a single story* [Video]. TED. https://www.ted.com/ talks/chimamanda_ngozi_adichie_the_danger_of_a_single_story?language=en

BLOGS

- O'Neil, J. F. (2019, February 28). Rembering Ira Progoff. Who? Memories of a Time. https:// memoriesofatime.blog/2019/02/28/remembering-ira-progoff-who
- Andrews Rob. (2020, February 12). Total performance leadership blog post #3: Engagement-stakeholders. *Allen Austin.* https://allenaustin.com/ building-peak-performance-cultures-part-three-stakeholder-engagement

PODCASTS

- Brown, B. (Host). (2020, January). Introducing: Unlocking Us [Audio podcast episode]. In *Unlocking Us.* https://brenebrown.com/podcast/introducing-unlocking-us
- Brown, B. (Host). (2020–present). *Dare to lead with Brene Brown* [Audio podcast]. https://brenebrown.com/dtl-podcast
- Grant A. (Host). (2018–present). *Work life with Adam Grant* [Audio podcast]. TED. https://www.adamgrant.net/podcast
- Leonard, K. (Host). (2016–present). *Getting to yes, and* [Audio podcast]. Second City Works. https://www.secondcityworks.com/podcast
- Recinos, C. (Host). (2020–present). Nurse leader network with Chris Recinos [Audio podcast]. https://www.listennotes.com/podcasts/nurse-leader-network-chris-recinos
- Meier, L. (Host). (2021, February 22). *Revisioning the image of nursing* [Audio podcast episode]. In *Once a Nurse, Always a Nurse: Exploring the World of Nursing with Leanne Meier, BSN, RN.* VoiceAmerica. https://www.voiceamerica.com/episode/128707/ revisioning-the-image-of-nursing

YOUTUBE

- Grigoriadic, J. (2011, May 28). *Power of words* [Video]. YouTube. https://www.youtube.com/watch?v=Lw9bct2n04I
- American Psychiatric Nurses Association. (2017, December 19). *A conversation with Hildegard Peplau* [Video]. YouTube. https://www.youtube.com/watch?v=Fdx5Dw-dkBg
- Punk Rock HR with Laurie Ruettimann. (2018, December 17). *The Feedback Fix with Joe Hirsch* [Video]. YouTube. https://www.youtube.com/watch?v=dC9BhS62aMg

WEBSITES

- *Warm-Ups*: http://www.impactbydesigninc.org/our-best-warmup-activities-for-virtual-meetings
- *Forgiveness Quiz*: https://greatergood.berkeley.edu/quizzes/take_quiz/forgiveness
- *Organizational Gratitude Survey*: https://greatergood.berkeley.edu/quizzes/take_quiz/grateful_organizations

A robust set of instructor resources designed to supplement this text is located at http://connect.springerpub.com/content/book/978-0-8261-7795-7. Qualifying instructors may request access by emailing textbook@springerpub.com.

REFERENCES

Agrawal, R. (2018). *Belonging*. Workman Publishing.

American Nurses Association. (n.d.). *Nurses in the workforce*. https://www.nursingworld.org/practice-policy/workforce

Appelbaum, N. P., Lockeman, K. S., Orr, S., Huff, T. A., Hogan, C. J., Queen, B. A., & Dow, A. W. (2020). Perceived influence of power distance, psychological safety, and team cohesion on team effectiveness. *Journal of Interprofessional Care, 34*(1), 20–26. https://doi.org/10.1080/13561820.2019.1633290

Clarke, C. (2019). The essential power of belonging [Video]. *TEDxBeaconStreetSalon*. https://www.ted.com/talks/caroline_clarke_the_essential_power_of_belonging

Crocker, A. F., & Smith, S. (2019). Person-first language: Are we practicing what we preach? *Journal of Multidisciplinary Healthcare, 12*, 125–129. https://doi.org/10.2147.JMDH.5140067

Cross, R., Dillion, K., & Greenberg, D. (2021). *The secret to building resilience*. https://hbr.org/2021/01/the-secret-to-building-resilience

Dickinson, J. K., Guzman, S. S., Maryniuk, M.-D., O'Brien, C. A., Kadohiro, J. K., Jackson, R. A., D'Hondt, N., Montgomery, B., Close, K. L., & Funnell, M. M. (2017). The use of language in diabetes care and education. *Diabetes Care, 40*(12), 1790–1799. https://doi.org/10.2337/dci 17-0041

Dziados, V. (2019). *Top 10 soft skills for nurses*. https://www.nursingcenter.com/ncblog/march-2019/top-10-soft-skills-for-nurses

Fulton, J. (2019). Professional citizenship. *Clinical Nurse Specialist, 33*(4), 153–154. https://doi.org/10.1097/NUR.0000000000000463

Goldsmith, M. (2012). *Feedforward*. Round Table Companies.

Granello, D. H., & Gibbs, T. A. (2016). The power of language and labels: "The mentally ill" versus "people with mental illness." *Journal of Counseling and Development, 94*(1), 31–40. https://doi.org/10.1002/cad.12059

Guillaumie, L., Boiral, O., & Champagne, J. (2017). A mixed-methods systematic review of the effects of mindfulness on nurses. *Journal of Advanced Nursing, 73*(5), 1017–1034. https://doi.org/10.1111/jan.13176

Gwande, A. (2010). *Checklist manifesto: How to get things right*. Holt.

Hagerty, B. M., Williams, R. A., Coyne, J. C., & Early, M. R. (1996). Sense of belonging and indicators of social and psychological functioning. *Archives of Psychiatric Nursing, 10*(4), 235–244. https://doi.org/10.1016/s0883-9417(96)80029-x

Hirsch, J. (2017). *The feedback fix: Dump the past, embrace the future and lead the way to change*. Rowman & Littlefield.

Jacob, K., Unerman, S., & Edwards, M. (2020). *Belonging*. Bloomsbury.

Kapitan, A. (2017). *On person first language: It's time to actually put the person first*. https://radicalcopyeditor.com/2017/07/03/person-centered-language

Koloroutis, M. (2020). Relational proficiency: What it is and why it matters. *Nursing Management, 5*(5), 52–54. https://doi.org/10.1097/01.NUMA.0000659444.30746.3e

Kroning, M. (2015, February 4). Fostering soft skills is a must for nurse leaders. *American Nurse, 10*(2). https://www.myamericannurse.com/fostering-soft-skills-must-nurse-leaders

Lazare, A. (2004). *On apology*. Oxford Press.

Lemieux-Charles, L., & McGuire, W. (2006, June). What do we know about health care team effectiveness? A review of the literature. *Medical Care Research and Review, 63*(3), 263–300. https://doi.org/10.1177/1077558706287003

Louis, M. (2017). Integrating Millennials into the workplace. *Harnessing the power of a multigenerational work force*. Executive Summary SHRM Foundation. https://www.shrm.org/foundation/ourwork/initiatives/the-aging-workforce

Lutz, D. W. (2009). African *Ubuntu* philosophy and global management. *Journal of Business Ethics, 84*, Article 313 (2009). https://doi.org/10.1007/s10551-009-0204-z

Malone, B. (2021). A perspective on the state of the world's nursing report. *Nursing Administration Quarterly, 45*(1), 6–12. https://doi.org/10.1097/NAQ.0000000000000443

Manion, J., & Bartholomew, K. (2004). Community in the workplace. *Journal of Nursing Management, 34*(1), 46–53. https://doi.org/10.10.1097/00005110-200401000-00010

Mann, A. (2018). *Why we need best friends at work*. https://www.gallup.com/workplace/236213/why-need-best-friends-work.aspx

Martin, A. D. (2020). The SHAPE framework: Empowering millennials to lead the future of healthcare. *Nursing Administration Quarterly, 44*(2), 166–178. https://doi.org/10.1097/NAQ.0000000000000410

Maslow, A. H. (1943). A theory of human motivation. *Psychology Review, 50*(4), 370–396. https://doi.org/10.1037/h0054346

McMaster, C. (2014). Elements of inclusion: Findings from the field. *Kairaranga, 15*, 42–49. https://files.eric.ed.gov/fulltext/EJ1040134.pdf

Modic, M. B. (2016a). Steppingstones: Reflecting on your professional career. *Journal for Nurses in Professional Development, 32*(3), 163–165. https://doi.org/10.1097/NND.0000000000000259

Modic, M. B. (2016b). Warm-up exercises are not only for running. *Journal for Nurses in Professional Development, 32*(4), 221–222. https://doi.org/10.1097/NND.0000000000000276

Montross-Thomas, L. P., Scheiber, C., Meier, E. A., & Irwin, S. A. (2016). Personally meaningful rituals: A way to increase compassion and decrease burnout among hospice staff and volunteers. *Journal of Palliative Medicine, 19*(10), 1043–1050. https://doi.org/10.1089/jpm.2015.0294

Murthy, V. (2020). *Together*. Harper Collins.

National Academy of Medicine. (2021). *The future of nursing 2020–2030: Charting a path to achieve health equity*. National Academies Press. https://doi.org/10.17226/25982

Nolte, A., & Downing, C. (2019). Ubuntu—The essence of caring and being: A concept analysis. *Holistic Nursing Practice, 33*(1), 9–11. https://doi.org/10.1097/HNP0000000000000030

Nurse Organization. (n.d.). *List of professional nursing organizations*. https://nurse.org/orgs.shtml

Peplau, H. E. (1952). *Interpersonal relations in nursing: Offering a conceptual frame of reference for psychodynamic nursing*. G.P. Putnam's Sons.

Peplau, H. E. (1991). *Interpersonal relations on nursing: A conceptual framework for psychodynamic for nursing*. Springer Publishing Company.

Peplau, H. E. (1994). Quality of life: An interpersonal perspective. *Nursing Science Quarterly, 7*(1), 10–15. https://doi.org/10.1177/089431849400700107

Smith, P. (2012). *Lead with a story*. Amacom.

Stichler, J. F. (2013). Healthy work environments for the ageing nursing workforce. *Journal of Nursing Management, 21*(7), 956–963. https://doi.org/10.1111/jonm.12174

Vogl, C. H. (2016). *The art of community*. Berett-Koehler Publishers.

Windover, A., Boissy, A., Rice, T., Gilligan, T., Velez, V. J., & Merlino, J. (2014). The REDE model of healthcare communication: Optimizing relationship as a therapeutic agent. *Journal of Patient Experience, 1*(1), 8–13. https://doi.org/10.1177/237437431400100103

Waldinger, R. (2015). What makes a good life? Lessons from the longest study on happiness [Video]. *TedxBeaconStreetSalon.* https://www.ted.com/talks/robert_waldinger_what_makes_a_good_life_lessons_from_the_longest_study_on_happiness

CHAPTER | 5

EMOTIONAL INTELLIGENCE

Mary T. Quinn Griffin and Lauraine Spano-Szekely

"Great leaders move us. They ignite our passion and inspire the best in us. When we try to explain why they are so effective, we speak of strategy, vision, or powerful ideas. But the reality is much more primal: Great leadership works through the emotions."

Goleman et al. (2013, p. 3)

LEARNING OBJECTIVES

- Differentiate between the emotional intelligence (EI) models presented.
- Analyze the benefits of EI.
- Design EI programs for effective nurse leaders and teams using the EI domains and competencies.
- Formulate strategies to enhance EI.

INTRODUCTION

Emotional intelligence (EI) is a concept that was developed in the 1990s. Its definition has changed and adapted over time. Many EI models have evolved and today there are four major models. Each model has its own definition for EI, but each has similar components. The main EI components are self-awareness, self-management, social awareness, and relational management (Boyatzis & McKee, 2005). EI skills or competencies have been developed for each of these components. EI competencies are learned and continue to develop over time.

EI has been identified as a key concept for frontline professional caregivers, particularly leaders. It is a critical component for successful effective nurse leaders, particularly using the five practices of exemplary leadership: modeling the way, challenging the process, inspiring a shared vision, enabling others to act, and encouraging the heart (Posner & Kouzes, 2011). EI is highly valued in the workplace as it is associated with transformational leadership and high performance. Emotionally intelligent nurse leaders have the skills to recognize, understand, and manage their own emotions and those of others. These skills enable nurse leaders to have an optimistic, open, transparent, transformational leadership style. These visionary leaders initiate and lead change in organizations while building teams and nurturing collaboration and cooperation. Emotionally intelligent nurse leaders mentor and coach their staff, leading to increased staff satisfaction and retention. EI is a salient leadership skill and its benefits to nurse leaders in their personal and professional lives are great. Through EI they are adaptable, inspirational, influential, high performing, transformational nurse leaders.

DEFINITIONS AND MODELS OF EMOTIONAL INTELLIGENCE

The definition of EI has evolved over time. The term EI is defined differently depending on the EI model. There are three major models of EI: the Mayer and Salovey's EI model, the Bar-On model of EI, and the Goleman–Boyatzis model of EI. The definition of EI and the frameworks for each of these three models are described in this section.

MAYER AND SALOVEY'S MODEL OF EMOTIONAL INTELLIGENCE

Salovey and Mayer (1990) defined EI as "the ability to monitor one's own and other's feelings and emotions, to discriminate among them and use this information to guide one's thinking and actions" (p. 189). In their conceptualization, EI had three components "appraisal and expression of emotion, regulation of emotion, and utilization of emotion" (p. 190). The ability of an individual to appraise and express emotion accurately allows the individual to perceive and respond to their emotions more quickly. Therefore, they can express their emotions more accurately to others. EI individuals can regulate emotions in themselves and others. Regulation of emotions in oneself involves reflective practice. Also, individuals have the ability to regulate the emotions of others through their own behavior. Salovey and Mayer (1990) believed that individuals can develop skills to become emotionally intelligent. In 1997, Mayer and Salovey developed the four branch EI ability model, accepted as the first EI model. The branches of the model represent the four problem-solving areas required for emotional reasoning (Mayer & Salovey, 1997). The four branches are: (1) perceiving emotions, (2) facilitating thought using emotion, (3) understanding emotions, and (4) managing emotions (Mayer & Salovey, 1997). These four branches are ordered, with branches 1 and 2—perceiving and facilitating—requiring lower order cognitive processes than branches 3 and 4—understanding and managing emotions. Within each branch there is a set of problem-solving skills going from simple to more complex. Scholars have questioned the ordering of the four. Zeidner et al. (2003) propose that branch abilities—for example, perceiving and facilitating—are not necessarily developed in the sequence of the ability model but may be developed together. Over the years, researchers using factor analysis have challenged the four-branch model. One criticism leveled at the authors is that the model is a three-factor model rather than having four factors (Fiori et al., 2014). Branch 2 does not appear to be a distinct factor (Fiori & Vesely-Maillefer, 2018). In 2016, Mayer and Salovey responded to these observations and reviewed and updated the model (Mayer et al., 2016). They added more problem-solving skills within each of the branches. They agree that branch 2 does not appear to have its own factor. However, they suggest this could be due to poor test construction or that individuals solve branch 2 problems with abilities in the other branches (Mayer et al., 2016). They decided to keep branch 2 in the model but that the cognitive skills involved in branch 2, facilitating thought using emotion, remain to be determined (Mayer et al., 2016). The Mayer-Salovey-Caruso Emotional Intelligence Test (MSCEIT; Mayer et al., 2003) is an ability based 141-item instrument measuring EI as it tests abilities in each of the four branches of the Mayer-Salovey model (Fiori & Vesely-Maillefer, 2018). It is widely used by researchers, administrators, executive leaders, and many others to measure EI.

THE BAR-ON MODEL OF SOCIAL AND EMOTIONAL INTELLIGENCE

The Bar-On model is classed as a mixed EI model as it measures traits, social skills, and competencies (O'Connor et al., 2019). Bar-On has described social and emotional intelligence (ESI) as "an array of interrelated emotional and social competencies, skills and behaviors" that determine the degree to which individuals can understand and express themselves and understand and interact with others (Bar-On, 2013). The social and emotional competencies, skills, and behaviors are made up of 15 factors divided into five broad areas: (1) interpersonal, (2) intrapersonal, (3) stress management, (4) adaptability, and (5) general mood (Bar-On, 2013). Two examples from the 15 factors are self-regard and emotional self-awareness. The Bar-On Emotional Quotient Inventory is the measurement instrument to measure emotional-social EI as conceptualized according to Bar-On (1997). This instrument and similar versions of it are used by academics, researchers, clinicians, and executive leaders to measure emotional-social EI.

THE GOLEMAN–BOYATZIS MODEL OF EMOTIONAL INTELLIGENCE

In 1995, Goleman popularized EI with publication of his book *Emotional Intelligence* (Goleman, 1995). He suggested that EI was much more important than cognitive intelligence in predicting career success and performance. Goleman described EI as the ability to identify, assess, and manage one's own emotions as well as the emotions of others and of groups (Goleman, 1995). Goleman's original EI model had 25 competencies. Later Goleman collaborated with Boyatzis, integrating their works, and they developed a new definition for EI: "emotional intelligence is observed when a person demonstrates the competencies that constitute self-awareness, self-management, social awareness, and social skills at appropriate times and ways in sufficient frequency to be effective in the situation" (Boyatzis et al., 2000, p. 345). Goleman and Boyatzis developed new competencies and revised existing ones to mirror the new EI definition (Boyatzis et al., 2000). The new Boyatzis–Goleman model has four domains with 18 competencies within the domains. The four domains are self-awareness, self-management, social awareness, and relationship management (Boyatzis & McKee, 2005). The self-awareness and self-management domains govern one's understanding and awareness of self. The social awareness and relationship management domains define our knowledge and management of the emotions of others (Boyatzis & McKee, 2005). Examples of the competencies include emotional self-awareness, and empathy. The Emotional Competence Inventory was developed to measure the competencies in each of the four domains of the Goleman–Boyatzis model (Boyatzis & Sala, 2004). This inventory is extensively used by academics, researchers, executive leaders, and many others. It is a popular inventory in leadership development programs.

DEVELOPING EMOTIONAL INTELLIGENCE IN NURSE LEADERS

EI is critical to the success and performance of nurse leaders in all aspects of life, personal and professional. It will enable the nurse leader to recognize and understand their own feelings and emotions, and how they respond to them. This skill will not only increase nurse leaders' own performance and success, but it will also contribute to the success of their staff. High EI is associated with high performance in the workplace. How does a nurse leader develop EI in oneself? First, reviewing the EI models is a good place to start. In this section, the Goleman and Boyatzis model (Boyatzis & McKee, 2005), the one most used in leadership programs, has been selected as a guide when nurse leaders are working to develop their EI. This model has four domains: self-awareness, self-management, social awareness, and relationship management (Boyatzis & McKee, 2005) with 18 competencies or skills that can be learned to develop EI.

Take the first domain, self-awareness, which governs how well nurse leaders can understand themselves and their emotions. In a fast-paced stressful working environment, the presence of self-awareness can assist nurse leaders to make the most of their strengths and manage their emotions. How can nurse leaders develop self-awareness? A first step is to take time to reflect on themselves taking time to answer a few questions; for example, who do they think they are? How do they see themselves? Time is precious for nurse leaders, so this exercise does not need to take too much time. The goal can be achieved within a short, dedicated, uninterrupted time. During this time, here are some prompts nurse leaders can use: How they see themselves in different situations? in the workplace? in the home? with friends? with colleagues? with peers, with superiors? Recognizing and understanding emotions is a major component of self-awareness. The next step will help nurse leaders to recognize and understand their emotions. To achieve this goal, the nurse leaders can arrange an EI assessment test from a reputable company to gather anonymous feedback from their peers, their direct reports, and their superiors that they work with on a regular basis. For this exercise, the nurse leaders will identify a list of peers, direct reports, and their superiors and ask them to complete the EI assessment once it is sent to them from the assessment company. The purpose of this assessment is to identify the nurse leader's areas of strengths and those that need improvement. The third step is to schedule a professional coaching session to get feedback from this assessment. The professional coach will assist the nurse leaders in the interpretation of the assessment survey. The assessment survey results will give the nurse leaders objective feedback about their strengths and limitations as perceived by others. Based on this feedback, they may decide to continue with a series of one-on-one coaching sessions to help them work on the areas that need improvement as well as acknowledging and capitalizing on their strengths. It is strongly recommended that the nurse leaders schedule a series of one-on-one coaching sessions to yield the benefits from the assessment survey.

When cultivating self-awareness, nurse leaders will want to understand their negative emotions also. Nurse leaders will need to identify their triggers for stress and negative emotions. These triggers are important as they identify the flashpoints for "flying off the handle" or having inappropriate responses to situations. After the fact, it can be difficult to recall the exact trigger for a specific event. Therefore, it is recommended to keep a reflective journal in real time identifying daily instances of times nurse leaders exhibited negative thoughts, feelings, and actions in the workplace. In the journal, write about the things that led up to each interaction, along with the feelings experienced during and after the interaction. Finally, identify the trigger. This is a good exercise to continue to do until the instances appear repetitive and it appears all or most of the triggers have been identified. Review the journal and identify the recurring emotions. Now for the hard part; EI is not easy. Nurse leaders need to manage the identified triggers and negative emotions so that they become effective high-performing leaders and are less likely to become stressed. This is where self-management comes into play.

Self-management is the second domain in the Goleman and Boyatzis model (Boyatzis & McKee, 2005). Emotionally intelligent nurse leaders can manage their emotions in all situations. This is an important leadership EI competency. One way to manage recurring negative emotions is to break the cycle of negative emotional activity in the brain. To do this, take a deep breath or take a 6-second pause to change the chemical reaction of the emotion. To break the chemical reaction, engage the analytical part of the brain with an activity for 6 seconds (e.g., name six of your friends). Six seconds is all it takes to change or slow your negative emotion. Now that the emotional landscape has changed, evaluate the situation. Having regained self-control, the nurse leader can make an appropriate response. Another strategy to regain and maintain self-control of emotions is to think before speaking, or perhaps asking to have something rephrased or to write it down as it is said. It is important to avoid saying anything that one will regret.

Mindfulness meditation practice is another strategy to develop EI and a way to become aware of your feelings, as well as understand and manage your emotions during the workday. Practicing mindfulness can help nurse leaders get in the moment and to be consciously and actively engaged in situations. Nurses should get into a routine of having a regular short mindfulness practice at the start of the day to remind themselves to be consciously mindful and present in all situations. Mindfulness practice can be as short as a minute or two, and nurse leaders can employ this short practice when they feel negative emotions are interfering with their performance. Short mindfulness exercises can help nurse leaders experience positive emotions and complete the task at hand. Regular time and space for mindfulness can increase EI, making the nurse leader more productive and transformational. Writing a reflection journal daily is another good strategy to become aware of emotions and the way they are handled. Regular review and reflection of the journal entry is important to develop EI.

◆ CASE SCENARIO

NURSE MANAGER AND EMOTIONAL INTELLIGENCE— SELF-AWARENESS AND SELF-MANAGEMENT DOMAINS

SITUATION

There are five new orientees on the unit that started together and are receiving the same orientation. Four out of the five are doing well. The remaining one now has made a second medication error and does not seem to be learning the hospital procedure and policy. This second error was a similar mistake to the first error where the orientee did not use the bar code to scan the medication as per hospital policy. After the first error, the preceptor had reviewed the policy again with the orientee and emphasized the safety issue with not using the bar code scanning process.

APPROACH

The nurse manager comes onto the unit and sees the orientee at the automated dispensing machine, which triggers some anger (**lack of self-awareness**). The nurse manager shouts at the new orientee (**poor self-management**), telling them to "use your head" and adhere to hospital policy when administering medications. The nurse manager tells the orientee that otherwise they are creating a safety issue on the unit.

OUTCOME

The nurse manager's demeanor, tone of voice, and way of telling the orientee of the nurse manager's concerns and risks to patient safety become too much for the new orientee and they begin to cry. Already fueled by anger, the nurse manager loses control, moves closer to the orientee, and proceeds to shout, telling the orientee that they should not be crying but that they should be listening and following policy! This outburst occurs in front of the entire staff on duty during that shift.

While most nurse managers probably do not have a temper like this nurse manager, there have probably been times when they have exhibited negative emotions and behaviors in the workplace. When this happens, it often can have negative consequences, not only for the nurse manager and the affected staff member, but for those around them as well.

DISCUSSION QUESTIONS

1. Is this nurse manager emotionally intelligent?
2. What happened in this scenario?
3. What was the response elicited by the orientee following the nurse manager's outburst?
4. What could have been done differently?

SELF-AWARENESS AND SELF-MANAGEMENT KEY POINTS

- Knowing our "triggers" can allow us to manage our reactions.
- Managing our reactions can help us to handle stress well and make good decisions. The nurse manager could have managed the situation better by identifying the trigger to their negative behavior, and then pausing before they responded to the situation.

Social competence includes the third and fourth domains of the Goleman and Boyatzis model: social awareness and relationship management (Boyatzis & McKee, 2005). Empathy, the ability to sense the other person's emotions and respond to them, is a key competency in this section. Nurse leaders need to become aware of the verbal and nonverbal cues they provide during interactions with peers and staff. This involves having a focus on understanding others' perspectives. Nurse leaders can develop EI by practicing empathy by being in the moment with the conversations and interactions they are having. Do not multitask while listening to another person. Listen to them and become aware of the verbal and nonverbal cues the other person provides during the interaction. When interacting with other individuals, the nurse leader can be empathetic but should remember everyone is responsible for one's own actions.

It is important to develop a positive outlook and engage in positive thinking. Having positive emotions (e.g., joy, hope) will keep negative emotions in check and allow the nurse leader to see the positive side of events in the workplace. Perhaps the nurse leader will start looking at things from different perspectives and objectively. This will help with creating a new vision, initiating change, and leading in a new direction. A leader's mood coupled with their influence are key drivers in the performance, success, and satisfaction of the staff and ultimately the organization. Increasing the nurse leader's mood involves paying attention to self-awareness and self-management. Managing work stress and ensuring a good work–life balance is important also. Some would argue that "balance" is not the correct term to use as it implies that work and personal time are in an equilibrium. This is never the case for nurse leaders as there are always competing work responsibilities creating imbalance. Mullen (2021) is of the opinion that work–life balance is an outdated term from a time when individuals had 9 a.m. to 5 p.m. employment and it was easier to balance or arrange relaxation time outside these hours. All of this changed with the advent of mobile technologies and the expectation that workers were available outside work hours (Mullen, 2021). Nurse leaders and particularly nurse executives are tied to their mobile technologies 24 hours a day with an inherent expectation that one is always available. To extract oneself from this line of thinking, conceptualize work–life balance in a new way: think of a new term, "work–life negotiation" (Mullen, 2021). Now, rather than trying to balance everything 50–50, nurse leaders can negotiate with themselves to perhaps work more today or this week and have more time to relax later. Taking a long-term approach works well when negotiating with oneself. This concept takes getting used to as it involves a seismic shift where the nurse leader is acknowledging the extra work up front but negotiating with oneself for less work later. This involves being strict with oneself to make sure the nurse leader takes the downtime and does not renege on the negotiation. With this new approach, nurse leaders may empower themselves and their staff to take some worktime to attend to personal issues, particularly if there is an expectation to attend to work issues during personal time. Taking care of oneself with regular time to relax and renew is important to increase one's energy to be an empathetic effective transformational nurse leader. Strategies to help reduce workplace stress include listening to music, engaging in activities that bring joy and happiness, making friends with positive supportive individuals, and trying new things. Close healthy relationships are important for EI. Regular exercise, which has been identified as a strategy to increase and maintain high EI, is thought to increase emotional clarity, emotional attention, and emotional repair (Acebes-Sánchez et al., 2019). EI will continue to develop over time, and you can build and enhance it as you continue to address the EI competencies and employ strategies for them.

⬡ | **CASE SCENARIO**

NURSE EXECUTIVE AND EMOTIONAL INTELLIGENCE— SOCIAL COMPETENCE AND RELATIONSHIP MANAGEMENT DOMAINS

SITUATION

A nurse executive has been invited to a staff meeting where there have been some issues on the unit related to staffing and work environment. The staff do not believe that they have an adequate number of staff to care for patients, or the supplies and equipment they need to deliver safe care. The nurse executive walks onto the unit and uses social awareness to pick up on the environment and milieu of the workplace. As they look around, the nurse executive realizes that the unit is busy, and staff are looking down and not making eye contact or connecting with the nurse executive. This has the nurse executive concerned. As soon as the nurse executive reaches the meeting room, however, the facial expression of worry and concern they felt after experiencing the mood on the unit disappears. The nurse executive is able to flip the switch on their positive emotions to greet the staff with confidence, smiling and welcoming despite the nurse executive's internal anxieties. Thus, it is evident that the nurse executive can recognize and skillfully manage their emotions at critical moments to succeed.

APPROACH

As the nurse executive enters the meeting, they scan and read the room and see angry staff, sullen, without smiles or acknowledgment. The body language is clear as the nurse executive notices the staff are slumped in their seats with arms crossed, seeming bored and closed off. The nurse executive greets the staff by name, establishing a relationship with them, and tells them that the nurse executive is happy to be there to support them. By doing this, the nurse executive acknowledges who the staff are and that they are in distress. The nurse executive uses the knowledge picked up when scanning the room to determine the best approach to take when facilitating the meeting. After picking up on the no-nonsense vibe, they decide to use honesty, earnestness, and humor to demonstrate awareness and dedication to addressing the staff's issues. The nurse executive knows exactly how to field the tough questions and lets their empathy and dedication to this staff shine through, despite the circumstances.

OUTCOME

The nurse executive's ability to accurately pick up on the emotional and behavioral cues when walking through the unit and then entering the meeting, and their awareness of their own emotions, allowed the nurse executive to determine the best approach to take in the meeting. As a result, the nurse executive was able to make the most of the situation, gain the trust of the unit staff, and leave a positive, hopeful impression on them.

DISCUSSION QUESTIONS

1. What indicators did the nurse executive pick up on when reading the milieu of the unit staff members?
2. What indicators did the nurse executive pick up on in the meeting?
3. How did the nurse executive handle the interaction with the staff to build a relationship and have the staff engage in conversation?
4. How does the nurse executive establish a relationship with the staff on the unit?

SOCIAL AWARENESS AND RELATIONSHIP MANAGEMENT KEY POINTS

- Reading social cues and others' emotions as well as taking time to understand their perspectives can impact the bottom line as well as the nurse executive's success solving problems and resolving conflicts.
- Reading the situation correctly allows the nurse executive to make better decisions and see and seize opportunities.
- The nurse executive's ability to manage their emotions affects how others perceive them.
- How others perceive the nurse executive can impact their relationships and networks.

USING EMOTIONAL INTELLIGENCE TO DEVELOP EFFECTIVE TEAMS AND ORGANIZATIONS

Emotionally intelligent nurse leaders and nurse executives are equipped with the EI skills to develop effective teams and organizations. They are self-confident and aware of their own strengths and weaknesses. They can manage their own emotions and thus are able to mentor, manage, and support their staff. They are socially competent sensing others' emotions and providing timely feedback when needed. Emotionally intelligent nurse leaders are good listeners and welcome feedback on any issue and on their personal performance. They are effective communicators and are skilled in conflict resolution. The nurse leaders role model the EI competencies in all situations. They encourage EI development in their staff and support use of EI strategies in the workplace; for example, a short mindfulness practice at the beginning of team meetings. Cooperation, collaboration, and team building are valued. The nurse leader will have a transformational leadership style with the ability to effectively communicate a clear vision for the staff. With these EI skills, how can nurse leaders develop effective teams and organizations? When developing effective teams, the nurse leader must ensure the team members have a strong sense of trust with each other, a group team identity, and robust beliefs about the ability of the team to perform their tasks effectively (Rampton, 2021). The team members must trust and respect the nurse leader. To gain this respect, the nurse leader must respect each team member, be willing to admit mistakes, and offer help when needed (Rampton, 2021). A commitment from the nurse leader to provide mentorship and coaching indicates the value the team leader places on the team members. Nurse team leaders must ensure that each team member has opportunities to offer their suggestions and recommendations for the project or task. Often team members are afraid to speak in the team meeting as they fear that their contribution will not be on the right track or may not be valued. To help team members contribute, the nurse leader can identify some ground rules for communicating and contributing within the meeting. Also, emotionally intelligent nurse leaders can use their excellent communication skills to promote and develop team members' communication skills including active listening, as well as verbal and nonverbal communication (Rampton, 2021).

Creating the correct team for the task may prove challenging. Team members must be enthusiastic, have the correct skills for the task, and, most importantly, maintain a strong commitment to the organization (Rampton, 2021). Nurse leaders can make the selection of the team members easier on themselves if they have developed strategies to get to know their staff outside the work situation. In these situations, the team leader may have identified specific strengths and weaknesses among the staff that may prove useful when creating teams for specific projects (Rampton, 2021). Once the team has been created, it may be beneficial to continue to have social events at intervals throughout the project. These events may foster team building, increase the group team identity, and strengthen the sense of trust among team members as well as provide time to relax and unwind from the project. At the first team meeting, the nurse leaders and the team members must develop some ground rules for the teamwork. Discussions must occur related to project management, timeline, and team meeting schedules. Time management during meetings and for project deadlines must be addressed also.

It is important that team members are rewarded and recognized for achievements within the team and organization. This recognition will help to build relationships with the nurse leader and within the team members. All nurse leaders have a responsibility to develop teams and organizations, but the emotionally intelligent nurse leaders are equipped with the EI skills to build teams and organizations that are effective and will be ahead of the curve.

◆ CASE SCENARIO

NURSE LEADERS AND EMOTIONAL INTELLIGENCE— USING EMOTIONAL INTELLIGENCE AND TEAMSTEPPS TO IMPROVE TEAMWORK BETWEEN THE EMERGENCY DEPARTMENT AND INPATIENT UNITS

SITUATION

Hospital X, a 400-bed teaching hospital, improved the timeliness of admitting patients from the ED to the inpatient units after implementing TEAMSTEPPS team training tools based on results from a culture of safety survey. These results indicated that there was a lack of trust and poor communication between units which affected the perception of safety during handoffs.

APPROACH

Two nurse leaders from the ED and inpatient divisions met to discuss the survey results and barriers to smooth handoffs, transitions, and teamwork across units. They developed an action plan with the first rule of business to develop a cross-functional team between the ED and inpatient units to discuss their issues and concerns. Both nurse leaders attended the meeting. They agreed to leave their own biases aside **(personal competence)** in preparation for the meeting to ensure that they can support the greater good and joint goal of smooth and safe transitions. They facilitated the team meetings on a weekly basis. The first priority was to understand how each set of nurses felt about the process. To do this, they conducted several "get to know you ice breakers" and "team building exercises" to foster building relationships **(social competence)**. They explained the "why" that what they are working together on is important to get the group to connect to the purpose of the meetings. They used a "walk-in-your-shoes" approach to see things in the eyes of the other department, which allowed them to appreciate what they were dealing with and the realization that they are all nurses with a common goal: care of the patients. They were alert to and managed triggers on both sides, which could lead to deterioration of the meetings and lack of development of mutual understanding and consideration, which could further erode their relationships. They allowed the staff to express their frustrations, understanding, and empathy and vowed to develop a process together to support both sides.

OUTCOME

Following this, the meetings were able to progress to understand and map the workflow from the ED to inpatient care, analyzing the workflow for opportunities to streamline the process. They found it vital to focus on process issues to avoid personal and departmental defensiveness. This approach proved both helpful and successful in getting staff members to come together as a team. The teams came to understand and appreciate the roles of different parts of the hospital. The result has been better patient care and improved intra-hospital relations as well as safer care with improved communication.

DISCUSSION QUESTIONS

1. What was the first key step that the nurse leaders took to ensure a successful outcome?
2. Which EI domains does this demonstrate?
3. What strategies did the nurse leaders employ to enable the teams to develop mutual understanding of each other's positions and develop a relationship which allowed the solution to occur?

4. Based on the previous text, what EI domains can you use to understand and manage your own biases?

5. What EI domain do you use to understand another person or group of people's needs?

6. What EI domains do you use to manage and develop relationships?

BACKGROUND

Nurse researchers have conducted studies on EI and its relationships to nursing leadership and nursing practice. The studies on EI and nurse leadership have included those on leadership styles, nurse leaders, and nurse managers. Researchers have examined EI in nurses working in different specialties globally. Studies have included EI, and many concepts related to nurses' work environment such as job satisfaction, nurse turnover, professionalism, competence, workplace bullying, conflict strategies, stress and coping, burnout, nurse well-being, and patient outcomes.

EMOTIONAL INTELLIGENCE AND NURSING LEADERSHIP

EI is a concept that is critical for nurse leaders if they are to be effective in their positions. In the literature, there were several studies focusing on nurse managers, leadership styles, and EI. The literature strongly supports the importance of EI for transformational leadership among nurse managers. Tyczkowski et al. (2015) and Echevarria et al. (2016) reported significantly positive relationships between EI and transformational leadership in nurse managers. Also in 2016, EI among frontline acute care nurse managers was significantly positively correlated with transformational leadership, as well as the outcome measures of extra effort, effectiveness, and satisfaction (Spano-Szekely et al., 2016). Interestingly, EI was not significantly related to transactional or *laissez-faire* leadership styles (Tyczkowski et al., 2015) while Spano-Szekely et al. (2016) found EI was significantly negatively correlated with *laissez-faire* leadership.

Tyczkowski et al. (2015) noted in their work that almost two-thirds of the nurse managers had previous EI training and education while over three-quarters of them reported having previous leadership training. This prior education and training may have influenced their responses. Echevarria et al. reported that all their nurse managers were members of the American Organization of Nurse Executives (AONE); this may have influenced the results (Echevarria et al., 2016). The best practices of transformational leadership positively impact patient outcomes and quality of care. Education programs in EI and transformational leadership for nurse managers are critical to meet the needs of these nurse leaders as they support healthy work environments and ensure high-quality patient care in healthcare systems. The findings of Echevarria et al. (2016) included the relationship between EI and education, and thus provided support for nurse managers to engage in EI programs to help them understand and increase their EI abilities. Increasing their understanding of EI will help them to have an effective leadership style.

Crowne et al. (2017) in an intervention study examined the effectiveness of a 3-year EI and leadership development education program among nurse leaders working in nursing homes. Almost half of the nurse leaders completed the 3-year program. They indicated that the EI educational development was effective in providing support for a long-term program, while the personal leadership development was not. There was a positive significant relationship between EI and transformational leadership. All the nurse managers were members of the AONE, possibly skewing the results. As nurse executives review the work of Crowne et al. (2017), they will have to consider the cost implications of a 3-year program as less than half of the nurse managers completed the program. Perhaps future work could include evaluation of shorter programs with different delivery modalities such as on-site and virtual.

Prufeta (2017) found that among nurse managers there were no differences in EI based on age and gender. However, nurse managers with less than 2 years of experience had a significantly lower "using emotions" branch score and strategic EI than those with 3 to 5 years of experience. It is interesting to note that nurse managers with a master's degree in nursing scored significantly higher in the "using emotions" branch score than did those with a master's degree in a related field. This indicates the importance of continuing education in nursing as opposed to pursuing degrees from other disciplines based on the results, Prufeta (2017) recommended developing and implementing EI programs for nurse managers to promote their EI abilities. She recommended that EI training should be included in the orientation of nurse managers with frequent ongoing education and support to enhance their EI levels.

EMOTIONAL INTELLIGENCE AND NURSING PRACTICE

EI has been studied among nurses in different care settings globally including EI and psychiatric-mental health nurses (PMHNs), critical care nurses, and neonatal intensive care nurses. Sims (2017) compared PMHNs' EI scores to a normed population. The PMHNs in the study had a higher mean EI compared with that of the normed sample. The higher mean scores for the PMHN were not unexpected as the PMHN would have had education related to communicating with patients, as well as self-reflecting and self-awareness of their own emotions and behaviors, and those of their patients. However, only one PMHN scored in the "Expert" range; more would have been expected based on their professional education and experience. This finding may be due to testing or lack of knowledge about EI. Therefore, education related to components of EI may be a way to improve the overall EI scores in the PMHN. In a South African study, Nagel et al. (2016) described the EI of RNs commencing work in critical care units. Most of the sample had less than 2 years' experience as RNs. The global EI score was in the higher range of global EI. Four EI factors were measured; the well-being factor scored the highest, followed by the emotionality factor. The third factor was self-control, and the sociability factor scored the lowest. Nagel et al. (2016) recommended that EI assessment should be included in the orientation program for newly hired nurses. The results could be used to identify EI areas where the nurse may benefit from further EI education and mentoring. Supporting newly hired nurses in this way may result in increased retention of staff.

Lewis (2019) conducted an integrative review to explore the relationship between EI, moral distress in NICU nurses, end-of-life care, and other priority nurse and patient outcomes. The work environments for nurses in NICUs can be very stressful due to the nature of the intensity of the patient care required. In many situations, they are involved in providing end-of-life care. NICU nurses are faced with moral issues on almost a daily basis, and prolonged exposure may lead to stress and burnout. In the studies retrieved, higher EI scores in nurses in different settings were associated with decreased stress, burnout, moral distress, performance, and competence. However, no research studies on EI and NICU nurses had been conducted within the time frame of the review. Lewis (2019) concluded that results from studies in other settings provided evidence to support the efficacy of EI in bedside nurses as a method of improving key nurse and patient outcomes, and that EI can be improved by training interventions. Lewis (2019) recommended that EI be included in staff development sessions.

EMOTIONAL INTELLIGENCE AND THE WORK ENVIRONMENT

EI is a critical component of a healthy work environment. Several nursing researchers have conducted studies on EI and negative work environment concepts such as conflict management, bullying, workplace incivility, intent to stay, and turnover intentions. Nurse leaders have a critical role in creating healthy positive work environments. Effective nurse managers create and maintain work environments where nurses enjoy coming to work, have professional development opportunities, and turnover is low. However, many nurses experience suboptimal or negative work environments and are exposed to workplace incivility and bullying. In some instances, nurses experience bullying through email and text communications as well as face-to-face. These negative acts can be overt or covert, meaning that the person doing the bullying may give the outward appearance of being open, honest, and friendly, although the person being bullied knows this is not the case.

Basogul and Ozgur (2016) in Turkey examined EI levels and nurses' conflict management strategies and the relationship between them. The nurses' mean EI score was ranked medium. Conflict management strategies such as integration, obliging, dominating, and compromising were positively correlated with EI whereas the strategy of avoidance was negatively correlated with EI. These results indicate that EI is related to effective conflict management. There is a need for training and professional development programs in EI and conflict management to assist nurses with conflict resolution. Workplace conflicts were identified as issues for nurse leaders with negative implications for patient care. They can be defined as a persistent pattern of inappropriate behaviors, for example, hostility, harassing, or sabotaging behaviors causing emotional or physical harm to another person or persons. Incivility, a related concept, can be defined as being rude, disrespectful, or impolite to another person (Meires, 2018). Incivility and bullying can lead to low staff job satisfaction, increased staff turnover, and eventually to suboptimal patient care and increased patient errors. EI strategies have been identified as a means to manage incivility and bullying in the workplace. Meires (2018) identified how implementing programs to increase EI can reduce or curtail bullying in the workplace. EI can provide situational awareness and model professional behaviors when behaviors and emotions are inappropriate (Meires, 2018). Nurse executives could develop case studies to demonstrate examples of healthcare settings where EI was used as a method to reduce incivility and bullying, and those that did not use EI.

EMOTIONAL INTELLIGENCE AND TURNOVER INTENTIONS

Globally there is a shortage of nurses. Many millions of dollars are spent each year recruiting and orienting newly hired nurses. Nurses leaving their positions and/or the profession is a growing global problem that directly impacts patient outcomes. In the United States, the nursing shortage is extremely acute, with a projected shortage of 1.1 million nurses stemming from the fact that 2020 saw the largest numbers ever of nurses retiring, coupled with estimates of 500,000 planning to retire in 2022 (Love & Pianko, 2021). The shortage of nurses across the specialties results in nurses feeling stressed and hurried, more likely to have medical errors, and needing more workarounds, all leading to reduced quality of care, burnout, and increased turnover.

Hong and Lee (2016) reported that EI did not directly affect turnover intention of full-time general nurses working in a South Korean university hospital for more than 1 year. However, EI had significant effects on turnover intention through job stress and burnout (Hong & Lee, 2016). These results may indicate that EI should be a component of staff development programs geared to reduce job stress and burnout. In China, Wang et al. (2017) reported that transformational leadership and staff nurse EI were significant predictors of nurse intention to stay. Wang et al. (2017) concluded that nurse leaders should develop educational programs to improve nurse manager transformational leadership style and increase staff nurse EI. Nurse managers could develop EI training and professional development for staff nurses. In the current climate of nurse shortages, however, EI and transformational leadership programs may be one cost effective way to increase retention and reduce turnover while improving EI and promoting transformational leadership.

EMOTIONAL INTELLIGENCE AND COMMUNICATION

EI is a significant skill for effective communication, particularly in nursing. Zhu et al. (2016) in a Chinese study indicated that the EI scores of clinical nurses was significantly lower than the international norm. However, the clinical communication competency of nurses was positively correlated with EI. Zhu et al. concluded that nursing administrators can improve the clinical communication ability of nurses by increasing EI. Development of continuing education EI programs or modules could assist with improving clinical communication ability and in turn could lead to better patient handover, and patient outcomes.

In Spain, Gimenez-Espert and Prado-Gasco (2018) investigated the relationship between empathy and EI as a predictor of nurses' attitudes toward communication. Results indicated that EI and empathy were predictors of nurses' attitudes toward communication. These researchers recommend that the results may be used to identify educational needs and to assess new interventions to promote attitudes regarding communication, empathy, and EI. Each of the EI domains of self-awareness, self-management, social awareness, and relationship management are crucial for effective communication.

EMOTIONAL INTELLIGENCE AND INTERVENTIONS

Kozlowski et al. (2018) conducted an intervention study to test whether a single training session on EI behaviors in the workplace together with an additional session of one-on-one coaching would result in increased EI from a 3-month post-training. They found that there was a significant increase in EI scores over baseline levels for the trained group while scores for the control did not increase. The results from this pilot study provide evidence that introducing a low-cost training intervention for nursing staff would be beneficial for increasing EI. In another intervention study in Israel, Bamberger et al. (2018) examined the association between EI training and a change in EI and patient satisfaction. The sample comprised physicians and nurses working on a hospital pediatric team. The training program included group discussions, simulations, and case studies. The results indicated interesting differences between the physicians and nurses. The overall EI score increased significantly for the physicians whereas the increase in the nurses' scores was not significant. In the intervention group, physicians reported a significant increase in scores related to intrapersonal EI, adaptability, and stress management. However, the nurses had a significant increase in stress management only. Patient satisfaction increased significantly among the post-intervention physicians but not the nurses. Bamberger et al. (2018) suggest that differences between the post-intervention physician and nurses' scores may be related to job expectations and demands. Physicians may have had more opportunities to experiment with the strategies learned during the intervention. The small increases in nurses' EI may be related to increased stress and burnout compared to physicians. Perhaps EI programs for nurses should be included with programs on stress reduction, decreasing burnout, increasing engagement, and personal well-being. Based on this study, perhaps nurse executives could consider dedicated EI training programs for nurses as opposed to including the nurses in generic programs for healthcare workers. It appears there is some evidence to include specific modules with a laser focus on the nurses' work environment including more education on intrapersonal EI and adaptability. Evaluation studies are needed to identify the ideal length of EI training programs, and the specific content required for nurses to increase all of the EI competencies. Overall, a critical observation from the literature is that there are few nursing interventional studies on EI, indicating a crucial need for future work in this area.

SYNOPSIS

In summary, there are some key findings that are important for nurse leaders. EI is correlated with transformational leadership. Higher levels of education in nursing are correlated with high EI. Higher levels of EI are correlated with lower stress and related to effective conflict management. EI programs appear to increase EI. From the interventional studies reviewed there is evidence that EI programs enhance and increase EI. Therefore, as EI is positively associated with transformational leadership, EI programs should be included for all emerging and current nurse leaders. However, nurses at all levels should work on improving EI through the EI domains and competencies at all times throughout their careers.

For those nurse leaders seeking more detail, here is an overview on the studies reported in this section. Almost all the studies employed descriptive correlational designs. The sample sizes were small, and most were nonrandom in nature with differing inclusion criteria. It is difficult to compare the EI results as different measures are used in the studies. Most studies include different outcome variables, making it difficult to compare outcome results and EI between studies. Although EI studies have been conducted with nurses in different specialties, there were none in NICU nurses. Only a few of the studies had interventions testing the impact of education programs on EI. Again, the results of these interventional studies cannot be compared as the interventions differ in length and type of program.

BENEFITS OF EMOTIONAL INTELLIGENCE

The presence of EI transforms a leader into an exemplary transformational leader. EI is a core leadership skill and has many critical leadership benefits for nurses, nurse leaders, nurse executives, and for organizations. In this section, the benefits of EI are framed within the four domains and the competencies of the Boyatzis–Goleman model: self-awareness, self-management, social awareness, and relational management (Boyatzis & McKee, 2005). Emotionally intelligent leaders have emotional self-awareness. The self-awareness domain encompasses recognition of one's own feelings, knowledge of the reasons these feelings happened, and understanding of one's own emotions. Self-aware leaders are self-confident and have a positive sense of their leadership capabilities.

Self-management competencies provide the nurse leader with the EI skills to exhibit emotional self-control. The emotionally intelligent nurse leader is transparent, trustworthy, and honest. A major benefit of EI for nurse leaders is the ability to adapt to changing workplace scenarios and lead change. The nurse leader demonstrates flexibility and uses initiative to take advantage of opportunities.

The third EI domain in the Goleman–Boyatzis model is social awareness. Empathy is an important benefit of EI within the social awareness domain. Emotionally intelligent nurse leaders are empathetic to their staff, are interested in them as individuals, take time to listen to their points of view, and value their contributions. They have a service orientation, and they understand and are responsive to the needs of their staff and their clients. Being socially aware includes having organizational awareness. Here the emotionally intelligent nurse leader will have an in-depth understanding of the political and cultural landscape of the healthcare organization. This will include knowledge of the principal decision makers and an understanding of how decisions are made within the organization.

Relationship management is the fourth domain in the Goleman–Boyatzis model. Within this domain, the emotionally intelligent nurse, nurse leaders, and nurse executives have many competencies. They will demonstrate an inspirational vision for their system or unit and communicate that vision effectively. They are optimistic and have a positive outlook regardless of the challenges they may encounter. Emotionally intelligent leaders can guide, motivate, coach, and mentor their staff. They provide timely feedback to staff coupled with recommendations for professional development. They recognize and reward staff for their achievements and successes. Their work environment will be positive, exciting, and trusting with an engaged workforce. EI among nurse leaders and their staff helps to promote a healthy work environment with compassionate staff; open, honest, and effective communication; and respect for each other. The presence of high levels of EI in nurses has been linked to increased job satisfaction, reduced conflict and bullying, and increased collaboration among staff (Davidson, 2017). In turn, the increased job satisfaction and healthy working environment can lead to increased retention and low turnover of staff.

The emotionally intelligent nurse leader will have the ability to resolve conflicts successfully and have tough conversations when needed. A hallmark of the emotionally intelligent nurse leader is expertise in successful team building, collaboration, and teamwork, coupled with developing and maintaining relationships. In conclusion, the benefits of EI are tremendous; the presence of EI results in emotionally intelligent nurse leaders and nurse executives that are strong effective transformational inspirational leaders with vision and influence.

EMOTIONAL INTELLIGENCE AND HEALTH AND WELL-BEING

EI has the potential to influence health and well-being positively. It can help nurses and nurse leaders to recognize their own feelings and can manage their emotions. This self-awareness enables them to deal with negative emotions (for example, stress, anger) and instead experience positive emotions such as joy, hope, and inspiration. Often nurse leaders work in stressful environments and the workplace stressors they experience as well as personal stress can lead to poor performance, decrease in work engagement, and lack of vision and initiative. EI may help reduce stress as emotionally intelligent nurse leaders will be more in tune with their behaviors. Effective management of emotions leads to more effective coping with stress and conflict. Unaddressed stress will ultimately lead to deterioration in physical and mental well-being. Mindfulness and self-reflective practices are strategies to increase EI. Mindfulness meditation provides opportunities to take time out to become aware of your feelings, as well as understand and manage your emotions. Regular time and space for mindfulness can increase EI, making the nurse leader more productive and transformational. Mindfulness practice can be as short as a minute or two and nurse leaders can employ this short practice when they feel negative emotions are interfering with their performance. Short mindfulness exercises can help nurse leaders experience positive emotions and complete the task at hand.

Karimi et al. (2021) investigated EI, psychological empowerment, and general well-being in a sample of 78 Australian nursing and personal care assistants working in an aged-care facility. Results indicated that psychological empowerment was significantly related to EI while high EI scores were related to lower illness levels. Karimi et al. (2021) suggest that programs to enhance EI by providing opportunities to learn and practice EI skills may enhance both psychological empowerment and staff well-being, and in turn quality of care. Researchers have reported the association of EI with social support and coping (Perera & DiGiacomo, 2015). Nurse leaders can develop the relational management EI competencies to build personal social support networks. Building good work teams and encouraging collaborations will help reduce the burden on the nurse leader and reduce work stress. EI is a valuable resource in the workplace.

Increasing EI in nurse leaders and staff through leadership programs will promote well-being, reduce stress, and foster a healthy empowered work environment.

◻ WHAT EVERY NURSE MANAGER NEEDS TO KNOW ABOUT EMOTIONAL INTELLIGENCE

EI is a key tool for nurse managers and contributes decisively to the achievement of effective management in healthcare. Analysis of several studies have shown that EI is associated with the exercise of transformational leadership. Transformational leaders exert a high level of influence over their constituents, which results in the accomplishments of organizational goals. EI is a high-level skill that contributes to effective relationship management necessary to engage and motivate employees. Regarding management functions, EI becomes an important "virtue" in the hands of nurse managers who must be equipped with skills to successfully meet the growing demands of the modern healthcare system. Management skills, such as negotiating resources, building trusting relationships, encouraging partnership development, and making evidence-based decisions, require a strong foundation of EI. Nurses who aspire to leadership and want to progress to a nurse manager role need to know that EI abilities will be strongly considered for the attainment of that goal. They must evaluate and advance their EI skills just as they do their clinical skills and managerial tasks. Nurse manager candidates who are seen as well rounded in all of these areas will rise to the top in the selection process.

In the nurse manager role, it is important to understand one's own personal strengths and weaknesses, to manage one's own emotions, and to read other's emotions to become successful. EI skills allow the nurse manager to be open to listening to their employees, approach situations with empathy and understanding, and allow them to move forward. The most successful nurse managers continually explore their roles and performance and work to seek opportunities to grow and develop in all areas of leadership, not the least of which is EI.

The primary reason most people leave their jobs is that they have a poor relationship with their boss. Therefore, it is important for nurse managers to possess EI competencies and not just IQ or technical competencies. EI competencies can be learned and developed; therefore, it is important for nurse managers to explore opportunities to work on this skill. Today's healthcare environment is ever-changing. It requires agility and resilience to continue to transform the work environment to meet the increasing demands. Utilizing EI skills to manage your own stress during these times will allow you to strengthen your leadership and build confidence with your team. This is what is needed to create practice environments and work climates that are healthier and safer to lead the change and transformation that is necessary to face and tackle these challenges.

WHAT EVERY NURSE MANAGER NEEDS TO KNOW

- EI is a learned skill needed for effective leadership.
- High EI is linked to transformational leadership style.
- High EI is associated with high performance.
- Leadership skills for nurse managers need to include EI and transformational leadership.

WHAT EVERY NURSE EXECUTIVE NEEDS TO KNOW ABOUT EMOTIONAL INTELLIGENCE

EI is a critical fundamental learned skill needed for leadership in today's complex, volatile, and unpredictable healthcare environment. Leadership during these times requires adaptive thinking abilities. High EI is linked to a transformational leadership style. Emotionally intelligent leaders are highly effective, strategic, and visionary and can achieve the organizational goals. They have excellent communication skills and can get their message across. They are transparent, trustworthy, optimistic, and goal oriented. They have abilities to build and influence effective collaborative teams that excel at getting the task at hand completed. They are passionate about their work and their motivation is conveyed through their actions. The Institute of Medicine (IOM) 2010 report called for nurses to lead and partner in the transformation of healthcare (IOM, 2011). *The Future of Nursing 2020–2030* IOM report with a focus on achieving health equity is calling on nurses to work in teams across disciplines, to provide patient care reducing disease burden, and to improve health outcomes as they deal with the social determinants of health (National Academies of Sciences, Engineering, and Medicine [NASEM], 2021). The American Nurses Association (ANA) supports the premise that leadership is a fundamental component of the scope of nursing practice (ANA, 2015). Of particular importance is the vital leadership role of the nurse manager who has direct influence over RN performance and, therefore, patient outcomes. To achieve positive patient outcomes, nurse managers are expected to influence RN job satisfaction, create a positive work environment, and empower staff to heightened professionalism, thus encouraging commitment to the highest quality of patient care. Most nurse manager development is from on-the-job experiences, training, and coaching/mentoring. In addition, while some larger healthcare organizations have invested in broader organizational development programs, most still have traditional education departments that focus on clinical skills and processes and are bereft of business and strategic essentials necessary for leadership development.

The traditional priorities that are used to select nurse managers for their roles are based on clinical expertise and years of experience. The leadership skills that need to be focused on now for nurse managers include both EI and transformational leadership. Nurse executives should lead the way in partnering with human resources (HR) professionals to consider EI characteristics when hiring nurse managers. They must utilize their expertise and knowledge of the leadership competencies needed for nurse managers, to collaborate and inform academic nursing programs at all levels to ensure that the goals for educators are linked to organizational needs and the needs of today's nursing leaders.

Now more than ever, working in teams and developing and motivating staff to come together around a shared vision is paramount to success. Nurse leaders at all levels must possess EI characteristics to enable development and management of relationships. These relationships at a nurse executive level need to be developed to influence public policy, as well as board and senior executive decision-making. Nurse executives must place themselves at the table and utilize EI skills to have a voice to shape the future of nursing locally and nationally.

WHAT EVERY NURSE EXECUTIVE NEEDS TO KNOW

- Nurse executives must possess EI characteristics to manage relationships.
- Nurse executives must utilize EI skills to have a voice to shape the future of nursing locally and nationally.
- It is important for nurse executives to not only have high levels of technical competence and IQ, which are important for task accomplishment, but to have EI competence, which governs how we relate to others.

KEY POINTS

- EI is the ability to identify, understand, and manage one's own emotions and those of others. This is a critical attribute of high-performing leaders and is associated with a transformational leadership style.
- There are multiple models of EI. Three of the most common are the Mayer and Salovey EI model, The Bar-On model of ESI, and the Goleman–Boyatzis model of EI.
- EI consists of four domains with multiple competencies. These domains are self-awareness, self-management, social awareness, and relational management. The self-awareness and self-management domains manage one's understanding and awareness of self. The social awareness and relationship management domains identify our knowledge and management of the emotions of others. To successfully manage relationships, a nurse leader needs self-awareness, self-management, and social awareness.
- There are strategies that can be learned and practiced to develop and improve EI skills and competencies.

SUMMARY

EI is one of the most sought-after skills among leaders. It can be learned but continues to develop and evolve. Leaders need to continue to nurture and practice it. The definition of EI is dependent on the EI model used; however, the definitions are similar. The Boyatzis–Goleman model (Boyatzis & McKee, 2005) is the most popular model used in leadership programs and healthcare organizations. This model has four domains: self-awareness, self-management, social awareness, and relationship management (Boyatzis & McKee, 2005). There are 18 competencies aligned with these domains and these can be learned.

EI is a critical component for successful effective nurse leaders. It is highly valued in the workplace as it is associated with transformational leadership and high performance. Emotionally intelligent nurse leaders can recognize, understand, and manage their own emotions and those of others. They are adaptable, inspirational, influential, high performing, transformational nurse leaders. They have the ability to far exceed in their professional and personal activities and are always out ahead of the curve.

END-OF-CHAPTER RESOURCES

◆ DISCUSSION QUESTIONS

1. Great leadership works through the emotions (Goleman et al., 2013, p. 3). Discuss.
2. EI skills are challenging. Discuss.
3. Nurse executive role models inspire us. Discuss.

◆ ADDITIONAL RESOURCES

- Six Seconds, The Emotional Intelligence Network. (2020, June 13). *How to stop and think before reacting* [Video]. YouTube. https://www.youtube.com/watch?v=rS2BEB_-dFM
- TEDx Talks. (2016, June 2). *What's love go to do with it? Leadership in new era of healthcare | Susan Carter | TEDxNashville* [Video]. YouTube. https://www.youtube.com/watch?v=Ut0vgq3zbiY
- Key Step Media. (2012, July 18). *Daniel Goleman on the importance of emotional intelligence* [Video]. YouTube. https://www.youtube.com/watch?app=desktop&v=7uQs1NxluKE

◆ GLOSSARY OF KEY TERMS

- **Emotional intelligence:** The ability to recognize, understand, and manage one's own emotions, as well as others' feelings and emotions.

A robust set of instructor resources designed to supplement this text is located at http://connect.springerpub.com/content/book/978-0-8261-7795-7. Qualifying instructors may request access by emailing textbook@springerpub.com.

REFERENCES

Acebes-Sánchez, J., Diez-Vega, I., Esteban-Gonzalo, S., & Rodriguez-Romo, G. (2019). Physical activity and emotional intelligence among undergraduate students: A correlational study. *BMC Public Health, 19*, 1241. https://doi.org/10.1186/s12889-019-7576-5

American Nurses Association. (2015). *Nursing: Scope and standards of practice* (3rd ed.). Author.

Bamberger, E., Genizi, J., Kerem, N., Reuven-Lalung, A., Doley, N., Srugo, I., & Rofe, A. (2018). A pilot study of an emotional intelligence training intervention for a paediatric team. *British Medical Journal, 102*, 159–164. https://doi.org/10.1136/archdischild-2016-310710

Bar-On, R. (1997). *The Bar–On Emotional Quotient Inventory (EQ-i): A test of emotional intelligence.* Multi-Health Systems.

Bar-On, R. (2013). Reuven BAR-ON.org. https://www.reuvenbaron.org/wp/37-2

Basogul, C., & Ozgur, G. (2016). Role of emotional intelligence in conflict management strategies of nurses. *Asian Nursing Research, 10*, 228–233. https://doi.org/10.1016/j.anr.2016.07.002

Boyatzis, R. E., Goleman, D., & Rhee, K. S. (2000). Clustering competence in emotional intelligence: Insights from the Emotional Competence Inventory. In R. Bar-On & J. D. A. Parker (Eds.), *The handbook of emotional intelligence: Theory, development, assessment, and application at home, school, and in the workplace* (pp. 343–362). Jossey-Bass.

Boyatzis, R. E., & McKee, A. (2005). *Resonant leadership.* Harvard Business School Press.

Boyatzis, R. E., & Sala, F. (2004). The Emotional Competence Inventory (ECI). In G. Geher (Ed.), *Measuring emotional intelligence: Common ground and controversy* (pp. 147–180). Nova Science Publishers.

Crowne, K. A., Young, T. M., Goldman, B., Patterson, B., Krouse, A. M., & Proenca, J. (2017). Leading nurses: Emotional intelligence and leadership development effectiveness. *Leadership Health Service (Bradford England), 30*(3), 217–232. https://doi.org/10.1108/LHS-12-2015-0055

Davidson, B. T. (2017). Emotional intelligence in heart failure nursing. *Heart and Lung, 46*(4), 338. https://doi.org/10.1016/j.hrtlng.2017.05.007

Echevarria, I., Patterson, B., & Krouse, A. (2016). Predictors of transformational leadership of nurse managers. *Journal of Nursing Management, 25,* 167–175. https://doi.org/10.1111/jonm.12452

Fiori, M., Antonietti, J. P., Mikolajczak, M., Luminet, O., Hansenne, M., & Rossier, J. (2014). What is the ability emotional intelligence test (MSCEIT) good for? An evaluation using Item Response Theory. *PLoS One, 9*(6), e98827. https://doi.org/10.1371/journal.pone.0098827

Fiori, M., & Vesely-Maillefer, A. K. (2018). Emotional intelligence as an ability: Theory, challenges, and new directions. In K. Keefer, J. Parker, & D. Saklofske (Eds.), *Emotional intelligence in education* (pp. 23–48). Springer. https://doi.org/10.1007/978-3-319-90633-1_2

Gimenez-Espert, M., & Prado-Gasco, V. J. (2018). The role of empathy and emotional intelligence in nurses' communication attitudes using regression models and fuzzy-set qualitative comparative analysis models. *Journal of Clinical Nursing, 27,* 2661–2672. https://doi.org/10.1111/jocn.14325

Goleman, D. (1995). *Emotional intelligence.* Bantam Books.

Goleman, D., Boyatzis, R., & Mc Kee, A. (2013). *Primal leadership: Unleashing the power of emotional intelligence.* Harvard Business Review Press.

Hong, E., & Lee, Y. S. (2016). The mediating effect of emotional intelligence between emotional labour, job stress, burnout and nurses' turnover intention. *International Journal of Nursing Practice, 22*(6), 625–632. https://doi.org/10.1111/ijn.12493

Institute of Medicine. (2011). *The future of nursing: Leading change, advancing health.* National Academies Press. https://www.ncbi.nlm.nih.gov/books/NBK209880

Karimi, L., Leggat, S. G., Bartram, T., Afshari, L., Sarkeshik, S., & Verulava, T. (2021). Emotional intelligence: Predictor of employees' wellbeing, quality of patient care, and psychological empowerment. *BMC Psychology, 9,* 93. https://doi.org/10.1186/s40359-021-00593-8

Kozlowski, D., Hutchinson, M., Hurley, J., & Browne, G. (2018). Increasing nurses' emotional intelligence with a brief intervention. *Applied Nursing Research, 41,* 59–61. https://doi.org/10.1016/j.apnr.2018.04.001

Lewis, S. L. (2019). Emotional intelligence in neonatal intensive care unit nurses: Decreasing moral distress in end-of-life care and laying a foundation for improved outcomes: An integrative review. *Journal of Hospice and Palliative Nursing, 21*(4), 250–256. https://doi.org/10.1097/NJH.0000000000000561

Love, R., & Pianko, D. (2021). *America's nurse shortage is a crisis in the making. Training nurses to be leaders could solve it.* https://fortune.com/2021/05/18/nurse-shortage-retirement-crisis-covid-training-leadership

Mayer, J. D., Caruso, D. R., & Salovey, P. (2016). The Ability Model of Emotional Intelligence: Principles and updates. *Emotion Review, 8*(4), 290–300. https://doi.org/10.1177/1754073916639667

Mayer, J. D., & Salovey, P. (1997). What is emotional intelligence? In D. J. Sluyter (Ed.), *Emotional development and emotional intelligence: Educational implications* (pp. 3–34). Basic Books.

Mayer, J. D., Salovey, P., Caruso, D. R., & Sitarenios, G. (2003). Measuring emotional intelligence with the MSCEIT V2.0. *Emotion, 3*(1), 97–105. https://doi.org/10.1037/1528-3542.3.1.97

Meires, J. (2018). The essentials: Using emotional intelligence to curtail bullying in the workplace. *Urologic Nursing, 38*(3), 150–153. https://doi.org/10.7257/1053-816X.2018.38.3.150

Mullen, C. (2021). *Work-life balance is a thing of the past: Now it's all about work-life negotiation.* https://www.forbes.com/sites/forbescoachescouncil/2021/03/16/work-life-balance-is-a-thing-of-the-past-now-its-all-about-work-life-negotiation/?sh=656d4f7f51ab

Nagel, Y., Towell, A., Nel, E., & Foxall, F. (2016). The emotional intelligence of registered nurses commencing critical care nursing. *Curationis, 39*(1), e1–e7. https://doi.org/10.4102/curationis.v39i1.1606

National Academies of Sciences, Engineering, and Medicine. (2021). *The future of nursing 2020–2030: Charting a path to achieve health equity.* The National Academies Press. http://doi.org/10.17226/25982

O'Connor, P. J., Hill, A., Kaya, M., & Martin, B. (2019). The measurement of emotional intelligence: A critical review of the literature and recommendations for researchers and practitioners. *Frontiers in Psychology, 10,* 1116. https://doi.org/10.3389/fpsyg.2019.01116

Perera, H. N., & DiGiacomo, M. (2015). The role of trait emotional intelligence in academic performance during the university transition: An integrative model of mediation via social support, coping, and adjustment. *Personal and Individual Differences, 83,* 208–213. https://doi.org/10.1016/j.paid.2015.04.001

Posner, B. Z., & Kouzes, J. M. (2011). *The five practices of exemplary leadership.* Wiley.

Prufeta, P. (2017). Emotional intelligence of nurse managers. *The Journal of Nursing Administration, 47*(3), 134–139. https://doi.org/10.1097/NNA.0000000000000455

Rampton, J. (2021). 7 ways to create emotionally intelligent teams. *The Economist: Executive Education Navigator.* https://execed.economist.com/blog/guest-post/7-ways-create-emotionally-intelligent-teams

Salovey, P., & Mayer, J. D. (1990). Emotional intelligence. *Imagination, Cognition and Personality, 9*(3), 185–211. https://doi.org/10.2190/DUGG-P24E-52WK-6CDG

Sims, T. T. (2017). Exploring an emotional intelligence model with psychiatric mental health nurses. *Journal of the American Psychiatric Nurses Association, 23*(2), 133–142. https://doi.org/10.1177/1078390316687024

Spano-Szekely, L., Quinn Griffin, M. T., Clavelle, J., & Fitzpatrick, J. J. (2016). Emotional intelligence and transformational leadership in nurse manager. *The Journal of Nursing Administration, 46*(2), 101–108. https://doi.org/10.1097/NNA.0000000000000303

Tyczkowski, B., Vandenbouten, C., Reilly, J., Bansal, G., Kubsch, S., & Jakkola, R. (2015). Emotional intelligence (EI) and nursing leadership styles among nurse managers. *Nursing Administration Quarterly, 39*(2), 172–180. https://doi.org/10.1097/NAQ.0000000000000094

Wang, L., Tao, H., Bowers, B. J., Brown, R., & Zhang, Y. (2017). When nurse emotional intelligence matters: How transformational leadership influences intent to stay. *Journal of Nursing Management, 26*, 358–365. https://doi.org/10.1111/jonm.12509

Zeidner, M., Matthews, G., Roberts, R. D., & MacCann, C. (2003). Development of emotional intelligence: Toward a multi-level investment model. *Human Development, 46*, 69–96. https://doi.org/10.1159/000068580

Zhu, B., Chen, C.-R., Shi, Z.-Y., Liang, H.-X., & Lui, B. (2016). Mediating effect of self-efficacy in relationship between emotional intelligence and clinical communication competency of nurses. *ScienceDirect, 3*, 162–168. https://doi.org/10.1016/j.ijnss.2016.04.003

CHAPTER 6

RELATIONSHIP-BASED LEADERSHIP THEORIES

Rosanne Raso and Rae Jean Hemway

> *"Leadership is a relational and ethical process of people together attempting to accomplish change."*
>
> *Komives et al. (2007, p. ix)*

LEARNING OBJECTIVES

- Compare relationship-based leadership theories including outcomes and measurement.
- Apply relationship-based leadership principles to case scenarios in nursing professional practice.
- Differentiate relationship-based leadership from traditional leadership theories and models.
- Construct relational leader development strategies for future applications.

INTRODUCTION

This chapter addresses the state of the science about relationship-based leadership, building on the importance of relationships as covered in Chapter 4, "The Importance of Relationships." The reader will discover that it is not about "being nice"; true relational leaders have solid attributes such as shared decision-making and purposefulness that result in effective leadership and outcomes. In this chapter, the reader will also learn about relationship-based leadership theories; how they differ from traditional, "old school" methods; and how they compare to each other.

Relational leadership (RL) is built on complex, three-dimensional relationships with followers and other disciplines, which is more advanced than simple contact based on virtual meetings and emails. This type of leadership is fundamentally positive, particularly in terms of nurturing employee engagement and healthy practice environments. According to Cathcart (2014), one cannot become an expert leader without mastering the skills of interpersonal engagement, and only through those connections do nurse leaders create trust and influence (Cathcart, 2014). The ultimate goal of effective RL is positive patient outcomes.

This chapter includes reviews of the effectiveness and outcomes of RL, describing the specific theories of transformational, authentic, and servant leadership (SL), plus emerging theories such as human-centered leadership (HCL). Relational leaders develop trusting relationships with their followers to influence behavior, as reflected in the American Organization for Nursing Leadership (AONL) nurse executive and nurse manager competencies. Development of related competencies is a lifelong journey of professional growth at every level and is foundational to demonstration of this type of leadership.

Workplace diversity, inclusion, and belonging continue to challenge organizational leaders. RL embodies an inclusive leadership philosophy, facilitating a sense of belonging among employees. Creating a culture where people feel empowered, supported, and receive fair and equal treatment brings innovation, a sense of belonging and fosters collaboration and diversity of thought.

The importance of effective leadership is also reflected in the recommendations of the National Academies of Science, Engineering, and Medicine *Future of Nursing 2020–2030: Charting a Path to Health Equity* report (Wakefield et al., 2021), particularly in regard to implementing structures and systems to ensure nurses' health and well-being, and competency in interprofessional teamwork to advance health equity. "New and established nurse leaders— at all levels and in all settings—are needed to lead change that results in achieving equity in health and health care" (Wakefield et al., 2021, p. 291). Relational leaders are well positioned to influence these imperatives.

RELATIONAL LEADERSHIP

RL is exactly what the words suggest—those leadership styles based on relationships and social connections. After many decades of positional leadership based on formal, top-down power, the evolution from an industrial economy to the complexity of a knowledge economy led to different, relatively new, RL paradigms that enable workers to learn and adapt. Public failures of bureaucratic systems and top-down management in all industries supported a change to a more dynamic leadership as well.

Although studying leader influence and social exchange is dated back to the 1950s, one of the earliest references to RL was in 1998 by three non-healthcare leadership scholars (Komives et al., 1998). Relationship-based leadership is based on positive psychology, the branch of psychology science that focuses on helping people to find meaning and purpose, live meaningful lives, and search for personal strength and value (Snyder et al., 2020). RL is therefore "positive" leadership, grounded in optimism, integrity, building positive emotions, and employee growth and development. The link to nursing leadership is obvious—ethics, positive change, purpose, growth, and social connection are all part of who we are as nurses and nurse leaders. Creating healthy practice environments and staff engagement are outcomes we seek for clinical nurses and all the practice and support disciplines which we may lead. In turn, a positive workforce and practice environment provides the foundation for positive patient outcomes.

The five main components of RL as defined by the Komives et al. (1998) study are inclusion, empowerment, purposefulness, ethical behaviors, and process orientation (Figure 6.1). Relational leaders empower others, building on strengths and improving weaknesses. They have a clear purpose, which they are able to communicate to others. RL is process oriented, focusing on the "how," as opposed to viewing leadership as coming from positional power. These components intersect with the attributes of several prevalent relational styles which we will expand on in this chapter (Box 6.1).

FOLLOWERSHIP AND ENGAGEMENT

An important aspect of RL is that it leads to followership and followers' engagement, which is not seen in nonrelational styles. Without relationships there are no followers, and without followers there are no leaders. This leader–follower relationship is vital, based on mutual goals, and is interwoven with the important workforce outcome, especially for nursing, of staff engagement. Gallup, a global analytics and advice firm, has conducted decades of organizational research on employee engagement. Their "Q12" engagement survey contains 12 key questions reflecting their research on the foundational elements of engagement that predict high performance, and several of them relate to RL (Table 6.1; Gallup, n.d.). The importance of the progression from using hierarchical power to relational influence is evidenced in Gallup's work validating that those employees with higher levels of engagement produce better outcomes, are more likely to be retained, and are less likely to experience burnout (Harter, 2020).

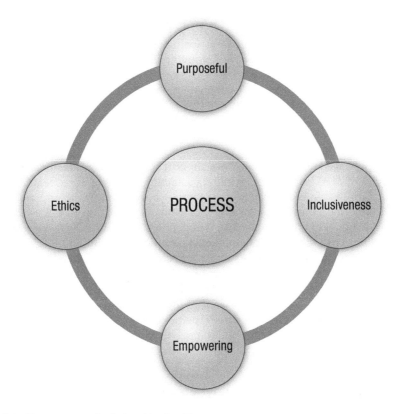

FIGURE 6.1: Components of relational leadership.

- Authentic
- Human-centered
- Resonant
- Servant
- Transformational

TABLE 6.1: Selected Gallup Employee Engagement "Q12" Survey Questions

Gallup "Q12" Engagement Survey Question	Relational Leadership Component
In the last 7 days, I have received recognition or praise for doing good work.	Process-oriented
My supervisor, or someone at work, seems to care about me as a person.	Inclusion
There is someone at work who encourages my development.	Empowering
At work, my opinions seem to count.	Empowering
The mission or purpose of my company makes me feel my job is important.	Purposefulness

Source: Data from Gallup. (n.d.). *The power of Gallup's Q12 employee engagement survey.* https://www.gallup.com/access/323333/q12-employee-engagement-survey.aspx.

NURSING AND RELATIONAL LEADERSHIP

There are nursing-specific engagement surveys which focus on the professional practice environment such as the National Database of Nursing Quality Indicators (NDNQI) RN Satisfaction Survey or the Practice Environment Scale of the Nursing Work Index. Measurement domains typically include autonomy/participation, staffing adequacy, leadership support, interdisciplinary relationships, and quality of care (Norman & Sjetne, 2017). The connection of nurse engagement to outcomes is evident in the literature as both patient and nurse experience are linked to it (Dempsey & Assi, 2018). Relational nurse leadership is a driving force behind nurse engagement.

Nursing thought leaders and researchers support RL models. Cathcart states that relational work is the core of leadership: creating, sustaining, and managing relationships with staff, patients, families, interdisciplinary colleagues, peers, and organizational executives (Cathcart, 2014). Shirey's systematic literature review on leadership practices for a healthy work environment (HWE) concluded that relational leaders contribute to higher nurse satisfaction and better work environments, boosting employee health and well-being (Shirey, 2017). A systematic review of 129 papers was conducted to study leadership styles and outcomes, finding that relational styles promote over 120 different positive nursing workforce and organizational outcomes. The authors conclude that RL practices need to be encouraged to enhance nursing job satisfaction, retention, productivity, and work environment factors in healthcare (Cummings et al., 2018). The imperative to promote relational nurse leadership is evident, understanding that the resulting positive workforce supports positive patient outcomes.

NONRELATIONAL LEADERSHIP STYLES

The Cummings et al. (2018) systematic review compared results between relational styles and "task-oriented" styles, finding that nonrelational styles were insufficient to achieve optimal outcomes for nursing. Task-oriented and other styles of leadership, which we will call "non relational," or without focus on connections, are very different from, although not the opposite of, RL. It is not that there is no relationship with followers, or an opposing one, or even that it is not effective; nonrelational could be characterized as neither "connected" nor empowering.

One of the nonrelational styles is *task-oriented* leadership, which focuses on the job to be done and completing responsibilities. For example, when running a command center for an unscheduled regulatory survey, the incident commander may resort to that style in order to get the required checklist of documents to the waiting surveyors quickly. Another example is the provider-in-charge of a cardiac arrest response who directs the team with orders to be immediately enacted. These autocratic, directive, task-oriented roles are appropriate in those situations, although clearly not a relational style.

Transactional leadership is often referred to as an opposing style to transformational leadership (TL). This style also focuses on task completion; the "transactional" aspect is the use of rewards and punishment as employee motivators. For example, a nurse manager may deny first choice vacation to a staff member for failure to use the sign-up sheet on time. This may be an organization policy, but it is still transactional in nature. So is adding "consequences" for any deviation from following patient safety processes. If we were to differentiate leadership (focus on inspiration and empowerment) from management (focus on execution), then the transactional style would be management. Both can be needed for effective operations. This style can be useful for short-term goals, simple processes, and when a clear chain of command and structure are needed. A systematic review to synthesize current evidence on nursing leadership styles, nurse satisfaction, and patient satisfaction suggested that RL traits contribute to greater nurse satisfaction, whereas task-oriented styles may decrease nurse satisfaction (McCay et al., 2018).

In the 1930s, psychologist Kurt Lewin and his team of researchers described another nonrelational style still seen today, *laissez-faire*. These leaders give little guidance and expect employees to solve their own problems. Self-motivated, creative staff may thrive under this style in certain industries; however, the fast-paced, dynamic healthcare environment is generally not conducive to hands-off leadership. A successful *laissez-faire* leader was Steve Jobs, who as chief executive officer (CEO) of Apple had his brilliant, out-of-the-box ideas and then left it to his employees to figure out. It is theorized that transformational and *laissez-faire* leadership are on a continuum with one on each end, with the transactional style in the middle (Bass & Avolio, 1994), known as Full Range Leadership Theory (FRLT).

Just as new graduates approach beginning their professional practice as a clinical nurse with a task-oriented focus, novice nurse leaders may approach their management practice with a task-oriented style. As growth in the role ensues, along with confidence, self-awareness, learning and feedback, the new leader should move along the continuum to a more relational style aligned with employee and organizational needs. This complexity requires more than tools and tasks; it is leadership that creates meaning about how and why we work together (Davidson, 2020, p. 107).

TRANSFORMATIONAL LEADERSHIP

TL is prevalent in nursing literature and recognized in the American Nurses Credentialing Center (ANCC) Magnet Recognition Program® as one of the five components of their model for nursing excellence (ANCC, n.d.). The origin of TL dates back to 1978 when Burns identified "transforming" leadership in a political context, contrasting it to transactional leadership (Burns, 1978). Bass built upon Burns's work and first described TL in 1985, establishing its place in organizational psychology. He found these leaders influence and motivate followers, offering them an inspiring mission and vision (Bass, 1985). This is the first distinct RL model in the literature.

BASS AND AVOLIO'S "FOUR I's"

Management scholars identified and recognized the characteristics of transformational leaders, framing them as the "Four I's": individualized consideration, intellectual stimulation, inspirational motivation, and idealized influence (Table 6.2; Avolio et al., 1991). Descriptions

TABLE 6.2: Transformational Leadership Attributes/Practices

Bass and Avolio: The "Four I's" Measurement: Multifactor Leadership Questionnaire (MLQ)	Kouzes and Posner Practices Measurement: Leadership Practices Inventory (LPI)
Individualized consideration: Everyone is respected and supported; mentoring	*Encourage the heart:* Recognition and appreciation *Enable others to act:* Collaboration and development
Intellectual stimulation: Open to innovation	*Challenge the process:* Open to innovation
Inspirational motivation: Convincing communication Charisma	*Inspire a shared vision:* Convincing communication
Idealized influence: Role modeling Charisma	*Model the way:* Role modeling

Source: Avolio, B. J., Waldman, D. A., & Yammarino, F. J. (1991). Leading in the 1990s: The four I's of transformational leadership. *Journal of European Industrial Training, 15*(4). https://doi.org/10.1108/03090599110143366; Kouzes, J. M., & Posner, B. Z. (2007). *The leadership challenge* (4th ed.). Jossey-Bass.

of these characteristics are relational in nature and are applicable to healthy nursing practice environments. *Individualized consideration* is the personalized connections the leader makes with followers, treating each as a unique individual, within a work environment that is safe and supportive. *Intellectual stimulation* is how the leader is open-minded and promotes creativity and innovation. *Inspirational motivation* is reliant on the leader's ability to communicate a compelling vision and high standards with subsequent follower enthusiasm and motivation to exceed expectations. *Idealized influence* is both the role modeling and follower respect the leader generates from their behaviors. The measurement tool used for this model is the Multifactor Leadership Questionnaire (MLQ), which is a 45-item questionnaire measuring the three leadership styles in the FRLT: transformational, transactional, and *laissez-faire* (Bass & Avolio, n.d.).

Followers may ascribe extraordinary capabilities to the transformational leader. An element of charisma is part of the leader's influence in this model. In nursing we easily see how the "Four I's" translate to a desired practice environment where professional development, staff engagement, and visionary leadership flourishes.

These scholars from organizational psychology continued to develop the theory including the influence of organizational culture on leadership and vice versa. If the organization values autonomy and trust in its people and shared decision-making, then the transformational leader can build on it using the "Four I's." The converse is true as the leader can influence organizational culture with their behaviors, beliefs, and expectations (Bass & Avolio, 1993). Shirey describes positive organizational culture as the "cement" between leadership and HWEs (Shirey, 2009). We have all seen failed leaders who did not "fit" into the organizational culture, and the opposite—transformational leaders who have contributed to positive change in the organizational culture and leave lasting legacies (Figure 6.2).

 CASE SCENARIO

TRANSFORMATIONAL LEADERSHIP: DIRECTOR LEVEL

SITUATION

MP is a director of women and children's nursing in a community hospital. The ED is experiencing frequent surges in adolescent psychiatric patients needing admission; however, there is a lack of psychiatric pediatric beds in the community. The patients are being held in the ED for days waiting for a bed.

APPROACH

MP works with all stakeholders to develop MP's vision of finding an innovative approach to meet the immediate needs of these patients and families, to include the ED, providers, inpatient nurses, social work, child life, and others, using a multimodal approach. MP meets individually and collectively in-person and via electronic communication, always focusing on the collective purpose of the patient and family needs of this vulnerable population.

OUTCOME

The group lands on the decision to admit to inpatient pediatrics while awaiting the appropriate psychiatric bed despite the challenges of caring for these patients. Plans to make the environment and care plan safe for all are finalized. Several patients are managed safely in this manner, and the group is enthusiastic about the outcome.

DISCUSSION QUESTIONS

1. Using the "Four I's," which attributes of TL is MP using in their approach?
2. If MP's sole approach was to give the directive to move the patients to inpatient beds, what could have resulted?

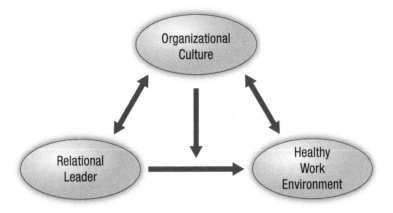

FIGURE 6.2: Relationship among leadership, work environment, and organizational culture.

KOUZES AND POSNER'S FIVE LEADERSHIP PRACTICES

These attributes were further developed by Kouzes and Posner, who described five leadership practices of the transformational leader: model the way, inspire a shared vision, challenge the process, enable others to act, and encourage the heart (Kouzes & Posner, 2007; Table 6.2). These practices relate to the "Four I's" and are worded in an understandable, conversational way that led to wide acceptance by the nursing community. *Modeling the way* for defined expectations and shared values with the leader consistently setting the example; *inspiring a shared vision* for the future that appeals to and motivates followers; *challenge the process* by being open to improvement through innovation, risk-taking, and learning along the way; *enable others to act* through collaboration, teamwork, and development; and *encourage the heart* by leader recognition, appreciation, and celebration of accomplishments both individually and as a team. All five of these practices are relationship-based. The measurement tool used for this model is the Leadership Practices Inventory (LPI), a 30-item questionnaire that assesses behaviors with six questions about each of the five practices (Kouzes & Posner, n.d.).

NURSING AND TRANSFORMATIONAL LEADERSHIP

Florence Nightingale can be considered the first nursing transformational leader. She was innovative, influential, respected, and role-modeled modern nursing. Aligning TL to the Magnet Recognition Model catapulted its significance in nursing. ANCC notes that the intent of this model component is not only for leaders to solve problems, but actually transform the organization through vision, influence, expertise, and innovation to meet the future demands of the healthcare system (ANCC, n.d.). TL's place as an essential characteristic of Magnet® organizations with HWEs has not wavered in decades.

Using the LPI as a self-assessment, a study of the TL practices of 56 Magnet chief nursing officers (CNOs) found the top two TL practices of these CNOs are enabling others to act and modeling the way, followed by inspiring a shared vision (Prado-Inzerillo et al., 2018). Buck and Doucette also studied the TL practices of CNOs, this time in Pathway to Excellence (PTE)-designated organizations, finding that the TL practice domains enable others to act and encourage the heart were the highest self-ranked practices (Buck & Doucette, 2015). In both studies, enabling others to act was the top-ranked practice, underscoring the importance of empowerment to CNOs. Exemplary practice environments require professional governance structures with shared decision-making, collaboration, and teamwork, hallmarks of enabling others to act.

Just as CNO TL practices can significantly contribute to the creation and maintenance of healthy practice environments, there is a positive influence of nurse managers' TL behaviors on empowerment, job satisfaction, and the self-reported frequency of adverse patient outcomes (Boamah et al., 2018). Merrill also found TL was a contributor to a safety climate (Merrill, 2015). The potential impact of TL on engagement and positive patient outcomes is a strong rationale to develop this style in nurse leaders. Several studies have found a positive relationship between emotional intelligence (EI) and TL (Echevarria et al., 2017; Spano-Szekely et al., 2016). Development of EI competency may contribute, or even predict, the nurse leader's ability to practice as a transformational leader.

POTENTIAL DISADVANTAGES

Along with the potential and actual effects of TL, there are downsides to this style. In the highly regulated world of healthcare and nursing, there are many detail-oriented tasks that need attention. The transformational leader may need to partner or delegate those overall responsibilities to ensure the focus is not only on their big picture vision, but also on the management elements of their role. Using the same comparison of transformational to transactional, some employees may be task-oriented and not willing or able to contribute more broadly to "greater things." As long as defined job responsibilities are met, this would be considered acceptable in most organizations, garnering a "meets standard" performance evaluation; however, to the transformational leader, it could be considered indifference if the employee is not reaching higher levels of contribution. This tendency should be avoided.

 CASE SCENARIO

TRANSFORMATIONAL LEADERSHIP: CHIEF NURSING OFFICER LEVEL

SITUATION

The energetic CNO of a specialty orthopedic hospital was told by the CEO that the board of trustees wanted the hospital to become Magnet-designated. The CNO had not been a huge supporter of the Magnet journey in the past as designation did not seem to be an adequate return on investment for the work and expense.

APPROACH

The CNO took on the challenge and began creating a vision for nursing reflecting excellence in patient care, the basis for the standards. The CNO inspired both their nurse leaders and staff with the vision, holding rousing town halls and Magnet fairs. The CNO was very convincing, and everyone rallied around their vision. Nurse leaders set up structure and processes to meet all the model components and standards.

OUTCOME

During the 4-year journey, practice was transformed, clinical outcomes edged above national standards, and staff engagement was at an all-time high. The CNO continued to inspire, using their charismatic personality to maintain everyone's motivation and willingness to keep pushing forward. Their efforts were a success, and the organization achieved Magnet designation.

DISCUSSION QUESTIONS

1. Which TL practices from Kouzes and Posner were used by this CNO?
2. "Encourage the heart" strategies were not mentioned in the case scenario. Is it possible to have this outcome without recognition and appreciation?
3. The CNO did not value the Magnet program prior to this experience. How did that affect the TL they demonstrated?

AUTHENTIC LEADERSHIP

Historically, the origins of authentic leadership (AL) are based on multiple business scandals seen in the early 2000s, such as Enron, which led to interest in a shift from "arrogant" leadership to genuine leaders who instill hope, trust, optimism, and resiliency (Avolio et al., 2004). Authenticity was noted to be on a continuum, rather than an either/or, and that the truer the leader is to their core values, the more authentic the leader becomes. Authentic leaders were described as having high moral character, acting in alignment with their personal values, building credibility and the positive emotions of respect, hope, and trust of followers, resulting in positive behaviors such as satisfaction, motivation, and performance. Contextual factors are noted to influence the relationship such as organizational culture, politics, and structure, as discussed earlier in the interaction between the leader and organizational culture (Figure 6.2).

Four core elements of AL were identified: self-awareness, balanced processing, relational transparency, and an internalized moral perspective. *Self-awareness* is the leader's continuous self-reflection and willingness to seek feedback; *balanced processing* is seeking differing perspectives and analyzing information objectively, which is also described as being "open-hearted"; *relational transparency* is the open sharing of thoughts, feelings, and beliefs, easily connecting with others; and an *internalized moral perspective* refers to a strong ethical foundation and acting in accord with one's values (Avolio & Gardner, 2005); in nursing, this is the "nursing compass" and may also be referred to as moral courage (Table 6.3). Authentic leaders are anchored by their own inner core values and deep sense of self; they know where they stand on important issues, values, and beliefs. Their positive relationships with followers lead to positive individual and organizational outcomes. This style can be measured by the Authentic Leadership Questionnaire (ALQ), which is a 16-item instrument that assesses the four attributes of AL (Walumbwa et al., 2008).

NURSING AND AUTHENTIC LEADERSHIP

As a complement to the 2005 landmark publication by the American Association of Critical-Care Nurses (2005), *Standards for Establishing and Sustaining Healthy Work Environments (HWEs): A Journey to Excellence,* Shirey describes in a stepwise way how AL influences outcomes—first through nurse engagement, leading to an HWE and then potential patient outcomes. This framework captures the importance, scope, and significance of AL. Shirey proposes that AL is the preferred style of leadership for creating and sustaining HWEs as the "glue that holds it together" (Figure 6.3; Shirey, 2006).

TABLE 6.3: Authentic Leadership Attributes

Authentic Leadership Four Attributes	Authentic Nurse Leadership Five Attributes in Three Domains
Self-awareness	Personal integrity: Self-awareness Moral-ethical courage
Internalized moral perspective	
Balanced processing	Transparency: Shared decision-making Relational integrality
Relational transparency	
	Altruism: Caring

Source: Avolio, B. J., & Gardner, W. L. (2005). Authentic leadership development: Getting to the root of positive forms of leadership. *The Leadership Quarterly, 16*(3), 315–338. https://doi.org/10.1016/j.leaqua.2005.03.001; Giordano-Mulligan, M., & Eckardt, S. (2019). Authentic nurse leadership conceptual framework: Nurses' perception of authentic nurse leader attributes. *Nursing Administration Quarterly, 43*(2), 164–174. https://doi.org/10.1097/NAQ.0000000000000344.

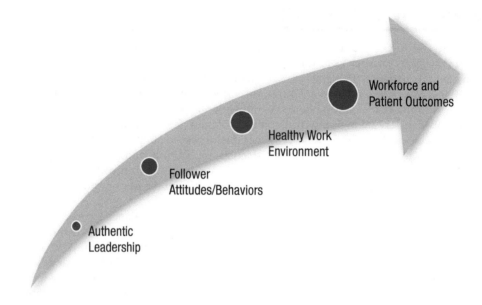

FIGURE 6.3: Model for authentic leadership, followership, and outcomes.

Source: Adapted from Shirey, M. R. (2006). Authentic leaders creating healthy work environments for nursing practice. *American Journal of Critical Care, 15*(3), 256–267. https://doi.org/10.4037/AJCC2006.15.3.256.

Nursing researchers have conducted multiple studies focused on AL, staff engagement, and job satisfaction, all with positive findings on the relationship between AL and workforce outcomes; for example, the role AL plays in retaining new graduate nurses (Fallatah et al., 2017), in decreasing new graduate burnout (Laschinger et al., 2012, 2013), and in influencing staff nurses' structural empowerment (Wong & Laschinger, 2013). In a scoping review of the literature from 2017 to 2019, Wong identified 27 studies focused on AL in nursing. Although the majority of these studies were conducted in the United States and Canada, there were 11 other countries in which AL among nurses was studied. Several personal and organizational variables were linked to AL including job satisfaction, turnover, work attitudes and behaviors, and staff empowerment (Wong & Walsh, 2020). Alilyyani and colleagues (2018) published a systematic review of antecedents, mediators, and outcomes of AL in healthcare, predominantly in acute care settings. Review of 136 manuscripts found associations with 43 positive outcomes including work satisfaction, work environment, health and well-being, and job performance, with 23 mediators such as incivility and burnout affecting the relationship between AL and the positive outcomes, illustrating the complexity of factors which can influence leadership effectiveness for the nurse leader. There was one patient outcome—a relationship with falls (Alilyyani et al., 2018).

AUTHENTIC NURSE LEADERSHIP

Giordano-Mulligan and Eckardt (2019) conceptualized the authentic *nurse* leadership model which was developed to be congruent with current nursing leadership attributes. These researchers created, implemented, and validated an instrument for their model, finding that nurses perceived a significant relationship between authentic nurse leaders' attributes, nurse engagement, and nurse work–life balance (Giordano-Mulligan & Eckardt, 2019). Previous nursing studies utilized the AL models that were developed and validated in disciplines other than nursing.

The authentic nursing leadership (ANL) model modifies the four historical attributes to align with contemporary nursing concepts and adds a fifth, caring (Figure 6.4). The five attributes of ANL are moral and ethical courage, self-awareness, relational integrality, shared decision-making, and caring (Table 6.3) in three domains: personal integrity, transparency,

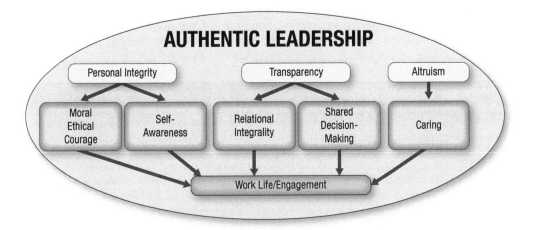

FIGURE 6.4: Giordano-Mulligan/Eckardt's authentic nurse leadership conceptual framework.

Source: Giordano-Mulligan, M., & Eckardt, S. (2019). Authentic nurse leadership conceptual framework: Nurses' perception of authentic nurse leader attributes. *Nursing Administration Quarterly, 43*(2), 164–174. https://doi.org/10.1097/NAQ.0000000000000344.

and altruism. *Moral and ethical courage* is akin to the "internalized moral perspective" of authentic leaders who have sound moral convictions aligned with their deeply held values, even under pressure. *Self-awareness* describes resilient leaders with personal insight. *Relational integrality* refers to open and honest leaders. *Shared decision-making* is the skill of evaluating all alternatives and being open to all ideas. It is the new attribute of *caring* which especially differentiates the ANL model from historical AL. Giordano-Mulligan and Eckardt note that caring is one of the metaparadigm concepts in nursing and important to the discipline; authentic nurse leaders care for themselves and others (Giordano-Mulligan & Eckardt, 2019). The measurement tool used for this model is the Authentic Nurse Leadership Questionnaire (ANLQ), a 29-item questionnaire that rates overall perception of ANL and its five attributes (Giordano-Mulligan & Eckardt, 2019).

Raso and colleagues conducted two correlational studies using the ANL model (2020, 2021), finding a positive relationship between perceptions of ANL and HWE in both studies. In the first study, nurses rated the ANL of their manager as present most of the time and as perceptions of ANL increased, so did perceptions of HWE, highlighting that AL matters. In the second study during the COVID-19 pandemic, over 5,000 U.S. nurses perceived ANL and HWE were present despite a high level of pandemic impact, signaling that nurse leaders authentically rose to meet frontline leadership needs at a time of extreme stress on the nursing workforce (Raso et al., 2020, 2021).

DIFFERENCE BETWEEN TRANSFORMATIONAL AND AUTHENTIC LEADERSHIP

Being an authentic leader does not necessarily mean that the leader is transformational, and transformational leaders are not necessarily anchored in their own deep sense of self and where they stand on important values (Avolio & Gardner, 2005). TL is often described as being charismatic, differentiated from AL by the ability to transform through a powerful vision and clear sense of purpose. Moral courage is not generally emphasized in TL as it is in AL. The difference may be a distinction between character and charisma.

Both styles contribute to positive outcomes. Wei et al.'s (2020) systematic review found that nurse leadership plays a significant role in reducing nurse burnout. The major influencing leadership styles include AL and TL, through empowering and promoting nurse engagement and creating an HWE (Wei et al., 2020). Banks et al.'s meta-analysis (2016) found empirical redundancy in AL and TL, evident by a strong correlation between the two constructs. There were two distinctions: AL was dominant over TL to predict organizational performance such as task performance and citizenship behaviors, and TL outperformed AL in regards to attitudinal behaviors such as follower satisfaction (Banks et al., 2016). Further exploration between these and other relational styles is warranted.

⬡ CASE SCENARIO

AUTHENTIC NURSE LEADERSHIP

SITUATION

Mercy General, a 150-bed community hospital, was recently merged into a neighboring large healthcare system. Mercy did not have a robust shared governance structure except for a few units with local staff committees. The chief nurse executive (CNE) of the large system expected Mercy to adopt their shared governance model which included multiple hospital councils, a co-ordinating council, and local unit-based councils.

APPROACH

The nursing leadership team of Mercy sought to implement the model. As a first step, they held focus groups with staff for their perceptions of current professional practice decision-making and their ideas on how to proceed and implement the model. Staff already had appreciation for their leaders' support and were enthusiastic about greater collaboration. They requested paid time for governance activities, which was granted. Leaders and staff partnered to get the councils up and running, with defined charters and a clear path for structure, process, and goals. Clinical council chairs were nurtured by leaders in their new roles.

OUTCOME

Staff attendance was at least 80% at all meetings and most of the councils worked on two projects to completion in the first year after implementation, both at the hospital and local levels. Positive impact on workforce or patient outcomes was achieved in 75% of the projects. The nursing leadership team presented the results to the system CNE, who congratulated them on exceeding expectations.

DISCUSSION QUESTIONS

1. Which elements of authentic nurse leadership are represented in this scenario?
2. Why were these leaders able to implement the new shared governance model so successfully in a relatively short period of time?

SERVANT LEADERSHIP

SL was first identified in 1970 by Robert Greenleaf in *The Servant as Leader*, writing "[t]he servant-leader is servant first. . . . focus[ing] primarily on the growth and well-being of people and communities to which they belong" (Greenleaf Center for Servant Leadership, n.d., paras. 2, 4). The concept of SL dates to centuries-old leadership categorized as the service of people and country. Greenleaf (1977) often refers to religious philosophies such as Jesus Christ as the exemplar for his concept of the servant leader, recognizing the feasibility of uniting the positions of servant and leader in one being. Greenleaf states "[t]he servant-leader is servant first. . . . then [a] conscious choice brings one to aspire to lead" (Greenleaf Center for Servant Leadership, n.d., para. 2).

SL reverses the organizational pyramid, creating an environment where everyone has the potential to serve as a leader. In the SL model, the most senior leaders are situated at the bottom of the pyramid with employees and customers (patients) situated at the top, which is

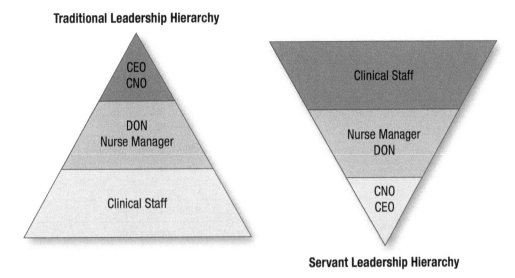

FIGURE 6.5: Traditional/servant leadership hierarchy.

CEO, chief executive officer; CNO, chief nursing officer; DON, department of nursing.

TABLE 6.4: "Old School" Traditional Leadership Versus Servant Leadership

	"Old School"	Servant
Motivation	Leading	Serving
Approach	Top-down	Bottom-up
Focus	Business	People
Self-awareness	Not important	Important
People development	May not develop	Definitely will develop

a significant shift in the organizational pyramid (Figure 6.5). This service component is what differentiates SL from other leadership styles as highlighted in Table 6.4, which shows the contrast between traditional and servant leaders. The servant-leader shares power, places the needs of others first, and helps people grow and perform as highly as possible (Greenleaf Center for Servant Leadership, n.d.).

CHARACTERISTICS AND BEHAVIORS

Larry Spears, a prominent SL theorist, draws upon Greenleaf's literature highlighting 10 characteristics of SL: *actively listening, being empathetic, providing a healing environment, EI and self-awareness,* using *powers of persuasion* rather than coercive power, *conceptualization* to focus on the bigger picture, foresight, *stewardship, commitment to the growth of people,* and *building a sense of community* among the staff (Spears, 1998; Table 6.5).

Laub (1999), another well-known SL theorist, highlighted six main characteristics important to the development of a servant leader, which when well demonstrated yields a successful work culture. These characteristics/behaviors are *displaying authenticity, valuing people, sharing leadership, providing leadership, developing people,* and *building community* by developing strong collaborative and personal relationships (Table 6.6). Laub developed the Organizational Leadership Assessment (OLA) to assess organizational health, which measures SL as a six-factor construct (Laub, n.d.).

TABLE 6.5: Servant Leadership Characteristics and Behaviors—Aligning of Spears, Laub, and Coetzer, Bussin, and Geldenhuys

Spears (1998) Ten Characteristics	Laub (1999) Six Behaviors	Coetzer, Bussin, and Geldenhuys (2017) Eight Characteristics and *Four Competencies
Listening	Displaying authenticity	Listening
Awareness		Authenticity, Humility
Empathy	Valuing people	Compassion
Healing		
Persuasion	Sharing leadership	*Empowerment
Conceptualization	Providing leadership	*Compelling vision
Foresight		
Stewardship		Accountability *Stewardship
Commitment to the growth of people	Developing people	Altruism
Building community	Building community	*Building relationships
		Courage, Integrity

Source: Spears, L. C. (1998). Tracing the growing impact of servant leadership. In L. C. Spears (Ed.), *Insights on leadership: Service, stewardship, spirit, and servant leadership* (pp. 1–12). John Wiley and Sons; Laub, J. (1999). *Assessing the servant organization: Development of the servant organizational leadership (SOLA) instrument* (Doctoral thesis). Florida Atlantic University; Coetzer, M. F., Bussin, M., & Geldenhuys, M. (2017). The functions of a servant leader. *Administrative Sciences*, 7(1), 5. https://doi.org/10.3390/admsci7010005.

TABLE 6.6: Servant Leader Outcomes at Individual Level

Positive Outcomes	Positive Impact on Negative Outcomes
Work engagement Organizational citizenship behaviors Creativity and innovation Trust Job satisfaction	Turnover intention Burnout

Source: Data from Coetzer, M. F., Bussin, M., & Geldenhuys, M. (2017). The functions of a servant leader. *Administrative Sciences*, 7(1), 5. https://doi.org/10.3390/admsci7010005.

Spear's (1998) 10 characteristics of SL serve as the starting point for leaders to develop as servant leaders, whereas Laub's model, as previously discussed, simplifies it. What differentiates the two is that Spears's model focuses primarily on the general characteristics of servant leaders and Laub's model focuses primarily on the behaviors of servant leaders (Laub, 2018). In addition, Coetzer et al. identified eight characteristics of SL in a systematic review—*authenticity, humility, compassion, accountability, courage, altruism, integrity,* and *listening* (Coetzer et al., 2017)—and four competencies—*empowerment, stewardship, building relationships,* and *compelling vision.* The connections between the three researchers are highlighted in Table 6.5.

The defining attribute of SL is its emphasis on service to others. The servant leader places employees first and supports their well-being and growth, which is unique among the RL styles. Servant leaders engage others, including all members of the care team, in establishing policies and practices that advance the mission (Dye, 2017). SL engages others in decision-making, grounded in ethical and caring behavior, enriching growth while cultivating the quality of organizational life.

NURSING AND SERVANT LEADERSHIP

Neville et al.'s concept analysis identified a linkage among SL characteristics, caring theories, and the profession of nursing (Neville et al., 2021). The attributes of empowerment, altruism, compassion, and relationships clearly relate to nursing values. Both clinical and formal leaders need valuable leadership skills, and SL priorities align with all levels of nursing whether a charge nurse, manager, or executive (Savel & Munro, 2017). SL permits an individual to demonstrate leadership without requiring the spotlight. It is the combination of humility, collaboration, and a meaningful work experience that leads to positive results. SL allows people who may not have a classic leadership personality (e.g., outgoing, or take-charge) to step forward and support the organization and support each other.

Berwick, the former CEO of the Institute for Healthcare Improvement (IHI), noted the irony of healthcare where caring should be the focus, yet many healthcare professionals are experiencing burnout and a loss of joy in their work. As frontline nurses endure challenging times, a nurse leader with an SL style can serve to combat burnout, disengagement, and turnover (Sherman, 2019).

SERVANT LEADERSHIP OUTCOMES

SL is positively correlated with follower outcomes. The best test of the leader is whether those served grow as individuals and, while being served, do they become healthier, wiser, and in a better position to become servant leaders themselves (Greenleaf, 1977).

Coetzer et al. identified eight characteristics of SL in a systematic review—*authenticity, humility, compassion, accountability, courage, altruism, integrity,* and *listening*—and four competencies—*empowerment, stewardship, building relationships,* and *compelling vision* (Coetzer et al., 2017). The connections between the three researchers are highlighted in Table 6.5. The outcomes associated with SL were grouped by Coetzer et al. (2017) into individual outcomes, team outcomes, and organizational outcomes. On an individual level, SL positively affected work engagement, organizational citizenship behavior, creativity and innovation, organizational commitment, trust, self-efficacy, job satisfaction, person–job fit or person–organizational fit, leader–member exchange, and work–life balance (Table 6.6). Additionally, SL was negatively correlated with burnout and turnover intention. On a team or group level, group organizational citizenship behavior, group identification, service culture or climate, and the procedural justice climate were positively influenced by SL. Lastly, on an organizational level, SL was positively correlated with customer service and sales performance. The outcomes were applied to categorize four overall functions of a servant leader grouped into strategic servant and operational SL. Each function was maintained by the competencies and characteristics of a servant leader as described in Table 6.5. These findings provided a theoretical contribution to the body of knowledge related to SL as well as a potential framework to develop servant leaders within organizations (Coetzer et al., 2017).

ADVANTAGES AND DISADVANTAGES OF SERVANT LEADERSHIP

Servant leaders value people, enabling them to develop and flourish, putting the concept of caring into leadership. One disadvantage is that servant leaders disturb the concept of hierarchy, with the nomenclature of "servant" possibly seen as detrimental to nurses. Humility can be perceived as a weakness, and some workers may not respond to this approach. It also can be perceived as a "religious" concept, which is alienating to some people.

In summary, SL is a management style that produces favorable outcomes, enhances morale, focuses on people, and generates support for the leaders (Dye, 2017). SL is conceptualized as a relationship-focused style that followers identify as being considerate and understanding and not necessarily prescriptive with regard to how work should be done.

CASE SCENARIO
SERVANT LEADERSHIP

SITUATION

The CNO at a world-renowned medical center was alarmed that, despite the hospital's reputation for excellence, the Hospital Consumer Assessment of Healthcare Providers and Systems (HCAHPS) patient experience scores were not on par with its clinical results. The CNO, CEO, and chief human resources officer (CHRO) on leadership rounds were surprised to hear concerns expressed by staff about feeling underappreciated and undervalued. Gallup was hired to conduct an employee engagement survey and the results were not encouraging.

APPROACH

As employee engagement has been shown to correlate with patient satisfaction, the executive leadership team focused on local level engagement strategies. The nurse manager on a high-performing unit was asked to help with three lower performing units. The nurse manager explained to their colleagues that they have a unit-based recognition program to acknowledge staff mentioned in patient compliments and HCAHPS reports, as well as other accomplishments or collaborative work. In addition, the nurse manager regularly meets with every employee at least twice a year to review their professional goals and progress. The other managers started using these nurturing and caring staff strategies in a structured way.

OUTCOME

Six months later, the three lower performing units started to see a steady upward trend in their nursing-sensitive HCAHPS outcomes.

DISCUSSION QUESTIONS

1. Was there a direct correlation between the newly used strategies for employee engagement and the HCAHPS results?
2. How is SL reflected in this case scenario?

HUMAN-CENTERED LEADERSHIP

HCL is a relatively new nursing leadership theory, based on complexity science that focuses on the satisfaction and effectiveness of the leader. The premise of HCL theory is "it starts with you, but it's not all about you." The human-centered leader recognizes the importance of self-care, self-compassion, self-awareness, and mindfulness. The HCL visual framework reflects an innovative approach to leadership in healthcare that starts with the leader's mind, body, and spirit as the locus of influence within local and larger complex systems. Through appreciation of humanity and nurturing the growth in others, the human-centered leader realizes success in connecting leadership attributes of the *connector, awakener*, and *upholder* to cultures of excellence, caring, and trust (Leclerc et al., 2021). The *awakener* is described as an architect who creates structure and processes, setting the vision that motivates the team to develop a culture of excellence in achieving patient outcomes. The *connector* focuses on building a community which supports an HWE and a culture of trust. The *upholder* supports the culture of caring for the team, recognizing the humanity in others while creating an exceptional experience for all.

Characteristics of the *awakener* are motivator, coach, mentor, architect, and advocate. Characteristics of the *connector* are collaborator, supporter, edge-walker (leader who walks the edge between the way things have always been done), and the innovation engineer (sees strengths in each person so their strengths will motivate the team; an authentic communicator who will walk the talk). Characteristics of the *upholder* include personal well-being and mindfulness (leader demonstrates these practices to their team, which has a huge impact), others-oriented mindset (leading means serving), and emotional awareness (Leclerc et al., 2020). HCL aligns with the characteristics of a RL style.

RESONANT LEADERSHIP

Resonance is a concept that involves the use of emotional, financial, environmental, social, and cultural intelligence to inspire followers to convey their best in all circumstances to achieve desired results (Boyatzis & McKee, 2005; Cummings, 2004). Resonant leadership is a relationally focused leadership style that is unique from other leadership theories by its foundation on EI. Resonant leaders use their EI skills to manage their emotions and the emotions of those they work with. Resonant leaders develop positive work environments and are mindful of organizational needs that contribute to positive organizational outcomes. These qualities make them effective leaders (Boyatzis & McKee, 2005). The characteristic of resonant leaders is the ability to work with their teams, creating positive work environments that encourage employee engagement resulting in improved job satisfaction and staff retention (Cummings et al., 2010). Nursing practice flourishes when relationships between managers and nurses are collaborative, and managers exhibit the EI fundamentals of self-awareness, self-management, social awareness, and relationship management (Wagner et al., 2013). A Canadian study of over 1,200 nurses found that resonant leadership is instrumental in creating empowering work environments and higher job satisfaction (Bawafaa et al., 2015).

Boyatzis and McKee (2005), Cummings et al. (2005), and Squires et al. (2010) call for robust RL skills for nurse leaders precisely, skills that involve high levels of EI known as resonant leadership. These skills include team support, mentorship, relationship building, and engaging others in organizational goals that are key attributes of resonant leaders (Boyatzis & McKee, 2005).

RELATIONAL LEADER DEVELOPMENT

The best approach to developing nurse leaders is not known. The paths are varied, including self-development, 1:1 coaching/mentoring/precepting, organizational home-grown programs, continuing education courses, content and fellowships from professional organizations, and academic programs at every level from generic to post-doctorate curriculums. The latest American Association of Colleges of Nursing *Core Essentials* includes a domain, *personal, professional, and leadership development*, described as "participation in activities and self-reflection that foster personal health, resilience, and well-being, lifelong learning, and support the acquisition of nursing expertise and assertion of leadership" (American Association of Colleges of Nursing, 2021, p. 11). Specific entry and advanced level leadership skills are identified in the document. A synthesis of 27 nursing leadership development studies supported the importance of evidence-based program content including academic education (Galuska, 2014).

Onboarding programs for nurse managers are inconsistent. Structured and mentored onboarding practices are suggested for training and retention such as a 100-day plan with an experienced mentor using the American Organization of Nurse Executives (AONE) nurse manager competency framework (Sherman & Saifman, 2018). Pedersen and colleagues developed a 3-month intensive residency program for emerging leaders using role exposure, didactic learning sessions, written materials, and a nurse executive coach. Of the 34 individuals who completed the program, 88% transitioned to leadership roles and there was a 97% retention rate at the 10-year mark (Pedersen et al., 2018). In another study of nurse managers, self-assessed competencies improved after a professional development program that included a project (McGarity et al., 2020). These papers are not specific to relational behaviors.

Frasier studied AL development in nurse managers (2019) using a longitudinal design before and after a formal educational program based on AL theory. Although there were increases in all domains, there was only a significant difference in one self-awareness indicator. Alexander studied the leader behaviors that nurse executives use to create and sustain HWEs that support the American Association of Colleges of Nursing standard of AL, stating that AL can be learned and simulated in leadership development programs in the academic and practice setting (Alexander & Lopez, 2018). There are very few empirical studies on AL development, underscoring a gap in nursing knowledge. Non-empirically, Shirey has noted that becoming an authentic leader involves a personal journey of self-discovery, self-improvement, and reflection (Shirey, 2006), and that relationally focused leadership "can be learned, but requires time, effort, and dedicated practice" (Shirey, 2017, p. 48).

For TL, Fischer's concept analysis (2016), in addition to evidence of the influence of TL on organizational culture and patient outcomes, concluded that TL can be defined as a set of teachable competencies to include EI, communication, collaboration, coaching, and mentoring. Buck and Doucette (2015) state that training does not have to start and stop at executive or senior-level leaders; aspiring leaders should be taught what to do and how to practice TL behaviors. Another study on TL practice development used LPI self-assessments for 261 CNOs, directors, and managers and found managers and those below would benefit most from additional education, with upper levels mostly benefiting from content on challenge the process and inspire a shared vision (Herman et al., 2015).

Although not specific to RL, the importance of diversity was successfully addressed with a 4-month nursing leader mentorship program tailored to 16 Black nurses in a New York City academic medical center. More improvement is recommended through mentorship, networking, sponsorship, and a direct career path (Brown-DeVeaux et al., 2021). A more diverse nursing leadership pool will encourage new ideas and workplace improvements, which are hallmarks of RL.

A deeper understanding and empiric evidence of successful ways to teach RL competencies and behaviors needs further exploration. Programming based on transactional functions, which is typical of new manager onboarding sessions, will not develop a leader's relational competencies. Development plans can be based on feedback of observed behaviors in addition to self-assessments using available instruments. Structured curriculum, peer support, self-reflection, experiential learning, coaching, mentoring (see Chapter 7, "The Coaching and Mentoring Process"), and supportive practice environments will support nurses in their lifelong journey of leader development, from aspiring leaders to CNOs and from the bedside to the boardroom. Both structure and nurture are indicated.

◆ CASE SCENARIO

LEADERSHIP DEVELOPMENT

SITUATION

JP is a new nurse manager of a 30-bed medical–surgical unit. JP was an assistant nurse manager on the night shift for 1 year on a smaller, adjacent unit and is in the first half of a master's program in nursing administration. They expressed fear and anxiety to their director as the unit's nursing-sensitive quality outcomes were below target and JP did not feel confident to take on unit leadership.

APPROACH

JP's director enrolled them in a hospital-based leadership program which included content to help JP meet the position responsibilities. In addition, a peer mentor volunteered to work with JP, and the quality department assigned a specialist to assist with the action plan for the quality indicators. JP developed a quality unit committee to engage staff in the plan.

OUTCOME

After 1 year, the unit's quality outcomes began to trend in a positive direction. The quality committee met monthly, focused on best practices and both process and outcome measures. JP
expressed joy at their progress as a leader and pride in their unit to the director, and was named
a Rising Star Leader in the organization.

DISCUSSION QUESTIONS

1. What skills and experience did JP develop prior to their promotion to the role?
2. Did peer mentoring and structured content contribute to JP's development as a leader?

◻ WHAT EVERY NURSE MANAGER NEEDS TO KNOW ABOUT RELATIONSHIP-BASED LEADERSHIP

A nurse manager's role is critical to providing day-to-day operations with 24-hour
responsibility of patient care unit(s), holding the link between the organizational
strategic plan and the point of care, in addition to providing inspiration and leadership
to nurses and other members of the healthcare team. New nurse managers may start
out as task-oriented; however, over time, they develop a balance between management
and RL. When it comes to balancing management versus leadership, it is just that—a
balancing act where nurse managers need to find the balance. Nurse managers need
to possess both: being inspirational (leadership) while concurrently managing care
delivery, often down to the strategy for the next hour (management; Raso, 2015).

Nurse managers set the tone for the unit, supporting an environment where nurses
are engaged and empowered. There is evidence of the effect of nurse managers' RL
behaviors on job satisfaction, engagement, empowerment, and patient safety outcomes.
Nurse managers are in a position to influence the nurses' professional practice
environment. Effective RL and HWE have been linked to positive patient and staff
outcomes. Evidence has shown that unless work environments are healthy, patient
safety is threatened. With nurses as the largest healthcare frontline workforce, the
nurses' work environment is critical. In a healthcare environment of value-based care
and high-performance expectations, leadership that influences outcomes is vital. Use of
RL styles such as authentic, transformational, resonant, and SL are regularly applied in
nursing management. AL is when the leader "walks the talk," provides the leadership
needed by the nursing staff, and believes and contributes to the promotion of an HWE.
The potential impact of RL on engagement and positive patient outcomes is a strong
rationale to develop this style in nurse leaders.

Relational work is the core of leadership practice. The use of individual and
professional values is significant in the practice of inspiring collaborative leadership
styles, such as TL and AL. When healthy relationships with staff members exist, they
are engaged, motivated, and willing to work with you. Developing these important
relationships is vital to the success of the nurse manager. As seen in most relationships,
it takes time, effective communication, and energy to develop trust. Nurse managers
must be available, authentic, self-confident, and respectful in order to develop trusting
relationships.

The nurse manager is responsible for creating safe, healthy environments that
support the work of the healthcare team and contribute to patient engagement. The
role is influential in creating a professional environment and fostering a culture where
interdisciplinary team members are able to contribute to optimal patient outcomes and
grow professionally. Nursing leadership is important at every level in healthcare, and
being a full partner necessitates RL skills and competencies. To make certain that nurses

are able to take on leadership roles, leadership competencies should be advocated for nurses of all educational levels (American Association of Colleges of Nursing, 2021). The AONL Nurse Manager competencies outline the knowledge and skills that guide the practice of nurse leaders. The successful nurse manager must achieve proficiency in RL principles aligned with leading the people and creating the leader within (AONE & AONL, 2015b).

WHAT EVERY NURSE MANAGER NEEDS TO KNOW

- Novice nurse managers may begin their leadership practice in a task-oriented manner; however, over time, they should develop a balance between management and RL.
- The potential impact of workforce engagement and positive patient outcomes is a strong rationale to develop relational styles in nurse leaders.
- Relational work is the core of leadership practice.
- The successful nurse manager must achieve proficiency in RL principles aligned with the AONL competencies of leading the people and creating the leader within.

WHAT EVERY NURSE EXECUTIVE NEEDS TO KNOW ABOUT RELATIONSHIP-BASED LEADERSHIP

The nurse executive holds the most senior administrative role in a nursing organization, and with it comes tremendous influence and responsibility for the practice discipline and its strategic direction. Accordingly, the AONL nurse executive competencies reflect the need for relationship-based leadership in several categories including relationship management, influencing behaviors, diversity, foundational thinking skills, personal journey discipline, and succession planning (AONE & AONL, 2015a). Learning and applying relational leader skills can lead to success in these competencies, and more importantly to employee engagement and patient outcomes. Engagement surveys should be used regularly to assess for areas of strength and opportunity in the workforce.

Exemplary practice environments require professional governance structures with shared decision-making, collaboration, teamwork, balanced processing, shared power, and enabling others to act, which are all relational attributes. Empowerment is and should be a top practice of Magnet and PTE CNOs. Balancing RL and everyday management is key for nurse executives who are accountable for both big picture vision and organizational operations. CNOs also have to consider the influence of organizational culture on their leadership and outcomes (Figure 6.2).

The nurse executive should encourage relational leader practices at all levels, including clinical nurses, and sponsor emerging nurse leader and new leader onboarding programs. They can sponsor research on the impact of RL on patient outcomes, which is sorely needed. Both of these strategies can be in collaboration with an academic partner, professional organization, outside expert, or internal resources. CNOs must mentor directors and managers as their experience matters in succession planning and relational leader development. Commitment and appreciation of lifelong learning are essential.

RL supports the work needed to bring *The Future of Nursing 2020–2030* (Wakefield et al., 2021) to fruition. The role modeling, vision, listening, moral courage, caring, transparency, and other relational attributes of the nurse executive will position nursing well to achieve the imperatives of interprofessional teamwork, health equity, and nurses' health and well-being.

WHAT EVERY NURSE EXECUTIVE NEEDS TO KNOW

- Balancing RL and everyday management is key for nurse executives who are accountable for both big picture vision and organizational operations.

- The AONL nurse executive competencies reflect the need for RL in several categories including relationship management, influencing behaviors, diversity, foundational thinking skills, personal journey discipline, and succession planning.

- The nurse executive should encourage relational leader practices at all levels, including clinical nurses, and sponsor emerging nurse leader and new leader onboarding programs.

- Commitment and appreciation of lifelong learning are essential.

- RL supports the work needed to bring *The Future of Nursing 2020–2030* (Wakefield et al., 2021) to fruition.

KEY POINTS

- RL outcomes include a positive workforce and practice environment and nurse engagement, providing the foundation for positive patient outcomes.

- TL practices include modeling the way, inspiring a shared vision, challenging the process, enabling others to act, and encouraging the heart. Transformational leaders may need complementary detail-oriented partners for the "management" aspects of their role.

- AL is anchored by inner core values. Attributes of authentic leaders include self-awareness, moral courage, balanced processing, and relational transparency.

- Servant leaders put people first, prioritizing and nurturing the needs of others in their professional development.

- Nurses need to be prepared for leadership roles at every level. Structured curriculum, peer support, self-reflection, experiential learning, coaching, mentoring, and supportive practice environments are needed for leadership development.

SUMMARY

RL is "positive" leadership, grounded in optimism, integrity, building positive emotions, and employee growth and development, a driving force behind nurse engagement and HWE. The links to ethics, positive change, purpose, growth, and social connection are all part of who we are as nurses and nurse leaders. The leader–follower relationship is vital, and the subsequent engaged workforce and healthy practice environment provides the foundation for positive patient outcomes. *The Future of Nursing 2020–2030* report (Wakefield et al., 2021) recommends implementing structures and systems to ensure nurses' health, well-being, and competency in interprofessional teamwork to advance health equity. Relational leaders are well positioned to influence these imperatives. At times, nonrelational styles may be needed to advance organizational needs.

TL, authentic leadership, and SL are the most frequently studied relationship-based styles found in nursing literature. Transformational leaders are visionary and convincingly communicate that vision to followers. TL practices of modeling the way, inspiring a shared vision, challenging the process, enabling others to act, and encouraging the heart can lead to positive staff, patient, and organizational outcomes. Authentic leaders

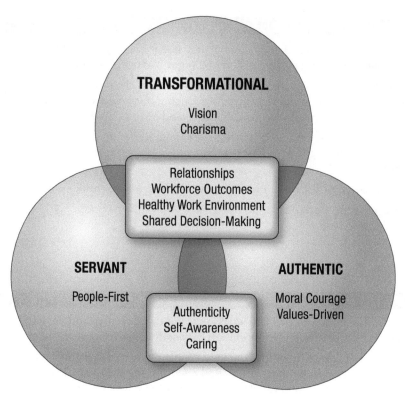

FIGURE 6.6: Intersections among transformational, authentic, and servant relational leadership styles.

are anchored by inner core values, with attributes of self-awareness, moral courage, balanced processing, and relational transparency. Authentic *nurse* leadership builds on historical models and adds a domain of altruism with caring, a nursing metaparadigm concept, as an important attribute. AL correlates with HWEs and workforce engagement, which is foundational for positive patient outcomes. Servant leaders put people first, prioritizing and nurturing the needs of followers in their professional development. Through sharing power, SL also produces favorable outcomes and enhances morale. The impact of organizational culture on leadership and outcomes is recognized, as depicted in Figure 6.2.

There are more similarities than differences in these styles (Figure 6.6). All are relationship-based, share power and decision-making, and influence work environment and workforce outcomes. Authenticity and a general sense of high character are shared between AL and SL, as well as self-awareness and caring (in the ANL model). The transformational leader is known for vision and charisma. It is not suggested that a leader should limit oneself to one or the other; characteristics of all styles in this chapter, and those not even covered, may be demonstrated by a leader along the continuum of one's career. The differences are about what drives the leader—in TL it is the vision for change, in AL/ANL it is values-driven, and in SL it is people first.

Leadership development is a lifelong journey and nurses need to be prepared for leadership roles at every level. Programming based on transactional functions will not develop a leader's relational competencies. Structured curriculum, peer support, self-reflection, experiential learning, coaching, mentoring, and supportive practice environments are all needed. Leadership learning is recognized as necessary from the core nursing curriculum through advanced practice and into the future of nursing.

END-OF-CHAPTER RESOURCES

◼ DISCUSSION QUESTIONS

1. Reflecting on your own leadership style, which elements of RL are you demonstrating and/or desiring in your self-development?
2. What are research priorities for nursing leadership and leader development?
3. Are RL styles effective in your organization? Why or why not?
4. In your experience, do relationships between leaders and followers matter? Can unconscious biases interfere with that relationship?
5. How is leadership learned in your organization, and is it effective?

◼ ADDITIONAL RESOURCES

- Sinek, S. (2009, September). *How great leaders inspire action* [Video]. TEDxPuget Sound. https://www.ted.com/talks/simon_sinek_how_great_leaders_inspire_action?language=en
- Widener University. (2014, March 25). *Leadership as a way of being: Dr. Susan R. Komives* [Video]. YouTube. https://www.youtube.com/watch?v=DTtc7rxcu-8
- Generate Insights. (2019, October 23). *SIMON SINEK: Leader versus manager* [Video]. YouTube. https://www.youtube.com/watch?v=nSUJwmPQEyg
- *Today in Nursing Leadership* [Audio podcasts]. American Organization for Nursing Leadership. https://www.aonl.org/nursing-leadership-podcast
- Swanwick, T. (Host). (2020, February 6). *Is followership a "thing"?* [Audio podcast]. BMJ talk medicine. https://soundcloud.com/bmjpodcasts/is-followership-a-thing
- *John Maxwell Leadership.* [Audio podcast]. The John Maxwell Company. https://johnmaxwellleadershippodcast.com

◼ LEARNING EXERCISES FOR STUDENTS

1. Identify leaders you admire. List why and then relate those reasons to the RL attributes in this chapter. Do they fit into one or more of the relationship-based theories? Do their behaviors influence followers? How?
2. Create an "elevator speech" for a project you are leading that needs stakeholder support. Practice it on peers and see if it influences their attitude toward the project.
3. Take a "personality survey" to discover your personality type. Use it to understand how it influences your RL behaviors and attitudes.

◼ GLOSSARY OF KEY TERMS

- **Authentic leadership:** Emphasizes a leader's transparency, genuineness, honesty, self-awareness, and moral courage within the workplace.
- **Authentic nurse leadership:** Adds altruism/caring to the authentic leadership definition.
- **Emotional intelligence:** Ability to recognize and manage one's emotions and recognize and influence the emotions of others.
- **Engagement:** Emotional state where individuals feel passionate, enthusiastic, and dedicated to their work.
- **Followership:** The capacity or willingness to follow a leader.
- **Healthy work environment:** A practice environment that promotes staff engagement and positive outcomes for patients and nurses.
- **Human-centered leadership:** A nursing leadership theory that puts people first, recognizing the importance of the leader's needs such as self-care, self-compassion, self-awareness, and mindfulness.

- ***Laissez-faire* leadership:** Characterized by nonparticipation from the leader, a hands-off approach.
- **Relational leadership:** Embodies an inclusive and positive leadership philosophy, creating a culture where people feel empowered and supported, bringing innovation, belonging, collaboration, and diversity of thought.
- **Resonant leadership:** Founded on emotional intelligence, whereby managers exhibit self-awareness, self-management, social awareness, and relationship management.
- **Servant leadership:** A "people-first" approach manifested through one-on-one prioritizing of follower needs and interests, and concern for others within the organization and the larger community.
- **Transactional leadership:** Focuses on the role of supervision, group performance, and specific tasks.
- **Transformational leadership:** Focuses on leader behaviors that create a vision for change and inspire and influence followers to perform at higher levels.

 SPRINGER PUBLISHING **CONNECT™** | A robust set of instructor resources designed to supplement this text is located at http://connect.springerpub.com/content/book/978-0-8261-7795-7. Qualifying instructors may request access by emailing textbook@springerpub.com.

REFERENCES

Alexander, C., & Lopez, R. P. (2018). A thematic analysis of self-described authentic leadership behaviors among experienced nurse executives. *JONA: The Journal of Nursing Administration, 48*(1), 38–43. https://doi.org/10.1097/NNA.0000000000000568

Alilyyani, B., Wong, C. A., & Cummings, G. (2018). Antecedents, mediators, and outcomes of authentic leadership in healthcare: A systematic review. *International Journal of Nursing Studies, 83*, 34–64. https://doi.org/10.1016/j.ijnurstu.2018.04.001

American Association of Colleges of Nursing. (2021). *The essentials: Core competencies for professional nursing education.* Author.

American Association of Critical-Care Nurses. (2005). AACN standards for establishing and sustaining healthy work environments: A journey to excellence. *American Journal of Critical Care, 14*(3), 187–197. https://doi.org/10.4037/ajcc2005.14.3.187

American Nurses Credentialing Center. (n.d.). *Organizational programs, Magnet recognition program.* https://www.nursingworld.org/organizational-programs/magnet/magnet-model/

American Organization of Nurse Executives and American Organization for Nursing Leardership. (2015a). *Nurse executive competencies.* Author. https://www.aonl.org/system/files/media/file/2019/06/nec.pdf

American Organization of Nurse Executives and American Organization for Nursing Leardership. (2015b). *Nurse manager competencies.* Author. https://www.aonl.org/system/files/media/file/2019/06/nurse-manager-competencies.pdf

Avolio, B. J., & Gardner, W. L. (2005). Authentic leadership development: Getting to the root of positive forms of leadership. *The Leadership Quarterly, 16*(3), 315–338. https://doi.org/10.1016/j.leaqua.2005.03.001

Avolio, B. J., Gardner, W. L., Walumbwa, F. O., Luthans, F., & May, D. R. (2004). Unlocking the mask: A look at the process by which authentic leaders impact follower attitudes and behaviors. *The Leadership Quarterly, 15*(6), 801–823. https://doi.org/10.1016/j.leaqua.2004.09.003

Avolio, B. J., Waldman, D. A., & Yammarino, F. J. (1991). Leading in the 1990s: The four I's of transformational leadership. *Journal of European Industrial Training, 15*(4). https://doi.org/10.1108/03090599110143366

Banks, G. C., McCauley, K. D., Gardner, W. L., & Guler, C. E. (2016). A meta-analytic review of authentic and transformational leadership: A test for redundancy. *The Leadership Quarterly, 27*(4), 634–652. https://doi.org/10.1016/j.leaqua.2016.02.006

Bass, B. M. (1985). *Leadership and performance beyond expectations.* Free Press. https://doi.org/10.1002/hrm.3930250310

Bass, B. M., & Avolio, B. J. (1993). Transformational leadership and organizational culture. *Public Administration Quarterly, 17,* 112–121. https://www.jstor.org/stable/40862298

Bass, B. M., & Avolio, B. J. (1994). *Improving organizational effectiveness through transformational leadership.* Sage Publications.

Bass, B. M., & Avolio, B. J. (n.d.). *Multifactor Leadership Questionnaire.* https://www.mindgarden.com/16-multifactor-leadership-questionnaire

Bawafaa, E., Wong, C. A., & Laschinger, H. (2015). The influence of resonant leadership on the structural empowerment and job satisfaction of registered nurses. *Journal of Research in Nursing, 20*(7), 610–622. https://doi.org/10.1177%2F1744987115603441

Boamah, S. A., Laschinger, H. K. S., Wong, C., & Clarke, S. (2018). Effect of transformational leadership on job satisfaction and patient safety outcomes. *Nursing Outlook, 66*(2), 180–189. https://doi.org/10.1016/j.outlook.2017.10.004

Boyatzis, R. E., & McKee, A. (2005). *Resonant leadership: Renewing yourself and connecting with others through mindfulness, hope, and compassion.* Harvard Business School Press.

Brown-DeVeaux, D., Jean-Louis, K., Glassman, K., & Kunisch, J. (2021). Using a mentorship approach to address the underrepresentation of ethnic minorities in senior nursing leadership. *JONA: The Journal of Nursing Administration, 51*(3), 149–155. https://doi.org/10.1097/NNA.0000000000000986

Buck, S., & Doucette, J. N. (2015). Transformational leadership practices of CNOs. *Nursing Management, 46*(9), 42–48. https://doi.org/10.1097/01.NUMA.0000469313.85935.f1

Burns, J. M. (1978). *Leadership.* Harper and Row.

Cathcart, E. B. (2014). Relational work: At the core of leadership. *Nursing Management, 45*(3), 44–46. https://doi.org/10.1097/01.NUMA.0000443943.14245.cf

Coetzer, M. F., Bussin, M., & Geldenhuys, M. (2017). The functions of a servant leader. *Administrative Sciences, 7*(1), 5. https://doi.org/10.3390/admsci7010005

Cummings, G. G. (2004). Investing relational energy: The hallmark of resonant leadership. *Canadian Journal of Nursing Leadership, 17*(4), 76–87. https://doi.org/10.12927/CJNL.2004.17019

Cummings, G. G., Hayduk, L., & Estabrooks, C. (2005). Mitigating the impact of hospital restructuring on nurses: The responsibility of emotionally intelligent leadership. *Nursing Research, 54*(1), 2–12. https://doi.org/10.1097/00006199-200501000-00002

Cummings, G. G., MacGregor, T., Davey, M., Lee, H., Wong, C. A., Lo, E., Muise, M., & Stafford, E. (2010). Leadership styles and outcome patterns for the nursing workforce and work environment: A systematic review. *International Journal of Nursing Studies, 47*(3), 363–385. https://doi.org/10.1016/j.ijnurstu.2009.08.006

Cummings, G. G., Tate, K., Lee, S., Wong, C. A., Paananen, T., Micaroni, S. P., & Chatterjee, G. E. (2018). Leadership styles and outcome patterns for the nursing workforce and work environment: A systematic review. *International Journal of Nursing Studies, 85,* 19–60. https://doi.org/10.1016/j.ijnurstu.2018.04.016

Davidson, S. (2020). Hard science and "soft" skills: Complex relational leading. *Nursing Administration Quarterly, 44*(2), 101–108. https://doi.org/10.1097/naq.0000000000000406

Dempsey, C., & Assi, M. J. (2018). The impact of nurse engagement on quality, safety, and the experience of care: What nurse leaders should know. *Nursing Administration Quarterly, 42*(3), 278–283. https://doi.org/10.1097/NAQ.0000000000000305

Dye, C. (2017). *Leadership in healthcare: Essential values and skills* (3rd ed.). Health Administration Press.

Echevarria, I. M., Patterson, B. J., & Krouse, A. (2017). Predictors of transformational leadership of nurse managers. *Journal of Nursing Management, 25*(3), 167–175. https://doi.org/10.1111/jonm.12452

Fallatah, F., Laschinger, H. K., & Read, E. A. (2017). The effects of authentic leadership, organizational identification, and occupational coping self-efficacy on new graduate nurses' job turnover intentions in Canada. *Nursing Outlook, 65*(2), 172–183. https://doi.org/10.1016/j.outlook.2016.11.020

Fischer, S. A. (2016). Transformational leadership in nursing: A concept analysis. *Journal of Advanced Nursing, 72*(11), 2644–2653. https://doi.org/10.1111/jan.13049

Frasier, N. (2019). Preparing nurse managers for authentic leadership: A pilot leadership development program. *JONA: The Journal of Nursing Administration, 49*(2), 79–85. https://doi.org/10.1097/NNA.0000000000000714

Gallup. (n.d.). *The power of Gallup's Q12 employee engagement survey.* https://www.gallup.com/access/323333/q12-employee-engagement-survey.aspx

Galuska, L. A. (2014). Education as a springboard for transformational leadership development: Listening to the voices of nurses. *The Journal of Continuing Education in Nursing, 45*(2), 67–76. https://doi.org/10.3928/00220124-20140124-21

Giordano-Mulligan, M., & Eckardt, S. (2019). Authentic nurse leadership conceptual framework: Nurses' perception of authentic nurse leader attributes. *Nursing Administration Quarterly, 43*(2), 164–174. https://doi.org/10.1097/NAQ.0000000000000344

Greenleaf, R. K. (1977). *Servant leadership: A journey into the nature of legitimate power and greatness.* Paulist Press.

Greenleaf Center for Servant Leadership. (n.d.). *What is servant leadership?* https://www.greenleaf.org/what-is-servant-leadership

Harter, J. (2020, February 4). *4 Factors driving record-high employee engagement in U.S.* https://www.gallup.com/workplace/284180/factors-driving-record-high-employee-engagement.aspx

Herman, S., Gish, M., & Rosenblum, R. (2015). Effects of nursing position on transformational leadership practices. *JONA: The Journal of Nursing Administration, 45*(2), 113–119. https://doi.org/10.1097/NNA.0000000000000165

Komives, S., Lucas, N., & McMahon, T. (1998). *Exploring leadership: For college students who want to make a difference.* Jossey-Bass. https://doi.org/10.1353/csd.2015.0008

Komives, S., Lucas, N., & McMahon, T. (2007). *Exploring leadership: For college students who want to make a difference (2nd ed.).* Jossey-Bass.

Kouzes, J. M., & Posner, B. Z. (n.d.). *Leadership Practices Inventory.* https://www.statisticssolutions.com/leadership-practices-inventory-lpi/

Kouzes, J. M., & Posner, B. Z. (2007). *The leadership challenge* (4th ed.). Jossey-Bass.

Laschinger, H. K. S., Wong, C. A., & Grau, A. L. (2012). The influence of authentic leadership on newly graduated nurses' experiences of workplace bullying, burnout and retention outcomes: A cross-sectional study. *International Journal of Nursing Studies, 49*(10), 1266–1276. https://doi.org/10.1016/j.ijnurstu.2012.05.012

Laschinger, H. K. S., Wong, C. A., & Grau, A. L. (2013). Authentic leadership, empowerment and burnout: A comparison in new graduates and experienced nurses. *Journal of Nursing Management, 21*(3), 541–552. https://doi.org/10.1111/j.1365-2834.2012.01375.x

Laub, J. (1999). *Assessing the servant organization: Development of the servant organizational leadership (SOLA) instrument* (Doctoral thesis). Florida Atlantic University.

Laub, J. (2018). *Leveraging the power of servant leadership* (pp. 73–111). Palgrave Macmillan. https://doi.org/10.1007/978-3-319-77143-4_4

Laub, J. (n.d.). *Organizational Leadership Assessment.* https://www.servantleaderperformance.com/ola/instrument

Leclerc, L., Kennedy, K., & Campis, S. (2020). Human-centered leadership in health care: An idea that's time has come. *Nursing Administration Quarterly, 44*(2), 117–126. https://doi.org/10.1097/NAQ.0000000000000409

Leclerc, L., Kennedy, K., & Campis, S. (2021). Human-centred leadership in health care: A contemporary nursing leadership theory generated via constructivist grounded theory. *Journal of Nursing Management, 29*(2), 294–306. https://doi.org/10.1111/jonm.13154

McCay, R., Lyles, A. A., & Larkey, L. (2018). Nurse leadership style, nurse satisfaction, and patient satisfaction: A systematic review. *Journal of Nursing Care Quality, 33*(4), 361–367. https://doi.org/10.1097/NCQ.0000000000000317

McGarity, T., Reed, C., Monahan, L., & Zhao, M. (2020). Innovative frontline nurse leader professional development program. *Journal for Nurses in Professional Development, 36*(5), 277–282. https://doi.org/10.1097/NND.0000000000000628

Merrill, K. C. (2015). Leadership style and patient safety: Implications for nurse managers. *JONA: The Journal of Nursing Administration, 45*(6), 319–324. https://doi.org/10.1097/nna.0000000000000207

Neville, K., Conway, K., Maglione, J., Connolly, K. A., Foley, M., & Re, S. (2021). Understanding servant leadership in nursing: A concept analysis. *International Journal for Human Caring, 25*(1). https://doi.org/10.20467/HumanCaring-D-20-00022

Norman, R. M., & Sjetne, I. S. (2017). Measuring nurses' perception of work environment: A scoping review of questionnaires. *BMC Nursing, 16*, 66. https://doi.org/10.1186/s12912-017-0256-9

Pedersen, A., Sorensen, J., Babcock, T., Bradley, M., Donaldson, N., Donnelly, J. E., & Edgar, W. (2018). A nursing leadership immersion program: Succession planning using social capital. *JONA: The Journal of Nursing Administration, 48*(3), 168–174. https://doi.org/10.1097/NNA.0000000000000592

Prado-Inzerillo, M., Clavelle, J. T., & Fitzpatrick, J. J. (2018). Leadership practices and engagement among Magnet® hospital chief nursing officers. *JONA: The Journal of Nursing Administration, 48*(10), 502–507. https://doi.org/10.1097/NNA.0000000000000658

Raso, R. (2015). The leadership balancing act. *Nursing Management, 46*(8), 4. https://doi.org/10.1097/01.NUMA.0000469355.49071.7b

Raso, R., Fitzpatrick, J. J., & Masick, K. (2020). Clinical nurses' perceptions of authentic nurse leadership and healthy work environment. *JONA: The Journal of Nursing Administration, 50*(9), 489–494. https://doi.org/10.1097/NNA.0000000000000921

Raso, R., Fitzpatrick, J. J., Masick, K., Giordano-Mulligan, M., & Sweeney, C. D. (2021). Perceptions of authentic nurse leadership and work environment and the pandemic impact for nurse leaders and clinical nurses. *JONA: The Journal of Nursing Administration, 51*(5), 257–263. https://doi.org/10.1097/nna.0000000000001010

Savel, R. H., & Munro, C. L. (2017). Servant leadership: The primacy of service. *American Journal of Critical Care, 26*(2), 97–99. https://doi.org/10.4037/ajcc2017356

Sherman, R. O. (2019). The case for servant leadership. *Nurse Leader, 17*(2), 86–87. https://doi.org/10.1016/j.mnl.2018.12.001

Sherman, R. O., & Saifman, H. (2018). Transitioning emerging leaders into nurse leader roles. *JONA: The Journal of Nursing Administration, 48*(7/8), 355–357. https://doi.org/10.1097/NNA.0000000000000628

Shirey, M. R. (2006). Authentic leaders creating healthy work environments for nursing practice. *American Journal of Critical Care, 15*(3), 256–267. https://doi.org/10.4037/AJCC2006.15.3.256

Shirey, M. R. (2009). Authentic leadership, organizational culture, and healthy work environments. *Critical Care Nursing Quarterly, 32*(3), 189–198. https://doi.org/10.1097/CNQ.0b013e3181ab91db

Shirey, M. R. (2017). Leadership practices for healthy work environments. *Nursing Management, 48*(5), 42–50. https://doi.org/10.1097/01.NUMA.0000515796.79720.e6

Snyder, C. R., Lopez, S. J., Edwards, L. M., & Marques, S. C. (Eds.). (2020). *The Oxford handbook of positive psychology*. Oxford University Press. https://doi.org/10.1093/oxfordhb/9780199396511.001.0001

Spano-Szekely, L., Griffin, M. T. Q., Clavelle, J., & Fitzpatrick, J. J. (2016). Emotional intelligence and transformational leadership in nurse managers. *JONA: The Journal of Nursing Administration, 46*(2), 101–108. https://doi.org/10.1097/NNA.0000000000000303

Spears, L. C. (1998). Tracing the growing impact of servant leadership. In Spears, L. C. (Ed.), *Insights on leadership: Service, stewardship, spirit, and servant leadership* (pp. 1–12). John Wiley and Sons.

Squires, M., Tourangeau, A., Spence Laschinger, H. K., & Doran, D. (2010). The link between leadership and safety outcomes in hospitals. *Journal of Nursing Management, 18*(8), 914–925. https://doi.org/10.1111/j.1365-2834.2010.01181.x

Wagner, J., Warren, S., Cummings, G., Smith, D., & Olson, J. (2013). Resonant leadership, workplace empowerment, and "spirit at work": Impact on job satisfaction and organizational commitment. *Canadian Journal of Nursing, 45*, 108–128. https://doi.org/10.1177/084456211304500409

Wakefield, M. K., Williams, W. R., Le Menestral, S. & Flaubert, J. L. (Eds.). (2021). *The future of nursing 2020–2030: Charting a path to achieve health equity*. National Academies Press. https://doi.org/10.17226/25982

Walumbwa, F. O., Avolio, B. J., Gardner, W. L., Wernsing, T. S., & Peterson, S. J. (2008). Authentic leadership: Development and validation of a theory-based measure. *Journal of Management, 34*(1), 89–126. https://psycnet.apa.org/doi/10.1177/0149206307308913

Wei, H., King, A., Jiang, Y., Sewell, K. A., & Lake, D. M. (2020). The impact of nurse leadership styles on nurse burnout: A systematic literature review. *Nurse Leader, 18*(5), 439–450. https://doi.org/10.1016/j.mnl.2020.04.002

Wong, C. A., & Laschinger, H. K. (2013). Authentic leadership, performance, and job satisfaction: The mediating role of empowerment. *Journal of Advanced Nursing, 69*(4), 947–959. https://doi.org/10.1111/j.1365-2648.2012.06089.x

Wong, C. A., & Walsh, E. J. (2020). Reflections on a decade of authentic leadership research in health care. *Journal of Nursing Management, 28*(1), 1–3. https://doi.org/10.1111/jonm.12861

CHAPTER 7

THE COACHING AND MENTORING PROCESS

M. Lisa Hedenstrom and Susan M. Dyess

"What nurses expect from their leaders is changing. Gone are the days of command-and-control leadership when staff were expected to be grateful because they had a job."

Rose Sherman (2019, p. v)

LEARNING OBJECTIVES

- Identify principles of coaching and mentoring within a relational-based leadership model.
- Examine the context of relationships for coaching and mentoring.
- Investigate opportunities for coaching and mentoring to promote the career development of nurse leaders.
- Plan for coaching and mentoring utilization to lead peak performance within nurses and nursing teams.

A NOTE ON RELATED COMPETENCIES

Due to the opportunity for individual and team performance development, coaching and mentoring encompass all related competencies of the professional bodies advising nurse leaders including the American Organization for Nursing Leadership (AONL) and the American Association of Colleges of Nursing (AACN) essentials and domains, as well as the Association for Leadership Science in Nursing (ALSN) and Quality and Safety Education for Nurses (QSEN) competencies identified. Specifically, however, coaching and mentoring uniquely display AONL competencies of communication, leadership, and professionalism and are characterized within the domains of nurse executive, system chief nurse executive (CNE), post-acute care, and population health. In addition, the AONL nurse manager competencies are displayed that include leader within, creating leader in self and art, and leading the people. The AACN essentials are represented by the core competencies of interprofessional partnerships, professionalism, and personal, professional, and leadership development. Further, the AACN concepts of communication, clinical judgment, and evidence-based practice also can be exemplified within coaching and mentoring. Finally, the QSEN graduate level competencies of teamwork, collaboration, and quality improvement are aspects that are illustrated within coaching and mentoring approaches.

INTRODUCTION

Globally there is an increasing expectation for nurse leaders and nursing teams to accomplish more, often with fewer resources. Still, a myriad of challenges, frequent changing and competing priorities, and system complexities within healthcare demand peak performance from nurse leaders and nursing teams. Coaching and mentoring are useful as deliberate nurse leader strategies for tapping into the existing expertise, developing the potential, and shaping necessary peak performance for individual nurses and nursing teams. Depending on what outcomes are desired, nurse leaders may find value in using the strategies concurrently. This chapter explores coaching and mentoring as essential components of nurse leadership and management foundations for effective administration.

Depending on the perspective one holds, there can be an interchangeable utilization of the terms "coaching" and "mentoring." However, for this chapter, coaching and mentoring will be considered as distinct terms. Most authors agree that coaching "differs from mentoring, a more familiar term in that its focus is on specific aims rather than general professional development" (Waldrop & Derouin, 2019, p. 170). Fielden et al. (2009) posited that coaching can be incorporated into a long-term mentoring relationship.

For this chapter, coaching and mentoring skills are embedded within a positive—not punitive—framework. More clearly, coaching and mentoring are not euphemistic for performance improvement action plans that may be associated with a human resources (HR) situation. Simply defined, coaching used by nurse leaders is an agreed upon, formal relationship that addresses specific performance goals. Mentoring used by nurse leaders can be a formal or informal relationship that addresses professional developmental needs. Both coaching and mentoring are elements of talent capacity building within a nursing practice unit or healthcare organization.

Both coaching and mentoring are strategies that support the overall mission of an organization and support peak performance for individuals, groups, or teams, yet their use can be distinct, defined, and deliberately implemented. There is convergence with aspects of coaching and mentoring as both connect two or more people in conversation and written formats over time. In healthcare practice, coaching and mentoring are poised for utilization and require nurse leaders to be intentional, consider resource support, attend to executive presence, and lead with staff development and retention in mind.

INTENTIONALITY IN COACHING AND MENTORING

Successful nurse leaders and executives can adopt creative and strategic approaches that support longevity within their workforce, as well as ongoing career development and skillset acquisition. Coaching and mentoring as a strategy for achieving high performance will not occur without purposeful planning and action. Wilmoth and Shapiro (2014) suggest there is limited discussion about "when to begin cultivating nurses. . ., how to develop nurses. . ., or who should be responsible. . ." (p. 334) for the plan; and further, "the nursing profession can no longer afford to use this laissez-faire approach" (p. 337). The activities of coaching and mentoring will require leadership to engage in purposeful approaches for execution to occur. Intention is essential and so are resources.

RESOURCE SUPPORT

While nurse leaders certainly will require intentional energy to create an atmosphere that welcomes and encourages coaching and mentoring, there also should be a recognition of the necessary investment of resources, both time and talent. Time cannot be undervalued because there is a productivity cost associated with planning, executing, and evaluating coaching and mentoring initiatives. Coaching and mentoring are dependent on talent, too. The skills associated with coaching and mentoring may need sufficient knowledge development or take time away from other role responsibilities. Finally, coaching and mentoring initiatives are dependent upon organizational investment from senior leadership buy-in for sponsorship, collaboration, and facilitation of barrier removal (Brown-DeVeaux & Jean-Louis, 2021). Coaching and mentoring not only require leadership resource support but also a unique executive presence from the coach or mentor.

EXECUTIVE PRESENCE

Shirey (2013) asserts executive presence is an essential factor for guiding transformation in organizations but also acknowledges a dearth of conceptual clarity in nursing literature. The core of executive presence for a nurse leader is the capacity to portray poise and a dignified demeanor. Often executive presence is depicted by one making wise decisions and working well, despite pressure. Executive leaders have impeccable communication skills and give off the impression that they are confidently in charge. Executive presence is not only identified as illusive and imperative to project for successful leadership, but also, it is portrayed as something that can be developed (Beeson, 2018). Executive presence can be thought of as the ability to inspire confidence, engender trust, and build a workplace culture that promotes enjoyment and success for individuals and the team. Executive presence is necessary for leveraging coaching and mentoring influence.

DEVELOPMENT AND RETENTION

A commitment to a culture of coaching and mentoring will yield high performance from individuals, groups, and teams promoting development and retention. Researchers posit that nurse leaders are key to develop their staff as they empower collaboration, support quality patient care, and stabilize retention (Cziraki et al., 2020). Nurse leaders can use coaching and mentoring as deliberate strategies to create a culture that nurtures and equips their team. It will require a sensitivity to variability in relationships, the unique practice setting context, and ways of knowing, being, and existing within a healthcare system. To be sure, nurses within the workforce today expect their leaders will be able to lead with various skillsets that support individual and collective professional outcomes. Coaching and mentoring are part of those skillsets.

COACHING

Coaching is a proactive collaborative process that supports goal achievement and high performance through discourse and action. Often noted to be a formal process, coaching is accomplished within the boundaries of a trusted relationship and typically is time limited. Coaching celebrates the wisdom of the one coached and builds upon any strengths identified. Yet, coaching focuses on a performance improvement goal as defined by the coached. As a best practice in nursing, coaching is known to positively influence clinical problem-solving and the development of nurse leaders, individual staff, and teams (Cable & Graham, 2018; Dyess et al., 2017; Sherman, 2019). "Coaching is a way to promote self-discovery, allow for the expression of wisdom, increase clinical effectiveness, and encourage innovative thinking" (Dyess et al., 2017, p. 374).

Coaching as an intentional strategy for individual staff or teams can be actualized by utilizing various approaches. Dyess et al. (2017) illustrate three examples of coaching variations: Gallup Executive Coaching, Dartmouth microsystem healthcare improvement team coaching, and health and wellness coaching. Each of the three coaching approaches support professional development and are demonstrated to facilitate change that results in better employee and potential patient outcomes. However, numerous other frameworks exist and are utilized within and outside nursing realms. Some frameworks combine performance and life coaching; while other frameworks focus on executive presence or leadership skills only (Gray, 2018; Olson & Tan, 2018; Pandolfi, 2020; Withrow, 2020). Still, no matter what coaching framework is selected, there is potential for adaptation to any healthcare or clinical practice setting for achieving the purposes of an organization. All coaching frameworks begin with basic processes that guide and empower others to attain their goals, address challenges, and reach peak performance.

THE COACHING PROCESS

The coaching processes generally follow common guidelines despite arising from varied frameworks. Coaching is thought to be a creative process with ethical principles that often guide relationship conduct. Typically, there are three stages for coaching (Dyess et al., 2017) and each stage accomplishes a purpose, serving as a foundation for the next aspect of coaching. These stages include pre-coaching, active coaching, and follow-up coaching. Tables 7.1 and 7.2 consider the focus of the stage and targeted questions that can be used to facilitate the coaching processes. Coaching standards are considered after the review of literature that follows.

In the pre-coaching phase, the nurse leader invests in the developing relationship. Efforts are made to create an atmosphere of acceptance, trust, and an appreciation of strengths and opportunities for advancement. It is useful to incorporate a formal assessment but not required. Steps are taken to move to an active coaching stage.

TABLE 7.1: Coaching Stages and Focus

Stage	Focus
Pre-coaching	Build relationships. Assess strengths and opportunities.
Active coaching	Clarify goals. Plan and actualize commitment to reach goal.
Follow-up coaching	Reflect on outcomes. Identify new behaviors. Provide feedback.

TABLE 7.2: Sample Guiding Questions Within Phases

Stage	Sample Guiding Questions
Pre-coaching	What brings you professional joy? Is there a professional story you want to build for yourself? What do you want to happen? What change are you seeking? Can you identify any specific performance goals? How will it be possible to know if you achieved your goal?
Active coaching	What is your performance goal? What is important about your goal? How will you move forward? Can you consider your first step? What do you see as barriers? How might you address barriers? How might you handle internal or external resistance?
Follow-up coaching	What actions did you consider? Did these actions facilitate movement toward your goal? Why or why not? What other approach may be wise to consider? Are there next steps? What insights did you gain about yourself? Or others?

Within the active coaching stage, a mutual commitment is made to the coaching relationship and processes. Next, the coaching goals are determined. Initial timelines for action, appropriate steps necessary for accomplishing goals, and the identification of metrics for meeting goals are clarified. In addition, barriers to goal achievement and ways to overcome barriers are considered. This phase may last the longest as coaching sessions work to support goal attainment.

Finally, a follow-up phase is identified. In the follow-up phase, the goals are reviewed and modified, or the commitment to new behaviors, skills, and practices is discussed. Coaching input approaches for refinement and/or any desire to continue the coaching relationship are contemplated. Formal closure to a coaching relationship can be beneficial. The closure does not equate to an ending of the professional relationship, but rather a shift.

The framework from which the coaching is based may determine stylistic approach and questions for the coached to consider. In Table 7.2, there are suggested sample questions that might be appropriate for a relationship-based leadership paradigm. Each coaching situation will shape the questions more clearly. It is possible for coaching to be iterative and long-lasting or also possible for coaching to be accomplished quickly, even within a one-time process.

While the relationship framework for coaching is formal, the principles guiding the process of coaching are nonprescriptive and unstructured. Each coaching relationship will be uniquely developed. The experiential learning within a clinical healthcare coaching framework supports the construction of meaning as psychomotor development accompanies thinking and feeling within knowledge acquisition (Hugill et al., 2018). Coaching may also be useful to support the development of emotional intelligence (EI), self-awareness, reflection, and presence for the coach and the coached.

USES FOR COACHING

Coaching improves results like individual and team performance, job satisfaction, retention, conflict resolution, and goal alignment; as well as supports "intangible benefits such as improving integrity, compassion, and commitment to the organization" (Olson & Tan, 2018, p. 67). The uses for coaching are limitless; therefore, an organization may determine policy for their coaching services. Globally, coaching is utilized in vast types of organizations; according to Olson and Tan (2018), the acronym SIDE (strengthen bench talent, increase revenue streams, decrease operational costs, and enhance productivity) highlights the value added. With a slight modification added to the acronym shared by Olson and Tan, nurse leaders can easily recognize coaching uses for their healthcare teams (Box 7.1).

BOX 7.1: ACRONYM FOR COACHING BENEFITS

- S: Strengthen bench talent
- I: Increase revenue streams
- D: Decrease operational costs
- E: Enhance productivity

COACHING RESEARCH LITERATURE REVIEW

There is a small but growing body of evidence that focuses on coaching interventions as part of nursing leadership development. The adaptation of coaching for nursing leadership is a timely resource addition within a complicated healthcare backdrop. As healthcare responds to multifaceted forces that include, but are not limited to, recovery from a global pandemic, chronic illness management, aging populations, and other disruptive change, coaching may be an enduring tool that supports and develops a wide range of competencies.

Globally, researchers offer promising nurse leadership development outcomes associated with coaching (Cable & Graham, 2018; Hugill et al., 2018; Leigh et al., 2018, 2019; Waldrop & Derouin, 2019). Indeed, the effects for nurse leaders and nurse executives to consider utilizing coaching initiatives include the cocreation of long-term transformative, widespread, and targeted yet inclusive professional development. Selected studies published in the last 5 years point to promising opportunities to implement coaching as a practice enhancing strategy that includes an improvement in self-confidence and the capacity for reflection on and in practice (Cable & Graham, 2018); an improvement within relationships, amplified motivation for engagement in work, and increased exchanges that allowed for constructive feedback communication (Hugill et al., 2018); supporting the bench strength of nurse leaders in the present and for the future of the organization (Leigh et al., 2018, 2019); and the emergence of personal accountability (Waldrop & Derouin, 2019).

Although the current body of literature is limited, recent researchers suggest coaching outcomes for healthcare leadership development and well-being are promising. Findings indicate coaching supports skill acquisition and leadership development for nurses. Coaching is utilized widely within executive business development settings and research supports similar findings that are noted within nursing practice settings (Auerbach, 2021). Thus far, no experimental designs are noted within the literature. More robust research is warranted to demonstrate specific measurable outcomes attributed to nurse leadership coaching. Cases of career situations are shared in the text that follows.

STANDARDS OF COACHING

The utilization of coaching in professional healthcare settings is believed to enhance individual and team performance. As a nurse leader, you may want to consider coaching as a strategy to augment your team's performance or consider it as a skill to support your own career progression. Both options for coaching can provide you with an interesting skillset to consider.

Founded as an organization in 2001, the international coaching community exists wherein a commitment to high standards of practice is considered (International Coaching Community, n.d.). Still, numerous private coaching courses with standards and certification processes also exist that are nonrelated to the international community. There are many approaches to, and techniques associated with, coaching. Some of the coaching approaches require specialized education, supervised training, and/or certifications. There are face to face, virtual, and hybrid options available from numerous coaching and professional organizations. Due diligence of investigating the right coaching approach for the best organizational fit is necessary. Costs, requirements, and continuing education vary across the different approaches. There is no conclusive evidence that identifies one approach to be better than others or to manifest more promising outcomes. Also, no matter what type of coaching is undertaken, there is no authoritative body for direct oversight of the coach/coached relationship.

Coaching is best undertaken within the confines of a relationship that is established for the purposes of accomplishing defined goals. Typically, the approach is one-on-one. The cocreation of a partnership is forged that fosters the coached to process four broad attributes of any practice: to gain insight, to acknowledge their unique potential, to strengthen their expression of expertise, and to identify and take action (Figure 7.1). These four attributes are not exhaustive but serve as a helpful guide to optimal coaching and potential outcomes for ultimately achieving peak performance. There is no prescribed timing or linear order to achieve the attributes. All attributes support the attainment of peak performance. The following case examples are presented from a nonspecific coaching approach to highlight possible benefits within practice settings.

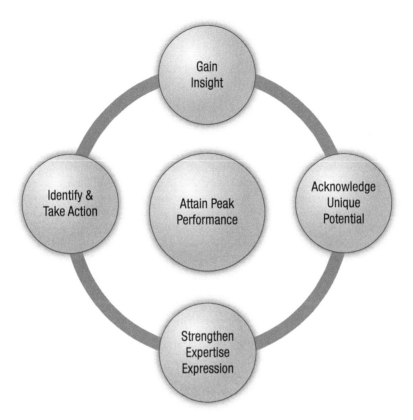

FIGURE 7.1: Key attributes of coaching.

COACHING CAREER SCENARIOS

Nurse leaders are afforded a nursing practice staging model of skill acquisition and demonstrated knowledge expertise advanced by Benner (1982). The stages correspond with proficiency in clinical practice and progress in critical decision-making for a nurse upon entry into the profession role until deemed an expert in the practice area. While Benner did not originally apply the stages to leadership, Titzer et al. (2014) affirmed Benner's staging from novice to expert to be an "effective framework for leadership development and competency measurement, mentoring programs, advanced nursing practice skill acquisition, and professional advancement ladders" (p. 38). While prescribing a stage label is not a process within coaching, coaching can be effectively implemented throughout the professional stages to support peak performance. Three examples are offered in the text that follows that correspond to Benner's stage for the staff and nurse leader most likely to be engaging in the coaching: novice- advanced beginner stage (new nurse manager), competent-proficient stage (nurse manager), and expert stage (nurse executive). The names and specifics of each scenario are altered to prevent identification of the parties involved.

⬡ **CASE SCENARIO**

EARLY CAREER COACHING FOR NOVICE, ADVANCED BEGINNER STAGE

SITUATION

KC is a new manager within a busy acute care medical–surgical services unit. KC was selected as a nurse manager because they were clinically superb, were well-liked among their peers, and held numerous council positions within the organizational shared governance structure. However, since becoming a new nurse manager, KC is feeling unprepared, unliked, and frazzled. KC is frequently missing report deadlines from their CNE. Also, KC finds their staff increasingly frustrated with KC's decision-making and scheduling approvals. At the beginning of their day, when KC came to work, they received three staff resignations in their inbox. KC reaches out to an organizational coach.

APPROACH

A relationship is established. The coach artfully guides KC through the coaching standards over five sessions. KC pinpoints their goals to be an effective nurse manager and experience feelings of preparedness and competence. KC is invited to reflect upon when they last experienced feelings of preparedness and competence. They easily recall their clinical prowess (gain insight). KC then is reminded of their capacity to be an extremely capable professional nurse who was selected because of recognized abilities (unique potential). KC considers how clinical skills are learned and refined and recognizes the same can occur with managerial and leadership skill sets (expression of expertise). Next, KC creates a reading list of leadership content, selects two nurse managers that they aspire to mirror, and creates a regular meeting time with both (take action). Within 6 months, KC makes weekly strides in not only feeling prepared but achieving a stable and productive practice unit (peak performance).

OUTCOME

Five 60-minute coaching sessions supported KC achieving peak performance as a nurse manager. The reading list KC creates is innovative and provides a great opportunity to hold discussions with their team about quality, safety, and patient outcomes. KC is adapting an evidence-based approach to leadership in the same manner they use evidence to guide clinical practice. KC recognizes their opportunity to invest time and energy in their team to develop their team's expertise, too. The morale within the unit is upbeat. The coaching process clearly impacted not only KC, but also the other employees and other practice units. It also enhanced safety and quality for patients and families. Coaching creates a positive difference in KC and their work performance.

DISCUSSION QUESTIONS

1. What evidence exists that supports pivoting from clinical expertise to leading teams?
2. How might KC's newly applied leadership approaches influence retention?
3. What question(s) could the coach use to create an environment for further reflection?

⬡ CASE SCENARIO

MID-CAREER COACHING FOR COMPETENT-PROFICIENT STAGE

SITUATION

JB is a seasoned nurse manager with 6 years' experience within a specialty genitourinary services unit. JB's track record as a nurse manager is superior. The CNE assigns the additional inaugural bariatric services unit to JB's portfolio of responsibilities. With the added responsibility, JB is unsure how or where to begin. JB desires the increased responsibility but is feeling extremely anxious about moving forward. The CNE requests a meeting in 1 month to discuss the progress. JB seeks out a coach for help.

APPROACH

Two coaching sessions meet the needs of this situation. The coach meets with JB and supports them to recognize their timid feelings as it relates to the bariatric assignment. Fear of failure is identified easily (gain insight). JB quickly pivots to acknowledge their track record of stellar leadership and their superior management abilities (unique potential). The coach invites JB to write down the necessary steps associated with the bariatric task. JB can easily recognize their ability to transfer the nurse management wisdom they hold from the genitourinary services unit to the bariatric project (expression of expertise). JB then identifies how they can begin and manage the project within the framework of their other responsibilities (take action). Soon JB creates a business plan that outlines the development and implementation of the bariatric unit. JB initiates meetings that will support the implementation and is eager to meet with the CNE to report their progress (peak performance).

OUTCOME

Within two 45-minute coaching sessions, JB was provided with the right amount of support to release anxiety, regain confidence, and create an action plan that would launch a bariatric unit successfully. JB easily identified their fear of failure and developed cognitive reframing phrases to combat negative self-talk. JB also created a detailed plan for the implementation of a successful bariatric unit that leveraged organizational resources. JB was prepared to meet with the CNE with confidence. Coaching assists JB to release anxiety and perform at their top level.

DISCUSSION QUESTIONS

1. Too often leaders take on assigned tasks as their sole responsibility. How might you avoid that trap?
2. How can you incorporate positive self-talk phrases into your leadership approach?
3. What resources are available to you for any given assigned task?

⬡ | CASE SCENARIO
LATE CAREER COACHING FOR EXPERT STAGE

SITUATION

AJ is a CNE with 15 years of community-based acute-care leadership experience. They hold a doctor of nursing practice (DNP) within executive healthcare. The healthcare system where AJ is employed is reorganizing, and the reporting structure is being altered. AJ finds themself in a difficult position of reporting to an executive who is nonsupportive of AJ's leadership and somewhat hostile to AJ's advocacy for nursing staff. AJ approaches the executive in a nonconfrontational manner to discuss these issues, but AJ's concerns are dismissed flippantly. The supervisor makes disparaging remarks and seems to unfairly berate AJ and their team for not meeting metrics. AJ seeks out input from trusted colleagues and recognizes they will not be able to work in an environment that is not supportive. AJ is defeated, they begin to disengage from their work, and their leadership oversight of projects begins to wane. A reliable friend encourages AJ to seek out coaching.

APPROACH

As a seasoned CNE, the coaching relationship is carefully vetted to ensure a trusted relationship can be developed. The coach invites AJ to complete a self-assessment tool in the first session. The comprehensive nature of the self-assessment provides valuable information from which the coaching can proceed. A thorough consideration of the self-assessment reveals that AJ is grossly unhappy in their professional role and is experiencing physical and mental impact from unhappiness (gain insight). Steps are taken within the coaching session to allow AJ to acknowledge their accomplishments, recover from the berating comments, and value their contributions made to the organization and the profession of nursing (unique potential). This work takes many coaching sessions, but progress is made. AJ is renewed in their own appreciation of their CNE abilities and begins engaging in professional organizations and collegial relationships (expression of exper-tise). AJ designs a 24-month action plan for their leadership team to accomplish a pathway to excellence survey (take action). In addition, AJ intentionally designs a health plan that focuses on life balance. Intermittent coaching sessions continue for 2 years and the pathway to excellence designation is achieved (peak performance). Meanwhile, the executive supervisor relocates and the newly appointed boss recognizes AJ's extraordinary contributions to the organization.

OUTCOME

A 26-month coaching relationship involving 30 coaching sessions provided the CNE with the support they needed. Coaching supports AJ to develop an acceptance of conflict with their supervisor. AJ incorporates a pause in their day, uses neutral language whenever possible, and agrees to disagree with the new supervisor. In addition, AJ begins intentional relationship devel-opment with members of their team. As AJ invests in team development, AJ's energy is renewed and their focus is redirected. AJ focuses on new initiatives with their team and does not overthink negative comments; rather, AJ reframes negativity to develop constructive solutions. Personal and organizational success is supported. Coaching allows AJ to achieve a higher level of performance.

DISCUSSION QUESTIONS

1. What types of conflict resolution skills were used?
2. How might you create space in your day to pause?
3. What strategies might be helpful to successfully advance job performance despite neg-ative feedback?

MENTORING

Mentoring has a variety of definitions in the literature which most commonly center on the relationship between mentee (protégé) and mentor (experienced leader) and the mentoring relationship (Hale, 2018). Mentoring is used in a variety of healthcare and nonhealthcare settings to help support leader professional development. The phases of the mentoring re-lationship can vary in the literature but are highlighted by having a beginning, middle, and end phase (Disch, 2018; Hale, 2018).

Mentoring is centered on a relationship between the mentee and mentor. Mentoring is an intentional relationship based on someone with more experience to guide and influence someone seeking the expertise of a mentor. In a mentoring relationship, mutual goals are es-tablished early in the relationship. The mentoring relationship is centered on the relationship between the mentee and mentor. Mentoring relationships often have core characteristics in-cluding well-defined goals for the relationship, mentee ability to hear and obtain feedback as well as mentor commitment to nurture and support mentee development through sharing of experience and providing feedback, ongoing communication to allow relationships to be formed and developed, and awareness that over time the relationship might evolve into a peer-to-peer phase or the mentee needs might necessitate a different mentor for the mentee (Disch, 2018; Hale, 2018; Vitale, 2018). The mentee drives the relationship. Success has been achieved in nurse leader mentoring with a structured, developed, and programmatic ap-proach to mentoring (Rich et al., 2015).

Mentors help develop their mentees by sharing their past experiences with them while also helping to develop them in broad ways to support overall professional development. The mentoring relationship often focuses on specific goals but can also include general de-velopment as well as support through challenges faced by a mentee in their role. Mentors may also suggest development opportunities for mentees including observing meetings or projects to help develop key skills that the mentor and mentee have identified as core competencies for nursing leadership roles. In addition, mentors often share their past experiences through stories and professional situations to share lessons learned with their mentee. Through this relationship building, the mentoring process has limitless potential to help support mentee development.

Mentoring programs can be formal and informal. Mutual goals and ongoing monitoring of progress toward goals support the development and success of the mentoring relationship. The mentee can identify what key skills and concepts they want to work on through the mentoring relationship. Together, the mentor and mentee can discuss action steps and activities to help support the mentoring goals. For example, the mentee might observe the mentor in leading various leadership activities (such as leading a staff or committee meeting).

Structured tools are helpful to initiate the relationship. These might include icebreaker discussion (background of mentor/mentee), current roles, sharing past experiences, strengths and weaknesses, and highlighting the needs of the mentee as initial work to start the mentoring journey.

THE MENTORING PROCESS

Mentoring has many identified approaches in the literature which range from seeking an individual mentor to having multiple mentors throughout your career to help you develop specific skill sets (Disch, 2018; Hale, 2018; Vitale, 2018). Key principles of the mentoring relationship are described in Table 7.3. Nurse leaders may assume the role of mentor and/or mentee in various phases of their career progression.

Tools and discussion are used to support the relationship and make progress toward reaching goals. In addition to defined goals, Hale and Phillips (2018) have outlined a nurse-to-nurse mentoring theory that includes the following phases: seeding, opening, laddering, equalizing, and reframing. Seeding and opening are the phases to begin the mentor/mentee relationship structure and process. As the relationship progresses, "laddering" occurs, where the bulk of the relationship and interactions with mentor and mentee take place. As the relationship develops over time, an equalizing phase occurs where the mentor and mentee might perceive themselves as equal. As the relationship evolves or ends, reframing is when the relationship is reevaluated (Hale & Phillips, 2018).

The mentoring process is not always a linear one, and there is often a point in time where the mentor and mentee become colleagues (Figure 7.2). In that case, the mentee can seek another mentor to develop new skills as well as become a mentor to others to help develop and support the profession of nursing.

TABLE 7.3: Mentoring Roles and Associated Principles

Mentoring Roles	Principles of the Mentoring Relationship
Mentee	Seeks expertise of the mentor and is open to feedback. Seeks out mentoring relationships. Takes the initiative for their own development. Sets goals with their mentor. Learns from the process and the experience mentoring offers. Is a mentor during their career.
Mentor	Offers expertise to support the mentee. Commits to the relationship. Shares their positive stories as well as lessons learned to help the mentee avoid leadership pitfalls.
Mentor and mentee	Commitment is made to the relationship.

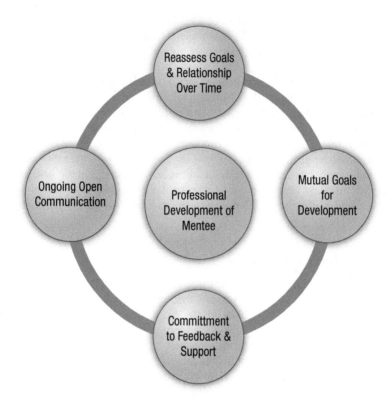

FIGURE 7.2: Key attributes of mentoring.

USES FOR MENTORING

Mentoring improves the skill sets and competencies of the mentee to help improve role performance as well as the benefits that are also noted in coaching relationships including job satisfaction and improving role effectiveness. Mentoring is often perceived to be broader than coaching as mentoring encompasses a wide scope of professional development and core competencies as the mentoring relationship evolves.

Mentoring is a way to develop and gain skills throughout your career from novice to expert in leadership roles. Having a mentor can help you develop skills as you progress in leadership roles, while offering you a skill set to become a mentor to others. By having and being a mentor, you can develop your skills as well as help others to develop key skills and leadership competencies.

A nurse leader can use mentoring to help determine career goals early in her career, seek mentoring upon transitioning to a new role, and obtain lifelong advice from expert colleagues throughout her career. The nurse leader can also contribute to the profession by becoming a mentor to support the development of colleagues who can benefit from their expertise and support. Lastly, the nurse leader who also mentors others to develop skills paves the way for succession planning, which could also benefit the mentor by allowing the mentor to seek their own development. (While doing succession planning for their role, they should position themselves for more complex and advanced roles simultaneously.)

RESEARCH LITERATURE REVIEW

Although there is research in the literature related to mentoring for clinical nurses, there is a dearth of research in the area of nurse leader mentoring (Hafsteinsdottir et al., 2017; Vitale, 2018). However, there have been a few studies related to nurse leader mentoring that are discussed in the text that follows.

The Veterans Health Administration (VHA) system held a pilot program to support development of leadership skills for mental health nurse leaders in the areas of strategic planning, HR, systems understanding, administrative operations and program evaluation, and professional and personal development (Kearney et al., 2018). Thirty-one new leaders participated, and significant improvement was found in all key areas. In addition, there was improvement in employee satisfaction as well (Kearney et al., 2018).

The New Jersey Organization of Nurse Leaders implemented a yearlong program to develop and mentor leaders with reported success in key areas (Rich et al., 2015; Wurmser & Kowalski, 2020). The New Jersey Organization of Nurse Leaders mentoring programs have reported on several cohorts of mentor/mentees in the literature highlighting the benefits of mentoring nurse leaders. Their goal was to establish a statewide mentorship program with a framework and model to support nurse leader mentoring (Rich et al., 2015). Programmatic information and feedback from the participants was acquired in some of the cohorts through qualitative research (Wurmser & Kowalski, 2020). The participants, both mentors and mentees, reported the program was positive and effective.

Nursing mentoring was a part of a nursing leadership development project by Ramseur et al. (2018). The nurse managers took a pre- and posttest as part of the program evaluation. A mentor was assigned to each participant during the program, which included monthly meetings. A statistically significant increase in all three subscales (managing the business, the art of leading people, and the leader within) of the nurse manager inventory tool were noted. In addition, Roth and Whitehead (2019) reported on the impact of a peer mentoring program for nurse managers on their job satisfaction and intent to stay in their positions. Fifteen nurse managers participated in the study of leadership practices inventory, and nurse manager practice environment scale, job satisfaction, intent to stay in the role, and leadership behaviors were evaluated. Leadership practices as well as nurse manager culture of generativity subscales were noted to have statistically significant differences between the pre- and posttest scores. This study used a peer mentoring process where peers enrolled in the study self-selected their mentors.

In summary, there are widely known benefits in the literature for mentoring clinical nurses while fewer studies focus on developing the process and science of nurse leader mentoring. As the field of nurse leader mentoring continues to develop through national programs such as AONL and Sigma Theta Tau (AONL, 2021; Sigma Theta Tau, 2021), there is a need for ongoing research examining the needs of nurse leaders engaged in mentoring relationships throughout their career. What are the long-term outcomes of nurse leader mentoring as they relate to job effectiveness, impact on staff and patient satisfaction, burnout of self, and impact on achieving organizational goals or other potential outcomes? Additional research in these areas can benefit further development of nurse leader mentoring programs and provide documentation of their impact on nursing.

MENTORING CAREER SCENARIOS

As it did in the previously noted coaching career scenario section, the use of Benner (1982) also applies to the scenarios presented in the text that follows. These scenarios are examples where mentoring can help a nurse leader gain the skills required for their role.

◆ CASE SCENARIO

EARLY CAREER MENTORING FOR NOVICE, ADVANCED BEGINNER STAGE

SITUATION

SS is a new graduate who has just completed formal orientation. SS feels minimally competent in their role, and then seeks support and guidance from an experienced nurse to help guide them in their professional development. SS is seeking to become a charge nurse or a new nurse manager and needs skills beyond technical competency in nursing for continued role transition and success.

APPROACH

SS can inquire to see if their organization has a formal mentoring program. If so, SS can become part of the formal mentoring program. If not, SS may seek out a mentor in the organization with the guidance of their preceptor or supervisor or another coworker. Finding a mentor who has the desired skills the mentee is seeking will be helpful to the mentee in the beginning to build their skill set for development.

OUTCOME

SS finds that their organization has a formal mentoring process applicable to new graduate nurses only. SS talks with their manager, leader, and colleagues to discuss potential mentors within the organization. SS then meets with the identified mentor to identify goals and a development plan. SS is technically competent but needs support and development on their leadership journey as they transition from a staff to a formal leadership role. SS and their mentor meet regularly over the next several months to discuss progress toward SS's goal as well as to share experiences. As the relationship progressed, SS and their mentor became colleagues who helped support each other as partners. SS moved on to a nurse manager role and left the organization but did stay in contact, at times informally, with their mentor over the next few years. As SS assumed their manager role, they sought a mentor in their new organization who could support SS's development as a nurse manager and the skills of financial management and other key skills SS wanted to develop.

DISCUSSION QUESTIONS

1. What is the process for mentoring in your organization?
2. How can a new nurse obtain formal mentoring support in your organization?
3. If you do not have a mentoring program, what can you do to help find a mentor as well as help support those seeking a mentor?

⬡ CASE SCENARIO

MID-CAREER MENTORING FOR COMPETENT-PROFICIENT STAGE

SITUATION

NJ is a medical–surgical unit nurse manager who has been promoted to a large scope nursing director role. NJ will be the nurse leader responsible for several medical–surgical and intermediate care units as well as oversight of quality, patient experience, and professional practice for the nursing organization. NJ will now have nurse managers of these areas reporting to them. NJ has been a mentor to other nurse managers, but now finds themself needing a mentor for the executive leadership role they will assume.

APPROACH

NJ is aware that their organization does not offer formal mentoring. NJ will be transitioned to their new role and report to the chief nursing officer (CNO) of the organization who has a broad role which will limit their ability to mentor NJ. NJ does a self-assessment of their strengths and opportunities for development and discusses the analysis with their leader. Together, they identify several core role competencies NJ will need to be successful in their new role. NJ seeks out two mentors who have strengths in the areas, which include financial management and how to steer the nursing leadership team they have oversight for to achieve organizational goals. NJ seeks out mentorship support from a former leader they worked with who has served as a nurse executive, and also seeks mentoring from a trusted HR colleague who has strengths in organizational development and leadership development. Over the next several months, NJ meets with them and works on developing strengths in these key areas.

OUTCOME

A mid-career mentor helps someone who is making upward progressive changes in leadership roles. Skills that an entry level manager needs are not the same skills a nurse executive needs, so a strong mentor can ensure success at this time. NJ is successful as they have the EI to recognize the need for continued development. At this stage of NJ's career, NJ feels they need two mentors who each have unique qualities and skills NJ wants to develop that will ensure NJ's success in their new role. NJ is successful as they have an intentional and thoughtful approach to seeking a mentor during this time. NJ also joins regional and national nursing leadership organizations and becomes certified in nursing leadership to help network as well as to increase and maintain leadership competencies for their executive role.

DISCUSSION QUESTIONS

1. What might be potential challenges for NJ in being promoted and supervising former peers?
2. How can NJ leverage potential sources for mentorship in the professional organizations they have joined?
3. What potential internal sources (formal or informal) of mentorship might be available for NJ in their new role? Could non-nursing mentors help them gain new skills? Describe.

● | CASE SCENARIO

LATE CAREER MENTOR COACHING FOR COMPETENT-PROFICIENT ROLE CHANGE MENTORING

SITUATION

For the purposes of this example, a former CNO who changes roles to become a nursing faculty member will be discussed. LM was a CNO for many years who is nearing retirement. LM has been approached by a nursing dean to join the faculty at a nearby public academic institution. LM makes the transition to a faculty role. However, they quickly realize that they have many years of practice in nursing leadership but lack the experience and core skills needed to be a successful professor. A late career mentor is someone who is either being mentored for a new role (second nursing career) or someone who changes fields at a late stage in their career. A late career mentor could be someone who transitions from a leadership position to a staff role or a high-level leadership position to a middle management role or a nurse who changes nursing fields at a late stage in their career.

APPROACH

LM approaches the dean to ask for a faculty mentor. The dean facilitates an introductory meeting with LM and an experienced faculty member. LM identifies their key experience and goals and sets up subsequent meetings with the mentor. LM outlines a personal development plan and has ongoing meetings with their mentor to review the key goals, skills, and competencies needed to become an effective leader. LM moves from a novice to a seasoned faculty member over the next year with the support of their mentor.

OUTCOME

LM initially struggles and feels frustrated as this new role is quite different from their leadership role in the acute-care setting. The structure and process are hugely different in the day-to-day work. LM enjoys the flexibility of their new role while also longing to feel like the expert they were seen as in their prior role. Being a neophyte in this setting is a humbling experience. After the first few months, LM dedicates time to meeting with a mentor who helps them. LM realizes that the autonomy in their new role necessitates that they identify their needs and seek help from esteemed colleagues who have expert knowledge of academia. By their sixth month in the new role, LM feels many rewards and is thankful that they made this change late in their career. LM feels professionally rewarded for the opportunity to influence the next generation of nurses while also feeling respected by students and academic peers for the knowledge of practice LM has brought into the department.

DISCUSSION QUESTIONS

1. What opportunities does the university have for formalizing a mentoring approach for new faculty? What do you think the next steps and possible approaches might be?

2. If someone late in their career was changing from a leadership role to another role in an organization (for example, a nurse director or manager role to a staff nurse or a role such as a quality control, education, or case manager role), what suggestions do you have for the organization and for the nurse leader making the transition?

3. What are the key mentoring needs for someone who is an expert in their current role who is moving to a new role and will be a novice?

◼ WHAT EVERY NURSE MANAGER NEEDS TO KNOW ABOUT COACHING AND MENTORING

Coaching and mentoring will manifest differently within organizations and are dependent upon relationships and performance intentions. Every nurse manager needs to know that coaching and mentoring will not happen without deliberate resources applied. First, nurse managers will need to invest time and energy in beginning their professional relationships to support themselves as a new leader to continue their professional development and growth. The scope of their oversight and long-term vision will vary for each position and utilization for coaching and mentoring, but relationships are crucially important. As discussed within Chapter 4 of this text, "The Importance of Relationships," relationships matter.

Another element of coaching and mentoring that is important to be cognizant of is the necessity to honor the professional wisdom and clinical expertise held by the coach and mentor. Trusting in others to know their job, their goals, and the steps necessary to reach the goals is essential for the nurse leader who is coaching. Nurse leaders will need to validate the professional wisdom that others hold, as well as celebrate and nurture the wisdom for it to be expressed fully.

A third crucial point for nurse managers to acknowledge is that coaching and mentoring require thoughtful, targeted, and timely development questions. Coaching questions assist others to gain clarity about their goals. Often the questions provoke personal awareness that supports performance growth. Samples of questions are provided in Table 7.2. Generally, the best questions are open-ended, personalized, and serve as a platform for a coaching session.

Finally, nurse managers must recognize that coaching and mentoring unlock potential in others and the universe. Hold space for possible outcomes that may emerge. Be prepared for affirming the accomplishments of the coached and mentored and honoring the contributions of the coached and mentored to overall goal attainment within a unit and/or team.

⬤ WHAT EVERY NURSE EXECUTIVE NEEDS TO KNOW ABOUT COACHING AND MENTORING

Coaching and mentoring are often not offered as a formal process or program in many institutions and settings. Often, the nurse seeks a mentor for support during various phases of their career development. Formal and informal coaching and mentoring can provide dedicated support to acquire key skills and competencies as coaches and mentors share their experiences and expertise with their mentee. First, as a nurse executive one must not only seek out these coaching and mentoring opportunities but to also guide their team into these relationships to support leader development and succession planning. Explore what is available in your institution or via a professional nursing organization. What are the key skills you need? What resources are available to you and your team? How can you partner with other organizational executives to develop and promote coaching and mentoring in your organization?

Second, throughout your career, take initiative for your own development. You can acquire strong mentors at different career phases based on your needs. You will need to think about what skills you need as you develop and plan for your career.

Third, once you find a coach and a mentor, have a formal mechanism to set goals and track progress. Identify early in the relationship what the short-term and long-term goals are for the mentoring relationship. How will you track and monitor your progress? How often will you meet? Will you meet in person, virtually, or both? As a nurse executive, how will you instill the skills you have learned to support and develop your team? How will you serve as a mentor and coach to others or provide leadership support to less experienced leaders?

Lastly, learn from the coaching and mentoring process. What experiences are helpful to you? Become a mentor to others as well during various phases of your career. You can be a mentor and a mentee simultaneously to help others develop their skills. Mentors often state great rewards and learning from their mentee as they serve as a mentor. Help develop mentoring processes and programs in your setting to help advance nursing leaders. In addition, identify coaches and coaching opportunities for your team members to support their development through role modeling of being coached and mentored, as well as through executive support of coaching and mentoring you and supporting your development as well as the success of your leadership team in their development.

KEY POINTS

- Coaching is often a formal, short-term skill development process and relationship. Coaching is goal oriented and has a specific time frame for achieving the goals identified. Coaches seek to highlight the wisdom that the person they are coaching has to help the person being coached identify solutions.

- Mentoring is often more information with direct access to expertise, driven by the mentee through goal setting. Mentoring roles and goals are mutually identified in the relationship. Most often, mentees drive the relationship as they seek guidance from their mentors.

- Coaching and mentoring might overlap in some situations as both involve collaborative directed relationships to help develop skills. Both are safe positive methods for leaders to collaborate with experts to share opportunities for their growth and development as a leader.

- It is important to define roles when entering coaching/mentoring relationships.

SUMMARY

Coaching and mentoring can be incorporated as deliberate strategies into any nurse leader or nurse executive's plan for reaching top performance in individuals, groups, and teams. The strategies of coaching and mentoring can be utilized to meet the performance needs of various professionals. At the same time, coaching and mentoring can improve healthcare quality and safety outcomes. While nonprescriptive, coaching generally is more short term, targeted, and goal driven, mentoring is a relationship that can last long term; it is multifaceted and crosses seasons of life.

Coaching and mentoring within a healthcare organization may hold overlapping elements but are distinct roles. The coach is trained to use specific skills to accomplish identified goals. A coach augments natural ability found within an individual, group, or team and supports the identification and removal of barriers, whereas a mentor may naturally and without training serve as a resource/role model to an individual, group, or team. A mentor is someone who is learned from to facilitate peak performance.

Coaching and mentoring allow the nurse leader/executive to honor diversity and be inclusive as they develop, form, and nurture peak performing teams comprised of peak performing individuals and groups. Bradley (2020) asserts that inclusive leadership seeks to embrace all healthcare staff, mitigates silos, and engages all perspectives. Further, Bradley notes,

> Attracting diverse people (diverse in perspectives, professional identities, and experiences) to the work, engaging the pluralism of ideas and perspectives to unearth new ways of seeing old problems, and channeling the inevitable conflict into creative problem solving takes strong leadership and commitment at all levels (p. 268).

It is likely apparent to any nurse leader or executive that different people present with different perspectives, performance capacities, and goals. Coaching and mentoring are adaptive to the uniqueness of whomever is involved. It is inherent to relational leadership approaches for a nurse leader/executive to authentically listen, seek to understand, and probe each member of the team to appreciate their goals. One nurse may desire more leadership responsibility, while another may desire to improve their clinical skills, or another may desire expanded communication skills. Utilizing coaching and mentoring in addition to an inclusive yet equitable style toward healthcare professional development leads to peak performance of individuals, groups, and teams.

Coaching and mentoring are enhanced with effective nursing leadership that is generally complemented by EI (Prezerakos, 2018). EI is also discussed in Chapter 6, "Relationship-Based Leadership Theories." It should be underscored that coaching and mentoring involve the ability to support and guide others; therefore, nurse leaders utilize their ability to manage their own emotions and responses as they nurture decision-making and actions of others. Being emotionally intelligent contributes to the transformational possibilities attained through coaching and mentoring for peak performance of individuals, groups, and teams.

END-OF-CHAPTER RESOURCES

DISCUSSION QUESTIONS

1. What are the benefits of coaching and mentoring?
2. What are the similarities and differences between coaching and mentoring?
3. How can a nurse leader support coaching and mentoring practices within the organization?
4. Describe how a nurse leader would seek out opportunities for coaching and mentoring.
5. How can you support your team through use of coaching or mentoring for yourself or your team?

◼ ADDITIONAL RESOURCES

PODCASTS

- *Coaching for Leaders* (multiple episodes; https://coachingforleaders.com/)
- *Natural Born Coaches* (multiple episodes; https://www.naturalborncoaches.com/)
- *The Art of Coaching* (multiple episodes; https://artofcoaching.com/podcast/)
- *The Coaching Life Podcast* (multiple episodes; https://www.philg.com/podcast/)
- *The Coaching Podcast* (multiple episodes; https://podcasts.apple.com/cg/podcast/the-coaching-podcast/id1189492103)

TED TALKS

- Gawande, A. (2017). *Want to get great at something? Get a coach* [Video]. 16 min 58 secs. Ted.com. (https://www.ted.com/talks/atul_gawande_want_to_get_great_at_something_get_a_coach
- Frei, F. (2018). *How to build and rebuild trust* [Video]. 14 min 57 secs. Ted.com. https://www.ted.com/talks/frances_frei_how_to_build_and_rebuild_trust
- Lyle, E. (2019). *How to break bad habits before they reach the next generation of leaders* [Video]. 12 min 3 secs. Ted.com. https://www.ted.com/talks/elizabeth_lyle_how_to_break_bad_management_habits_before_they_reach_the_next_generation_of_leaders
- Nelson, R. (2019). *The power of mentoring* [Video]. 15 min 17 secs. YouTube. https://www.youtube.com/watch?v=0W3d-PJ4-FM&t=1s
- Ortiz, K. (2019). *How to be a great mentor* [Video]. 14 min 34 secs. YouTube. https://www.youtube.com/watch?v=G3q8kEn_nsg
- Stanford, A. (2017). *Standing on the shoulders of giants* [Video]. 15 min 41 secs. YouTube. https://www.youtube.com/watch?v=WWoY8fabFck&t=8s
- Stewart, D. (2016). *5 ½ mentors that will change your life* [Video]. 17 min 47 secs. YouTube. https://www.youtube.com/watch?v=quhcyPpCaSk&t=2s
- Torres R. (2014). *What it takes to be a great leader* [Video]. 9 min 19 secs. Ted.com. https://www.ted.com/talks/roselinde_torres_what_it_takes_to_be_a_great_leader

WEB LINKS

- Ibarra, H., & Scoular A. (2019). The leader as coach: How to unleash innovation, energy, and commitment. *Harvard Business Review.* https://hbr.org/2019/11/the-leader-as-coach
- Hearne, M. (2019). Being direct without crossing the line. *The Institute for Life Coach Training.* https://www.lifecoachtraining.com//blog/entry/being_direct_without_crossing_the_line

◼ GLOSSARY OF KEY TERMS

- **Coach:** An individual who supports the coached achieve peak performance within a defined and committed relationship.
- **Coached:** An individual meeting with a coach to meet goals maximizing their own expertise.
- **Coaching:** A proactive collaborative process that supports goal achievement and high performance through discourse and action.
- **Mentee:** Someone who seeks to find help and support from a mentor to help themselves with professional development and future career goals.

- **Mentoring:** A process that supports and develops people to help them reach their potential.
- **Mentor:** An experienced nursing leader who is willing to support the development of the mentee through support and guidance.

A robust set of instructor resources designed to supplement this text is located at http://connect.springerpub.com/content/book/978-0-8261-7795-7. Qualifying instructors may request access by emailing textbook@springerpub.com.

REFERENCES

American Organization for Nursing Leadership. (2021). *Leader to leader member community.* https://www.aonl.org/membership/community

Auerbach, J. (2021). *The benefits of business coaching.* https://www.executivecoachcollege.com/research-and-publications/benefits-of-business-coaching.php

Beeson, J. (2018). Deconstructing executive presence. In A. J. Cuddy, D. Tannen, A. J. Su, & J. Beeson (Eds.), *Leadership presence (HBR Emotional Intelligence Series)* (pp. 1–11). Harvard Business Review Press.

Benner, P. (1982). From novice to expert. *American Journal of Nursing, 82*(3), 402–407. https://journals.lww.com/ajnonline/citation/1982/82030/from_novice_to_expert.4.aspx

Bradley, E. (2020). Diversity, inclusive leadership, and health outcomes. *International Journal of Health Policy and Management, 9*(7), 266–268. https://doi.org/10.15171/ijhpm.2020.12

Brown-DeVeaux, D., & Jean-Louis, K. (2021). Using a mentorship approach to address the underrepresentation of ethnic minorities in senior nursing leadership. *Journal of Nursing Administration, 51*(3), 149–155. https://doi.org/10.1097/NNA.0000000000000986

Cable, S., & Graham, E. (2018). Leading better care: An evaluation of an accelerated coaching intervention for clinical nursing leadership development. *Journal of Nursing Management, 26*(5), 605–612. https://doi.org/10.1111/jonm.12590

Cziraki, K., Wong, C., Kerr, M., & Finegan, J. (2020). Leader empowering behavior: Relationships with nurse and patient outcomes. *Leadership in Health Sciences, 33*(4), 397–415. https://doi.org/10.1108/LHS-04-2020-0019

Disch, J. (2018). Rethinking mentoring. *Critical Care Medicine, 46*(3), 438–441. https://doi.org/10.1097/CCM.0000000000002914

Dyess, S. M., Sherman, R. O., Opalinski, A., & Eggenberger, T. (2017). Structured coaching programs to develop staff. *Journal of Continuing Education in Nursing, 48*(8), 373–378. https://doi.org/10.3928/00220124-20170712-10

Fielden, S. L., Davidson, M. J., & Sutherland, V. J. (2009). Innovations in coaching and mentoring: Implications for nurse leadership development. *Health Services Management Research, 22*, 92–99. https://doi.org/10.1258/hsmr.2008.008021

Gray, J. (2018). Leadership coaching and mentoring: A research-based model for stronger partnerships. *International Journal of Education Policy and Leadership, 13*(12), 1–7. https://doi.org/10.22230/ijepl.2018v13n12a844

Hafsteinsdottir, T. B., van der Zwaag, A. M., & Schuurmans, M. J. (2017). Leadership mentoring in nursing research, career development, and scholarly productivity: A systematic review. *International Journal of Nursing Studies, 75*, 21–34. https://doi.org/10.1016/j.ijnurstu.2017.07.004

Hale, R. L. (2018). Conceptualizing the mentoring relationship: An appraisal of evidence. *Nursing Forum, 53*(3), 333–338. https://doi.org/10.1111/nuf.12259

Hale, R. L., & Phillips, C. A. (2018). Mentoring up: A grounded theory of nurse-to-nurse mentoring. *Journal of Clinical Nursing. 28*(1-2), 159–172. https://doi.org/10.1111/jocn.14636

Hugill, K., Sullivan, J., & Ezpeleta, L. (2018). Team coaching and rounding as a framework to enhance organizational wellbeing & team performance. *Journal of Neonatal Nursing, 24*(3), 148–153. https://doi.org/10.1016/j.jnn.2017.10.004

International Coaching Community. (n.d.). *International Coaching Community homepage*. https:// internationalcoachingcommunity.com

Kearney, L. K., Smith, C., Carroll, D., Burk, J. P., Cohen, J. L., & Henderson, K. (2018). Veterans' Health Administration's (VHA) national mental health leadership mentoring program: A pilot evaluation. *Training and Education in Professional Psychology, 12*(1), 29–37. https://doi.org/10.1037/ tep0000164

Leigh, J. A., Littlewood, L., & Heggs, K. (2018). Using simulation to test use of coaching in clinical placements. *Nursing Times, 114*(4), 44–46. https://www.nursingtimes.net/roles/nurse-educators/ using-simulation-to-test-use-of-coaching-in-clinical-placements-12-03-2018

Leigh, J., Littlewood, L., & Lyons, G. (2019). Reflection on creating a coaching approach to student nurse clinical leadership development. *British Journal of Nursing, 28*(17), 1124–1128. https://doi .org/10.12968/bjon.2019.28.17.1124

Olson, A., & Tan, S. C. (2018). Leadership coaching: A cross-cultural exploration. *Journal of Practical Consulting, 6*(1), 65–73. https://www.regent.edu/acad/global/publications/jpc/vol6iss1/ JPC_6-1_Olson_Tan_pgs65-73.pdf

Pandolfi, C. (2020). Active ingredients in executive coaching: A systematic literature review. *International Coaching Psychology Review, 15*(2), 6–30. https://www.trishturner.co.uk/wp-content/ uploads/2020/10/Active-ingredients-in-executive-coaching-A-systematic-literature-review -2020.pdf

Prezerakos, P. E. (2018). Nurse managers' emotional intelligence and effective leadership: A review of the current evidence. *Open Nursing Journal, 12*, 86–92. https://doi.org/10.2174/ 1874434601812010086

Ramseur, P., Fuchs, M. A., Edwards, P., & Humphreys, J. (2018). The implementation of a structured nursing leadership development program for succession planning in a health system. *Journal of Nursing Administration, 48*(1), 25–30. https://doi.org/10.1097/NNA.0000000000000566

Rich, M., Kempin, B., Loughlin, M. J., Vitale, T. R., Wurmser, T., & Thrall, T. H. (2015). Developing leadership talent: A statewide nurse leader mentorship program. *Journal of Nursing Administration, 45*(2), 63–66. https://doi.org/10.1097/NNA.0000000000000166

Roth, T., & Whitehead, D. (2019). Impact of a nurse manager peer mentorship program on job satisfaction and intent to stay. *Journal of Excellence in Nursing and Healthcare Practice, 1*, 4–14. https://doi.org/10.5590/JENHP.2019.1.1.02

Sherman, R. O. (2019). *The nurse leader coach: Become the boss no one wants to leave*. Author.

Shirey, M. (2013). Executive presence for strategic influence. *Journal of Nursing Administration, 43*(7/8), 373–376. https://doi.org/10.1097/NNA.0b013e31829d6096

Sigma Theta Tau. (2021). Mentoring cohort. https://www.sigmanursing.org/advance-elevate/ careers/sigma-mentoring-cohort

Titzer, J. L., Shirey, M. R., & Hauck, S. (2014). A nurse manager succession planning model with associated empirical outcomes. *Journal of Nursing Administration, 44*(1), 37–46. https://doi .org/10.1097/NNA.0000000000000019

Vitale, T. (2018). Nurse leader mentorship. *Nursing Management, 49*(2), 8–10. https://doi.org/10.1097/ 01.NUMA.0000529932.89246.ab

Waldrop, J., & Derouin, A. (2019). The coaching experience of advanced practice nurses in a national leadership program. *The Journal of Continuing Education in Nursing, 50*(4), 170–175. https://doi .org/10.3928/00220124-20190319-07

Wilmoth, M. C., & Shapiro, S. E. (2014). The intentional development of nurses as leaders. *Journal of Nursing Administration, 44*(6), 333–338. https://doi.org/10.1097/NNA.0000000000000078

Withrow, L. (2020). Fostering curiosity, asking powerful questions: Lessons of a leadership coach. *Journal of Religious Leadership, 19*(1), 69–82.

Wurmser, T., & Kowalski, M. O. (2020). Perceptions of a statewide nurse mentorship programme: A qualitative study. *Journal of Nursing Management, 28*(7), 1545–1552. https://doi.org/10.1111/ jonm.13104

SECTION III

INNOVATIVE AND EXPANDING MODELS OF CARE DELIVERY

CHAPTER 8

VALUE-BASED CONTRACTING

Kristine Adams and Nicholas Engelhardt

"... a comprehensive health program is required as an essential link in our national defenses against individual and social insecurity."

Franklin Delano Roosevelt, 1939

LEARNING OBJECTIVES

- Demonstrate understanding of the history of healthcare payment structures and their effect on healthcare delivery over the decades.
- Differentiate fee-for-service versus value-based care.
- Appraise how the different payment structures affect the care delivered and how nursing must adapt to the different structures.
- Evaluate the different types of alternative payment programs available in the United States market.
- Investigate the differences between government payor programs and commercial programs.

INTRODUCTION

Today's healthcare landscape in the United States is extremely complex and increasingly more difficult for patients to navigate. In the United States, there has not been an appetite for a single-payor health system to provide a basic safety net of care to our population. Instead, over the years fragmented approaches from both government and commercial payors, healthcare systems, private practices, and hospitals have all emerged to attempt to fill gaps for patients. What has resulted is a complex, multilayered system that has become difficult to navigate for both patients and providers alike.

As a nurse manager and executive leader, it has never really been the purview of nursing to get involved in the financial aspects of taking care of patients. As nurses, we have always prided ourselves on being "payor agnostic," meaning treating patients regardless of their insurance coverage and ability to pay. And as much as we can continue to do this, we must be mindful of the payor landscape in which we work. Different payors have different requirements for their members, and both the providers and consumers (also known as members) must understand the extent of their coverage and what requirements need to be met for payment.

It is an interesting time in our healthcare history and one as nurses we should capitalize on. For the very first time, payors and healthcare providers are actually on the same page in wanting to keep our populations healthy and well. For everyone, especially the patient, the health outcomes are the best in a value-based payment structure where good health is incentivized. And for the payor, the costs of care decrease if the patient can avoid worsening of illness. The provider/hospital side hopefully will get relief from constantly full beds and worsening mortality from chronic disease. As nurses, if we embrace these opportunities to partner with patients and payors, we can really achieve the best health outcomes for our populations. In this chapter we discuss the various payor landscapes that are attempting to do this and the programs driving these initiatives. Chapter 9, "Population and Community Health," discusses implementation of these initiatives. But healthcare starts where the money does: at the point of payment.

HEALTHCARE HISTORY

The financing of our healthcare system began after World War II when Harry Truman became president after the death of Franklin Delano Roosevelt. It was FDR who asked Congress for the Economic Bill of Rights that included the right to adequate healthcare for all Americans. This was never fulfilled by Congress, but Harry Truman continued his attempts by proposing a national healthcare program. The American Medical Association (AMA) denounced this proposal as a "communist plot" and thus it never did pass. This was a time, however, when Europe and many other industrialized nations were starting their own national healthcare programs.

In 1965, under ever-increasing healthcare costs, Social Security Act Amendments were passed by Congress to establish the Centers for Medicare & Medicaid Services (CMS), enacting the first and only source of socialized medicine in the United States. The program was designed to care for those citizens who were poor and older adults. Unfortunately, it suffered a benefit design that was taken from the many commercial plans that were also being developed during the 1960s and 1970s. Almost overnight, the federal government became the largest healthcare consumer and the effects on the federal budget have been felt ever since. None of these plans had any utilization management or cost containment strategies. A "moral hazard" was created by giving people open access to healthcare services, resulting in overutilization and increasing costs.

As the United States entered the 1980s and 1990s, healthcare costs began to soar. Much of this was due to the ever-advancing technologies that were very successful in treating cardiovascular disease and cancer. However, U.S. healthcare costs were 50% higher than other industrialized nations and the United States had a lower life expectancy and higher infant mortality rate compared to other peer nations around the world. Something had to be done; therefore, Medicare and Medicaid developed different types of healthcare plans including health maintenance organizations (HMOs) and prospective payment systems (PPS). In addition, 475 diagnostic-related groups (DRGs) were added, creating a capitated payment model. Simply put, a maximum dollar amount was allotted for each DRG, and the dollars left over after caring for the patient were kept by the hospital as profit. This is very similar to the bundle programs we often hear about today. Readmission penalties were assessed if patients returned to the hospital above acceptable levels. As an effect of this payment structure, hospitals began a care model redesign, putting into place functions such as utilization management that were intended to evaluate the necessity of medical care. Length of stay (LOS) within the hospitals became scrutinized because the longer a patient occupied a bed, the more money was spent caring for the patient, and thus less profit for the hospital. One extreme example of this LOS scrutiny took place in the maternity ward where "drive through deliveries" were commonplace. A mother delivered on a Saturday and mom and baby had to leave Sunday. Care paths, pharmacy formularies, consolidations, and partnerships of hospitals were all a part of a forced redesign by the payment structures that were attempting to reduce the cost of care. In 1999 the Core Measures were introduced by The Joint Commission (TJC) with implementation in 2001. This was the first large-scale attempt to start looking at the quality of care provided in a given organization (Moselely, 2008).

The next large-scale attempt to contain healthcare costs that also added the tenets of accessibility and quality outcomes was the Affordable Care Act (ACA). This was designed by a team of healthcare providers and stakeholders under President Barack Obama. In 2008 the national gross domestic product (GDP) cost of healthcare in the United States was 17%, the highest ever and far above peer nations which hovered around 9%. Many Americans were finding themselves underinsured or uninsured during the housing mortgage crises and subsequent economic downturn of 2008. In enacting the ACA in 2010, with full roll out in 2014, Americans had access to a free-market healthcare exchange, where they could purchase healthcare plans independent of an employer at an affordable cost. This was a first major attempt to improve healthcare access for Americans who increasingly could not afford it. It had many provisions for improving and building out primary care practices instead of investing in expensive hospitals. Efforts were put into more preventive care to prevent disease and increase life expectancy and quality. Another major and important provision was accountability for healthcare outcomes. This was being placed on health systems, hospitals, and primary care practices in increasing ways.

FEE-FOR-SERVICE VERSUS VALUE-BASED CARE

Historically in the United States, healthcare has been transactional. The care is episodic. From a patient perspective, one gets sick or injured, seeks healthcare, gets better, goes on with life, and receives a bill. The hope for the patient is always that the incident is over and that life can continue as it was with no further intervention needed. In a fee-for-service (FFS) world, profit is earned on the healthcare provider's side. The more often a person is sick and the more interventions performed, the more bills are generated, and the more money made. There is little regard for what happens to the patient in this scenario. If left unchecked, as has been done historically, healthcare providers can perform unnecessary and costly testing and interventions on an unknowing patient. For example, in a systematic review in 2017, Morgan et al. (2018) reviewed the top 10 overused and overperformed medical procedures. At the top of the list is advanced cardiac imaging, which has tripled in incidence over the last 10 years. Some of this is driven by consumer demand, but also by profit margins. Testing often leads to even more testing, invasive procedures, further complications, and higher costs of care. FFS thrives on independent practice where the ability of providers and healthcare systems to write their own paychecks went unmonitored. Now enter the solution: value-based care (VBC).

Conversely to FFS, VBC is not concerned with payment around volume; its payment structure lies in overall patient outcomes, promoting quality and safety (Table 8.1). In this payment model, all areas of the continuum of care must be seamlessly aligned and coordinated. This is accomplished through the functions of care coordination (CC), which often rely heavily on nurses, social workers, behavioral health caregivers, community health workers, and care navigators. Patients are often very confused about the complexities of navigating the fragmented and episodic healthcare system. Healthcare has become complicated with its many specialists, testing, complicated interventions, interpreting and obtaining results,

TABLE 8.1: Comparison of Fee-for-Service and Value-Based Care

Fee-for-Service	Value-Based Care
• Transactional care delivery	• Longitudinal health outcome consideration
• Episodic clinical decisions	• Incentivizing coordinated care delivery
• Can lead to overtesting	• Health outcomes closely tracked and measured
• Uncoordinated care delivery continuum	• Care coordination

and understanding next steps. Primarily, these functions of CC reside in the ambulatory or primary care space although they start in the transitions of care out of the hospital. Making that connection between the inpatient hospital and outpatient clinic for a seamless transition of care is more important than ever in a value-based contracting payment model. Outpatient evaluation and testing is far less expensive, and the constant push to provide interventions on an outpatient basis is even more paramount. The VBC reimbursement model puts the focus on preventing disease and keeping patients healthy—also widely known as population health. The ACA made many provisions to allow for this new reimbursement model, and incentivized both the CMS and commercial payors to adopt a new care model that supports these initiatives, which we will discuss later.

STRATEGIES OF VALUE-BASED CARE

In order to have a VBC model, there are key components that need to be a part of the care design. These key points are

- correct patient attribution;
- closed network of services that provides care throughout the life span and continuum with minimal leakage;
- data and analytics;
- risk stratification data, so a provider knows where to put their resources and who needs intense CC;
- wellness and prevention strategies for patients; and
- patient activation.

PATIENT ATTRIBUTION

Attribution of patients refers to being assigned a provider that is responsible for all of the care and can coordinate functions with specialists and other services as needed for seamless transitions and increased efficiencies. Attribution is also important in ensuring that the quality outcome metrics that are achieved by a provider relate to the panel of patients for whom the provider is responsible for care.

CLOSED NETWORK OF SERVICES

All these quality outcome metrics need to roll up for payment; thus, it is important to offer patients a closed network of services they may need for all their healthcare needs and not have them "leak" out of the system. Leakage causes fragmented care and often duplication of services, especially if a patient is moving across different healthcare systems, as it becomes difficult to determine who is to be credited for a patient's outcomes and who deserves payment. Therefore, many health benefit plans include different network tiers; accessing care outside the network will cost the patient more if they access outside the network. Critics of the value-based payment model argue that one cannot always control where a patient seeks care. To be successful, health systems must define their network and patients have to remain within those boundaries in order for accurate payment to be routed to a provider.

DATA AND ANALYTICS

Data and analytics are key components to perform successfully in a value-based contract. Identifying those patients who are "at risk" in a contract is important for front-line caregivers to know who may be in special payor arrangements that need to be addressed. This can be done through the electronic medical record if the health system has a team that can build and provide that artificial intelligence (AI). In addition, data and analytics can inform how a provider and health system are doing on any particular payor contract, and analysis of the data can illustrate performance metrics at any point during the de-fined contract year—also known as a "model year"—and guide necessary payment and adjustments.

RISK STRATIFICATION

Regardless of a health system's payment model, resources will always be limited. For this reason, "risk stratification" is important. Risk stratification allows the provider to understand which patients attributed to them need the most attention and care. Risk stratification can come through different avenues. There are data and analytics that can identify—based on age, comorbidities, even zip codes—who may really be at risk for high utilization costs. However, it is important to not lose the human touch: providers and their staff know attributed patients and their families well and understand the dynamics of any given individual who might need help. Consideration in adding those patients to the higher risk panels for closer monitoring is a sound strategy and speaks to the need of keeping the art of medicine and nursing in care delivery.

WELLNESS AND PREVENTION

Value-based contracting focuses on a wellness and disease prevention model of care. Providers and their attributed panels work together to achieve better identification and management of chronic disease through cancer screening, blood pressure control, diabetes management, atrial fibrillation, and stroke metrics (among many others) to prevent disease or slow the progression of chronic disease. Programs such as smoking cessation offerings, weight management, or diet and exercise may also be a part of value-based contracting to prevent illness and improve overall health.

PATIENT ACTIVATION

No initiatives are going to be successful if patients are not empowered and encouraged to be partners in their care. Patient activation refers to the patient having the knowledge, ability, skills, and confidence to manage their own health. Their active participation in following a plan of care, making positive changes in their health behaviors, taking their medications, and attending medical appointments for follow-up all factor in the success of their health outcomes (Green & Hibbard, 2011). A patient's ability can be measured and assessed using the validated tool of Patient Activation Measure (PAM). The PAM is a psychometric assessment that consists of 13 items that score a patient from 0 to 100, most falling within the 35- to 95-point range. The higher the score, the more able the patient is to manage their healthcare and affect their health outcomes. This can help healthcare providers gauge how to tailor interventions and assess changes (Hibbard et al., 2004)

SOCIAL DETERMINANTS OF HEALTH

The World Health Organization (WHO) defines the social determinants of health (SDOH) as the distribution of money, power, and resources at the global, national, and local levels that shapes the financial circumstances of our population (WHO, 2012). Intuitively, clinicians know that poverty brings poor health. It affects access to care, ability to act on recommended interventions, development of healthcare literacy, ability to purchase healthy food and medications, access to adequate shelter, and so on. Medical care accounts for only about 10% to 20% of the modifiable health factors that affect healthcare outcomes. The remaining 80% are rooted in a patient's understanding and financial ability to make the best choices possible for the best health outcomes. Healthcare systems often feel that this is not their area of clinical expertise and beyond the scope of their work as a medical provider (Magnan, 2017). However, value-based contracting pays on the health outcomes of patients, not on the process metrics. So, for healthcare systems to address the SDOH to achieve better health outcomes may be financially beneficial. Examples may include smoking cessation programs, obesity management programs, social workers embedded in practices to help patients manage behavioral health, and medically tailored food programs. These are just a few ways health systems are adding the resources to improve health outcomes.

◼ WHAT EVERY NURSE MANAGER NEEDS TO KNOW ABOUT VALUE-BASED CONTRACTING

A high-functioning nurse manager, who is tasked with initiatives such as throughput, LOS, total healthcare spend, or any other type of resource efficiency drivers, should be aware of the rules of the VBC world. They should, at a high level, be aware of which patients may fall into bundles, accountable care organizations (ACOs), or other value-based contracts that the healthcare system is a part of and how metrics like LOS, readmissions, and/or overall clinical outcomes may impact those contracts. Their staff should be well versed in appropriate clinical and social safety nets for all patients in order to buffer against negative outcomes, particularly for those patients who are in an at-risk contract with the network or system. Understanding the role of care management (CM) in the inpatient or ambulatory settings will be key in developing clear and safe discharge plans for your patients.

◆ CASE SCENARIO

HEALTHCARE ETHICS: A TALE OF TWO PATIENTS

RT is a 65-year-old who is a Medicare/Medicaid patient. This "dual eligible" status does not place them in a value-based contract. They are FFS for any hospital or provider who treats them. RT does not incur any out-of-pocket costs for medications. They have a primary care physician (PCP), but the PCP is private practice and is only loosely affiliated with several local hospitals. RT lives alone, is beginning to lose their sight, has no family close by, and has a case worker who runs their errands. RT has a history significant for chronic obstructive pulmonary disease (COPD) Gold Stage I, is on nebulizers at home as well as inhaled steroids, and goes on 3 L N/C of O₂ at night. RT continues to smoke 1 pack per day and has for the last 50 years. No one pays any penalty if RT's outcome metrics are poor. But Medicare/Medicaid incurs the cost of care, testing, medications, oxygen, transportation to repeat ED visits, and multiple hospital admissions as RT's chronic conditions continue to deteriorate.

FS is a 67-year-old who has traditional Medicare. They have a PCP strongly affiliated with a local healthcare system. This healthcare system has contracted with Medicare to be in an "ACO." This means that FS's PCP and the health system are accountable for FS's care and will only receive payment if FS stays out of the hospital and has good health outcomes. FS's history is also significant for COPD Stage I. FS is on nebulizers at home, takes an inhaled steroid, and uses 3 L O₂ prn. They smoke 1 pack per day as well and are starting to have some significant deterioration of their COPD. If FS were to enter the hospital, the hospital will only receive a "bundled payment," and if they re-enter the hospital in 90 days, the hospital will spend all the money they were given to care for FS just on this one episode. FS is also offered home care, respiratory therapy, and smoking cessation classes and coaching. FS says they cannot afford their inhaled steroid, so a pharmacist works with them to get the medications they need at a lower cost.

DISCUSSION QUESTIONS

1. Would a bedside nurse know the difference in these two patients' payor arrangements?
2. Should nursing be aware?
3. Should nursing continue to educate both patients on their disease?
4. What if these patients were on the same nursing unit? Would there be concern that these patients were being offered different levels of support at home going?
5. Clinically, what is the better way to care for the patient? Does that match the payor payment?

ORGANIZATIONAL IMPACT
AND OPERATIONAL DECISIONS

VBC—both in private insurance and through government programs—is the future of health-care in the United States. Although that sentiment has been around for years and even de-cades, the current healthcare landscape is beginning to push more and more into the VBC approach and introduce increasing numbers of programs designed to drive value to the payor, patient, and healthcare system. Generally, it is important to understand the time scale that each program takes place on. ACOs, for example, attribute patients to PCPs and mea-sure success and value creation over years while some specific episodic bundles measure value creation within 60 or 90 days. Some programs measure value created to the hospital, such as reduction in ED utilization or coordinating post-acute services to the inpatient spend, while other programs focus more on preventive care and testing in physician offices and/ or the ambulatory setting. When leaders in healthcare systems are beginning to research each of these programs and consider their implications within their own teams, they must consider a few key areas that will be critical to the success or failure of these new initiatives. Much of the approaches discussed in the chapter focus on philosophical differences between FFS models and value-based approaches (e.g., being payor agnostic or designing workflows around certain payor and patient groups for best value). However, certain cornerstones of nursing practice will be critical regardless of the approach chosen within the healthcare team or organization.

It is imperative that leaders have staff in place who understand the implications of a suc-cessful bundle episode or value-based contract and can identify operational deficiencies that stand in the way of that success as early as possible in a patient's stay. For certain programs, such as ACOs, patients may be attributed to PCPs who are responsible for supporting each patient's health in the ambulatory setting. "Success" for these patients could be improve-ment of quality metrics—like preventive screenings for colon cancer or blood pressure (BP) monitoring at home with a cuff—or could be measured in decreased utilization of hospital resources. Also critical is the alignment between the utilization management/utilization re-view (UM/UR) and clinical documentation improvement (CDI) teams with front-line care-givers in CM. All billing, and thus attribution to value-based programs, relies on the accurate coding of each case which, in turn, relies on the accurate documentation and charting on those patients at the bedside. The smooth and timely transfer of information from one team to the other allows for more accurate anticipation of bundle inclusion or patient attribution to PCPs. Both of which are critical, depending on the programs with which the health system is affiliated.

Finally, it would be impossible to measure the success and opportunities of any VBC program within a health system without the appropriate data analytics and information technology (IT) infrastructure. The ability to determine workflow efficacy and measure areas of improvement, with minimal data lag, allows leaders and their teams to pivot if necessary to tighten up the process or can alleviate the stresses of nursing and physician leaders by proving the early successes of the program and aid in expanding to other units, sites, bun-dle programs, or patient populations. These systems, either individual or working together, will all need to be considered when deciding what VBC strategies to employ at your health system or hospital.

CARE REDESIGN

When evaluating VBC models and programs, it may be advantageous to tweak workflows for program success. However, if a substantial portion of the patient population within a health system is part of these value-based programs, it may also be necessary for leaders to completely redesign the care delivery of the entire system. This is a strategy employed by teams working in hospital systems and has worked well in scaling these programs out to a large array of regional hospital sites, remote work teams, and ambulatory practices. Often, this work can be incentivized by contracts signed with various payors by including a CM fee in the per member per month (PMPM) charge. This fee should allow for increased revenue to be generated to support the expansion of the teams necessary to create a successful value-based program within a health system. Care redesign is the systematic restructure of workflows to align with evidence-based best practices as well as the continued monitoring of compliance of those best practices. This process is not the work of a single department, but instead requires buy-in from leadership within the nursing, physician, IT/data analytics, and CM teams. Without the clear and concise creation of best practices, typically monitored and recorded within the electronic health record (EHR), care redesign will be short-lived and relatively difficult to achieve. Care redesign typically starts with the identification of a known problem with measurable outcomes (e.g., COPD patients utilizing the ED too often). From there, a strategy is developed to ensure that an appropriate safety net of resources exists in the community to eliminate the need for ED utilization. In this case, COPD patients may need further education on symptom management and what they should consider an emergency. In conjunction with a connection to an engaged PCP, this can sometimes be enough to prevent future hospital utilization. Each hospital team and health system will need to develop clear and concise strategies to manage patients' utilization of inpatient resources to reduce cost and continue to improve outcomes for these chronic conditions. Care redesign is the process of considering how each member of the care team, both inpatient and ambulatory practices, may impact the outcome and success of that patient as well as the financial implications of that patient's ongoing healthcare needs. An argument can be made that a rising tide does raise all boats. Caring for each of the patients in the case study with the same level of CM intensity, education, and post-acute follow-up will yield the best outcome for the patients overall. Thus, everyone wins. At issue is the resources required to provide that intensity. However, with more and more payors moving to value-based contract payment structures, the compelling financial story is to treat all patients as if they were "at risk" and provide whatever support can be offered to ultimately have better outcomes. The following sections continue the discussion of care redesign by delving deeper into areas of consideration when beginning to undertake care redesign processes.

RESOURCE ALIGNMENT

Within the VBC world, as with most things, so many of the decisions made by leaders will be directly tied to the overall philosophy of their teams or where their organization has contractually aligned with payor partners. Aligning resources (i.e., staff, clinical space, physicians) to the areas that prevent future readmissions and allow patients to access the resources they need to be successful and healthy may look different depending on the patient population, needs of the community, and where the organization has chosen to pursue VBC models. In general, access to community resources or ambulatory care teams who can act as a support team tend to provide patients with the best value in staying healthy and managing their care independently. Overall, the goal of most VBC models is to prevent overutilization of the acute hospital spaces and, instead, find alternate or preventive care that allows patients to remain out of the hospital while still having a safety net for unexpected issues. It is critical to place support systems in the ambulatory space as points of contact, particularly for patients with chronic conditions; something many value-based programs focus on.

TRANSITIONAL CARE MANAGEMENT HUB

Many studies have confirmed that in older adults, healthcare needs are poorly managed as they are complex and involve multiple diseases and providers. Dr. Mary Naylor and her colleagues from the University of Pennsylvania studied the transitions of care in these complex patients and found that they had very poor outcomes and high healthcare utilization costs. Although her original model had master's prepared APRNs doing this work, today most health systems use registered nurses (RNs). Therefore, one resource alignment strategy is to create a transitional care management (TCM) hub that reaches out to patients when they leave the acute care setting. Oftentimes, this starts as a group of nurses who work in a centralized "hub" and contact patients telephonically after they are discharged from the hospital. The goal of this team is to ensure that the patients have what they need to succeed at home and have appropriate follow-up appointments with their PCPs as well as any specialists who are managing their care. It also serves as a touch point for any questions or support the patient may need. The CMS created the TCM program by creating a very specific, evidence-based set of questions that a licensed person must contact and reach out to the patient and assess within 2 business days of discharge from an acute care hospital. In turn, as an incentive to this work, providers are allowed to bill the follow-up visit post-discharge at a much higher rate as long as all the elements are met. This is one example of care redesign to prevent readmissions and utilization at higher costs of care (Box 8.1).

BOX 8.1: REQUIRED ELEMENTS TO BILL FOR A TRANSITIONAL CARE MANAGEMENT VISIT

- Contact the beneficiary or caregiver within 2 business days following a discharge. The contact may be via telephone, email, or a face-to-face visit. Attempts to communicate should continue after the first two attempts in the required business days until successful.

- Conduct a follow-up visit within 7 or 14 days of discharge, depending on the complexity of medical decision-making involved. The face-to-face visit is part of the TCM service and should not be reported separately.

- Medicine reconciliation and management must be furnished no later than the date of the face-to-face visit.

- Obtain and review discharge information.

- Review the need for diagnostic tests/treatments and/or follow-up on pending diagnostic tests/treatments.

- Educate the beneficiary, family member, caregiver, and/or guardian.

- Establish or re-establish referrals with community providers and services, if necessary.

- Assist in scheduling follow-up visits with providers and services, if necessary.

Source: Reproduced with permission from American Academy of Family Physicians. (n.d.). *Transitional care management.* https://www.aafp.org/family-physician/practice-and-career/getting-paid/coding/transitional-care-management.html.

The prevention of hospitalizations is a critical measure that is constantly monitored by executive leadership to better align resources to gaps in care across the healthcare spectrum.

CARE MANAGEMENT STRUCTURE

CM operates as a central figure in the VBC world, both in the inpatient setting—collaborating with physicians to create safe and effective discharge plans and finding resources in the post-acute space that can best help patients—and in the ambulatory setting, following up with patients and ensuring that those discharge plans remain the best course of care and that the patient has resources for questions or concerns about their care. More is being asked of the CM teams than ever before, and as organizations develop VBC strategies, inpatient CM can no longer be content to create a discharge plan, discharge the patient, and move on to the next room. It is imperative that CM act as an information conduit between inpatient and outpatient care teams, handing off complex cases to CC colleagues and participate in ongoing strategies to align the missions of various departments across the healthcare system.

Many VBC strategies stem from using the index admission as the beginning of a payment episode. Given this, the steps taken in that initial admission are critical to determining the success of the discharge and efficiently aligning resources during that episode. Without a clearly aligned inpatient and ambulatory CM/CC strategy, the time spent finding resources for patients would be wasted, as patients would not be handed off to those resources.

Another arm of CM is UM/UR. UM's primary responsibility is to package clinical information, known as "reviews," to send to the insurance provider. Those payors use the information about the patient's current medical condition to determine whether a patient is in the appropriate status or setting of care based on their healthcare needs. As the VBC programs have become more and more prevalent, UM has been increasingly relied on to proactively request information from the medical teams at the bedside in an effort to more accurately document the reason for that patient's admission and, in turn, their potential medical needs at discharge. UM/UR teams must be familiar with the VBC world so that they can act as an extra set of eyes for the bedside nursing teams in regard to bundle inclusion or value-based programs within the commercial payor landscape. Also, because a patient can sometimes admit and discharge quickly, the UM teams can act as a second set of eyes for inclusion in an at-risk contract. It is imperative that the UM team have an understanding of the active value-based programs to assist in catching potential cases and alerting the medical teams at the bedside of that potential.

Once the patients have been discharged from the hospitals, they are often handed off to care coordinators in the ambulatory space. They can be added to the CC work lists for a variety of reasons: program inclusion based on their PCP or ACO alignment, chronic conditions to be managed, episodic bundle inclusion, new diagnosis, and so on. Often patients are added to these work lists based on their risk stratification. Risk stratification is an algorithmic look at the patients' underlying medical conditions, any comorbidities they may have, their risk (or rising risk) of needing acute care, and other factors such as their age and SDOH. The CC team uses those factors to build prioritized lists for patients to ensure they have the appropriate follow-up appointments scheduled, have rides to those follow-ups, and receive any other support that patient may need. Like the TCM hub from earlier in the chapter, the ultimate goal of these ambulatory CC teams is to avoid unnecessary hospitalizations and keep their patients healthy using the resources available to them in the ambulatory setting.

These three teams make up CM and ambulatory services within the health system. In conjunction with physicians and bedside nursing staff, CM and care coordinators develop strategies to reduce the burden on the inpatient services and keep patients healthy and supported in their post-acute settings. This overarching goal perfectly dovetails with the goals of all VBC models. As the chapter continues, you will learn about specific strategies based on the various VBC programs.

BUDGETING STRATEGY

In VBC programs, there are a variety of ways leaders will be challenged to create value for their patients, system, or payor. These value-based agreements are either prospective or retrospective depending on the specific type. Prospective agreements will be awarded to the hospital based on the analytics of a certain group in a set period of time. Retrospective payments will be dispersed based on the performance of the hospital and attributed patient population based on a historical analysis. The details are covered in more depth later in the chapter; however, as leaders, there are several key terms to know in order to begin to evaluate each program and the potential value created within. Most commercial VBC initiatives use a PMPM incentive as a base figure for the cost of care analysis. Generally, this figure represents the potential value created for your organization in keeping those patients healthy and supported in the ambulatory setting. Each contract will be negotiated based on a variety of parameters ranging from specific results of lab tests and screenings to more broad criteria like PCP visits or follow-up appointments in a given period of time; this is referred to as the closure of care gaps. All of the negotiated parameters are based on reducing hospitalizations and proactively managing chronic conditions to ultimately reduce the cost of care for the payor to the hospital system over a number of months or even years. Unlike government programs, these value-based agreements often focus on longer periods of time. If the organization succeeds in meeting these criteria, they are awarded the PMPM amount. In this way, successfully navigating commercial value-based agreements can result in revenue generation (and cost reduction) for a health system.

This works slightly differently in the government payor space. For CMS-sponsored programs, just like commercial programs, there are criteria identified to determine the program's success. However, unlike commercial value-based agreements, these criteria are often much broader, like readmissions or acute bed days. Also different from commercial agreements is how the value is created or judged. Bundles are often 30, 60, or 90 days long and the goal is to manage the medical spend on that patient for the set duration of time. A certain amount of money is set aside to manage the patient's condition; if the health system spends less, they get to keep that amount, and if they spend more than that predetermined episode cost of care, they lose that money and are sometimes charged additional fees as a penalty. ACOs take place over a much larger time scale than bundle payment programs. This program could be judged on a year-over-year basis and involve a much larger patient population with significantly different initial healthcare conditions. Physician groups and hospital systems who enter ACOs can choose to take on a broader responsibility for their patients and their outcomes for the possibility of a larger financial reward, considered an "at-risk" model. They can also choose to adopt these practices while remaining financially separated from those outcomes, referred to as "not at risk."

The intricacies of each type of VBC agreement are covered later in the chapter. It is important as leaders to understand the implications of success and failure of each of these agreements and build a system that simultaneously is supporting the patients in the appropriate setting while also being mindful of the cost of care (and cost of resources) in order to capture the most value for patients and the health system. Data analytics and IT platforms allow leaders to accurately measure the progress of these programs as well as consider the implications of various VBC programs.

ANALYTICS AND KEY PERFORMANCE INDICATORS

As leaders evaluate the possibilities of taking on value-based agreements with either government or private insurance providers, it is important to align closely with data analytics and data science teams. These teams will assist in determining the gaps and opportunities within each of the programs and provide key insights along the way to continue to improve clinical outcomes and, in turn, contracting performance.

INFRASTRUCTURE, INFORMATION TECHNOLOGY PLATFORMS, SYSTEM STRUCTURE, AND DATA REPORTING

The ability to have timely and accurate measures of the process is essential to a successful VBC strategy. Without the IT infrastructure and/or data analytics platforms to assist in this process, it would be all but impossible to accurately assess and plan for taking on VBC programs. In addition to the EHR, which is imperative, the ability to extract discreet data points to measure progress in real time is valuable to track individual team metrics and identify areas for improvement before being penalized by the bundle contract or government agencies. It is also important to have a developed network for presenting and discussing data between teams and leaders. This allows for transparency in the contracting process and a cohesive vision for next steps and successes among the teams.

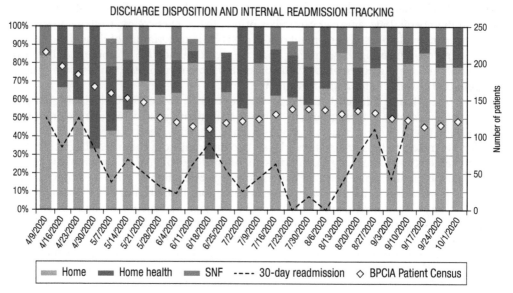

FIGURE 8.1: Example of weekly metric dashboard. Data around discharge disposition and internal readmission is tracked and reviewed weekly by the team.
BPCI-A, bundle payments for care improvement–advanced; CCU, coronary care unit; SNF, skilled nursing facility.

In addition to having the ability to pull appropriate and timely data related to the programs in which leaders are engaged, leaders in this space must have a clear and concise way of relaying the success and opportunities for improvement to their teams. Having a weekly data check in, or the ability for individual administrators to access their own data, graphs, charts, or some combination of them, may make the most sense. In our system, we have weekly working meetings where the data and stats are reviewed (Figure 8.1). In addition to those stats, the teams can discuss individual cases, ongoing concerns regarding the processes, handoffs, and so on.

The data that is tracked is always initially based on the contract stipulations and then developed further from there. Depending on the type of VBC agreement, it may be outcomes-based like readmissions, ED utilization, or whether care gaps are being closed as is stipulated in the contracts (e.g., PCP follow-ups). There are also process-based metrics that indicate whether our staff are taking the appropriate action while the patient is in their care. We track note types, number of contacts, referral types, and handoff documentation as well to ensure that we are putting appropriate safety nets around our patients that will translate to their success in the program. Each of these individual data points are combined to form the basis of a cohesive and comprehensive data reporting strategy in the VBC world. It allows us to have a top-down view of both process and outcomes to better understand whether certain performance within the patient population is an anomaly or a symptom of the workflow itself.

PREDICTIVE ANALYTICS AND OUTCOMES

The natural next step in producing data in real time and making operational decisions is using data that was gathered retroactively to make more informed and proactive decisions about patient care and patient inclusion. This can be done either manually with comprehensive analysis of the historical data or using software to draw out insights from that data. Creating these models using software is referred to as predictive analytics. More and more health systems are embarking on predictive analytics and AI-based modeling for either outcomes predictions—with the aim to more accurately plan budgets or sign more advantageous value-based agreements—or identify more subtle criteria for patient inclusion, thus more accurately capturing bundle inclusion at the time of the index admission or alignment of post-acute services for better patient outcomes during the bundle episode. Additionally, this process can provide valuable insight into patient behavior and patient activation for potential future programs. Both approaches come with some risk of "analysis paralysis" or making assumptions that patient behavior will not change between the reference patient population and the next bundle patient population.

DATA-DRIVEN OPERATIONS AND THE LEADERSHIP FEEDBACK LOOP

Throughout this section, the focus has been on using data and analytics as a method of establishing clear workflows and metrics for success in the VBC world. As a leader, it is important to take each of these areas into consideration in forming a strategy for the individual health system or hospital. While there are established best practices in the VBC world, there is no perfect solution for each system. Every leader must weigh the impacts of shifting work to various teams and setting up data and working meetings with collaborators across the health space to establish how and when to update the team and when to change course. Establishing a rhythm for when and how to approach teams with changes is for each leader to gauge and decide on their own. The remaining sections contain deeper dives into the variety of value-based programs, through both the CMS and some of the largest health plans in the United States. The important thing to recognize in the field of VBC is that there is no "one size fits all" solution; without the collaboration of the nursing, physician, data analytics, CM, and executive leadership teams, success will be very difficult if not impossible to come by.

GOVERNMENT PAYOR PROGRAMS

The CMS has partnered with health systems, private insurance payors, PCPs, and ancillary service providers in a number of ways to provide better care to their beneficiaries and coordinate services in an effort to reduce costs and improve healthcare outcomes. The next few sections will detail the current state of a variety of common programs focusing on generalized metrics, measures, and strategies for implementation. The CMS VBC landscape is constantly shifting to better meet the needs of patients and providers. This portion of the chapter should serve as a jumping off point for understanding the implications of these programs to a health system.

MEDICARE PAYOR PROGRAMS

Medicare is the national health insurance program that was started in 1966 under the Social Security Administration and is now administered by the CMS. It was designed to primarily provide insurance for retirees in the United States (age 65 and older) and currently insures roughly 60 million Americans. Traditional FFS Medicare is a great payor and considered very desirable by hospitals, private practice, and post-acute facilities. The premiums can be expensive, but the coverage is considered very good. No precertification of services is required by Medicare, so patients can seek care when and where they want to with few barriers. The Medicare coverage is divided into four parts: A, B, C, and D (Box 8.2).

BOX 8.2: DIVISIONS OF MEDICARE COVERAGE

- **Part A:** Covers inpatient hospital stays, skilled nursing stays (after a qualifying three midnight stay), and hospice services.

- **Part B:** Covers ambulatory and outpatient services including most PCP visits and prescription drugs that require a licensed professional to administer.

- **Part C:** Often referred to as "managed Medicare" or "Medicare advantage." This system allows a patient to select a commercially available health plan that serves to cover Parts A, B, and D and often offers additional services for their beneficiaries. Part C also has an out-of-pocket annual spend limit to help reduce additional burden. This is the VBC benefit design of Medicare.

- **Part D:** Covers most prescription drugs taken at home.

Often the programs discussed in the following sections will be designed to reduce Part A billing costs while increasing Part B or D. Part C billing and programs are administered by private insurance plans and often vary by state. Each managed Medicare or Medicare Advantage payor must follow the rules and regulations of the CMS and Medicare plans in order to continue to qualify and be available for enrollees to use. This is discussed in more detail later in the chapter.

ACCOUNTABLE CARE ORGANIZATIONS

An ACO is a healthcare organization that incentivizes providers and health systems by tracking identified quality metrics and reductions in the overall cost of care. By tying the financial incentives of the organization to the cost of care and those quality metrics, the ACO is responsible for delivering higher quality, more efficient and appropriate care to its patients. This differs dramatically from the Medicare FFS models that were common a number of years ago. In an ACO, providers are rewarded for coordinating care across the healthcare continuum and keeping patients healthy and engaged with their primary care providers. Of note: Although ACOs were created by government payors, they are also used in commercial and healthcare system designs as well to provide coordinated care at a lower cost and shared savings.

ACOs were first introduced in 2009 as part of the ACA. A group of 32 "pioneer" ACOs began operation in December of 2011 with a planned program end in 2016. Throughout the initial program life, 19 of the 32 pioneer ACOs showed a cost savings totaling an estimated $76M. In response to their research and the findings from the pioneer ACOs, several stakeholders responsible for developing ACO strategy within the U.S. government identified three core principles that contribute to the success of ACOs, including

1. provider-led organizations with a strong base of primary care that are collectively accountable for quality and per capita costs across the continuum of care,

2. payments linked to quality improvements and reduced costs, and

3. reliable and increasingly sophisticated performance measurement to support improvement and provide confidence that savings are achieved through care improvements (McClellan et al., 2010).

The creation of the ACO model was furthered solidified by the Medicare Shared Savings Program (MSSP), which was codified within the ACA. This established four reimbursement tracks for health organizations seeking to enter into an ACO. The tracks were labeled 1, 1+, 2, and 3. Track 1 provided no financial risk to the health system but did provide potential financial incentives for quality performance and was, therefore, often the first step in entering into an ACO. Each track has a set agreement period, often 3 to 5 years. During this time, the ACO organization may progress through a variety of risk levels based on its performance relative to the benchmark data. Through a Track 1 ACO, a provider network or health system had the opportunity to improve on several quality measures and metrics (e.g., increasing PCP appointments, reducing readmissions, reducing acute bed days) and, in turn, benefit from the shared savings of more closely monitoring those processes in their network and the reduction in Part A and Part B Medicare billing. Tracks 1+, 2, and 3 had similar benefits, but had the added pressure of sharing in any underperformance of the system itself (shared loss). This is known as the *downside risk* contracting model, also sometimes referred to as the two-sided model (shared savings/shared risk). As any ACO progresses through the track model, it will be exposed to greater potential financial risk while also earning higher shared savings percentages for continued performance and improvements of quality benchmarks.

◼ WHAT EVERY NURSE EXECUTIVE NEEDS TO KNOW ABOUT VALUE-BASED CONTRACTING

A nurse executive who manages teams such as CM, UM, bedside nursing, or ambulatory care teams should have a keen understanding of the financial impacts of maintaining the patient population within their system. They should understand the long-term goals of the VBC models present at their hospital and when a nursing team may need additional education, resources, or direction if they aren't meeting the demands of the at-risk patient population. A strong nurse executive has a plan for success in a value-based model and clear action steps to ensure patients' needs are being met and you are meeting the core criteria for success within those at-risk contracts.

⬡ CASE SCENARIO

CHIEF NURSING OFFICER CONSIDERS PARTICIPATING IN AN ACCOUNTABLE CARE ORGANIZATION

As a chief nursing officer (CNO), you are overseeing nursing practice at three smaller regional hospitals and a larger, centralized main campus. Your health system also has a network of private and employed physician partners in the community, specialty practices, and a preferred provider network of home care agencies, skilled nursing facilities (SNFs), and one acute rehab. You are in the boardroom and there is conversation from the finance team to consider starting an ACO within the four hospitals, medical practices, and post-acute networks affiliated within your healthcare system. Your colleagues on the executive team are evaluating the different options available and are reviewing the different tracks over the next 4 years. Model year one is looking pretty good, with defined quality metrics that you are already working on and do pretty well at, such as readmissions. In the first year there is no penalty for underperforming, and in fact, if your health system does better than expected they will receive a shared savings reward from the CMS. Year two has a few more metrics that are added, but by pivoting some key resources and adding in care coordinators and social workers, there is a reasonable chance of success in reducing ED utilization and improving some behavioral health services. This is great news because you have noted this need for a long time, and this is a great opportunity to get those needed services for patients. Concerning, however, are years three and four. There is increased focus on post-acute utilization and spending. You know you have a lot of physicians who are medical directors of SNFs and they like to keep the beds full. There is a lot of pressure to use that acute rehab because they are a joint venture partner and there are long-term financial contracts in place. The risk in these later model years is more "downside," and now penalties are going to be incurred if the metrics are not met. Everyone is very excited at the potential gains that can be made in this scenario, but you think there are some things that still need to be discussed, and you know that nursing will end up shouldering a large portion of this work.

DISCUSSION QUESTIONS

1. What type of analytics will be available to the provider teams to know if a patient is in the ACO?
2. If there are CM fees or a shared savings, where will those funds flow?
3. Is there support to increase CM and social work resources to be successful in this ACO?
4. How will the private practices be handled? Are they active partners with our hospitals in this?
5. Will we treat all patients the same, or for those who are in the ACO will there be different workflows and expectations?

CENTERS FOR MEDICARE & MEDICAID SERVICES UPDATES AND CHANGES TO ACCOUNTABLE CARE ORGANIZATIONS

In 2018, the CMS redefined the original tracks and timelines in order to encourage Track 1 ACOs to transition to performance-based risk more quickly and for ACOs already in downside risk contracts to incrementally increase savings opportunities for their organizations. The "Pathways to Success" went into effect July 1, 2019. The CMS stated that the Pathways to Success was designed to advance five goals: accountability, competition, quality, engagement, and integrity.

Using the first few years of data on ACO performance, Medicare determined that pushing organizations to take on financial risk more quickly will ultimately continue to push for improvements in the healthcare system in general. This rule change reduced the amount of time that an ACO can remain in the program without taking on financial risk, from 6 years in the previous model down to 2 years (*accountability* and *competition*). Simultaneously, the CMS expanded telehealth services for ACOs that are already taking on financial risk (*quality*), allowed for ACOs to offer incentive payments to beneficiaries for engaging in their healthcare decisions such as obtaining primary care services or necessary follow-up appointments (*engagement*), and re-established regional data benchmarks for Medicare spending, providing a more accurate comparison for evaluating ACO performance (*integrity*; CMS, 2018).

Overall the CMS eliminated Tracks 1, 1+, 2, and 3 and renamed them Basic (formerly 1, 1+, and 2) and Enhanced (formerly Track 3). Each ACO type (Basic or Enhanced) involves a 5-year agreement period with a progression from one-sided model beginning in year 2 with gradually increasing levels of risk, in exchange for additional performance incentives and administrative flexibility in years 3 through 5. ACOs eligible for Track 3 or Enhanced program inclusion are those determined to be experienced with performance-based risk (Figure 8.2).

The big change in 2018 and 2019 was based on data of the performance of ACOs within the most aggressive risk/shared savings plans that the CMS offered at the time. Of the 44 ACOs in this model, the shared savings totaled $164 million and showed strong quality metric performance. The thought was that the initial ACO program was too lenient on ACOs with no downside risk and therefore did not achieve the value and overall cost savings for the patients that was intended. The 2018 final rule change sought to correct that by pushing ACOs to perform better and more quickly than they had before.

ACOs are among the most common forms of VBC incentive programs across the U.S. healthcare landscape. While the changes made in 2018 and 2019 to encourage ACOs to take on greater levels of risk have not been fully vetted, it is expected that the number of ACOs will continue to grow each year.

	BASIC TRACK					ENHANCED TRACK
	Level A	Level B	Level C	Level D	Level E	
Risk	Upside Only		Two-Sided	Two-Sided	Two-Sided	Two-Sided
Shared Savings	Rate of **40%**	Rate of **50%**	Rate of **50%**	Rate of **50%**	Rate of **50%**	Rate of **75%**
Shared Losses	N/A	N/A	Rate of **30%**, not to exceed **2%** of revenue	Rate of **30%**, not to exceed **4%** of revenue	Rate of **30%**, not to exceed **8%** of revenue	Rate of 1 minus sharing rate, not to exceed **15%** of bechmark

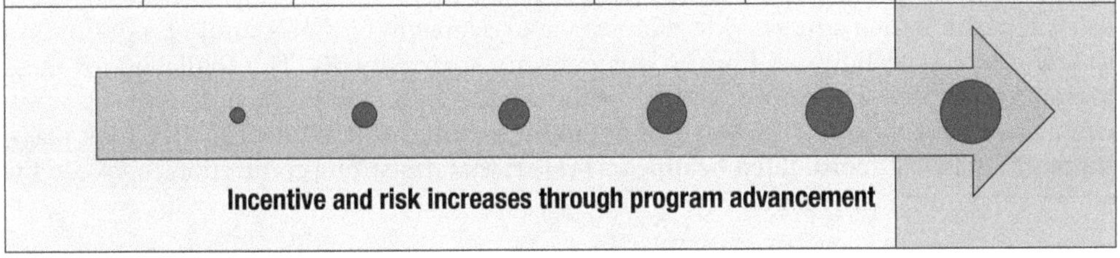

Incentive and risk increases through program advancement

FIGURE 8.2: Pathways to Success for accountable care organizations (ACOs) were designed to advance five goals: accountability, competition, quality, engagement, and integrity.

BUNDLE PAYMENTS FOR CARE IMPROVEMENT

The Bundle Payments for Care Improvement (BPCI) initiative began in 2013 with the goal of coordinating care and services for a specific episode of care across the healthcare spectrum and landscape, thereby reducing the total cost billed to Medicare Parts A and B. BPCI differs dramatically from an ACO and other types of value-based models in several ways. First, the BPCI model focuses on specific episodes and conditions of patients. Episode length can vary by program type (known Model 1-4) and clinical setting. For example, there are bundles for orthopedics, COPD/asthma exacerbation, and others. Participants in BPCI could choose up to 48 different clinical episodes to test in the model. Often, health systems would determine which clinical episodes to test based on their past performance related to the criteria the CMS used to determine success. They would also have the option of the bundle length—choosing between being at-risk for 30, 60, or 90 days for each clinical episode. There are also four different model types associated with BPCI based on the setting or settings that services are being performed (Box 8.3). All of the bundles operate under the same premise regardless of setting. Each model starts with the identification of a target clinical episode. A target price is then set for the clinical episode (set by the CMS based on historical costs associated with the identified DRG), and the health system or hospital is then awarded a percentage of the savings based on whichever model they are in and what level of risk they are accepting.

BOX 8.3: BUNDLED PAYMENT FOR CARE IMPROVEMENT MODEL TYPES

- Model 1: Acute care hospital stay only
- Model 2: Acute care and post-acute care episode
- Model 3: Post-acute care only
- Model 4: Prospective acute care hospital stay only

Bundle payment initiatives differ from ACOs in that the success and risk are attributed not to the PCPs but to the setting in which the patient is receiving care. Although coordination and care gap closure can benefit both the ACO and bundle payment programs, the timeline to judge success is dramatically shorter in bundles than in an ACO.

In 2018, the second iteration of the bundle payment model program was developed by the CMS, known as Bundle Payments for Care Improvement—Advanced (BPCI-A). This iteration brought about a few changes to the program that reduced flexibility to the health system while also increasing risk. Just like the ACO development, the CMS felt that the initial program was not aggressive enough in pushing physicians, care coordinators, and health systems in general to provide value for Medicare beneficiaries and the CMS. The biggest changes between BPCI and BPCI-A are the removal of bundle length options for the hospital and removing the phase-in period for financial risk. Each of these changes was designed to push the health systems to provide more concrete oversight of their bundle programs and increase the responsibility and health outcomes for their patients. The challenge for these programs is that the actual work caring for these patients occurs in the post-acute and outpatient space, but the dollars saved are sent to the hospital where the discharge took place. This requires a very coordinated healthcare system that has strong connections between the inpatient and outpatient realms.

STRATEGIES FOR SUCCESS

BPCI-A and all bundle payment models require a strong link between the inpatient and ambulatory care teams in order to succeed. As a patient transitions from an inpatient stay to their post-acute or ambulatory setting, identifying in bundle patients and understanding the target price for those episodes is critical. Partnering with resources in the community to assist in avoiding those costly readmissions during the bundle period is another sound strategy to bundle success. In general, most bundle target prices are designed around avoiding a readmission and the utilization of post-acute resources. The fewer resources that need to be utilized, the lower the bundle episode cost would be, obviously, but any readmission generally will increase the bundle cost to above the target price. Using post-acute resources such as congestive heart failure (CHF) clinics to keep patients who are fluid overloaded from going to an ED or leveraging engaged PCPs to ensure appropriate follow-ups will all reduce readmission risk to patients within a medical bundle. Health systems with clear communication, appropriate support in the post-acute and ambulatory space, and data infrastructure to appropriately capture the bundle patient as quickly as possible will have the highest chance of success in BPCI-A.

COMPREHENSIVE PRIMARY CARE PLUS

Comprehensive Primary Care Plus (CPC+) is a large-scale primary care payment and delivery reform project that was launched by the CMS in January 2017. This 5-year program partners with several payors and PCP practices and health IT platforms across the country to test whether enhanced CC and engagement with the PCP would improve clinical outcomes and reduce the overall Medicare spend for patients. The CMS partnered with private payors to assist in adopting systems that placed more of an emphasis on preventive care in the ambulatory space and PCP offices by offering alternative payment models that incentivize PCP engagement and wellness appointments. Physician practices were assessed on the utilization of inpatient resources, ED visits, and overall Medicare expenditures relative to patients who are not involved with a CPC+ PCP. CPC+ requires practices to transform across five care delivery functions: (a) access and continuity of care, (b) CM, (c) comprehensiveness and coordination, (d) patient and caregiver engagement, and (e) planned care and population health. Key performance metrics were established to measure effectiveness and growth in each of these areas. For physician practices that were affiliated with a large healthcare system, joining this program meant advocating for additional resources within their practices that would allow each physician team to be successful. CM follow-up became a particularly important issue that physicians advocated for upon engaging with the program. Often the payor partners that worked with the CMS would provide a PMPM CM fee to help offset the cost of hiring additional staff for this work, under the promise of overall reduced costs of care for patients who were more holistically supported in the ambulatory space. Additionally, CPC+ practices work with the CMS or other payor partners to prospectively pay and retrospectively reconcile a performance-based incentive structure on how well a practice performs on patient experience, clinical quality, and utilization measures that drive total cost of care. Lastly, for Track 2 practices, a portion of their payment model is shifted to a lump sum payment model on a quarterly basis to manage patients and practice costs. This further incentivizes physicians and their CC partners to remain in constant engagement with their attributed patients to ensure their needs are met in the lowest cost appropriate setting of care.

PHYSICIAN ALIGNMENT OUTCOMES

When CPC+ went live in 2017, 2,905 primary physician practices were approved to go live with the program at the outset. These practices often were part of the original CPC program (CPC Classic) and had seen success, and therefore wanted to expand and take on more risk for their patient's outcomes. At the outset, many physician offices had partnered with payor collaborators, the CMS, and IT health platforms to derive the areas of greatest opportunity and continued to leverage the CMS's support while striving to close care gaps with their patients. As of program year 3 (2019), most practices reported that they were likely to participate in CPC+ again if they could. While the most recent data findings show that there is an increased cost associated with caring for these patients, as practitioners and practices have grown into the workflows, they are beginning to have steady positive impact in key areas such as hospital readmissions, ED utilization, and unplanned acute hospitalizations. While additional years will continue to flesh out the total efficacy of this program, the positive changes are being felt by those practitioners who have taken on this program.

OTHER PAYMENT INNOVATIONS

The CMS is constantly evaluating current care delivery methods and reacting to changes in both the governmental policy space or within the provider space. It is important to maintain an eye toward upcoming programs or changes to existing programs as they occur and have a clear and concise method for communicating with internal and external partners in order to evaluate the efficacy of new or existing VBC agreements. There is no "one size fits all" approach to VBC. Medicare and Medicaid allow for a wide array of programs—short-term and episodic, or long-term and more population health driven—that allow health systems, providers, and practitioners of all shapes and sizes to take advantage of new and innovative care delivery strategies across the country.

CHRONIC DISEASE MANAGEMENT

Chronic disease management is a smaller program that incentivizes the documentation and education of patients with one or more chronic diagnoses. A primary care provider can document a chronic care management (CCM) code in the medical chart in order receive an additional payment for those patients. This relatively small change incentivizes practitioners to begin to more proactively manage chronic conditions with their patients with the goal to educate patients to avoid potential acute care utilization.

The CMS relies on the constant engagement of physicians, health systems, and managed care payors to continue to look for opportunities and challenges in creating value for the CMS and their beneficiaries. In an effort to continue to ensure these programs are helping and continuing to grow, the CMS allows for open comments on any and all new programs or pilots they are trying. As part of the open comment period, health systems, payor partners, and PCPs can voice concerns and bring up potential pain points prior to the CMS instituting large changes across the healthcare landscape.

MEDICARE ADVANTAGE

Medicare Advantage programs are the "Part C"; they are also called M/A programs. They are another way to get Parts A and B as part of a bundle in traditional Medicare but often at a lower monthly premium and other out-of-pocket costs. Some plans include things like dental care, vision checks and eyeglasses, hearing aids, and fitness programs which traditional Medicare does not cover. Like many other plans, these are administered by familiar commercial payor names such as Blue Cross and Blue Shield, Anthem, or Aetna, but they are actually led by rules and guidelines from Medicare. These administered plans are often within a very tight geographic network and the member must stay within a list of providers and a certain hospital network. The intent is to help make Medicare more affordable, especially for those who are pretty healthy and do not anticipate a lot of healthcare needs. The M/A plans behave a little more like a commercial payor does as described later in the chapter (Medicare.gov, 2017).

These programs are very attractive for seniors who are now often on a fixed income as they enter their retirement years. At the age of 65, the health of the member may be well preserved, but over time it is logical to assume that as one ages, health begins to decline and needed services and costs increase. The monthly premium and out-of-pocket costs are low in an M/A plan, but the coverage for needed services may not be a part of the plan, and the member has to really read about the program thoroughly. For example, most post-acute stays are not covered by a Medicare Advantage plan, and thus may be out-of-pocket costs or simply not covered. So if the patient is in need of post-acute services after an elective surgical procedure, they may incur costs, or plan to have other provisions for care in the home setting. This is often a surprise to patients and their families.

In addition, since hospitals and providers may be a part of a tight network, these patients are considered "attributed" and are "at risk" for the hospital system. Thus, the hospital or provider is truly in a value-based contract, and will only get paid if agreed upon outcome metrics are met. For hospitals, this means a capture of a market share, which can be good news if the population in the particular M/A plan is healthy and does not need a lot of expensive services. But if the population is frail, is older, and has a lot of social needs, these plans can make it very hard to get needed care for patients, especially in post-acute care.

⬡ CASE SCENARIO

CONSUMER QUESTIONS RELATED TO MEDICARE ADVANTAGE

JW is 64 years old and has been working at their job as a paralegal in a law firm for 40 years. They turn 65 in June (6 months away) and are looking forward to their retirement the following July. JW's children and grandchildren live all across the country, and JW is looking forward to visiting them often. JW has already noticed that in the mail they are receiving loads of information about Medicare, for which they become eligible on the first day of the month that they turn 65. This will be the first time JW has ever had health insurance coverage that is outside their employer. The options are simply overwhelming. Traditional Medicare has great coverage, and if anything happens while JW is visiting their grandchildren they will have coverage. But JW is healthy and the Medicare Advantage plan monthly payment is so much more affordable than traditional Medicare. JW is also a little anxious about being on a "fixed income." After losing their spouse, JW has found their job to be a safe financial net. The thought of living off their retirement savings is daunting to think about. The good news is that JW is fairly healthy. They are on two BP medications and one for their thyroid, and they exercise regularly, eat healthy, have a healthy weight, and have no comorbid conditions. JW's only concern lately is severe pain in their right shoulder that started after they were walking the dog and the dog chased a squirrel, pulling on JW's arm. JW's doctor thinks JW may have torn their rotator cuff and will need an MRI to determine the diagnosis. If there is a tear, that may mean surgery, which will limit JW's driving, and JW will need help for several weeks post-op. JW is undergoing physical therapy for 6 weeks, which is required by their commercial insurance before they can have the MRI. As JW prepares to change insurance and retire, what are the considerations that JW should be thinking about?

DISCUSSION QUESTIONS

1. Given that JW is facing a potential surgery, should they consider the traditional Medicare plan at a higher cost knowing they may need help at home for their recovery?

2. Should JW rush through the physical therapy and try to get the MRI and surgery scheduled and completed before they go off their commercial insurance, even though it may delay JW's retirement date?

3. Would the Medicare Advantage plan pay for home care nursing and physical therapy after the surgery?

4. Traditional Medicare has no prior authorizations or limitations. Should JW hold on while in pain until they are on Medicare to get anything done?

MEDICAID AND THE CHILDREN'S HEALTH INSURANCE PROGRAM

The CMS also serve to provide the blueprint for Medicaid services for the three main areas of Medicaid. This includes the healthcare access for low-income individuals through Medicaid, the Children's Health Insurance Program (CHIP) which ensures all children have access to healthcare to age 18, and the Basic Health Program which is available on the Health Insurance Marketplace in accordance with the ACA: www.medicaid.gov/basic-health-program/index.html

The Medicaid financing structure relies on both the federal and state budgets to support it. The Federal Medical Assistance Percentage (FMAP) is the "match rate" given to the states and is a provision in the ACA. Wealthier states receive a lower portion of federal dollars while poor states match to a higher number of federal dollars. Although states still have to pay their share, those 37 states who chose to take advantage of the Medicaid expansion had an improved "match rate" and received more dollars from the federal government without tapping into their state revenue (Allen & Sommers, 2020). This proved to be a win for those states that participated. Despite how the states receive funding, what is uniquely different with Medicaid versus Medicare is that it is administered at the state level with only guidance at the federal level. Thus, Medicaid will vary state by state in its design and offerings, making this coverage not always portable between the states and certainly not equal. Some states use a VBC design to ensure there are quality patient outcomes at a lower cost of care. One such example is the State of California. In the fiscal year of 2019 California voluntarily published quality outcomes data in 19 of the 21 domains of frequently reported healthcare quality measures in the CMS Medicaid/CHIP Child Core Set. The state also voluntarily reported 21 of 24 frequently reported healthcare quality measures in the CMS Medicaid Adult Core Set. This transparent reporting of outcomes data is in alignment with how value-based contracting works and supports a number of population health initiatives such as programs to combat the SDOH, increased access to care, support to areas of neighborhood disadvantage and desperate populations, and increasing wellness and preventive services. Thirty-seven other states have chosen to take a more open access approach by providing a "Medicaid Expansion." This expansion increased the income requirements for eligibility and allowed for more state residents to receive Medicaid coverage. The end result for these states was actually a reduction in cost of healthcare, because more residents were given access to preventive and wellness care such as mammograms, colonoscopies, and diabetes screening, thus allowing people to receive treatment before the disease was out of control and more expensive to treat. This became especially important in the COVID-19 pandemic in 2020. States who had put in place the Medicaid Expansion prior to the pandemic saw much lower death rates and better long-term outcomes with less disability and morbidity (Allen & Sommers, 2020).

States generally contract with local health insurance companies in the state who already have a structure and process in place to administer the care. States are not the expert on the delivery of healthcare services; therefore, these large companies can manage the benefit design, billing, claims data, and administrative tasks of healthcare. This is at great expense, however, to state budgets. As more and more of the state budget gets taken over by the healthcare costs, there is less money for other services such as roads and infrastructure, education, parks and recreation, and other services residents of states also consider essential. So the drive to these value-based products—the ongoing improvement of care at a lower cost—is very appealing to state governments who want to improve the overall quality of life of their residents.

Medicaid in many states is considered to be a very poor payor. They usually pay way below what the actual cost of care is, making many physician practices, health systems, SNFs, and home care options either not contract with a Medicaid network or extremely limit the population of Medicaid patients they will accept. This can be difficult when trying to move a patient out of the hospital if there are no facilities in the geographic area who will accept Medicaid. Federally Qualified Health Centers (FQHCs) are government-supported primary care practices to give access to patients with Medicaid or who are underinsured. These safety net health facilities are generally located in underserved communities and serve those communities despite a patient's ability to pay (Transamerica Institute, n.d.).

MEDICAID MANAGED CARE ORGANIZATIONS

What Medicare Advantage is to Medicare, Medicaid Managed Care Organizations (MCOs) are to Medicaid. These programs grew rapidly in the 1990s, and by 2004 had increased by 900% (Dick Cauchi, n.d.). These government programs are administered by private MCOs with familiar names such as Caresource, Aetna, and Blue Cross/Blue Shield. Because they use these commercial names, patients are not stigmatized by the use of Medicaid, which can be a distinct advantage. And, as in Medicare Advantage programs, the state and federal governments provide guidelines and oversight. Also, much like Medicare Advantage, non-traditional Medicaid services can be offered in these products to beneficiaries such as vision coverage, dental care, transportation services to appointments, and CM services. The state agencies will contract with these MCOs and offer payment on a PMPM basis (capitation). Again, as with any value-based contract the goal is to improve quality outcomes while holding down the cost of care (Medicaid, n.d.).

As with Medicare Advantage, these Medicaid managed care plans have some definite downsides. Patients are really expected to navigate the system on their own, as the physician or health system does not have as much opportunity to advocate for their health. This requires patients to be very active in their healthcare and have a high degree of health literacy. Also, many of the touted benefits such as dental care, transportation, and so on can actually be very hard to access, and patients often give up on trying to get those needed services. Despite having a commercial payor name, since they are still considered Medicaid, many private practices will not accept this insurance because the payment is lower than other health plans and is capitated, meaning if the patient needs a lot of services they may render care that is uncompensated. Patients who select these programs have to be aware of all the rules and networks affiliated with the type of plan.

COMMERCIAL PAYORS

Adding to the complexity of the healthcare system in the United States is the many commercial payors that patients have to choose from. Generally, these are purchased through employers, limiting a member's selection, but commercial plans may also be accessed through the healthcare marketplace initiated by the ACA. Also, unlike government payors, the commercial plans have less cost-sharing with hospitals and providers. These plans tend to engage the consumers, also known as "members," in the copays, deductibles, and co-insurance. This is with the intent to lower the healthcare costs, but does so by incentivizing the consumer, not the healthcare system.

This section discusses the various commercial payors and how they add value-based contracting (often called cost-sharing) as a part of their benefit design to offer to their members. Many of the concepts are very similar to those discussed in the government payor section, but often the terminology may be slightly different.

BENEFIT DESIGN

Benefit designs are the rules that structure health insurance plans. They determine how consumers can gain access to healthcare services and providers. In particular, they dictate which services will be covered by the health plan, from which providers a consumer can seek care (also known as a "network"), and the types and amount of cost-sharing for which the consumer or member is responsible. Almost all benefit designs in the commercial space leverage cost-sharing to shift a portion of the financial responsibility for care onto consumers through out-of-pocket cost. The costs that the consumer or member must pay is often at the point of service, such as in the ED when seeking care or as a co-pay at the doctor's office. The theory is that this helps to avoid the "moral hazard" described earlier in the chapter. It aims to curb or dis-incentivize unnecessary and high expense levels of care and encourages consumers to seek lower, less expensive levels of care.

Employers who are purchasing these plans for their employees are increasingly using benefit designs with a VBC incentive to encourage the use of a less expensive but quality level of care. Employers are trying to save dollars on their bottom line and reserve profits. Healthcare costs are a large portion of their annual budget, and cost-sharing or value-based contracting with commercial payors is a common way to keep employees healthy while controlling costs. There are several different benefit designs used by commercial payors; the most commonly used to shape consumer behavior are high-deductible health plans, tiered networks, reference pricing, centers of excellence (COEs), narrow networks, value-based insurance designs, and benefit designs for alternative sites of care.

HIGH-DEDUCTIBLE HEALTH PLANS

High-deductible health plans are those plans that require consumers to cover 100% of their healthcare costs up to a certain amount of money, known as the deductible. At that point, other cost-sharing arrangements, such as co-pays or co-insurance, become available to the consumer or member. The consumer may make some very different decisions on how to access healthcare and spend their deductible dollars. They may put off needed care in a calendar year to wait until they have several issues so they can meet the deductible all at once. Elective procedures go way up at the end of the year in surgery centers, so patients can take advantage of meeting the deductible and get procedures done before the end of the year.

TIERED NETWORKS

Tiered networks are another way to direct the care of a consumer or member. Groups of network providers such as hospitals and physician practices are designated into levels, or tiers, based on the cost savings they can provide. Consumers' out-of-pocket costs will vary so that they pay less if they get care from a designated group by their commercial payor. The cost of care is negotiated up front by the payor and the provider, and the savings are passed onto the employer. If the networks or insurance change frequently, or the member changes employers, they may lose access to the healthcare provider with whom they have a relationship.

REFERENCE PRICING

Reference pricing is very similar to the bundled programs described earlier in the chapter. It establishes a standard price for any procedure, pharmacy costs, a service, or a bundle of services, and requires that the consumer pay out-of-pocket for any allowable charges above this price. An example would be the use of a formulary. On a smaller scale, the patient can receive a generic drug for a low price, but if they want the name brand they have to pay a higher cost. Similarly, a knee replacement may be offered to a member at a fixed price, but if there are complications the consumer has to pay the overages. This is very similar to bundle payments in the government payor space, except it is the consumer incurring the costs, not the hospital or provider.

CENTERS OF EXCELLENCE

COEs are similar to the tiered network concept. The member is allowed access to designated groups of providers that meet high standards for both the quality and cost of care for a particular service or set of services. The out-of-pocket expenses are generally much lower for the consumer or the member. An example may be a large employer uses only this provider for all hip and knee surgeries. The disadvantage is that other healthcare services may be in other COEs and run the risk of fragmenting care across several healthcare providers.

NARROW NETWORKS

Narrow networks use cost and quality criteria to select healthcare providers from a broader network and then establish strong incentives for consumers to seek care from that more limited set of providers (the narrow network). These incentives can include lower out-of-pocket costs for in-network care and higher out-of-pocket costs for care received from the broader network. This is becoming a more popular benefit design in certain areas of the country. It allows for a healthcare system to become an exclusive provider for an employer, driving patients to their health system and allowing them to capture a larger market share. A downside is that patients who travel outside the network and may become injured or ill may incur very high costs of out-of-pocket care if they are outside the network. Often, but not always, there are provisions to this in the design, but consumers should know what restrictions or out-of-pocket costs could be incurred if they must go outside the network.

VALUE-BASED INSURANCE DESIGN

Value-based insurance design (V-BID) is an attempt to avoid the "one size fits all" cost-sharing. It is a demand-based form of payment that attempts to drive patients to a lower cost but more high value care. For example, a primary care appointment may have no cost-sharing or co-pays associated with it, but an ED visit will have a $250 co-pay for the patient. This can also be done with procedures. For example, imaging for lower back pain is costly and has little effect on treatments for the patient. So, if the patient does want imaging it is going to have a high out-of-pocket cost. Conversely, physical therapy has known benefits to improve low back pain and thus may be at no cost to the patient.

BENEFIT DESIGNS FOR ALTERNATIVE SITES OF CARE

These are consumer incentives to seek care from locations where care is offered at a lower cost than at traditional venues, such as the hospital. For instance, consumers would have lower or no out-of-pocket costs for care received via telehealth or from an onsite clinic. As another example, one could utilize occupational health clinics located at worksites where nurse practitioners and physicians are available to access during work hours to help employees with preventive care, management of chronic disease, and wellness initiatives at little or no cost (Berenson et al., 2016).

KEY POINTS

- Payors, both government and private insurance, are moving from an FFS and episodic payment model to a value-centric long-term healthcare outcome model.

- Coordinated efforts to reduce hospitalization and/or increase support for patients outside the hospital are essential to continue to efficiently and effectively manage patients in a value-based healthcare system.

- Partnering with insurance companies to design insurance products that incentivize patient management of chronic conditions, or disease risk factors, could be of long-term benefit to both organizations.

- New payment models based in the hospital, primary care offices, ambulatory care centers, or even private service providers are constantly being researched, developed, and piloted. Change management is a key skill for nurse leadership to develop in order to continue to excel in the most updated VBC agreements.

- Healthcare leaders must learn the basics of VBC in order to effectively manage their resources to ensure they are providing the care their patients need in the most appropriate settings.

SUMMARY

"Payment reform promises to substitute value for volume, but value- and volume-based approaches typically are implemented together. All payment methods have strengths and weaknesses, and how they affect the behavior of health care providers depends on their operational design features and how they interact with benefit design."

Berenson et al. (2016, para. 1)

The healthcare and payment landscape in the United States is a complex web of providers, payors, and consumers who are all trying to receive high-quality care at an affordable cost. Doing this without a single-payor health system, but rather a system of differentiated payors, is hard to achieve, not to mention operationalize. As we face as a nation the struggle to care for people while also trying to preserve our state and national budgets to continue to provide for roads, education, and other important infrastructures, we have to grasp the urgency and act. As nurse leaders, we have to become educated and savvy on how payment models work, especially as we find ourselves in the very middle of the changing tide from volume to value. Understanding the implications of these payment models, how they affect consumers, and how they affect the business of healthcare will direct us in how we take care of patients going forward. There is no doubt that patients are going to have to take better care of themselves for this to be successful.

In a world where everything is politicized, recognize that healthcare has been one of the most politicized social issues in modern times, particularly in the United States. This only solidifies that nurses need to educate themselves on VBC and payment reform models so they are in a better position to advocate for their patients in this shifting landscape. Nurses need to stay true to their value system of patient advocacy and help both patients and our front-line caregivers navigate this new world. This will mean sitting in board rooms and asking difficult questions. It will mean balancing what is the right thing to do versus what is the lower cost option. Not all of these questions are easy, and injustice will exist. Being the conscience of our nation both in the boardroom and in the halls of policy and lawmaking will remain a critical role for nurses now and in the future.

END-OF-CHAPTER RESOURCES

◆ DISCUSSION QUESTIONS

1. What do you think are important factors and considerations when selecting a Medicare plan upon retirement?
2. As a nurse leader, would you support your organization going full risk in value-based contracts knowing your performance will be absolutely key in getting paid?
3. What do you think are some of the biggest challenges facing our national healthcare system in the next 10 years?
4. How do you think the global pandemic of SARS-COV-2 has changed the future on the delivery of healthcare? What we have learned, and what didn't we learn and should have?

◆ ADDITIONAL RESOURCES

- Medicare Advantage plans: https://www.healthcarefinancenews.com/news/disadvantages-medicare-advantage-plan
- Transitional Care Management: https://www.aafp.org/family-physician/practice-and-career/getting-paid/coding/transitional-care-management.html
- Social Determinants of Health: http://www.who.int/social_determinants/sdh_definition/en/
- Medicare ACO: https://www.cms.gov/Medicare/Medicare-Fee-for-Service-Payment/ACO

A robust set of instructor resources designed to supplement this text is located at http://connect.springerpub.com/content/book/978-0-8261-7795-7. Qualifying instructors may request access by emailing textbook@springerpub.com.

REFERENCES

Allen, H. L., & Sommers, B. D. (2020). Medicaid and COVID-19; at the center of both health and economic crisis. *The Journal of the American Medical Association, 324*(2), 135–136. https://doi.org/10.1001/jama.2020.10553

Berenson, R. A., Upadhyay, D., Delbanco, S. F., & Murray, R. (2016). *A typology of benefit designs.* Urban Institute Research Report. https://www.urban.org/research/publication/typology-payment-methods

Centers for Medicare & Medicaid Services. (2018, December 21). *Final rule creates pathways to success for the Medicare Shared Savings Program.* https://www.cms.gov/newsroom/fact-sheets/final-rule-creates-pathways-success-medicare-shared-savings-program

Dick Cauchi, A. G. (n.d.). *Managed care, market reports and the states.* Retrieved October 14, 2021, from https://www.ncsl.org/research/health/managed-care-and-the-states.aspx

Green, J., & Hibbard, J. H. (2011). Why does patient activation matter? *Journal of General Internal Medicine, 27*(5), 520–526. https://doi.org/10.1007/s11-1931-2.

Hibbard, J. H., Stockard, J., Mahoney, E. R., & Tusler, M. (2004). Development of the Patient Activation Measure (PAM): conceptualizing and measuring activation in patients and consumers. *Health Services Research, 39*(4 Pt 1), 1005–1026. https://doi.org/10.1111/j.1475-6773.2004.00269.x

Magnan, S. (2017). Social determinants of health 101 for health care: Five plus five. *NAM perspectives.* Discussion Paper, National Academy of Medicine. https://doi.org/10.31478/201710c

McClellan, M., McKethan, A. N., Lewis, J. L., Roski, J., & Fisher, E. S. (2010). A national strategy to put accountable care into practice. *Health Affairs (Millwood), 29*(5), 982–990. https://doi.org/10.1377/hlthaff.2010.0194

Morgan, D. J., Dhruva, S. S., Coon, E. R., Wright, S. M., & Korenstein, D. (2018). 2017 update on medical overuse: A systematic review. *JAMA Internal Medicine, 178*(1), 110–115. https://doi.org/10.1001/jamainternmed.2017.4361

Medicaid. (n.d.). *Managed care.* Retrieved October 14, 2021, from https://www.medicaid.gov/medicaid/managed-care/index.html

Medicare.gov. (n.d.). *What's Medicare?* Retrieved April 06, 2021, from https://www.medicare.gov/what-medicare-covers/your-medicare-coverage-choices/whats-medicare

Moselely, G. B. (2008). The US healthcare non-system, 1908–2008. *Virtual Mentoring, 10*(5), 324–331. https://doi.org/10.1001/virtualmentor.2008.10.5.mhst1-0805

Transamerica Institute. (n.d.). *Federally Qualified Health Centers (FQHCs).* Retrieved October 14, 2021, from https://www.transamericainstitute.org/health-wellness/health-care-guides/federally-qualified-health-centers

World Health Organization. (2012). *What are the social determinants of health?* http://www.who.int/social_determinants/sdh_definition/en

CHAPTER | 9

POPULATION AND COMMUNITY HEALTH: LEVERAGING LEADERSHIP AND EMPOWERING NURSES TO UNDERSTAND AND POSITIVELY IMPACT SOCIAL DETERMINANTS OF HEALTH

Natalia Cineas and Donna Boyle Schwartz

"I'm opposed to any policy that would deny in our country any human being from access to public safety, public education, or public health, period."

Kamala Harris, American politician and attorney, serving as the 49th and current vice president of the United States

LEARNING OBJECTIVES

- Demonstrate knowledge of the primary social determinants of health (SDOH) and the impact on individual, community, and population health.
- Describe the connection between governmental policies and the impact on SDOH.
- Define the role nurses and nurse leaders play in advocacy and aligning nurse assessments with SDOH.

INTRODUCTION

The terms "population health" and "community health" have become increasingly important in the past two decades. The healthcare industry has shifted its focus from simply treating the physical illness or injury of an individual patient to putting the patient's health into a broader context, encompassing the various physical, mental, social, and environmental factors that can positively or negatively impact individuals and communities. These factors have come to be identified as the "social determinants of health" (SDOH) that collectively impact population health, community health, and individual health, and form the basis for numerous national and international public health policies designed to mitigate widespread disparities in health and healthcare.

The concept of "population health" may be traced back to the earliest inception of the World Health Organization (WHO) in the 1940s, when the nascent group defined health in a broader sense as "a state of complete physical, mental, and social well-being and not merely the absence of disease or infirmity" in its constitution (WHO, 1946, p. 1).

Generally, the concept of population health is centered on improving the overall health of an entire human population, as opposed to a specific group or category of the population.

By many accounts, the United States is lagging behind other developed nations in terms of population health, and the decline is expected to continue: According to the U.S. Census Bureau, the United States had the 20th highest life expectancy among developed nations in 1960; that ranking dropped to 40th by 2015, and is expected to drop to 43rd by 2060 (Medina et al. 2020).

Many international and national organizations—including WHO, the U.S. Centers for Disease Control and Prevention (CDC), and the U.S. Department of Health and Human Services (DHHS)—have established the goal of achieving population health by reducing health disparities or health inequities. These inequities are due to the SDOH, which are loosely defined as a host of factors that have a measurable impact on the health of individuals, communities, and overall human populations, including economic, educational, social, environmental, cultural, and physical components. The CDC defines SDOH as the "conditions in the places where people live, learn, work, and play that affect a wide range of health and quality-of life-risks and outcomes" (n.d.-a, para. 1). Various industry associations and analyses have indicated that these factors may be responsible for more than 70% to 80% of all health outcomes (Moody's Analytics, 2017; Robert Wood Johnson Foundation, 2019); medical care is estimated to account for just 10% to 20% of outcomes. In fact, the impact of the SDOH on health outcomes and health disparities is considered to be so great that the Robert Wood Johnson Foundation sponsored a series of in-depth reports, town halls, site visits, and public meetings across the country in 2019, summarizing its findings for the *Future of Nursing 2020–2030* report by the National Academies of Sciences, Engineering, and Medicine (NASEM). This report, released in 2021, identifies and categorizes the myriad contributions of nurses and the nursing profession to addressing the SDOH and the goal of achieving health equity in the United States (Wakefield et al., 2021).

"Community health" is typically defined as a subset of population health, focusing on specific population groups, as defined by geographical factors, such as cities, towns, counties, or neighborhoods; demographic factors, such as children or Medicare recipients, specific racial or ethnic groups, and differing income echelons; and, in some cases, chronic disease factors, such as asthma sufferers, diabetes patients, cancer cases and other pervasive disease classifications. Community health is defined by WHO as the "environmental, social and economic resources to sustain emotional and physical well-being among people in ways that advance their aspirations and satisfy their needs in their unique environment" (Health Promotion International, 1986, pp. 73–76). Community health also is a subset of public health, spotlighting the role governmental policies and people play in their own health, as contrasted with "environmental health," which is primarily concerned with the physical environment.

Community health initiatives in the United States received increasing amounts of attention and funding following the passage of the Affordable Care Act (ACA) by the U.S. Congress in 2010. The ACA also is known as the Patient Protection and Affordable Care Act and nicknamed "Obamacare," for being championed by President Barack Obama, who signed the bill into law during his term. The ACA increased funding and expanded insurance coverage for Medicaid, representing the most comprehensive overhaul of this massive public health program since it was originally enacted in 1965.

This chapter examines the primary SDOH, providing concrete examples of each major factor and the associated subfactors, as well as addressing the roles that nurse leaders, nurse managers, and frontline nurses can play in addressing these issues, mitigating health disparities, promoting health literacy and wellness programs within communities, and thereby fostering enhanced overall population health.

CONSIDERING SOCIAL DETERMINANTS OF HEALTH

An essential tenet of the nursing profession is that nurses and nurse leaders are a driving force in promoting health and wellness within the communities they serve, thereby enhancing overall population health. Nursing, therefore, is the logical healthcare segment to take the lead in addressing population health and community health because nurses and nurse leaders traditionally take a broader view of the overall continuum of care. Rather than treating patients only when they are sick in acute care environments, nurses and nurse leaders address larger population and community health issues, focusing on preventive care, health education, and health literacy, and understanding and evaluating the SDOH as they relate to providing better and more comprehensive patient care (Carlson et al., 2016).

Nurses and nurse leaders also play a vital role in advocating for public policy changes that address the SDOH. Increased engagement by nurses and nurse leaders in public policy advocacy can help provide a framework for enhancing overall population health at the local, state, regional, national, and international levels.

Many thought leaders point out that it is essential for the nursing profession to incorporate the SDOH into professional practice and patient care to achieve improved overall community and population health (Wilson, 2019). *The Future of Nursing 2020–2030* report, for instance, calls for a strengthening of nursing capacity and expertise in pursuit of health equity in the United States (Wakefield et al., 2021).

One emergent strategy for identifying and addressing community health needs—and the SDOH specific to a particular population—grew out of 2010's ACA, which added a new Internal Revenue Service (IRS) requirement for hospitals to conduct a community health needs assessment that assesses and identifies the existing health resources and prioritizes the health needs of the community being served, and to develop and implement a plan to answer those needs (Stoto, 2013). The assessment typically leads to an "action plan," also known as a community health improvement plan, defined by the Public Health Accreditation Board (PHAB) as a "long-term, systematic effort to address public health problems on the basis of the results of community health assessment activities and the community health improvement process" (PHAB, 2012, p. 8).

The role of the SDOH in community health assessments and improvement plans has taken center stage as decades of evidence have demonstrated that economic, environmental, educational, community, and social context, as well as healthcare conditions, are the primary drivers of disease and health for individuals, communities, and the human population as a whole. The decennial *Healthy People* initiative launched in 1979 by the DHHS has steadily updated its definitions of the SDOH and has made eliminating health disparities a centerpiece of the program in its 2010, 2020, and 2030 incarnations.

The *Healthy People 2020* and *Healthy People 2030* updates to this initiative codified the "place-based" framework for the SDOH, organizing these factors into five key areas: neighborhood and built environment, social and community context, economic stability, education access and quality, and healthcare access and quality (DHHS, Office of Disease Prevention and Health Promotion [ODPHP], n.d.-a, n.d.-b; Figure 9.1). These five categories form the umbrella for a defined set of underlying factors that reflect the key issues and problems that can contribute to diseases, chronic illnesses, infections, maternal mortality and morbidity, situational emergencies and accidents, and domestic violence.

Each of the categories defined by the *Healthy People* initiative presents a unique set of situations and circumstances that can affect individual, community, and population health (Table 9.1). The category of "neighborhood and built environment," for instance, involves issues such as environmental crises; water, soil, and air pollution; aging and degraded housing stock; unsafe neighborhoods; and other physical characteristics affecting people where they live, work and play. "Social and community context" addresses the negative health impacts of discrimination, racism, sexism, the excessive and inordinate high rates of incarceration among minorities, and distrust of authority. The "economic stability" classification deals with the impact of poverty, unemployment, food insecurity and homelessness as contributors to health inequities. The

Social Determinants of Health

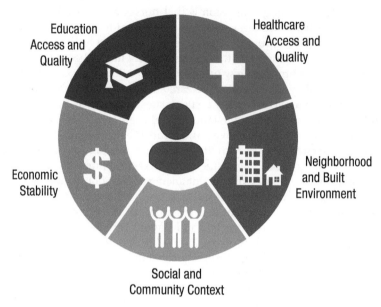

FIGURE 9.1: Social determinants of health.

Source: U.S. Department of Health and Human Services, Office of Disease Prevention and Health Promotion. (n.d.). *Social determinants of health.* https://health.gov/healthypeople/objectives-and-data/social-determinants-health.

TABLE 9.1: Social Determinants of Health and Key Influencers Within Each

Neighborhood and Built Environment	
Key Influencers	**Examples**
Environmental conditions	Water, soil, air quality, parks and recreation, transportation access
Quality of housing	Aging or degraded housing stock, vermin infestations
Crime and violence	Unsafe neighborhoods, unsafe family or social situations
Access to foods that support healthy eating patterns	Availability of grocery stores, farmers markets, locally grown fresh foods
Social and Community Context	
Key Influencers	**Examples**
Discrimination	Racism, poverty, sexism
Incarceration	Negative impact on minority families and communities
Civic participation	Voting, distrust of government, distrust of authority, including healthcare institutions
Social cohesion	Psychosocial impact, community health

(continued)

TABLE 9.1: Social Determinants of Health and Key Influencers Within Each (*continued*)

Economic Stability	
Key Influencers	**Examples**
Poverty	Income stress, access to healthy foods, adequate housing, transportation, healthcare
Employment	Fair employment, minimum/living wage
Food insecurity	Hunger and nutrition
Housing instability	Homelessness
Education Access and Quality	
Key Influencers	**Examples**
Language and literacy	Immigration status, english as a second language, health literacy
Early childhood education and development	Proper nutrition, exercise, stress
High school graduation	Role in poverty, joblessness, future success
Enrollment in higher education	Teenage dropout rates, teenage pregnancy
Health and Healthcare Access and Quality	
Key Influencers	**Examples**
Access to healthcare	Transportation, hospital/clinic closures, language barriers
Access to primary care	Lack of access/transportation, especially in rural areas, lack of physicians
Health literacy	Providing patient education, establishing trust, developing better communication strategies
COVID-19	Racial disparities in cases, hospitalizations and deaths, racial disparities in essential workers
COVID-19 vaccines	Vaccine hesitancy, racial disparities in hesitancy and access

area of "education access and quality" focuses on the importance of early childhood development, high school graduation rates, enrollment in higher education, and the problems of language and literacy in terms of delivering healthcare and wellness information to immigrant and impoverished populations. The "health and healthcare access and quality" segment engages with the problems of access to care in both urban and rural locations, and the overall challenges of improving health literacy and promoting wellness among minority and disadvantaged communities; this section also articulates many of the health disparities revealed by the COVID-19 global pandemic, including higher rates of cases, hospitalizations, and deaths among minority populations and the racial disparities in vaccine access and vaccine hesitancy.

In its *Future of Nursing 2020–2030* report, the NASEM point out that it is the role of nurse executives and nurse leaders to know and understand the collection, relevance, and interpretation of data on the SDOH in order to effectively communicate and lead frontline nurses on community health initiatives (Wakefield et al., 2021). Similarly, Wilson (2019) calls on nurse leaders and nurse informaticians to develop an expertise in the evaluation of data and programs concerned with the SDOH and their impact on patient care. Additionally, the American Organization of Nurse Executives (AONE) and the American Organization for Nursing Leadership (AONL) list "improving the health of populations" as an essential competency for all nurse executives (AONE & AONL, 2015, p. 3).

Each of the main categories of the SDOH and its attendant concerns represents an opportunity for engagement and interaction on the part of the nursing profession; therefore, it is incumbent upon nurse leaders to acquire expertise in all applicable categories.

NEIGHBORHOOD AND BUILT ENVIRONMENT

The impact of the "neighborhood and built environment" on individual, community, and population health is all around us. One only needs to look as far as today's news headlines to see the pervasive, far-reaching effects of location-based health consequences, especially when it comes to contamination of the water, soil, and air quality; a high prevalence of violence and crime; and the degradation of urban housing stock, home to many minorities, children, older adults, and low-income people.

From the contamination of Flint, Michigan's drinking water with lead and the third-largest outbreak of Legionnaires' disease recorded in U.S. history (Natural Resources Defense Council, 2018) to the ongoing chemical contamination from perfluorooctane sulfonate and perfluorooctanoic acid (PFAS/PFOA) at some 2,854 locations in 50 states and two territories (Environmental Working Group, 2021), it is clear that the places where many people live, work, and play are proving to be hazardous to their health. The main SDOH under this category include the following: environmental conditions, quality of housing, crime and violence, and access to foods that support healthy eating patterns (Table 9.2). Each of these subcategories has serious ramifications for the healthcare industry in general, and the nursing profession specifically, as these issues have a direct impact on the health and well-being of the patient population and the communities in which they reside.

TABLE 9.2: Neighborhood and the Built Environment—Social Determinants of Health

Examples	Negative Health Outcomes
Environmental Conditions	
• Climate and climate change • Water, soil, and air quality • Access to parks, gardens, and green spaces • Transportation access • Urban versus rural location	• Famine and food insecurity • Cardiovascular diseases • Respiratory diseases • Infections and parasitic diseases • Neonatal and maternal morbidity
Housing Quality	
• Aging or degraded housing stock • Lead and other contaminants • Heating, air conditioning, and appliances • Mold and mildew • Vermin infestations	• Injuries • Lead and carbon monoxide poisoning • Allergies • Asthma and respiratory illness • Cardiovascular diseases
Crime and Violence	
• Direct victimization • Witnessing crime and violence • Perceptions of unsafe neighborhood • Domestic violence	• Injuries and death • Mental trauma/post-traumatic stress • Behavioral disorders • Drug and alcohol abuse • Suicide • Sexual and reproductive disorders, including HIV/AIDS

(continued)

TABLE 9.2: Neighborhood and the Built Environment—Social Determinants of Health (*continued*)

Examples	Negative Health Outcomes
Access to Foods That Support Healthy Eating Patterns	
<ul><li>Food deserts</li><li>Prevalence of convenience stores</li><li>Lack of healthy foods</li><li>High prices</li><li>Distance and lack of transportation</li></ul>	<ul><li>Obesity</li><li>Cardiovascular diseases</li><li>Diabetes</li><li>High blood pressure</li><li>Cancer</li></ul>

ENVIRONMENTAL CONDITIONS

Some of the leading environmental elements that impact health include the overall climate in a particular region and the increasing impact of climate change worldwide, causing severe illness and death due to higher average temperatures as well as the increasing frequency and severity of cataclysmic storms such as hurricanes, typhoons, and monsoons, and the increasing frequency and severity of drought and desertification. According to the National Oceanic and Atmospheric Administration (NOAA; 2021), 2020 was the second hottest year on record since 1880, surpassed only by 2016; the 10 warmest years on record have all occurred since 2005. Extreme weather conditions and higher temperatures can cause heat-related disease and death, especially among children and older adults. Drought and floods caused by severe storms often lead to famine, contaminated water, insect infestations, and community displacement, all of which can cause disease and death. Because many impoverished people and racial and ethnic minorities live and work in areas susceptible to these extreme weather events, they are more at risk of climate-related disease and death.

The water, soil, and air quality in an area; availability or absence of parks, gardens, trees, grass, and other green spaces; and the accessibility of transportation alternatives, including public transportation, sidewalks, roads, and highways, also are all environmental conditions that have a major impact on health and healthcare, and can vary depending on the location. A significant geographical condition affecting health is whether the location is urban or rural. One of the most severe urban conditions that has been shown to have negative health impacts is air pollution, which can contribute to hypertension and high blood pressure; cardiovascular disease and stroke; lung diseases, including emphysema, asthma, chronic bronchitis, and chronic obstructive pulmonary disease (COPD); and cancer, leukemia, and non-Hodgkin lymphoma (National Institute of Environmental Health Sciences, 2021). A comprehensive literature review found that nearly nine out of 10 people living in urban areas worldwide suffer health issues caused by air pollution; the study also ranked air pollution as the ninth leading risk factor for cardiopulmonary mortality (Kurt et al., 2016). Excessive noise in the urban environment also has been linked to hypertension (Healthy People 2030; DHHS, ODPHP, n.d.-b) and cardiovascular disease (Münzel et al., 2018).

The rural environment has its own set of problems: air pollution sources in rural regions include factory farming and the spraying of insecticides/pesticides, and animal husbandry, where animal feed and waste can emit pollutants such as ammonia. Rural mining communities are subject to numerous air pollutants, leading to higher rates of respiratory illnesses and cancer (Hendryx et al., 2010; Shi et al., 2019). Rural residents also face higher rates of water contamination, due to a greater prevalence of wells as a primary water source, which can be impacted by contaminated groundwater and polluted runoff. An estimated one in three Americans get their drinking water from groundwater sources, which can be contaminated by agriculture chemicals and pesticides, landfill runoff, septic tanks, and leaking underground storage tanks containing hazardous materials, such as home heating oil (Healthy People 2030; DHHS, ODPHP, n.d.-b). A comprehensive study of public wells by the U.S.

Geological Survey found that 22% contained one or more chemical contaminants at levels above human-health benchmarks, and 80% contained one or more contaminants at concentrations greater than one-tenth of human-health benchmarks (Toccalino & Hopple, 2010). Follow-up studies by the U.S. Geological Survey found that an estimated 90% of 383 public supply wells across 35 states contained mixtures of two or more contaminants (Eberts et al., 2013).

Other toxic substances found in the natural environment in both urban and rural locations include lead, arsenic, asbestos, radon, and mercury, all of which cause negative health impacts in humans, including many forms of cancer; endocrine and reproductive system disruption; respiratory and lung diseases; neurological disorders, headaches, and dizziness; skin and eye irritation and allergic reactions; and glandular, hormonal, and DNA irregularities.

Minorities, people living in poverty, and those in economically disadvantaged communities are more likely to suffer adverse health outcomes due to environmental conditions (Evans & Kantrowitz, 2002). According to the U.S. Environmental Protection Agency (EPA), there are numerous currently identified relationships between exposure to environmental contaminants and disease, including radon and lung cancer, arsenic and cancer in several organs, lead and nervous system disorders, disease-causing bacteria (such as *Escherichia coli*) and gastrointestinal illness and death, and particulate matter and aggravation of cardiovascular and respiratory diseases (EPA, n.d.). It is therefore necessary for public and private nursing professionals to incorporate questions regarding environmental factors into routine health assessments and treatment plans to identify and target harmful environmental conditions that contribute to health disparities and poor patient outcomes.

QUALITY OF HOUSING

Aging or degraded housing stock is an additional environmental condition impacting health. Older houses and apartment buildings often lack modern heating and air conditioning systems to mitigate the effects of climate; may contain aging or damaged appliances and structural elements; are more susceptible to allergens such as mold and mildew; and may be subject to vermin infestations, including mice, rats, cockroaches, and other insects; these all lead to negative health consequences. Damaged, neglected, or inadequately vented appliances, for instance, can result in dangerous levels of carbon monoxide, which can lead to heart disease, neurological disorders, and death—according to the CDC, more than 50,000 people a year suffer from carbon monoxide poisoning (n.d.-b).

Several studies have attributed skyrocketing rates of childhood asthma and adult respiratory diseases to the conditions common to many low-income urban housing developments. One study found that 21.8% of children living in public housing had asthma, as compared to just 7% of children living in single-family homes (Northridge et al., 2010). The study also found 68.7% of public housing residents reported cockroaches, compared to 21% of residents in private homes. Similarly, a 2017 report from the nonprofit Urban Institute found that low-income renters receiving housing assistance suffered more from asthma than the general U.S. population; the report speculated that the higher prevalence of asthma was due to the renters' poor housing conditions, including dampness and mold, inadequate ventilation and temperature control, pest infestations, asbestos, and overcrowding (Ganesh et al., 2017).

Contaminants found in aging buildings can be harmful to human health. Lead poisoning, for example, is a huge health issue for children living in homes that were constructed prior to 1978, before lead was banned in residential paint. The CDC estimates that some 29 million housing units in the United States are contaminated with lead-based paint residue; aging or corroded plumbing also increases the risk of lead poisoning (CDC, n.d.-c).

Substandard or crumbling buildings can lead to injuries among older adults and young children; narrow hallways and buildings with steps can pose serious access issues for people with physical limitations; and old, brittle window glass and low windowsills can lead to severe cuts and falls.

Nurses and nurse leaders can and should play an important role in advocating for community-level interventions—including programs to replace aging plumbing, campaigns for better sidewalks and additional parks, and aesthetic improvements, such as better lighting and tree planting—to have a positive impact on population health.

CRIME AND VIOLENCE

Crime and violence can have significant and enduring consequences for both physical and mental health. Individuals may be directly victimized by violent acts; they may witness crime or violence against others or against property; or they may hear about crime and violence from others, creating a perception of an unsafe neighborhood. Domestic violence may directly impact individuals and create unsafe family and social situations.

Violence-related injuries kill 1.25 million people every year and millions more suffer from nonfatal injuries due to violence (WHO, 2021); violence is considered one of the world's leading causes of death for people aged between 15 and 44 years. Victims of violence may suffer immediate injury or premature death; survivors of violent crime often suffer from post-traumatic stress, mental trauma, and have higher rates of drug and alcohol abuse and suicide (WHO, 2010); individuals who are victims or exposed to violence in childhood can suffer from many long-term behavioral and mental health issues, including increased risk of social problems, anxiety, depression and aggression, as well as increased risk of mental illness, substance abuse, and suicide. These factors that are linked to violence in childhood can engender and prolong a cycle of violence in which traumatized victims of violence in childhood grow up to become perpetrators of violence as adults. Women who are victims of intimate partner violence (IPV) may suffer from multiple and severe injuries; sexual and reproductive health disorders, including sexually transmitted diseases, HIV/AIDS, and unintended pregnancy; and mental traumas leading to eating disorders, depression, anxiety, substance abuse, and suicide (Stockman et al., 2015). Victims of crime and violence also have higher rates of many chronic diseases, including heart disease, diabetes, and cancer (WHO, 2021).

Logically, therefore, nurses and other healthcare professionals should take crime and violence, and the perception of crime and violence, into account when considering how to improve community and local population health. Advocacy on behalf of vulnerable populations is an important part of the nursing toolbox when it comes to addressing this specific SDOH and is especially pertinent in the public health sphere.

ACCESS TO FOODS THAT SUPPORT HEALTHY EATING PATTERNS

Public health proponents have long decried the dearth of fresh food markets in urban locales, with some thought leaders calling cities "food wastelands" and "food deserts." Many low-income and minority communities are dominated by convenience stores and bodegas, which often charge a premium price for fruits, vegetables, and other healthy foods . . . if they carry these items at all. The paucity of full-service grocery stores, farmers' markets, and community gardens in urban areas make access to foods that support healthy eating patterns difficult, if not downright impossible. Instead, urban dwellers are faced with a seemingly limitless supply of processed convenience foods, many loaded with artery-clogging saturated and trans fats and packed with sodium and added sugars.

Rural communities also suffer barriers to access of healthy foods, most notably distance and lack of public transportation. People living in rural communities without convenient public transportation, those who do not have access to a personal vehicle, and those who are unable to drive due to age or disability face sharply limited choices in accessing healthy foods. A 2015 study conducted for the U.S. Department of Agriculture (USDA) found that the average distance from all U.S. households to the nearest supermarket that accepted Supplemental Nutrition Assistance Program (SNAP) benefits was 2.19 miles (Ver Ploeg et al., 2015).

Lack of access to healthy foods has been shown to have a suite of adverse health consequences, including obesity, cardiovascular disease, high blood pressure, diabetes, liver disease, and cancer. According to the USDA's *Dietary Guidelines for Americans 2020-2025*, 60% of adults have one or more chronic diseases that can be traced to dietary causes and more than 74% of American adults and 40% of children and youth are overweight or obese (USDA & DHHS, 2020). An earlier version of the Dietary Guidelines noted that chronic, diet-related diseases engender a high price tag, with $147 billion in estimated medical costs linked to obesity in 2008; and $245 billion in estimated medical costs linked to diagnosed cases of diabetes (DHHS & USDA, 2015).

Improving access to foods that support healthy eating patterns is vital to any effort to improve individual, community, and population health. Public health agencies, healthcare systems, governmental entities, and concerned individuals need public and private collaborative efforts to ascertain and implement programs to reduce reliance on processed convenience foods, curtail the proximity of fast-food restaurants to schools, and, overall, to address the scarcity of healthy food alternatives in both urban and rural environments. As the nursing profession has traditionally played a key role in educating patients and families about the importance of nutrition, healthy eating, and healthy food choices at every life stage, it is imperative that nurses and nurse leaders are active participants in programs designed to help lower the risk of chronic, diet-related diseases.

SOCIAL AND COMMUNITY CONTEXT

"Social and community context" covers the myriad ways in which individuals react to each other, both singly and in groups; and the ways in which individuals *and* groups react to institutions, beginning at the local municipal level and continuing up the governmental chain to the federal authorities and even global influences. This category of SDOH encompasses discrimination, including systemic and structural racism; entrenched sexism; and the social problems faced by the LGBTQ+ (lesbian, gay, bisexual, transgender, queer, plus) community, older adults, and disabled people. Related issues include incarceration and its impact on children, families, and communities; civic participation, including voting and trust or distrust of government and other authorities such as healthcare institutions; and social cohesion, including the psychological and sociological impacts and community health (Table 9.3).

Many social and community concerns are challenges that represent deep-rooted structural problems historically embedded in American society. Again, one need look no farther than contemporary news reports to find accounts of the deleterious effects, including the persistent discrimination and overt racism pervading community policing as evidenced by the 2020 killings of George Floyd, Breonna Taylor, and Ahmaud Arbery and the overly aggressive rates of incarceration among minority communities; the 2016 domestic terror incident targeting LGBTQ+ patrons at an Orlando nightclub that left 50 dead and more than 50 wounded; the 2021 mass murder of six Asian women in the Atlanta area; the prevailing sexist beliefs about women's "proper" roles and abilities that lead to persistent wage inequity and the "glass ceiling" effect; and the tsunami of voter suppression laws proposed in state and local governments to disenfranchise minority communities in the wake of the 2020 election.

These complicated and interdependent societal issues require a coordinated and collaborative response on the part of public and private institutions. The nursing profession is integral to any discussion within the social and community context, particularly because nurses are the most trusted profession in America. Nurses have ranked at the top of the Gallup Honesty and Ethics Poll for the past two decades, earning a record high/very high score of 89% in 2020, up 4 percentage points from the previous high score of 85% in 2019 (Saad, 2020). It is essential, therefore, that nurses and nurse leaders are well-informed and knowledgeable about these formidable societal problems in order to take an active role in interventions addressing the complex and multifaceted health impacts.

TABLE 9.3: Social and Community Context—Social Determinants of Health

Examples	Negative Health Outcomes
Discrimination	
• Systemic and structural racism • Sexism • LGBTQ+ social issues • Ageism • Disabled social issues	• Injuries and death • Mental and behavioral disorders • Drug and alcohol abuse • Suicide • Obesity • Cardiovascular diseases • Diabetes • Respiratory diseases • Infectious and parasitic-borne illnesses • Sexually transmitted diseases, including HIV/AIDS
Incarceration	
• Overpolicing of minority communities • Uneven legal and criminal justice • Broken homes and single parents • Poverty • Social support	• Mental and behavioral issues • Drug and alcohol abuse • High blood pressure • Tuberculosis • Hepatitis C • HIV/AIDS • Cervical cancer • Children with mental and behavioral problems
Civic Participation	
• Voting • Volunteerism • Church attendance • Community sporting and leisure activities	• Social isolation • Depression and anxiety • Mental and behavioral disorders • Distrust of authorities, including healthcare systems • Cardiovascular diseases
Social Cohesion	
• Interconnected relationships • Social networks • Mutual trust • Social support	• Isolation and depression • Anxiety • Cardiovascular diseases

DISCRIMINATION

Blatant, overt, and hostile instances of discrimination beleaguer minorities, women, and ethnic and social groups in the United States while insidious and subtle manifestations of discrimination result from implicit biases which many people may not even realize they possess. A 2011 study reported 31% of U.S. adults experienced at least one major occurrence of discrimination in their lifetimes, and nearly two-thirds (63%) reported facing discrimination every day (Luo et al., 2011).

With the advent of European colonization, many Native Americans perished from previously unknown diseases, including smallpox, measles, chicken pox, whooping cough, diphtheria, scarlet fever, trachoma, malaria, typhus fever, typhoid fever, influenza, cholera, and bubonic plague, leading to a massive population decline—historians estimate that the Native American population may have decreased an estimated 70% to 90%. Native Americans were forced to relocate to reservations; children were torn from their families and forced to go to assimilation boarding schools where they were prohibited from speaking their native languages or communicating with their families; many were abused and buried in unmarked graves, a practice that continued into the 1960s. Native Americans today suffer from higher rates of chronic liver disease and cirrhosis, diabetes mellitus, and chronic lower respiratory diseases, as well as deaths due to violence, injury, or suicide, leading to an average life expectancy that is 5.5 years less than the U.S. all-races average (Indian Health Service, 2019).

The experience of most Black Americans is a similarly grim one, as many of their ancestors were brought to the New World as slaves and endured horrific beatings, torture, rape, forced breeding programs, and murder. Black Americans have suffered from the effects of structural discrimination, including residential segregation, educational and employment inequities, and individual discrimination, including violence, threats, and harassment. Black Americans suffer disproportionately high rates of death from heart disease, stroke, high blood pressure, asthma, cancer, HIV/AIDS, influenza, pneumonia, diabetes, and kidney disease, leading to a projected average life expectancy of 76.2 years for Black Americans, versus an average life expectancy of 80 years for non-Hispanic White Americans (Medina et al., 2020).

The negative effects of discrimination also are felt by other racial and ethnic groups, leading to health disparities. Specific communities of Hispanics and Latinos in the border region between the United States and Mexico suffer from the highest rates of obesity and diabetes in the world, with obesity affecting 40% of adults and diabetes rates of more than 20% (Rosales et al., 2016). Mexican Americans living in the border region also face higher rates of tuberculosis, diabetes, hepatitis C, cervical cancer, and parasitic-borne illnesses such as Zika, dengue, chikungunya, rickettsial infections, West Nile, Rocky Mountain spotted fever, and Chagas disease; deaths by traffic accident and violence also are a recurring tragedy (Rural Health Information Hub, n.d.).

Asian Americans continue to be haunted by discrimination, including the harassment and violence endured by the early Chinese immigrants who came to the United States to build the transcontinental railway; the internment of Japanese Americans in concentration camps during World War II; the housing discrimination and denigration of Vietnamese immigrants as "boat people," and the more recent attacks against random Asian Americans fueled by politicians' misrepresentation of COVID-19 as the "Chinese virus" or "Kung Flu." According to the Office of Minority Health (2021), Asian Americans suffer from higher rates of COPD, hepatitis B, HIV/AIDS, and liver disease; Asian Americans also are most at risk from cancer, heart disease, stroke, and diabetes. Further, the CDC found that as of 2020 the rate of tuberculosis among Asian Americans was 33 times higher than that of non-Hispanic Whites (CDC, n.d.-d).

GENDER DISCRIMINATION

Gender discrimination, including pay and wage inequities, sexual harassment, and sexual assault, can affect both women and men, but is far more common against women. Studies published in 2017 by Pew Research Center found that 42% of working women have faced discrimination on the job and 25% say they have earned less than a man doing the same job (Parker & Funk, 2017).

Sexual harassment and sexual assault are some of the most egregious examples of gender discrimination, and many more instances have come to light in the wake of the #MeToo movement. A 2019 study found that 81% of American women reported sexual harassment and/or assault in their lifetime, with 38% of women reporting harassment at their workplace or school; 23% of women reported surviving sexual assault (Kearl et al., 2019).

LGBTQ+ DISCRIMINATION

LGBTQ+ individuals have the highest rates of tobacco, alcohol, and other drug use. LGBTQ+ youth are two to three times more likely to attempt suicide, and more likely to be homeless, due to social rejection, bullying, isolation, and verbal or physical abuse. Gay men and transgender individuals are at higher risk of HIV/AIDS and other sexually transmitted diseases, as well as mental health issues and suicide. The 2019 study found that 95% of lesbian and bisexual women reported being sexually harassed during their lifetime, and 47% reported sexual assault; 77% of gay or bisexual men reported a lifetime experience of sexual harassment and 21% reported sexual assault (Kearl et al., 2019).

AGE AND DISABILITY DISCRIMINATION

Aging adults are subject to many forms of discrimination and ageism, especially in the workplace. Indeed, instances of age discrimination reported to the Equal Employment Opportunity Commission (EEOC) average nearly 22,000 incidents a year (EEOC, n.d.-a). The health needs of older Americans may contribute to this workplace discrimination, as many employers may be reluctant to hire individuals who may require more sick leaves. At the same time, nonworking older adults face a host of other problems, including social isolation, depression, anxiety and loneliness, and the associated mental health issues.

Individuals with disabilities also face significant health inequities, including stigmatization, bullying, frequent institutionalization, and lack of access to healthcare services and healthcare facilities. The EEOC reports that instances of complaints filed under the 1990 Americans with Disabilities Act eclipse the number of charges filed in other categories, totaling 283,658 complaints from 2010 to 2020 (EEOC, n.d.-b).

According to the CDC, 61 million U.S. adults—or one in four—live with a disability, including issues with mobility, cognition, independent living, hearing, vision, and self-care activities. The problem is especially acute for older, disabled adults; the CDC reports that two in five adults aged 65 or older have a disability. An estimated 38% of disabled adults are obese, 28% of disabled adults smoke, 16% have diabetes, and 11.5% have heart disease (CDC, n.d.-e).

There is a compelling and urgent need for nurses and nurse leaders to advocate for proper and compassionate health service for the disabled, aged, LGBTQ+, and ethnic minorities who face discrimination, and it is incumbent upon healthcare systems and nurse leaders to create a workplace environment that fosters diversity and inclusion among frontline nurses and mentors a diverse demographic of future nurse leaders.

INCARCERATION

Overly aggressive policing of minority communities, uneven implementation of the criminal justice system, and massively inequitable incarceration rates are another form of structural discrimination contributing to health disparities in the United States. *The Future of Nursing 2020–2030* report calls mass incarceration "a public health crisis," with disproportionate impact on Black and Hispanic Americans, leading to greater incidence of chronic physical and mental health conditions (Wakefield et al., 2021). Incarcerated and formerly incarcerated individuals face substantially higher rates of both mental and physical problems, including infections and chronic diseases, hypertension and high blood pressure, asthma, arthritis, cervical cancer, and hepatitis (Binswanger et al., 2009; Cloud et al., 2014). Numerous studies have shown that incarcerated individuals also have high rates of tuberculosis, hepatitis C, and HIV/AIDS when compared to the general population (Restum, 2005), and many suffer from mental health problems and health concerns related to prior drug and alcohol abuse: in fact, an estimated 50% of incarcerated individuals have negative health outcomes due to drugs or alcohol; additionally, 16% of men and 31% of women who are incarcerated have serious psychiatric issues, compared with 5% of the general U.S. population (Cloud et al., 2014).

Beginning with the now-discredited federal "war on drugs" in the 1970s and continuing through to the present day, state and federal policies such as the "three strikes" laws, "stop and frisk" practices, "broken windows" policies, mandatory minimum sentences, racial profiling, and Draconian measures such as life without parole are taking a toll on minority populations. New research has found that these hardline policies have exacerbated health disparities among minorities. "Communities of color—particularly Black communities—are overexposed to these policing strategies and, by extension, the health harms they engender" (Esposito et al., 2021). One study found that the risk of being killed by a police officer is one of the leading causes of death for young men of color and reported that one in 1,000 Black men risk being killed by police, compared to the risk of one in 2,500 White males (Edwards et al., 2019).

The impacts of incarceration reach far beyond the prison walls, contributing to a pernicious cycle of broken homes, struggling single parents, and a life of poverty for many children, who in turn suffer negative health outcomes. Having an incarcerated parent has a negative impact on family income, increases a child's risk of being homeless, can have a deleterious effect on children's educational performance, and places children at greater risk of learning disabilities, developmental difficulties, behavioral problems, and attention disorders (Turney, 2014).

CIVIC PARTICIPATION

As previously noted, minority communities suffer from higher rates of discrimination, aggressive policing, and have higher percentages of incarcerated individuals; many minority communities also have higher crime rates, fewer parks and green spaces, and fewer recreational amenities. This can inhibit traditional forms of civic participation, such as voting, volunteerism, church attendance, and community activities, such as sporting and leisure pursuits, community gardening, adult education programs, and library visitation.

A wide variety of documented physical and mental health benefits of civic participation are noted. Voting, for example, allows individuals to have a say in local, state, and national government, which can enhance mental well-being. One international study of 44 countries found that people who voted and engaged in voluntary social activities reported better health than those who did not (S. Kim et al., 2015). Volunteerism provides a direct benefit to the community by weaving a stronger social fabric and creating shared bonds between members of that community. A 2015 study found that middle-aged and older adults who volunteer have lower rates of five common risk factors related to cardiovascular disease and metabolic syndrome (Burr et al., 2015) and a 2016 study found that "consistent civic engagement in old age is associated with lower risk of cognitive impairment" (Infurna et al., 2016).

Belonging to community groups can have benefits similar to volunteerism, promoting activity and social engagement and leading to better mental and physical health.

As the most trusted profession, nurses can play a major and important role in helping to integrate local healthcare establishments into community affairs, thereby minimizing or alleviating some of the inherent distrust among the patient population. Communities also can promote civic participation by starting early and getting children and young adults involved: one study found that adolescents who were involved in community activities were more likely to vote, participate in political campaigns, volunteer, donate blood, and be involved in service organizations as adults (Duke et al., 2009). A 2018 research project found that adolescents who form connections outside the family have a greater propensity for both political and nonpolitical civic engagement later in life (Hemer, 2018).

SOCIAL COHESION

Closely related to civic participation—in fact, sometimes causally linked to it—is the concept of social cohesion. Social cohesion as an SDOH is tied to the concept that the relationships we form with families, friends, neighbors, and even strangers in our communities strongly contribute to our individual and collective health. One of the key components to social cohesion is social capital, which is the "value" that is accrued during positive interactions between various individuals and groups. This value takes many forms, including coordination and cooperation for mutual benefit, perceived fairness and perceived helpfulness between people and organizations, membership in a group and sharing group benefits, and trust between individuals and members of a group. Individuals access their social capital through interconnected relationships, which are often called social networks.

Another aspect of social cohesion is social control, a phrase that is typically used to describe a community's ability to develop mutual trust and exercise control and adherence to informal "norms," such as neighborhood standards for acceptable behavior, satisfactory housekeeping and landscaping, and maintenance of common areas.

The connection between social ties and health contributes to both physical and psychosocial well-being. Individuals with strong social cohesion and social support often self-report more positive health outcomes; some studies have backed up this self-reporting with actual outcomes: a 2014 study found that a higher rate of neighborhood social cohesion is associated with lower rates of myocardial infarction (E. S. Kim et al., 2014). Another study found that high levels of social support corresponded to lower atherosclerosis levels in women who were at high risk for heart disease (Knox et al., 2000, the most recent available). Other studies have found that social support and strong social networks can help alleviate isolation and depression for older people and can help mitigate some of the negative health outcomes of discrimination.

ECONOMIC STABILITY

The "economic stability" category is one of the most far-reaching categories to impact the SDOH. More than one in 10 people—37.2 million, the first increase in poverty after five consecutive annual declines—live in poverty in the United States, according to U.S. Census figures for 2020; this represents the first increase in poverty after five consecutive annual declines (Shrider et al., 2021). People who are mired in poverty often cannot afford many of the essentials that allow them to live a healthy life, including fresh and healthy foods, health insurance and access to preventive healthcare, and adequate and safe housing. Many people struggle to find and keep steady employment that will support themselves and their families. The income chasm in America continues to widen, with the top 20% of the population earning nearly 52%—and the top 5% earning 23%—of the entire nation's income, and the bottom 20% only earning 3.1% of all U.S. income, according to the Census.

This category of SDOH encompasses issues related to poverty, including stress, anxiety, and pressure; access to healthy food; availability of adequate and affordable housing; access to either personal or public transportation; and healthcare. Housing issues include the quality of housing stock, which in many cases may be aging and degraded, or infested with insects, rodents, and other vermin; and housing instability, leading to homelessness. Many of these issues are tied to the lack of employment, or lack of a fair minimum wage that can support the costs of living in America. Poverty and unemployment, or underemployment, also contribute to food insecurity, leading to hunger and inadequate nutrition, especially for children (Table 9.4).

While nurses and nurse leaders cannot be expected to redress the sociological structures relating to these broad-based economic stability issues, they can and should be prepared to deal with the health-related results of these social determinants. Nurses must be prepared, through educational initiatives during schooling and throughout subsequent employment, to identify and address health outcomes related to poverty, food insecurity, and housing instability. New nurses should be encouraged to pursue employment with public hospitals and other safety net healthcare systems to provide services to the most fragile and vulnerable members of America's population.

TABLE 9.4: Economic Stability—Social Determinants of Health

Examples	Negative Health Outcomes
Poverty	
• Lack of education • Unemployment and underemployment • Lack of access to healthy foods • Lack of health insurance/access to preventive care • Lack of access to transportation • Substandard, low-quality housing • Homelessness and food insecurity	• Cardiovascular diseases • Diabetes • COPD and respiratory illnesses • Obesity • Psychological distress • Lower life expectancy/higher mortality
Quality of Housing	
• Aging, degraded, substandard housing stock • Air and water pollution • Hazardous waste and toxic materials • Traffic congestion • Overcrowding • Lack of health resources • Vermin infestations	• Injury and death • Lead poisoning and other toxicities • Poor mental health/behavioral issues • Cardiovascular diseases • Asthma, allergies, and respiratory diseases • Infectious diseases • Cancer
Employment	
• Unemployment • Underemployment • Poverty • Food and housing insecurity • Exposure to toxic substances • Access to health insurance	• Anxiety, depression, and social isolation • Poor mental health/behavioral issues • Cardiovascular diseases • Substance abuse • Suicide
Food Insecurity	
• Hunger • Childhood food insecurity • Access to healthy foods • Access to transportation	• Nutritional problems • Obesity • Cardiovascular diseases • Developmental and behavioral issues • Diabetes • Birth defects/low birth rate • Cognitive difficulties
Housing Instability	
• Homelessness • Lack of affordable housing • Substandard housing • Overcrowding • Frequent moves/lack of social cohesion	• Injury and death • Depression/behavioral issues • Drug and alcohol abuse • Tuberculosis • HIV/AIDS • Diabetes • Lack of access to healthcare • Poor oral health

COPD, chronic obstructive pulmonary disease.

POVERTY

Poverty in America is an intractable tragedy that defies easy solutions. Poverty is more prevalent among minorities, children, and older adults. The poverty rate in 2020 for Blacks was 19.5%; for Hispanics, 17%, and for Asians, 8.1%, compared to the poverty rate for Whites of 8.2%. The poverty rate for children under the age of 18 was 16.1%; and for adults aged 65 and older, 9% (Shrider et al., 2021).

A multitude of studies have identified poverty as a critical public health issue, showing a strong correlation between socioeconomic status and health. People living in poverty tend to suffer from higher rates of illness; chronic diseases including heart disease, stroke, diabetes, hypertension, COPD, and certain types of cancer; higher mortality; and lower life expectancy. One study found that men in the bottom 1% of U.S. income distribution had an expected age of death 14.6 years less than men in the top 1% of income distribution; women in the bottom 1% of income had an average age of death of 10.1 years less than women in the top 1% of income (Chetty et al., 2016).

Many factors contribute to poverty, including education; employment, or lack thereof; marital status; access to resources; and geographic location. Poverty is often correlated with other demographic factors, including race and ethnicity: the wealth of a typical White family registers about eight times more than the wealth of a typical Black family and about five times more than the wealth of a typical Hispanic family (Bhutta et al., 2020). People living in poverty also are less likely to have health insurance and face greater barriers to medical care; low-income workers are less likely to receive health insurance benefits through their employers and many may postpone or eschew medical care due to cost concerns (Khullar & Chokshi, 2018).

Perhaps the cruelest impact of poverty is on children: nearly one in six children lived in poverty in 2018, and nearly 73% of poor children were children of color (Semega et al., 2019). Children living in poverty face greater risks of housing and food insecurity and suffer academically; children living in poverty also lack health insurance, with an estimated 4.3 million children under 19 uninsured in 2018. Poor children also face a greater risk of being abused, neglected, or being placed in foster care, with more than 673,000 children suffering abuse or neglect in 2018, and more than 435,000 children in foster care in 2018. Poor children experience greater rates of juvenile incarceration; and are at greater risk of dying from gun violence, which is the leading cause of death for Black children and teens, and the second leading cause of death for those under age 19 (Children's Defense Fund, 2020). Poor children are more likely to remain poor in adulthood, perpetuating an intergenerational cycle of poverty.

QUALITY OF HOUSING

Poor people are typically crowded into areas laden with substandard, inadequately maintained housing stock and often in areas where there are serious environmental issues, including air and water pollution, hazardous waste, and traffic congestion. Many of these neighborhoods lack resources, such as supermarkets, parks, and playgrounds; have underresourced schools; and often have higher rates of violence and crime. The buildings themselves may be aging and deteriorated, with inadequate insulation, heating, and air conditioning systems, and may be contaminated with toxic building materials, including lead, asbestos, formaldehyde, polychlorinated biphenyls (PCBs), and mercury. Deteriorated housing stock also may be contaminated with mold and mildew, or infested with vermin.

The quality of housing as a social determinant encompasses the physical structure of housing, as well as the overall environment where the housing is located, all of which affect the mental and physical well-being of the residents. A 2016 policy brief by the MacArthur Foundation found that poor housing conditions and overcrowded neighborhoods are linked to poor mental health outcomes, including depression, anxiety, and hostility (Chambers et al., 2016).

Negative physical outcomes from poor quality housing are myriad: lead poisoning in children can cause impaired speech and hearing, decreased verbal ability, decreased learning and memory capability, hyperactivity, attention deficit disorder, and other mental issues. Lead poisoning in adults can cause headaches, tremors, irritability, abdominal pains, myalgia, seizures, paralysis, coma, and death. Asbestos exposure can lead to a compromised respiratory system, wheezing and shortness of breath, mesothelioma, lung cancer, laryngeal cancer, and ovarian cancer. Exposure to insect infestations, rodent droppings, or bird droppings can cause asthma, allergies, plague, murine typhus, leptospirosis, rickettsialpox, salmonella, dysentery, cholera, and many other diseases.

Substandard housing also can cause injury and death due to structural problems and poorly maintained appliances. Carbon monoxide poisoning can cause heart damage, neurological issues, and death. Homes with stairs, narrow doorways and narrow hallways, balconies, and low windows can cause injuries or death from falls, especially for older people and disabled individuals.

EMPLOYMENT

Employment is a cornerstone of economic stability: a steady job at a living wage helps keep families secure and out of poverty. Unfortunately, many people are either unemployed or underemployed, and many more have difficulty finding and keeping a job, leading to poverty, food insecurity, and housing insecurity.

There are many negative health impacts from unemployment, including mental health issues such as stress, anxiety, depression, low self-esteem, substance abuse, and suicide (Dooley et al., 1996; Robert Wood Johnson Foundation, 2013). Studies also have found that people who are unemployed may suffer from higher rates of high blood pressure, heart disease, stroke, and arthritis (Robert Wood Johnson Foundation, 2013).

Additionally, people who are unemployed are less likely to have health insurance. In 2020, employment-based insurance was the most common subtype of health insurance, with 54.4% of people getting coverage through employers; 8.6%, or 28 million people, did not have health insurance in 2020 (Keisler-Starkey & Bunch, 2021).

Although negative health outcomes have been linked to unemployment, employment also can be a source of illness or injury. According to the Bureau of Labor Statistics (BLS; 2021a, 2021b), there were 4,764 fatal work injuries and 2.7 million nonfatal workplace injuries and illnesses in 2020; workers aged 55 and over accounted for 36.2% of workplace fatalities and Hispanic or Latino workers accounted for 22.5% of fatal workplace injuries. Workers also may be exposed to toxic or harmful chemicals such as lead, asbestos, or pesticides, which can have long-term negative health consequences.

FOOD INSECURITY

One appalling consequence of poverty and unemployment is hunger and the closely related concept known as "food insecurity," which the USDA defines as "a household-level economic and social condition of limited or uncertain access to adequate food" (USDA, 2020, "CNSTAT Review and Recommendations"). Hunger is the result of food insecurity and refers to the individual's condition of inadequate food intake to live a normal, active, and healthy life. More than 37 million Americans—or about one in nine—experienced food insecurity in 2018, including more than 11 million children (Coleman-Jensen et al., 2019). The COVID-19 global pandemic exacerbated the problem of food insecurity, with some estimating that more than 45 million people experienced food insecurity in 2020, including 15 million children (Feeding America, 2021a, 2021b).

Food insecurity impacts communities across the United States, including both urban and rural neighborhoods. According to Feeding America, rural communities have higher levels of food insecurity, with an estimated 2.2 million households in rural communities facing hunger; according to a USDA breakdown by county, rural communities represent 63% of U.S. counties but account for 87% of the counties with the highest rates of food insecurity (Coleman-Jensen et al., 2019).

Older Americans, children, Blacks, and Latinos also have higher rates of food insecurity, including an estimated 5.3 million senior citizens; 21.6% of the Black community, including one in four Black children; and one in six Latinos. The problem is especially acute for children because children experiencing food insecurity are more likely to experience developmental impairment in language and motor skills; are more likely to have to repeat a grade in elementary school; and have more reported social and behavioral problems (Feeding America, 2021a).

In rural areas, lack of transportation options and the physical distance to full-line supermarkets contribute to food insecurity, while in urban areas shopping options may be limited to convenience stores, which often offer less variety of healthy food and lower quality foods at higher prices. Food insecurity causes a variety of negative health outcomes in both adults and children, including obesity, diabetes, metabolic syndrome, cardiovascular disease, hypertension, stroke, cancer, hepatitis, asthma, arthritis, COPD, and kidney disease; negative psychological health outcomes include stress and depression (Gregory & Coleman-Jensen, 2017; Holben & Pheley, 2006; Laraia, 2013; Nagata et al., 2019). In adults, households reporting very low food security were 15.3 percentage points more likely to experience any of 10 major chronic illnesses than adults in households reporting high food security (Gregory & Coleman-Jensen, 2017). In children, food insecurity has been associated with birth defects and low birth weight, cognitive difficulties, anemia, aggression and behavioral problems, asthma, and poor oral health (Gundersen & Ziliak, 2015).

HOUSING INSTABILITY

At the most basic level, housing instability encompasses myriad ways in which individuals and families may have difficulty finding and keeping adequate shelter, including not being able to afford housing, spending the bulk of household income on housing, overcrowding, moving frequently, staying with relatives, and being forced to live in subpar segregated neighborhoods due to discrimination. At its most extreme, housing instability leads to homelessness, which affected more than 580,000 people in the United States in 2020 (U.S. Department of Housing and Urban Development [HUD], 2020). The problem is especially acute for single-parent families with children; children represent an estimated one in five homeless people (Children's Defense Fund, 2020).

Studies have found that people who experience homelessness are at increased risk for premature death, mental health issues, and many chronic diseases. One 2007 study of people newly experiencing homelessness in New York City found that 53% had a substance abuse disorder, 35% experienced depression, 17% had hypertension, 17% had asthma, and 6% had diabetes (Schanzer et al., 2007, the most recent study of the newly homeless). Other studies have found that homeless people have higher rates of tuberculosis and HIV/AIDS, and that "nearly one in three homeless deaths were due to causes amenable to timely and effective health care" (Aldridge et al., 2019, "Conclusion").

Housing instability also can take a toll on health outcomes even when it does not result in homelessness. Households that spent more than 30% of income on housing are defined as "cost-burdened"; those that spend more than 50% of income on housing are "severely cost-burdened." According to the Harvard Joint Center for Housing Studies (JCHS), nearly half of all renter households were cost-burdened (JCHS, 2021).

Cost-burdened households are more likely to have trouble keeping up with rent or mortgage payments, leading to eviction or foreclosure; they may move more frequently or experience overcrowding, with multiple families living in the same residence and more than one person per bedroom; they may be forced to live in substandard, poorly maintained, or vermin-infested housing; may be discriminated against due to racial or ethnic characteristics or previous record of incarceration; and may not form lasting connections within a neighborhood, leading to a loss of social cohesion. Children who move frequently and are part of cost-burdened households may suffer academically and may not have access to adequate healthcare.

Discrimination and segregation also contribute to housing instability. A 2021 analysis found that 81% of U.S. metropolitan regions with more than 200,000 residents were more segregated in 2019 than they were in 1990, and that neighborhood poverty rates were three times higher in segregated communities of color (21%) compared to segregated White neighborhoods (7%; Menendian et al., 2021).

EDUCATION ACCESS AND QUALITY

According to the *Healthy People 2030* initiative, education is strongly correlated with health and life expectancy (DHHS, ODPHP, n.d.-b). Conversely, lack of educational opportunities can have negative health effects, beginning in childhood and continuing into adulthood. Children from low-income families, those who live in neighborhoods with underresourced schools, children who do not have access to healthy foods, and those who suffer from food insecurity or housing instability often have substantially shorter life expectancy and are more at risk from chronic diseases including diabetes, circulatory diseases, liver diseases, and mental disorders; people with less than high school education "are 2.4 times as likely as high school graduates and 4.1 times as likely as those with postsecondary education to rate their health as poor" (Hahn & Truman, 2015, p. 7).

This category encompasses numerous concerns relating to education and educational achievement, including language and literacy, which is impacted by immigration status, primary spoken language versus English as a second language, and health literacy, including the accessibility and understandability of health information. Other major issues that fall under the education category include early childhood education and development, encompassing proper nutrition, exercise, and the role of stress in children; the high school graduation rate, which often has been shown to be a determining factor in poverty, unemployment, and future success; and enrollment in higher education, which is negatively impacted by teenage dropout rates and teenage pregnancy (Table 9.5).

TABLE 9.5: Education Access and Quality—Social Determinants of Health

Examples	Negative Health Outcomes
Language and Literacy	
• Speaking and language skills • Reading and writing comprehension • Understanding/working with numbers • Limited English proficiency	• Barrier to accessing health information • Problems following provider instructions • Difficulty following medication instructions • Diabetes • Cancer • Lack of preventive care
Early Childhood Education and Development	
• Proper nutrition • Brain development • Access to healthcare • Preventive care • Education • Physical activity	• Hunger/inadequate nutrition • Developmental delays/behavioral issues • Cognitive impairment • Smoking, drug, and alcohol abuse • Physical abuse • Obesity • Cardiovascular diseases • Diabetes • Lack of access to healthcare

(continued)

TABLE 9.5: Education Access and Quality—Social Determinants of Health (*continued*)

High School Graduation	
• Reading proficiency • Employment • Housing • Access to healthcare	• Unemployment/underemployment • Depression/behavioral issues • Drug and alcohol abuse • Cardiovascular diseases • Teen pregnancy/parenthood • Diabetes • Hepatitis
Enrollment in Higher Education	
• Employment/income • Adult success • Access to healthcare • Longer life expectancy	• Depression/behavioral issues • Drug and alcohol abuse • Shorter life expectancy • Poorer self-reported health • Cardiovascular diseases

One of the earliest opportunities for nursing intervention in education comes from school and public health nurses, who can play an important role in identifying these SDOH in children and help families access programs to alleviate health disparities. *The Future of Nursing 2020–2030* report calls school nurses "frontline health care providers, serving as a bridge between the healthcare and education systems and other sectors," and notes that school and public health nurses can have a huge impact on advancing health equity by helping identify and address food and housing insecurity, poverty, access to healthcare, safety issues, and other factors that impact childhood health (Wakefield et al., 2021). In some cases, school nurses may be the *only* healthcare provider that a child sees, heightening the importance of continuing training and education for this segment of the nursing profession.

LANGUAGE AND LITERACY

On the surface, language and literacy may not seem to be relevant to health outcomes but can be vitally important to helping people understand how to take care of themselves, how to access and follow provider instructions, and, in general, how to live healthier lives. Literacy in this context is different from but related to health literacy, which is categorized as part of the "health and healthcare access and quality" category. Low levels of literacy are associated with lower levels of educational attainment, leading to the associated negative health outcomes.

Immigrants and others who have limited English proficiency may not be able to adequately access, understand, or navigate the complicated healthcare landscape. According to the U.S. Census Bureau 2020 American Community Survey, more than 66 million U.S. residents—or 21.5% of the U.S. population—spoke a language other than English at home, a number which has doubled since 1990 and tripled since 1980 (U.S. Census Bureau, 2020a).

Studies have found that limited English proficiency can be a barrier to accessing proper healthcare, following provider instructions, and understanding health information; this information includes discussions between patients and healthcare providers, consent forms, instructions, proper medication use, health promotional literature, and many other forms of communication, all of which have negative health consequences and lead to more chronic conditions, including diabetes and cancer (Nielsen-Bohlman et al., 2004; Raynor, 2016).

Individuals with limited literacy and limited English proficiency also may have difficulty accessing mental healthcare services, due to the complexity of symptoms. A dearth of interpreter services and lack of cultural competency translate to overall lower quality of patient care.

EARLY CHILDHOOD EDUCATION AND DEVELOPMENT

The first years of a child's life are crucial in terms of brain development, yet far too many children lack proper nutrition, are born into poverty, and face a variety of stressors that have a negative impact on their physical and mental development, including developmental delays that persist into adulthood. These stressors can include food insecurity, housing instability, having one or more parents who are incarcerated, physical abuse, and unsafe neighborhoods with underresourced schools. Exposure to environmental health hazards—such as lead—has both immediate and long-term negative health consequences, including developmental delays, cognitive impairment, and behavioral and mental health issues.

Early child development and education has been shown to have long-range consequences for adult health. The Carolina Abecedarian Project, which tracked individuals from childhood to adulthood, revealed that those children who had access to early childhood healthcare, nutrition, and education had better health in adulthood, including lower rates of obesity, high blood pressure, elevated blood sugar, and high cholesterol, lowering their risk of heart disease (Muennig et al., 2011).

According to the *Healthy People 2030* initiative, "Early childhood programs are a critical outlet for fostering the mental and physical development of young children" (DHHS, ODPHP, n.d.-b), including federally funded programs like Head Start as well as state-based programs such as school breakfast and lunch, and full-day kindergarten. However, the Children's Defense Fund found that in 2018, the Early Head Start program served just 8% of eligible infants and toddlers, and the Head Start program served just 50% of eligible 3- and 4-year-olds. The Children's Defense Fund also asserted that "America's schools have slipped backwards into patterns of deep racial and socioeconomic segregation, perpetuating achievement gaps," including in reading and math, where 74% of low-income, 79% of Black, and 72% of Hispanic fourth and eighth grade public school students did not achieve reading or math proficiency in 2019 (Children's Defense Fund, 2020).

HIGH SCHOOL GRADUATION

Racial, ethnic, and income disparities continue to impact children as they move through the school system, setting up poor and minority students for failure in high school, and subsequent problems finding and maintaining employment in adulthood. The U.S. Census Bureau's American Community Survey for 2020 found that 24.1% of adults who did not graduate high school were living in poverty (U.S. Census Bureau, 2020b).

The Children's Defense Fund revealed that less than 81% of Black, Hispanic, and American Indian/Alaska Native public school students graduated on time during the 2016 to 2017 school year (Children's Defense Fund, 2020). The Save the Children Foundation estimates that the pandemic may cause as many as 1 million students to drop out of high school (Save the Children Foundation, 2021a, 2021b).

High school graduation has profound consequences for future adult employment, earnings, and health outcomes, as a high school diploma is considered a requirement for most jobs in America. According to the BLS (2019), workers without a high school diploma typically earn between 55% and 62% of the earnings of all workers, compared to the earnings of high school graduates, which range between 77% and 85% of the earnings of all workers.

Teen pregnancy and teen parenthood cause many young women to drop out of high school, resulting in adverse health outcomes throughout life. One study found that only 51% of teen mothers earned a high school diploma, versus 89% who did not give birth as teens (Steinka-Fry et al., 2013).

Students who drop out of high school are at risk of poverty, poor adult health, and premature death; many self-report suffering from at least one chronic health condition, including asthma, high blood pressure, heart disease, stroke, diabetes, and hepatitis as compared to high school graduates, indicating that improving the high school graduation rate has the potential to improve community and population health.

ENROLLMENT IN HIGHER EDUCATION

Just as a high school diploma is a strong predictor of future adult success and positive health outcomes, enrollment in higher education can lead to higher lifetime earnings potential and, in turn, contribute to better health and longer life expectancy. According to the BLS (2019), a worker with a bachelor's degree earned more than double what a worker without a high school diploma earned; and a worker with an advanced degree earned more than double what a high school graduate earned.

The term "higher education" encompasses any post-high-school formal educational programs, including advanced certificate programs, 2-year community colleges, 4-year colleges and universities, and graduate and professional programs. A 2018 study revealed that the lack of higher education among poor and minority communities is leading to greater health disparities, noting that "American youth have experienced increasingly unequal educational opportunities that depend on the schools they attend, the neighborhoods in which they live, the color of their skin, and families' financial resources" (Zajacova & Lawrence, 2018, p. 174).

Many underresourced high schools in poor or segregated neighborhoods lack the funding, assets, teachers, and guidance counselors to adequately prepare children for higher education; students from impoverished and minority families may not even be aware of the availability of scholarships and financial aid. Black and Hispanic students have lower college enrollment and college graduate rates than White students. A 2019 report by the American Council on Education found that 40.1% of all associate degrees and 31.5% of bachelor's degrees were earned by people of color (Espinosa et al., 2019).

Enrollment in higher education has been shown to have a positive benefit on self-reported health later in life. An international study published in 2020 found that individuals with higher education enjoyed longer life expectancy; lower levels of mortality, morbidity, and disability; and overall better physical and mental health than individuals with low educational attainment (Raghupathi & Raghupathi, 2020). Conversely, a lack of educational achievement is associated with shorter life expectancy and self-reported poorer health. Other researchers have found that individuals with higher educational attainment were more likely to engage in preventive health measures, such as exercise, avoiding alcohol and illegal drugs, and having regular health screening, leading to lower incidence of diabetes, heart disease, and high blood pressure, as well as fewer mental health issues, including depression and anxiety.

HEALTH AND HEALTHCARE ACCESS AND QUALITY

The United States spent more than $3.6 trillion on national health expenditures in 2018, representing 17.7% of the gross domestic product and $11,172 per capita (NCHS, 2019). This is about double what other developed nations spend—on average, other wealthy countries spend $5,697 per capita (Kamal et al., 2020). And yet, in spite of this outsized spending, average life expectancy dropped to 40th among developed nations in 2015 and is expected to drop to 43rd by 2060 (Medina et al., 2020). Why? The answer may be due to the issues raised in the "health and healthcare access and quality" category of SDOH.

According to the *Healthy People 2030* initiative, many Americans don't get the healthcare they need due to a combination of factors, including a lack of health insurance; the high cost of healthcare and medications; a lack of access to healthcare services due to location or inadequacy of transportation; a shortage in the numbers, availability, and access to primary care physicians (PCPs) and other healthcare professionals; distrust of the healthcare system; and

TABLE 9.6: Health and Healthcare Access and Quality—Social Determinants of Health

Examples	Negative Health Outcomes
Access to Healthcare	
• Health insurance • Cost of doctor visits, medications, equipment, tests • Transportation barriers • Lack of healthcare facilities • Shortages of physicians, providers	• Lack of preventive care • Cardiovascular disease • Diabetes • Cancer • Childhood immunizations • Dental care
Access to Primary Care	
• Preventive care • Health information • Screenings • Immunizations • Health insurance • Management of chronic conditions • Transportation • Cost • Lack of providers	• Cardiovascular disease • Diabetes • Asthma and respiratory illnesses • Lack of screenings • Lack of immunizations
Health Literacy	
• Access to health information • Reading and understanding health information • Comprehension of health information • Recognize/understand common medical conditions • Management of chronic conditions	• Poor compliance with provider instructions • Problems with medication management • Cardiovascular diseases • Diabetes • Lack of preventive healthcare • Lack of immunizations • Lower life expectancy

poor communication about the need for, importance of, and connection between preventive care and better health (Table 9.6). These factors are exacerbated by other SDOH, including discrimination, environmental and housing conditions, poverty, language and literacy, education, and other interrelated circumstances (DHHS, ODPHP, n.d.-b).

Massive income, racial, ethnic, and social disparities exist in the U.S. healthcare system, preventing a large swath of the population from getting necessary, timely, high-quality, and compassionate care. For instance, the 2019 National Healthcare Quality and Disparities Report by the Agency for Healthcare Research and Quality (AHRQ) found that Blacks, American Indians, and Alaska natives received worse care than Whites for 40% of quality measures; Hispanics and Native Hawaiians/Pacific Islanders received worse care than Whites for more than one-third of quality measures. Racial disparities were further illuminated by the COVID-19 pandemic, with disproportionately high numbers of Blacks and Hispanics across the country being struck down by the disease.

The "health and healthcare access and quality" category comprises issues related to access to healthcare, such as location, transportation, hospital and clinic availability and closures, and language barriers. A separate but connected grouping involves access to primary care, again addressing transportation issues, which can be especially applicable in rural areas and for older adults and disabled individuals, as well as a national shortfall in the number of physicians and other healthcare providers. Health literacy also comes into play in this category, including establishing trust, providing patient education, and developing better communication strategies. Finally, although not technically part of the DHHS definition of SDOH, we examine the impact of the COVID-19 pandemic, including racial disparities in cases, hospitalizations and deaths, racial disparities in the definition of essential workers, and the racial disparities in vaccine hesitancy and vaccine access.

Nurses play an indispensable and growing role in addressing the issues in the health-care category, and are requisite participants in any effort to alleviate health inequities in the United States. The *Future of Nursing* report noted, "The nation cannot achieve true health equity without nurses, which means it must do better for nurses" (Wakefield et al., 2021, pp. x–xi). Innovations in nursing modalities, including increasing the focus on screening for SDOH and forming collaborative partnerships within the practice setting as well as in the community, is a necessary evolution in the role of nurses in society, and a key component to eliminating or reducing health disparities.

ACCESS TO HEALTHCARE

Barriers preventing access to healthcare may prevent many people from getting the preven-tion and treatment they need to live longer, healthier lives. One of the biggest barriers is not having health insurance: in spite of the gains made since the passage of the ACA, some 28 million people in the United States did not have health insurance in 2020 (Keisler-Starkey & Bunch, 2021).

The high cost of doctor visits, medications, equipment, and screening tests and other pro-cedures may cause many people to postpone or forego necessary healthcare. Even people who do have health insurance may find out-of-pocket costs to be prohibitive: according to a 2018 study, medical debt from chronic or adverse health conditions can push families into bankruptcy or cause them to do without necessities such as food, heat, or rent (Richard et al., 2018). People without health insurance, or those with inadequate health insurance, are less likely to have preventive care and health screenings, and therefore are at higher risk of cardiovascular disease, diabetes, and cancer; children without health insurance are less likely to receive well-child visits, dental care, and immunizations.

Lack of health insurance is not the only barrier to care. A major problem, especially for rural communities, older adults, and disabled people is inconvenient, unreliable, or erratic transportation alternatives. A 2018 study found that transportation barriers can cause pa-tients to postpone care, miss or frequently reschedule appointments, and delay or skip med-ications; these problems were particularly acute for vulnerable, low-income populations and contribute to poorer management of chronic diseases (Syed et al., 2013).

Another barrier to healthcare access is a lack of healthcare facilities and shortages of phy-sicians and other providers. The U.S. Government Accountability Office (GAO) found that more than 100 rural hospitals closed from January 2013 to February 2020, increasing the median distance for patients to travel to access general inpatient services by more than 20 miles—from 3.4 miles in 2012 to 23.9 miles (GAO, 2021).

Language difficulties and limited English proficiency, as detailed in the "Education Access and Quality" section of this chapter, also are barriers to care. Studies have found that speaking a language other than English at home can prevent individuals from accessing primary care and health screening programs. For instance, a study of women whose primary language was Spanish, Cantonese, or Japanese found that they were less likely to be screened for cervical cancer or breast cancer (Jacobs et al., 2005). A subsequent study found that Chinese Americans with limited English proficiency and limited health literacy were less likely to have requisite health screenings for colorectal and breast cancer, despite the fact that cancer is the leading cause of death among Asian Americans (Sentell et al., 2015). Similarly, a 2021 study found significant disparities in clinical trial screening and engagement, use of genetic counseling, and communication via electronic patient portals in breast cancer screenings between in-dividuals with limited English proficiency compared to English-speaking patients; native Spanish speakers were the least likely to engage in an electronic patient portal among all non-native English-speaking subgroups (Roy et al., 2021). Language barriers and limited English proficiency often prevent patients from understanding and following provider instructions, following guidelines for proper medication use, and understanding other forms of health information, all of which may contribute to poor health outcomes.

ACCESS TO PRIMARY CARE

A lack of or inadequate access to primary care can also be a significant barrier to proper healthcare, due to the fact that primary care is the main source of health information and preventive health services such as blood pressure screenings, cancer screenings, flu shots, and other immunizations, as well as early detection and treatment of disease and management of chronic health conditions such as cardiovascular disease, diabetes, and asthma.

There are a variety of barriers to primary care access, including a lack of or inadequate health insurance; cost of physician visits, screenings, and medications; location and transportation difficulties; language-related barriers; and limited provider hours.

Additionally, numerous reports have cited a shortage of PCPs in the United States. The Health Resources and Services Administration (n.d., 2022) notes that some 96 million people live in Health Professional Shortage Areas (HPSA) for primary care, and 154 million people live in HPSAs for mental health; as of June 2022, approximately 65.49% of primary care HPSAs were located in rural areas. In addition to shortages of PCPs, the United States can expect a shortage of nurses: a 2015 study predicted that more than 1 million registered nurses will retire before 2030, leading to shortages in most regions of the country, but particularly in rural communities (Auerbach et al., 2015).

Vulnerable populations such as older adults and individuals with disabilities have need of regular health screenings and management of chronic conditions yet may have significant obstacles to seeing a PCP. The CDC notes that one in three adults with disabilities aged 18 to 44 years do not have a usual healthcare provider; furthermore, one in four adults with disabilities aged 45 to 64 years old did not have a routine checkup in the past year; yet people with disabilities are more likely to smoke, be obese, have heart disease, and have diabetes than nondisabled individuals (CDC, n.d.-e).

Creative approaches, including implementing telehealth and artificial intelligence and utilizing more nurse practitioners, physician assistants, and other clinicians could be a solution, with some researchers suggesting this could be equivalent to adding 44,000 new PCPs (Kerns & Willis, 2020). However, physician and nursing shortages are likely to be a problem for the foreseeable future: The 2019 National Healthcare Quality and Disparities Report notes that, "[h]ealthcare access and quality can be affected by workforce shortages, which can be an issue especially in rural areas" (AHRQ, 2020, p. O8). Improving access to primary care is therefore of critical importance to reducing health disparities and improving overall population health.

HEALTH LITERACY

Health literacy is a separate issue from language and literacy, which is categorized under the "Education Access and Quality" category. It is nonetheless an important issue to consider. Health literacy is defined by the DHHS as being able to "obtain, process and understand basic health information needed to make appropriate health decisions" (DHHS, ODPHP, 2010, p. iii). The agency estimates that nearly nine out of 10 adults have difficulty using everyday health information (DHHS, ODPHP, 2010).

Examples of health literacy include being able to read and understand preventive health information, provider instructions, medication labels, consent forms, and other materials. Much of today's current medical and healthcare information requires some degree of both print literacy, including the ability to read, write, and comprehend written material; and oral literacy, including speaking and listening skills. Low levels of literacy are associated with negative health outcomes; to complicate matters further, even individuals with high overall literacy can have low health literacy; especially as healthcare information becomes ever more complex and complicated.

A 2018 study found an estimated 80 million Americans have limited health literacy (Prince et al., 2018). This means that millions of Americans may not recognize the signs and symptoms of common medical conditions, such as heart disease or stroke; they may not know about, understand, or manage their medical conditions, such as high blood pressure and diabetes; they may not understand how or when to take their medications properly, or use medical devices correctly, such as asthma inhalers. Another 2018 study suggests that older adults, men, racial and ethnic minorities, and people of low socioeconomic status have the lowest levels of health literacy among all population subgroups, leading to higher morbidity and mortality (Hickey et al., 2018). Patients with lower health literacy also may seek care in the ED more frequently and be more likely to be hospitalized; children whose parents have low health literacy may not receive preventive care, immunizations, or well-child screenings.

Healthcare providers and systems can address health literacy and establish greater trust by embracing patient-centered care models, avoiding medical jargon, and developing better communication strategies.

One 2018 study recommends that patient education be tailored specifically to each patient's needs, limiting the focus of a visit to three key points, and providing printed material written at or below a sixth-grade reading level (Wittink & Oosterhaven, 2018). Other options include asking open-ended questions and asking patients to repeat information and instructions in their own words, to assess their level of understanding.

COVID-19 AND COVID-19 VACCINE HESITANCY

The devastating COVID-19 global pandemic revealed the cavernous fissures fracturing American society, as communities of color were devastated by the disease. The toll on Black and Hispanic populations brought into sharp relief the horrific health disparities plaguing American society. According to the CDC, racial and ethnic minorities are disproportionately represented among COVID-19 cases; Blacks and Hispanics of all age groups were hospitalized with COVID-19 at a rate 2.3 and 2.2 times higher than the White population, respectively. Hispanics were 1.8 times more likely to die of COVID-19, Blacks were 1.7 times more likely to die, and American Indian or Alaska Native, non-Hispanic people were 2.1 times more likely to die as Whites (CDC, 2022).

The pandemic also disproportionately affected dense urban neighborhoods, rural communities with lack of access to healthcare, and essential workers in frontline jobs, including nurses and other healthcare personnel. Undocumented immigrants and immigrants held in detention centers as well as incarcerated individuals also suffered higher rates of COVID-19 cases, hospitalizations, and deaths. The crisis exacted a huge toll on employment and income in communities of color, with higher rates of pandemic-related job losses among Blacks and Hispanics. Poor and minority children also were unduly impacted by the situation: Save the Children reported that the poorest families were 15 times more likely to struggle with hunger, four times more likely to lack internet access for remote education, and nine times more likely to have difficulty paying bills as wealthier families during the pandemic (Save the Children Foundation, 2021a, 2021b).

COVID-19 also exposed the disparities inherent in the workplace, where nurses and other healthcare practitioners struggled to secure enough personal protective equipment (PPE). Approximately 50 million U.S. workers—or 34.5% of all workers—are classified as frontline and essential workers, working in fields such as healthcare, transportation, emergency services, and certain retail establishments, including grocery stores and pharmacies. A 2021 health policy brief pointed out that "[w]omen, people of color, and those of lower socioeconomic status are the most likely among all workers to hold frontline positions that require in-person work and the least likely to have paid sick leave. These groups have disproportionately experienced the negative health and economic consequences of COVID-19" (Wolfe et al., 2021, Key point #3).

The COVID-19 vaccination program also revealed cultural, racial, ethnic, and age disparities in terms of access and vaccine hesitancy. Initially, Blacks and Hispanics were among the population segments most likely to report vaccine hesitancy, and minority communities were the most likely to report difficulties in accessing COVID-19 vaccines. Many thought leaders attributed this vaccine hesitancy to a legacy of medical experimentation, medical injustices, and fear of an unknown, rapidly developed vaccine; many cited the now infamous and unethical "Tuskegee Study of Untreated Syphilis in the Negro Male" as a reason for vaccine hesitancy among Black Americans. By March of 2021, however, a survey by the Kaiser Family Foundation showed that Black adults who had either received a COVID-19 vaccine shot or wanted one as soon as possible rose to 55%, up from 41% in February. By May of 2021, vaccine hesitancy had shifted, to being less about race or ethnicity, and more about political affiliation and age. An analysis of polling by the Kaiser Family Foundation by *The New York Times* found that 29% of Republicans said they definitely would not get a COVID-19 vaccine, or only if required, compared to 8% of Democrats; the same analysis showed that 20% of Blacks, 19% of Whites, and 16% of Hispanics definitely would not get a COVID-19 vaccine, or only if required (Leonhardt, 2021).

The COVID-19 crisis clearly illustrated the vital role that nurses play in disaster response and emergency preparedness . . . and also illuminated many challenges for the future. *The Future of Nursing* report pointed out that future disasters, infectious disease outbreaks, and other public health emergencies will most likely create significant burdens for the nursing profession and have a major impact on individual, community, and population health (Wakefield et al., 2021). However, the report stated that the nursing profession is woefully unprepared to meet these challenges, calling for "a bold and expansive effort, executed across multiple platforms," including nursing education, practice policy, and research.

◼ WHAT EVERY NURSE MANAGER NEEDS TO KNOW ABOUT POPULATION HEALTH

Nurse managers have a unique opportunity to witness the impact of SDOH of patients firsthand in clinical settings. Nurse managers need to understand the respective elements of SDOH resulting in hospital readmissions and the impact on discharge plans. Nurse managers can assess the underlying factors contributing to hospital admissions, medication, and chronic disease management. Nurse managers can influence the care patients receive by advocating for resources, ensuring adequate patient education, and assisting with health literacy (Carlson et al., 2016).

Nurse managers are able to educate frontline staff of the importance of gaining comprehensive knowledge of their patients' social status, where patients live, whether they have access to food, and the social support available to ensure success in their communities (National Advisory Council on Nurse Education and Practice, 2019).

WHAT EVERY NURSE MANAGER NEEDS TO KNOW

- Nurse managers need to know the elements of SDOH impacting patients in their settings.
- Nurse managers can have an impact on discharge plans by collaborating with members of the team and training frontline nurses to advocate for resources within the patient's community.
- SDOH can impact the lives of patients in a significant manner overriding the care provided in the clinical setting.
- Addressing SDOH is critical to ensuring population health.

◻ WHAT EVERY NURSE EXECUTIVE NEEDS TO KNOW ABOUT POPULATION HEALTH

Nurse executives can create the systems that can help hospitals and healthcare organizations address SDOH, thereby creating opportunities to improve population health through community-based initiatives (Sullivan, 2019). Nurse executives can ensure nurse leaders and nurses participate in forums to address SDOH by establishing the infrastructure to learn and recommend resources. Nurse executives also play a key role in assessing and applying for grants to assist organizations in addressing the SDOH; many international, national, and state philanthropic institutions—including the Robert Wood Johnson Foundation, Rose Community Foundation, Humana Foundation, Kresge Foundation, Michael and Susan Dell Foundation, Conrad N. Hilton Foundation, New York Community Trust, and General Mills Foundation, among others—offer grants specifically tailored to address SDOH, such as food insecurity and housing instability (Health Affairs, 2019).

As senior members of executive teams, nurse executives can advocate for health systems to take a risk to care for disadvantaged (i.e., uninsured, undomiciled, and foster care) patients. Nurse executives have the financial acumen to address the impact on caring for the underserved and the impact it has financially on organizations, as well as how current and future methods of paying providers can incentivize addressing the SDOH as part of an overall healthcare delivery strategy (NASEM, 2019). Nurse executives can provide insight on the impact of not caring for these patients by assessing the financial ramifications on hospital readmissions, which have been shown to lead to decreased profitability over time (Upadhyay et al., 2019). A 2020 report by the Centers for Medicare & Medicaid Services (CMS) states that hospital readmissions account for billions of dollars in annual Medicare spending and notes that hospital readmissions often are considered a key indicator of quality of care, with significant impact on overall health outcomes. The report also reveals that vulnerable populations face an increased risk of hospital readmissions, known as "readmission disparity," pointing out that racial and ethnic minorities account for a disproportionate percentage of hospital readmissions (CMS Office of Minority Health, 2020).

WHAT EVERY NURSE EXECUTIVE NEEDS TO KNOW

- The nurse executive should create systems to ensure frontline staff are learning about SDOH.

- The nurse executive can demonstrate the need to care for patients impacted by SDOH.

- Financial acumen of hospital readmissions and risk of not caring for patients impacted by SDOH can be shared to other executives of the team by nurse executives.

⬡ CASE SCENARIO

EVALUATION OF HEAD TRAUMA

SITUATION

DR is a 56-year-old patient admitted via ambulance to a 120-bed community care hospital. DR was brought in by ambulance for evaluation of head trauma due to a fall in a local subway station. Upon evaluation, DR is transferred to the neurological intensive care unit for evacuation of a subdural hematoma. The RN in charge of the night shift, NJ, assigns DR to a second-year nurse,

SJ. Nurse SJ takes DR to CT scan upon arrival to the unit. Post-CT scan, Nurse SJ gets DR settled and begins administering a presurgical checklist for a planned procedure in the morning. Nurse SJ gives report to the operating room (OR) and prepares for handoff to the day nurse, MW. Day Nurse MW attempts to complete the 24-hour admission note post-procedure. DR is responsive and expresses they have been undomiciled for the past 10 years due to alcohol dependency; DR is unemployed and has no insurance.

During interdisciplinary rounds, Nurse MW expresses the need for housing, treatment, and insurance for DR. Medical Resident Dr. JM reads the patient's past medical notes and mentions during interdisciplinary rounds that DR is known to the hospital and frequently visits the ED. Social Worker RT mentions the need to ensure a safe discharge plan to prevent readmission.

APPROACH

Interdisciplinary rounds act as a forum that allows members of the team to discuss critical aspects of patient care. Communication allowed during interdisciplinary rounds is instrumental to learning best practice for various members of the team. Interdisciplinary teams can have a fundamental impact on safe, effective, and efficient patient care, and many healthcare organizations are formalizing the team approach to enhance care management, including adding care coordinators or care navigators to facilitate the process (Mosher et al., 2014).

In this scenario, all members of the team are instrumental in facilitating discharge planning at the interdisciplinary rounds. The medical team can focus on health progression by ensuring surgical healing and addressing alcohol abuse and physical therapy. Nurses during rounds can provide insight on patient concerns regarding discharge. Case management and social workers can provide context to determine the resources required and means to ensure a safe discharge. Patient involvement in interdisciplinary rounds is an opportunity to ensure the patients are aware of discharge plans.

OUTCOME

DISCHARGE PLANNING

A lack of interdisciplinary collaboration and inadequate communication can have adverse consequences for patients, including increased length of stay, medical errors, hospital-acquired infections, post-discharge adverse medication episodes, and readmission (Ryan et al., 2017).

A report from the AHRQ found that nearly 20% of patients experience an undesirable outcome within 30 days of discharge and noted that an estimated three-quarters of these adverse events could have been prevented or ameliorated (AHRQ, n.d.).

To assist healthcare systems with discharge planning, the AHRQ developed the IDEAL tool for teams to use during the process. The main components are:

(I) Include the patient and family as full partners in the process.

(D) Discuss five key areas to prevent post-discharge problems:

1.   What life at home will be like
2.   Medication review
3.   Warning signs and problems
4.   Review and explain test results
5.   Make follow-up appointments

(E) Educate the patient and family about the condition and steps to follow.

(A) Assess and use teach-back techniques to determine how well doctors and nurses explain the diagnosis, condition, and next steps in the patient's care to the patient and family.

(L) Listen to and honor the patient's and family's goals, preferences, observations, and concerns.

Discharge planning beginning at the patient's admission allows for appropriate preparation for a safe discharge. Physicians, nurses, physical and occupational therapists, social workers, and case managers all contribute their respective patient knowledge and expertise to ensure patients are discharged appropriately. Communication with members of the team, including the patient and family members, is key to minimize readmissions. The creation of a discharge checklist can ensure factors such as transportation, patient belongings, insurance, and post-discharge placement are all addressed prior to discharge and bottlenecks are prevented.

DISCUSSION QUESTIONS

1. Upon arrival to the ED, what are some potential resources to consider due to SDOH?
2. What discharge planning resources should be considered during admission?
3. What aspects of the plan of care should be considered for DR?

◆ CASE SCENARIO

REDUCING AVOIDABLE EMERGENCY VISITS

SITUATION

Hospital K is a 400-bed trauma level one academic medical center providing care to the community for more than 30 years. The level of ED visits has led administrators to investigate other mechanisms to ensure appropriate utilization of the ED. Hospital K has decided to open up an express care clinic to provide patients the mechanism of receiving care expeditiously.

PB, a 73-year-old patient, has recently been admitted due to fainting at home. PB admits to avoiding the ED because of fear of contracting COVID-19 during the global pandemic. Upon arrival, Dr. RJ assesses PB's neurological, urinary, and endocrine systems. PB reports taking water pills without appropriate follow-up care and experiencing periods of confusion and abdomen pain. Dr. RJ plans to admit PB with a diagnosis of acute kidney failure.

APPROACH

COVID-19 led to patients becoming ill at home and not seeking medical help. A study by the CDC comparing March 31 to April 27, 2019, prior to the pandemic, to the similar 4-week period March 29 to April 25, 2020, during the early phase of the pandemic, found that U.S. ED visits were 42% lower in 2020, indicating that some people were delaying care for potentially serious conditions, including nonspecific chest pain and acute myocardial infarction (Hartnett et al., 2020).

As COVID-19 numbers decline across the country, health systems saw the number of patients visiting the ED trend resume to pre-COVID numbers. An August 2021 survey by global management consulting firm McKinsey & Company reported that ED and inpatient volumes had returned to 2019 levels and projected that volumes would rise 5% to 6% higher in 2022 (Berlin et al., 2021). Minority patients across the country tend to visit EDs versus going to see a PCP. Studies have found that the use of EDs is particularly high among Black and Hispanic patients and women, as well as Medicare and Medicaid beneficiaries (Hanchate et al., 2019; Marcozzi et al., 2018). The increase of ambulatory clinics has emerged as a result of patients needing access to reduce ED utilization.

Patient education regarding the mechanisms to access care is integral to improving SDOH. Because there are myriad socioeconomic and racial disparities that create barriers to healthcare access, vulnerable populations often turn to EDs for non-emergency care (Marcozzi et al., 2018). Educational efforts focused on these vulnerable populations can help patients understand that there are other avenues to attain the care they need in a timely fashion, without having to resort to EDs. The American Academy of Family Physicians (AAFP) recommends a team-based approach to addressing the SDOH, urging physicians and medical practices to ask patients about their circumstances, identify resources within their communities to assist them, and act to connect patients with those resources, thereby helping to educate patients about their options (AAFP, 2018).

The establishment of ambulatory clinics necessitates the need to educate patients about the mechanisms by which they can obtain care. A comprehensive marketing plan is necessary to ensure patients understand the new service and methods to begin receiving care.

INTERPRETATION

A March 2021 report to Congress by the Office of the Assistant Secretary for Planning and Evaluation, DHHS, found that there are many issues surrounding the perceived overuse or inappropriate use of EDs, including a lack of understanding on the part of patients about what constitutes an actual emergency, a lack of access or long wait times for PCPs or other alternative avenues for care, and a lack of insurance coverage and concerns about ability to pay (DHHS, 2021). The same report pointed out that over-utilization of EDs creates many challenges for the U.S. healthcare system, including the significantly higher cost for emergency care as compared to ambulatory or other care settings, as well as other factors, such as over-crowding, long wait times, a lack of continuity of care, and a deficit in preventive care services, all of which can lead to higher patient mortality (DHHS, 2021). It is therefore incumbent upon healthcare providers to study and understand the factors driving patient usage of EDs and develop plans to educate and inform those patients about care alternatives.

ACCESS TO CARE

The SDOH have major implications on patients' access to care and preventive screenings, which can be especially troubling when it comes to serious illnesses such as cardiovascular disease, respiratory disease, and cancer, where lack of preventive and follow-up care can lead to significantly higher mortality rates. Despite this fact, many healthcare organizations are not addressing SDOH in their patient assessment process. A 2021 study from researchers at New York-Presbyterian and Weill Cornell Medicine pointed out that only 15.6% of U.S. physician practices and 24.4% of U.S. hospital systems screen patients for multiple SDOH, including food insecurity, housing instability, utility needs, transportation needs, and interpersonal violence; the study reported that the top barriers in access to care reported by cancer patients were economic instability, education and low health literacy, and community and social context, including bias, stigma, and cultural misconceptions (Jou et al., 2021).

OUTCOME

Stakeholders should work to determine a business plan and communication plan. The business plan should include assessment of ED utilization and readmissions. The communication plan should focus on internal and external success.

DISCUSSION QUESTIONS

1. What activities and considerations would you include in communicating new primary care clinics at your organization to the community?
2. What factors should leadership take into account to determine whether express care clinics can be beneficial for their patient population?
3. What are some key elements to be used by the patient upon discharge?

KEY POINTS

- Nurses and nurse leaders are essential to achieving broad population and community health goals. The history of the nursing profession is based on a commitment to community health and wellness, as well as actions and advocacy to promote social justice and alleviate health disparities.

- It is vitally important for nurses and nurse leaders to understand and address the SDOH when implementing evidence-based professional practice, as well as providing quality and compassionate patient care.

- Decades of research has shown that economic, environmental, educational, community and social context, and healthcare conditions are the primary drivers of disease and health for individuals, communities, and the human population as a whole.

- The SDOH are organized into five key areas: neighborhood and built environment, social and community context, economic stability, education access and quality, and health and healthcare access and quality. Each of these categories presents a unique set of situations and circumstances that can affect individual, community, and population health, reflecting the key issues and problems that can contribute to diseases, chronic illnesses, infections, maternal mortality and morbidity, situational emergencies and accidents, and domestic violence.

- Nurses and nurse leaders are a critical link in the chain connecting healthcare organizations and the patient populations they serve. As the most trusted profession, nurses are uniquely positioned to address the SDOH and thereby help promote health equity and enhance overall community and population health.

SUMMARY

Nurses occupy a unique role within the healthcare landscape, spending more time with patients than any other healthcare professionals. A 2018 study of patient care times using motion and location sensors found that nurses accounted for more than 86% of patient care times, compared to 9.9% of physicians and 8.14% of critical support staff such as respiratory therapists and pharmacists (Butler et al., 2018). It is therefore incumbent upon nurses and nurse leaders to be fully conversant with the concepts of population health, community health, and the SDOH in order to effectively and competently treat their individual patients and contribute constructively to the health of the community and overall population health.

Nurses are exceptionally well-positioned to use their expertise and judgment to advocate for patient-centered care policies to positively impact the larger healthcare ecosystem. Today and in the future, nurses and nurse leaders must be knowledgeable and practiced in the art of gathering and interpreting both individual patient and overall community healthcare trends and information. Additionally, nurses need to use their clinical skills and practical experience to analyze and utilize this data to help promote continuity of care, health screenings, and wellness and disease prevention programs within the community, thereby positively impacting overall population health.

Nurse managers and nurse executives have an even greater responsibility to raise their voices and advocate for policies that empower frontline nurses and thereby shape the way healthcare systems approach individual, community, and population health. Nurse leaders formulate organizational policies that facilitate and inspire collaboration, communication, mentorship programs, shared governance, interprofessional teamwork, quality management, and continuous care improvements using evidence-based professional practice models. Nurses and nurse leaders are indispensable to improving, outlining, and creating new policies to ensure that healthcare systems achieve the mission of providing culturally competent, responsive, high-quality patient care.

In the final analysis, nurses need to be better prepared, in both education and clinical practice settings, to identify, address, and mitigate the impact of the SDOH in order to alleviate health disparities, achieve better health equity, and collectively impact the health of individuals, communities, and the overall population. Nurses are the engine propelling population health progress forward into the future.

END-OF-CHAPTER RESOURCES

● DISCUSSION QUESTIONS

1. What are the primary SDOH, and how do these factors impact individual, community, and population health?
2. What role do nurses and nurse leaders play in addressing the SDOH? Why are nurses and nurse leaders ideally suited to this role?
3. How important are nursing advocacy, community action, and policy campaigns in addressing the SDOH? How can nurses and nurse leaders promote better population and community health through these activities?

● ADDITIONAL RESOURCES

- *Healthy People 2030* Launch—August 18, 2020, U.S. Department of Health and Human Services (DHHS): https://www.youtube.com/watch?v=atDcD86ChC8

  This decade, *Healthy People 2030* continues its focus on health data, SDOH, and health equity with a new set of 355 measurable health objectives with 10-year targets.

- Dr. Koh Presents at *Healthy People 2020* Launch—July 17, 2012, Office of Disease Prevention and Health Promotion (ODPHP): https://www.youtube.com/watch?v=qAx8nyaeT9g

  Dr. Howard Koh, assistant secretary for health, discusses the *Healthy People 2020* initiative and how it hopes to improve the health of all Americans in the next decade. *Healthy People* provides science-based, 10-year national objectives for improving the health of all Americans.

- *Healthy People 2020*: Determinants of Health (ODPHP)—February 8, 2012, IQ Solutions: https://www.youtube.com/watch?v=5Yb3B75eqbo

- Creating a Better Normal: Improving Population Health for Everyone—October 15, 2020, University of Washington: https://www.youtube.com/watch?v=6Vv8I9Naw3g

  The pandemic has highlighted the racial, social, and economic inequities that shape the health and well-being of all people in the United States and throughout the world. As we look forward to a post-COVID-19 world, how can we create a future in which we are all healthier—as individuals and entire populations? How do we enhance the resilience of the environment we rely on? And how do we address the factors perpetuating the inequities that harm so many? Join the University of Washington for a discussion with leaders who are envisioning how we will improve population health for everyone. Featuring panelists Cecilia Bitz, Renee Cheng, Pamela Collins, Julio Frenk, and Toni Hoover, it is moderated by Hanson Hosein.

- Population Health Management: Improving Health Where We Live, Work, and Play—June 29, 2015, Centers for Disease Control and Prevention (CDC): https://www.youtube.com/watch?v=1sJDit8zsPI

  Healthcare costs continue to soar, taking large portions of business, government, and consumer budgets. While costs are rising, health and well-being are declining. Dr. Ron Loeppke and Dr. Jeanette May help participants recognize the social, economic, and physical factors that contribute to health and learn how employers and communities can work together to control healthcare spending and improve health using a population health management approach.

■ What Is Population Health?—August 24, 2018, Mount Sinai Health System: https://www.youtube.com/watch?v=f9JbT0eK81g

Learn more about population health by following our patient Joe on his healthcare journey in our "What Is Population Health?" video. Joe's experience should feel familiar as he faces the same barriers many patients encounter in New York City and across the United States. This video tells the story of Joe's experience in the current healthcare system and provides insight into how a population health approach can improve his experience and outcomes. This video is meant to support staff in the transition to population health and value-based payments.

■ Population Health: Crash Course Sociology #43—February 5, 2018, Crash Course: https://www.youtube.com/watch?v=D9SWRByzDSo

We are continuing our unit on health with a discussion of some of the indicators that help us measure health for different populations. We will also explore three contributors to health disparities: individual factors like genetics, physical factors like pollution, and social factors like stress.

■ Understanding Public Health as Community Health—October 15, 2018, Littlefield Lecture Series, School of Nursing, University of Wisconsin–Madison: https://www.youtube.com/watch?v=KYZ9qP8m0X8

Deputy Surgeon General Rear Admiral Sylvia Trent-Adams, PhD, RN, FAAN, challenges us to shift our thinking and our reality to move from a healthcare system to a system of health for all. As deputy surgeon general, RADM Trent-Adams advises and supports the surgeon general in communicating the best available scientific information to advance the health of the nation. Throughout her career, RADM Trent-Adams has worked to improve access to care for poor and underserved communities. She spent over 25 years working within the federal government, including 3 years as chief nursing officer for the U.S. Public Health Service Commissioned Corps.

■ Community Health, Population Health and Public Health: Understanding the Differences—May 12, 2017, Renown Health: https://www.youtube.com/watch?v=_ag3g_iHzuM

Many people use the terms "population health," "public health," and "community health" interchangeably, even though these words speak to unique concepts. Dr. Anthony Slonim, CEO and president of Renown Health, describes the differences between these three important healthcare concepts.

■ Social Determinants of Health: Claire Pomeroy at TEDxUCDavis—July 12, 2012: https://www.youtube.com/watch?v=qykD-2AXKIU

Claire Pomeroy is the president and chief executive officer of the Albert and Mary Lasker Foundation. She is a professor emeritus at the University of California Davis. During her academic career, her research focused on HIV/AIDS.

■ Taking Health Care to the Streets: Dr. Cheryl Whitaker at TEDxNashvilleSalon—December 4, 2017: https://www.youtube.com/watch?v=cfNPHQRvBb4

Healthcare in underserved communities has poor results due to lack of access and engagement. To succeed, it is necessary to innovate. What works? Borrowing a page from the community organizer's playbook and hitting the streets, the answer is using care consultants who are from the community. They understand the conditions and the lifestyles that pertain to their community's residents and are armed with mobile technology and know-how that can make a difference. How do you assess a patient's neighborhood? None of the 81 measures health plans use to measure performance do, yet studies show that social determinants are up to 50% of what impacts health, and the care patients receive. Cheryl Whitaker, MD, co-founded NextLevel Health (NLH) in 2014 because government-funded healthcare programs often fail to reach their intended beneficiaries. This innovative for-profit health insurance company helps the underserved access and manage Medicaid services by borrowing a page from the community organizer's playbook. NLH provides extensive patient services with a geographically based Care Management Team model. Cheryl is a Washington University- and Stanford-trained physician with a Harvard MPH. After practicing medicine, consulting for the government and NGOs, and founding NLH, she has a 360° view of the healthcare system as a patient, provider, and now payor. This informs her conviction that payors need a new model of patient-centric engagement. This talk was given at a TEDx event using the TED conference format but was independently organized by a local community.

- The Social Determinants of Health: Dr. Thomas Ward at TEDxSpringHillCollege— November 14, 2018: https://www.youtube.com/watch?v=tuYRY0XKw9c

  In *The Social Determinants of Health*, Historian Dr. Tom Ward identifies the factors that led to social inequalities in the Deep South during the Civil Rights era. Poverty had a tremendous impact on an individual's health, then and now. Thomas J. Ward, Jr., is professor and chair of the history department at Spring Hill College in Mobile, Alabama, where he teaches a variety of courses in American history. A native of Annapolis, Maryland, Dr. Ward received his BA at Hampden-Sydney College, his MA at Clemson University, and his doctorate at the University of Southern Mississippi. Before coming to Spring Hill College in 2007, Dr. Ward taught at Rockhurst University in Kansas City, Missouri. Dr. Ward has written numerous articles on African American history and the history of medicine in the American South. In 2003, the University of Arkansas Press published his first book, *Black Physicians in the Jim Crow South*. His most recent work, *Out in the Rural: A Mississippi Health Center and Its War on Poverty*, was released by Oxford University Press in 2017. Dr. Ward is currently working on a book project on African American prisoners of war. He lives in Spanish Fort, Alabama, with his wife and three sons. This talk was given at a TEDx event using the TED conference format but was independently organized by a local community.

A robust set of instructor resources designed to supplement this text is located at http://connect.springerpub.com/content/book/978-0-8261-7795-7. Qualifying instructors may request access by emailing textbook@springerpub.com.

REFERENCES

Agency for Healthcare Research and Quality. (n.d.). *IDEAL discharge planning overview, process, and checklist*. Retrieved September 27, 2021, from https://www.ahrq.gov/sites/default/files/wysiwyg/professionals/systems/hospital/engagingfamilies/strategy4/Strat4_Tool_1_IDEAL_chklst_508.pdf

Agency for Healthcare Research and Quality. (2020, December). *2019 National healthcare quality and disparities report*. AHRQ Pub. No. 20(21)-0045-EF. https://www.ahrq.gov/sites/default/files/wysiwyg/research/findings/nhqrdr/2019qdr-cx061021.pdf

Aldridge, R. W., Menezes, D., Lewer, D., Cornes, M., Evans, H., Blackburn, R. M., Byng, R., Clark, M., Denaxas, S., Fuller, J., Hewett, N., Kilmister, A., Luchenski, S., Manthorpe, J., McKee, M., Neale, J., Story, A., Tinbelli, M., Whiteford, M., Wurie, F., & Hayward, A. (2019). Causes of death among homeless people: A population-based cross-sectional study of linked hospitalisation and mortality data in England. *Wellcome Open Research, 4*, 49. https://doi.org/10.12688/wellcomeopenres.15151.1

American Academy of Family Physicians. (2018). *Addressing social determinants of health in primary care: Team-based approach for advancing health equity*. https://www.aafp.org/dam/AAFP/documents/patient_care/everyone_project/team-based-approach.pdf

American Organization of Nurse Executives & American Organization for Nursing Leadership. (2015). *AONL nurse executive competencies*. https://www.aonl.org/system/files/media/file/2019/06/nec.pdf

Auerbach, D. I., Buerhaus, P. I., & Staiger, D. O. (2015, October). Will the RN workforce weather the retirement of the Baby Boomers? *Medical Care, 53*(10), 850–856. https://doi.org/10.1097/MLR.0000000000000415

Berlin, G., Bueno, D., Gibler, K., Schulz, J., & Wexler, J. (2021, August 12). *Survey: US hospital patient volumes move back towards 2019 levels*. McKinsey & Company. https://www.mckinsey.com/industries/healthcare-systems-and-services/our-insights/survey-us-hospital-patient-volumes-move-back-towards-2019-levels

Bhutta, N., Chang, A. C., Dettling, L. J., & Hsu, J. W. (2020, September 28). *Disparities in wealth by race and ethnicity in the 2019 survey of consumer finances*. FEDS Notes. Board of Governors of the Federal Reserve System. https://doi.org/10.17016/2380-7172.2797

Binswanger, I. A., Krueger, P. M., & Steiner, J. F. (2009, November). Prevalence of chronic medical conditions among jail and prison inmates in the United States compared with the general population. *Journal of Epidemiology and Community Health, 63*(11), 912–919. https://doi.org/10.1136/jech.2009.090662

Burr, J. A., Han, S. H., & Tavares, J. L. (2015, April 15). Volunteering and cardiovascular disease risk: Does helping others get "under the skin"? *Gerontologist, 56*(5), 937–947. https://doi.org/10.1093/geront/gnv032

Butler, R., Monsalve, M., Thomas, G. W., Herman, T., Segre, A. M., Polgreen, P. M., & Suneja, M. (2018). Estimating time physicians and other health care workers spend with patients in an intensive care unit using a sensor network. *The American Journal of Medicine, 131*(8), 972.e9–972.e15. https://doi.org/10.1016/j.amjmed.2018.03.015

Carlson, E., Kline, M., & Zangerle, C. M. (2016, April). AONE competencies: Preparing nurse executives to lead population health. *Nurse Leader, 14*(2), 108–112. https://doi.org/10.1016/j.mnl.2016.01.004

Centers for Disease Control and Prevention. (n.d.-a). *Social determinants of health: Know what affects health*. Retrieved June 6, 2022, from https://www.cdc.gov/socialdeterminants/index.htm

Centers for Disease Control and Prevention. (n.d.-b). *Carbon monoxide poisoning (CO)*. Retrieved April 22, 2021, from https://www.cdc.gov/dotw/carbonmonoxide/index.html

Centers for Disease Control and Prevention. (n.d.-c). *Childhood lead poisoning prevention: Lead in paint*. Retrieved June 6, 2022, from https://www.cdc.gov/nceh/lead/prevention/sources/paint.htm

Centers for Disease Control and Prevention (n.d.-d). Tuberculosis: TB and Asian persons. Retrieved June 6, 2022, from https://www.cdc.gov/tb/topic/populations/tbinasians/default.htm

Centers for Disease Control and Prevention. (n.d.-e). *Disability impacts all of us*. https://www.cdc.gov/ncbddd/disabilityandhealth/infographic-disability-impacts-all.html

Centers for Disease Control and Prevention. (2022, June 2). *Risk for COVID-19 infection, hospitalization, and death by race/ethnicity*. https://www.cdc.gov/coronavirus/2019-ncov/covid-data/investigations-discovery/hospitalization-death-by-race-ethnicity.html

Centers for Medicare & Medicaid Services Office of Minority Health. (2020, September). *Impact of hospital readmissions reduction initiatives on vulnerable populations*. Centers for Medicare & Medicaid Services; U.S. Department of Health and Human Services. https://www.cms.gov/files/document/impact-readmissions-reduction-initiatives-report.pdf

Chambers, E., Fuster, D., Suglia, S. A., & Rosenbaum, E. (2016). *The link between housing, neighborhood, and mental health*. MacArthur Foundation, How Housing Matters to Families and Communities Research Initiative, John D. and Catherine T. MacArthur Foundation. https://www.macfound.org/media/files/hhm_brief_-_reverse_mortgages.pdf

Chetty, R., Stepner, M., Abraham, S., Lin, S., Scuderi, B., Turner, N., Bergeron, A., & Cutler, D. (2016, April 26). The association between income and life expectancy in the United States, 2001–2014. *Journal of the American Medical Association, 315*(16), 1750–1766. https://doi.org/10.1001/jama.2016.4226

Children's Defense Fund. (2020, February). *The State of America's Children® 2020*. https://www.childrensdefense.org/wp-content/uploads/2020/02/The-State-Of-Americas-Children-2020.pdf

Cloud, D. H., Parsons, J., & Delany-Brumsey, A. (2014, February 12). Addressing mass incarceration: A clarion call for public health. *American Journal of Public Health, 104*, 389–391. https://doi.org/10.2105/AJPH.2013.301741

Coleman-Jensen, A., Rabbitt, M. P., Gregory, C. A., & Singh, A. (2019, September). *Household food security in the United States in 2018*. ERR-270, U.S. Department of Agriculture, Economic Research Service. https://www.ers.usda.gov/webdocs/publications/94849/err-270.pdf?v=963.1

Dooley, D., Fielding, J., & Levi, L. (1996). Health and unemployment. *Annual Review of Public Health*, *17*, 449–465. https://doi.org/10.1146/annurev.pu.17.050196.002313

Duke, N. N., Skay, C. L., Pettingell, S. L., & Borowsky, I. W. (2009, February). From adolescent connections to social capital: Predictors of civic engagement in young adulthood. *Journal of Adolescent Health*, *44*(2), 161–168. https://doi.org/10.1016/j.jadohealth.2008.07.007

Eberts, S. M., Thomas, M. A., & Jagucki, M. L. (2013). *The quality of our nation's waters—Factors affecting public-supply-well vulnerability to contamination—Understanding observed water quality and anticipating future water quality.* U.S. Geological Survey Circular 1385. http://pubs.usgs.gov/circ/1385/

Edwards, F., Lee, H., & Esposito, M. (2019, August 20). Risk of being killed by police use of force in the United States by age, race–ethnicity, and sex. *Proceedings of the National Academy of Sciences*, *116*(34), 16793–16798; first published August 5, 2019. https://doi.org/10.1073/pnas.1821204116

Environmental Working Group. (2021, August). *PFAS chemicals.* Retrieved July 20, 2022, from https://www.ewg.org/areas-focus/toxic-chemicals/pfas-chemicals

Espinosa, L. L., Turk, J. M., Taylor, M., & Chessman, H. M. (2019). *Race and ethnicity in higher education: A status report.* American Council on Education. https://1xfsu31b52d33idlp13twtos-wpengine.netdna-ssl.com/wp-content/uploads/2019/02/Race-and-Ethnicity-in-Higher-Education.pdf

Esposito, M., Larimore, S., & Lee, H. L. (2021, April 30). *Aggressive policing, health, and health equity.* Health Affairs, Health Policy Brief, Culture of Health. https://www.healthaffairs.org/do/10.1377/hpb20210412.997570/full

Evans, G. W., & Kantrowitz, E. (2002, May). Socioeconomic status and health: The potential role of environmental risk exposure. *Annual Review of Public Health*, *23*(1), 303–331. https://doi.org/10.1146/annurev.publhealth.23.112001.112349

Feeding America. (2021a). *The impact of the coronavirus on food insecurity in 2020 and 2021.* https://www.feedingamerica.org/sites/default/files/2021-03/National%20Projections%20Brief_3.9.2021_0.pdf

Feeding America. (2021b). *The impact of the coronavirus on food insecurity in 2020 and 2021.* https://www.feedingamerica.org/sites/default/files/2021-03/Local%20Projections%20Brief_3.31.2021.pdf

Ganesh, B., Scally, C. P., Skopec, L., & Zhu, J. (2017, October). The relationship between housing and asthma among school-age children: Analysis of the 2015 American Housing Survey. *The Urban Institute Research Report.* https://www.urban.org/sites/default/files/publication/93881/the-relationshi-between-housing-and-asthma_1.pdf

Gregory, C. A., & Coleman-Jensen, A. (2017, July). *Food insecurity, chronic disease, and health among working-age adults.* ERR-235. U.S. Department of Agriculture, Economic Research Service. https://www.ers.usda.gov/webdocs/publications/84467/err-235.pdf?v=9837.9

Gundersen, C., & Ziliak, J. P. (2015, November). Food insecurity and health outcomes. *Health Affairs*, *34*(11), 1830–1839. https://doi.org/10.1377/hlthaff.2015.0645

Hahn, R. A., & Truman, B. I. (2015, May 19). Education improves public health and promotes health equity. *International Journal of Health Services: Planning, Administration, Evaluation*, *45*(4), 657–678. https://doi.org/10.1177/0020731415585986

Hanchate, A. D., Dyer, K. S., Paasche-Orlow, M. K., Banerjee, S., Baker, W. E., Lin, M., Xue, W. D., & Feldman, J. (2019, March). Disparities in emergency department visits among collocated racial/ethnic Medicare enrollees. *Annals of Emergency Medicine*, *73*(3), 225–235. https://doi.org/10.1016/j.annemergmed.2018.09.007

Hartnett, K. P., Kite-Powell, A., DeVies, J., Coletta, M. A., Boehmer, T. K., Adjemian, J., & Gundlapalli, A. V., & National Syndromic Surveillance Program Community of Practice. (2020, June 12). Impact of the COVID-19 pandemic on emergency department visits—United States, January 1, 2019–May 30, 2020. *Morbidity and Mortality Weekly Report*, *69*, 699–704. https://doi.org/10.15585/mmwr.mm6923e1

Harvard Joint Center for Housing Studies. (2021). *The state of the nation's housing 2021.* Harvard University Graduate School of Design, Harvard Kennedy School. https://www.jchs.harvard.edu/sites/default/files/reports/files/Harvard_JCHS_State_Nations_Housing_2021.pdf

Health Affairs. (2019, September). Grant watch: Funding to improve social determinants of health. *Health Affairs*, *38*(9), 1589–1590. https://doi.org/10.1377/hlthaff.2019.01013

Health Promotion International. (1986, May). A discussion document on the concept and principles of health promotion. *Health Promotion International*, *1*(1), 73–76. https://doi.org/10.1093/heapro/1.1.73

Health Resources & Services Administration. (n.d.). *Shortage areas: Explore HPSAs.* Retrieved July 20, 2022, from https://data.hrsa.gov/topics/health-workforce/shortage-areas

Health Resources & Services Administration. (2022, August 8). Designated health professional shortage areas statistics: *Third quarter of fiscal year 2022 designated HPSA quarterly summary*. Retrieved July 20, 2022, from https://data.hrsa.gov/Default/GenerateHPSAQuarterlyReport

Hemer, K. M. (2018). *Civic engagement in young adulthood: Social capital and the mediating effects of postsecondary educational attainment*. Graduate Theses and Dissertations. 16591. https://lib .dr.iastate.edu/etd/1659

Hendryx, M., Fedorko, E., & Halverson, J. (2010, July 6). Pollution sources and mortality rates across rural-urban areas in the United States. *The Journal of Rural Health, 26*(4), 383–391. https://doi .org/10.1111/j.1748-0361.2010.00305.x

Hickey, K. T., Masterson Creber, R. M., Reading, M., Sciacca, R. R., Riga, T. C., Frulla, A. P., & Casida, J. M. (2018, August). Low health literacy: Implications for managing cardiac patients in practice. *The Nurse Practitioner, 43*(8), 49–55. https://doi.org/10.1097/01.NPR.0000541468.54290.49

Holben, D. H., & Pheley, A. M. (2006, July). Diabetes risk and obesity in food-insecure households in rural Appalachian Ohio. *Preventing Chronic Disease, 3*(3). http://www.cdc.gov/pcd/issues/2006/jul/05_0127.htm

Indian Health Service, U.S. Department of Health and Human Services. (2019, October). *Indian health disparities fact sheet*. https://www.ihs.gov/newsroom/factsheets/disparities

Infurna, F. J., Okun, M. A., & Grimm, K. J. (2016, October 3). Volunteering is associated with lower risk of cognitive impairment. *Journal of the American Geriatrics Society, 64*(11), 2263–2269. https://doi .org/10.1111/jgs.14398

Jacobs, E. A., Karavolos, K., Rathouz, P. J., Ferris, T. G., & Powell, L. H. (2005). Limited English proficiency and breast and cervical cancer screening in a multiethnic population. *American Journal of Public Health, 95*(8), 1410–1416. https://doi.org/10.2105/AJPH.2004.041418

Jou, K., Sterling, M. R., Ramos, R., Antoine, F., Nanus, D. M., & Phillips, E. (2021). Eliciting the social determinants of cancer prevention and control in the catchment of an urban cancer center. *Ethnicity & Disease, 31*(1), 23–30. https://doi.org/10.18865/ed.31.1.23

Kamal, R., Ramirez, G., & Cox, C. (2020, December 23). *How does health spending in the U.S. compare to other countries?* The Peterson Center on Healthcare and KFF (Kaiser Family Foundation). https://www.healthsystemtracker.org/chart-collection/health-spending-u-s-compare-countries/#item-start

Kearl, H., Johns, N. E., & Raj, A. (2019, April). *Measuring #MeToo: A national study on sexual harassment and assault*. University of California San Diego Center on Gender Equity and Health, Stop Street Harassment, Promundo, and California Coalition Against Sexual Assault. https://gehweb.ucsd .edu/wp-content/uploads/2019/05/2019-metoo-national-sexual-harassment-and-assault-report.pdf

Keisler-Starkey, K., & Bunch, L. N. (2021, September). *Health insurance coverage in the United States: 2020*. U.S. Census Bureau Current Population Reports. P60-274. U.S. Government Publishing Office, Washington, DC. https://www.census.gov/library/publications/2021/demo/p60-274 .html

Kerns, C., & Willis, D. (2020, March 16). The problem with U.S. health care isn't a shortage of doctors. *Harvard Business Review*. https://hbr.org/2020/03/the-problem-with-u-s-health-care-isnt-a -shortage-of-doctors

Khullar, D., & Chokshi, D. A. (2018, October 4). Health, income, and poverty: Where we are and what could help. *Health Affairs Health Policy Brief*. https://doi.org/10.1377/hpb20180817.901935

Kim, E. S., Hawes, A. M., & Smith, J. (2014). Perceived neighbourhood social cohesion and myocardial infarction. *Journal of Epidemiology & Community Health, 68*, 1020–1026. https://doi.org/10.1136/jech-2014-204009

Kim, S., Kim, C.-Y., & You, M. S. (2015, January 27). Civic participation and self-rated health: A cross-national multi-level analysis using the world value survey. *Journal Preventive Medicine & Public Health, 48*(1):18–27. https://doi.org/10.3961/jpmph.14.031

Knox, S. S., Adelman, A., Ellison, C. R., Arnett, D. K., Siegmund, K. D., Weidner, G., & Province, M. A. (2000, November 15). Hostility, social support, and carotid artery atherosclerosis in the National Heart, Lung, and Blood Institute Family Heart Study. *American Journal of Cardiology, 86*(10), 1086–1089. https://doi.org/10.1016/S0002-9149(00)01164-4

Kurt, O. K., Zhang, J., & Pinkerton, K. E. (2016, March). Pulmonary health effects of air pollution. *Current Opinion in Pulmonary Medicine, 22*(2), 138–143. https://doi.org/10.1097/mcp.0000000000000248

Laraia, B. A. (2013, March). Food insecurity and chronic disease. *Advances in Nutrition, 4*(2), 203–212. https://doi.org/10.3945/an.112.003277

Leonhardt, D. (2021, May 24). The vaccine class gap. *The New York Times*. https://www.nytimes.com/2021/05/24/briefing/vaccination-class-gap-us.html

Luo, Y., Xu, J., Granberg, E., & Wentworth, W. M. (2011, December 14). A longitudinal study of social status, perceived discrimination, and physical and emotional health among older adults. *Research on Aging, 34*, 275–301. https://doi.org/10.1177/0164027511426151

Marcozzi, D., Carr, B., Liferidge, A., Baehr, N., & Browne, B. (2018). Trends in the contribution of emergency departments to the provision of health care in the USA. *International Journal of Health Services, 48*(2), 267–288. https://doi.org/10.1177/0020731417734498

Medina, L., Sabo, S., & Vespa, J. (2020, February). *Living longer: Historical and projected life expectancy in the United States, 1960 to 2060, population estimates and projections*. U.S. Census Bureau, U.S. Department of Commerce. https://www.census.gov/content/dam/Census/library/publications/2020/demo/p25-1145.pdf

Menendian, S., Gambhir, S., & Gailes, A. (2021). *The Roots of Structural Racism Project*. Othering and Belonging Institute. https://belonging.berkeley.edu/roots-structural-racism

Moody's Analytics. (2017, December 14). *The health of America report: Understanding health conditions across the U.S.* BlueCross BlueShield Association. https://www.bcbs.com/the-health-of-america/reports/understanding-health-conditions-across-the-us

Mosher, H., Lose, D., Leslie, R., & Kaboli, P. (2014, May). *Interdisciplinary rounding toolkit: A guide to optimizing interdisciplinary rounds on inpatient medical services*. VA Quality Scholars (VAQS) Fellowship Program, Center for Comprehensive Access and Delivery Research and Evaluation (CADRE), Iowa City VA Healthcare System, U.S. Department of Veterans Affairs. https://www.cadre.research.va.gov/docs/IDR_Toolkit_Final.pdf

Muennig, P., Robertson, D., Johnson, G., Campbell, F., Pungello, E., & Neidell, M. (2011, March). The effect of an early education program on adult health: The Carolina Abecedarian Project Randomized Controlled Trial. *American Journal of Public Health, 101*, 512–516. https://doi.org/10.2105/AJPH.2010.200063

Münzel, T., Sørensen, M., Schmidt, F., Schmidt, E., Steven, S., Kröller-Schön, S., & Daiber, A. (2018). The adverse effects of environmental noise exposure on oxidative stress and cardiovascular risk. *Antioxidants & Redox Signaling, 28*(9), 873–908. https://doi.org/10.1089/ars.2017.7118

Nagata, J. M., Palar, K., Gooding, H. C., Garber, A. K., Bibbins-Domingo, K., & Weiser, S. D. (2019). Food insecurity and chronic disease in US young adults: Findings from the national longitudinal study of adolescent to adult health. *Journal of General Internal Medicine, 34*, 2756–2762. https://doi.org/10.1007/s11606-019-05317-8

National Academies of Sciences, Engineering, and Medicine. (2019). *Integrating social care into the delivery of health care: Moving upstream to improve the nation's health*. National Academies Press. https://doi.org/10.17226/25467

National Advisory Council on Nurse Education and Practice. (2019). *Integration of social determinants of health in nursing education, practice, and research. 16th report to the secretary of health and human services and the U.S. Congress*. Health Resources and Services Administration. https://www.hrsa.gov/sites/default/files/hrsa/advisory-committees/nursing/reports/nacnep-2019-sixteenthreport.pdf

National Center for Health Statistics. (2019). *Table 44. Gross domestic product, national health expenditures, per capita amounts,% distribution, and average annual% change: United States, selected years 1960–2018.* https://www.cdc.gov/nchs/data/hus/2019/044-508.pdf

National Institute of Environmental Health Sciences, National Institutes of Health. (2021). *Air pollution and your health*. https://www.niehs.nih.gov/health/topics/agents/air-pollution/index.cfm

National Oceanic and Atmospheric Administration National Centers for Environmental Information. (2021, January). *State of the climate: Global climate report for annual 2020*. https://www.ncdc.noaa.gov/sotc/global/202013

Natural Resources Defense Council. (2018, November 8). *Flint water crisis: Everything you need to know*. https://www.nrdc.org/stories/flint-water-crisis-everything-you-need-know#sec-summary

Nielsen-Bohlman, L., Panzer, A. M., & Kindig, D. A. (Eds.). (2004). *Health literacy: A prescription to end confusion*. National Academies Press. https://pubmed.ncbi.nlm.nih.gov/25009856

Northridge, J., Ramirez, O., Stingone, J., & Claudio, L. (2010, January 9). The role of housing type and housing quality in urban children with asthma. *Journal of Urban Health: Bulletin of the New York Academy of Medicine, 87*, 211–224. https://doi.org/10.1007/s11524-009-9404-1

Office of Minority Health, U.S. Department of Health and Human Services. (2021, October 12). *Profile: Asian Americans*. https://www.minorityhealth.hhs.gov/omh/browse.aspx?lvl=3&lvlid=63

Office of the Assistant Secretary for Planning and Evaluation, U.S. Department of Health & Human Services. (2021). *Report to Congress: Trends in the utilization of emergency department services, 2009–2018*. https://aspe.hhs.gov/pdf-report/utilization-emergency-department-services

Parker, K., & Funk, C. (2017, December 14). Gender discrimination comes in many forms for today's working women. *Pew Research Center*. https://www.pewresearch.org/fact-tank/2017/12/14/gender-discrimination-comes-in-many-forms-for-todays-working-women

Prince, L. Y., Schmidtke, C., Beck, J. K., & Hadden, K. B. (2018, April/June). An assessment of organizational health literacy practices at an academic health center. *Quality Management in Health Care, 27*(2), 93–97. https://doi.org/10.1097/QMH.0000000000000162

Public Health Accreditation Board. (2012). *Acronyms and glossary of terms* (Version 1.0). https://www.phaboard.org/wp-content/uploads/PHAB-Acronyms-and-Glossary-of-Terms-Version-1.02.pdf

Raghupathi, V., & Raghupathi, W. (2020, December). The influence of education on health: An empirical assessment of OECD countries for the period 1995–2015. *Archives of Public Health, 78*, 20. https://doi.org/10.1186/s13690-020-00402-5

Raynor, E. M. (2016, February). Factors affecting care in non-English-speaking patients and families. *Clinical Pediatrics, 55*(2), 145–149. https://doi.org/10.1177/0009922815586052

Restum, Z. G. (2005, April 26). Public health implications of substandard correctional health care. *American Journal of Public Health, 95*(10), 1689–1691. https://doi.org/10.2105/AJPH.2004.055053

Richard, P., Walker, R., & Alexandre, P. (2018, June 25). The burden of out of pocket costs and medical debt faced by households with chronic health conditions in the United States. *PLOS One, 13*(6), e0199598. https://doi.org/10.1371/journal.pone.0199598

Robert Wood Johnson Foundation. (2013, March). How does employment—Or unemployment—Affect health? *Health Policy Snapshot 2013*. http://www.rwjf.org/content/dam/farm/reports/issue_briefs/2013/rwjf403360

Robert Wood Johnson Foundation. (2019, February 1). *Medicaid's role in addressing social determinants of health*. https://www.rwjf.org/en/library/research/2019/02/medicaid-s-role-in-addressing-social-determinants-of-health.html

Rosales, C. B., Carvajal, S. C., & De Zapien, J. E. G. (2016). Emergent public health issues in the US–Mexico border region. *Lausanne: Frontiers Media*. https://doi.org/10.3389/978-2-88945-047-3

Roy, M., Purington, N., Liu, M., Blayney, D. W., Kurian, A. W., & Schapira, L. (2021). Limited English proficiency and disparities in health care engagement among patients with breast cancer. *JCO Oncology Practice, 17*(12), e1837–e1845. https://doi.org/10.1200/OP.20.01093

Rural Health Information Hub. (n.d.). *Rural border health*. Retrieved May 28, 2021, from https://www.ruralhealthinfo.org/topics/border-health

Ryan, L., Scott, S., & Fields, W. (2017, October/December). Implementation of interdisciplinary rapid rounds in observation units. *Journal of Nursing Care Quality, 32*(4), 348–353. https://doi.org/10.1097/NCQ.0000000000000250

Saad, L. (2020, December 22). *U.S. ethics ratings rise for medical workers and teachers*. Gallup. https://news.gallup.com/poll/328136/ethics-ratings-rise-medical-workers-teachers.aspx

Save the Children Foundation. (2021a). *Childhood in the time of COVID: U.S. complement to the global childhood report 2021*. https://www.savethechildren.org/content/dam/usa/reports/advocacy/2021-us-childhood-report.pdf

Save the Children Foundation. (2021b). *When high school—and childhood—is cut short in America*. https://www.savethechildren.org/us/charity-stories/high-school-drop-out-rate-in-america

Schanzer, B., Dominguez, B., Shrout, P. E., & Caton, C. L. (2007, January 31). Homelessness, health status, and health care use. *American Journal of Public Health, 97*(3), 464–469. https://doi.org/10.2105/AJPH.2005.076190

Semega, J., Kollar, M., Creamer, J., & Mohanty, A. (2019). *Income and poverty in the United States* [U.S. Census Bureau Current Population Reports, P60-266(RV). U.S. Government Printing Office. https://www.census.gov/content/dam/Census/library/publications/2019/demo/p60-266.pdf

Sentell, T. L., Tsoh, J. Y., Davis, T., Davis, J., & Braun, K. L. (2015). Low health literacy and cancer screening among Chinese Americans in California: A cross-sectional analysis. *BMJ Open, 5*(1), e006104. https://doi.org/10.1136/bmjopen-2014-006104

Shi, R., Meacham, S., Davis, G. C., You, W., Sun, Y., & Goessl, C. (2019, November 8). Factors influencing high respiratory mortality in coal-mining counties: A repeated cross-sectional study. *BMC Public Health, 19*, 1484. https://doi.org/10.1186/s12889-019-7858-y

Shrider, E. A., Kollar, M., Chen, F., & Semega, J. (2021). *Income and poverty in the United States: 2020*. U.S. Census Bureau Current Population Reports, P60-273(RV). U.S. Government Printing Office. https://www.census.gov/content/dam/Census/library/publications/2021/demo/p60-273.pdf

Steinka-Fry, K. T., Wilson, S. J., & Tanner-Smith, E. E. (2013, December 31). Effects of school dropout prevention programs for pregnant and parenting adolescents: A meta-analytic review. *Journal of the Society for Social Work and Research, 4*(4), 373–379. https://doi.org/10.5243/jsswr.2013.23

Stockman, J. K., Hayashi, H., & Campbell, J. C. (2015). Intimate partner violence and its health impact on ethnic minority women [corrected]. *Journal of Women's Health, 24*(1), 62–79. https://doi.org/10.1089/jwh.2014.4879

Stoto, M. A. (2013, February 21). *Population health in the Affordable Care Act era*. Academy Health. https://www.academyhealth.org/files/AH2013pophealth.pdf

Sullivan, H. R. (2019, March). HEALTH LAW: Hospitals' obligations to address social determinants of health. *AMA Journal of Ethics, 21*(3), E248–E258. https://journalofethics.ama-assn.org/sites/journalofethics.ama-assn.org/files/2019-02/hlaw1-1903.pdf

Syed, S. T., Gerber, B. S., & Sharp, L. K. (2013, October). Traveling towards disease: Transportation barriers to health care access. *Journal of Community Health, 38*(5), 976–993. https://doi.org/10.1007/s10900-013-9681-1

Toccalino, P. L., & Hopple, J. A. (2010). *The quality of our nation's waters: Quality of water from public-supply wells in the United States, 1993–2007: Overview of major findings* [U.S. Geological Survey Circular 1346]. https://pubs.usgs.gov/circ/1346/pdf/circ1346.pdf

Turney, K. (2014). Stress proliferation across generations? Examining the relationship between parental incarceration and childhood health. *Journal of Health and Social Behavior, 55*(3), 302–319. https://doi.org/10.1177/0022146514544173

Upadhyay, S., Stephenson, A. L., & Smith, D. G. (2019, January–December). Readmission rates and their impact on hospital financial performance: A study of Washington hospitals. *Inquiry: A Journal of Medical Care Organization, Provision and Financing*. https://doi.org/10.1177/0046958019860386

U.S. Bureau of Labor Statistics. (2019, October 21). *Median weekly earnings $606 for high school dropouts, $1,559 for advanced degree holders*. The Economics Daily. https://www.bls.gov/opub/ted/2019/median-weekly-earnings-606-for-high-school-dropouts-1559-for-advanced-degree-holders.htm

U.S. Bureau of Labor Statitics. (2021a). *Census of fatal occupational injuries (CFOI) – Current*. Retrieved June 7, 2022, from https://www.bls.gov/iif/oshcfoi1.htm

U.S. Bureau of Labor Statitics. (2021b). Survey of occupational injuries and illness data. Retrieved June 7, 2022, from https://www.bls.gov/iif/soii-data.htm

U.S. Census Bureau. (2020a). *American Community Survey: Characteristics of people by language spoken at home [2018: ACS 1-year estimates subject tables]*. https://data.census.gov/cedsci/table?q=language%20spoken%20at%20home&tid=ACSST5Y2020.S1603

U.S. Census Bureau. (2020b). *American Community Survey: Educational attainment [2019: ACS 1-year estimates subject tables]*. https://data.census.gov/cedsci/table?q=high%20school%20graduation,%20poverty

U.S. Department of Agriculture, Economic Research Service. (2020). *Definitions of food security*. https://www.ers.usda.gov/topics/food-nutrition-assistance/food-security-in-the-us/definitions-of-food-security.aspx

U.S. Department of Agriculture, & U.S. Department of Health and Human Services. (2020, December). *Dietary guidelines for Americans, 2020–2025* (9th ed.). https://www.dietaryguidelines.gov/sites/default/files/2021-03/Dietary_Guidelines_for_Americans-2020-2025.pdf

U.S. Department of Health and Human Services, Office of Disease Prevention and Health Promotion. (n.d.-a). *Healthy People 2020: Social determinants of health*. https://www.healthypeople.gov/2020/topics-objectives/topic/social-determinants-of-health

U.S. Department of Health and Human Services, Office of Disease Prevention and Health Promotion. (n.d.-b). *Healthy People 2030: Social determinants of health*. https://health.gov/healthypeople/objectives-and-data/social-determinants-health

U.S. Department of Health and Human Services, Office of Disease Prevention and Health Promotion. (2010). *National action plan to improve health literacy*. Author. https://origin.health.gov/sites/default/files/2019-09/Health_Literacy_Action_Plan.pdf

U.S. Department of Health and Human Services, Office of the Assistant Secretary for Planning and Evaluation. (2021, March 2). Trends in the utilization of emergency department services, 2009-2018. Author. https://aspe.hhs.gov/sites/default/files/migrated_legacy_files/199046/ED-report-to-Congress.pdf

U.S. Department of Health and Human Services & U.S. Department of Agriculture. (2015, December). *Dietary guidelines for Americans 2015–2020* (8th ed.). https://health.gov/sites/default/files/2019-09/2015-2020_Dietary_Guidelines.pdf

U.S. Department of Housing and Urban Development. (2020, December 15). *HUD 2020 continuum of care homeless assistance programs homeless populations and subpopulation*. Homelessness Data Exchange (HDX), Versions 1.0 and 2.0. https://files.hudexchange.info/reports/published/CoC _PopSub_NatlTerrDC_2020.pdf

U.S. Environmental Protection Agency. (n.d.). Connection between environmental exposure and health outcomes. Retrieved September 2, 2021, from https://www.epa.gov/report-environment/ connection-between-environmental-exposure-and-health-outcomes

U.S. Equal Opportunity Employment Commission. (n.d.-a). *Age Discrimination in Employment Act (charges filed with EEOC) (includes concurrent charges with Title VII, ADA, EPA, and GINA) FY 1997– FY 2020*. Retrieved May 12, 2021, from https://www.eeoc.gov/statistics/age-discrimination -employment-act-charges-filed-eeoc-includes-concurrent-charges-title

U.S. Equal Opportunity Employment Commission. (n.d.-b). *Americans with Disabilities Act of 1990 (ADA) charges (charges filed with EEOC) (includes concurrent charges with Title VII, ADEA, EPA, and GINA) FY 1997–FY 2020*. Retrieved May 12, 2021, from https://www.eeoc.gov/statistics/ americans-disabilities-act-1990-ada-charges-charges-filed-eeoc-includes-concurrent

U.S. Government Accountability Office. (2021, January 21). *Rural hospital closures: Affected residents had reduced access to health care services*. GAO-21-93. https://www.gao.gov/products/gao-21-93

Ver Ploeg, M., Mancino, L., Todd, J. E., Clay, D. M., & Scharadin, B. (2015, March). *Where do Americans usually shop for food and how do they travel to get there? Initial findings from the National Household Food Acquisition and Purchase Survey, Economic Information Bulletin-138*. U.S. Department of Agriculture, Economic Research Service. https://www.ers.usda.gov/webdocs/publications/43953/ eib138_errata.pdf?v=9776.2

Wakefield, M. K., Williams, D. R., Le Menestrel, S., & Flaubert, J. L. (Eds.). (2021). *The future of nursing 2020–2030: Charting a path to achieve health equity*. National Academies Press. https://doi.org/ 10.17226/25982

Wilson, M. L. (2019). Incorporating social determinants of health into patient care. *Nursing Management (Springhouse), 50*(12), 13–15. https://doi.org/10.1097/01.numa.0000605188.82349.3c

Wittink, H., & Oosterhaven, J. (2018). Patient education and health literacy. *Musculoskeletal Science & Practice, 38*, 120–127. https://doi.org/10.1016/j.msksp.2018.06.004

Wolfe, R., Harknett, K., & Schneider, D. (2021, June 4). Inequalities at work and the toll of COVID-19. *Health Affairs: Health Policy Brief*. https://doi.org/10.1377/hpb20210428.863621

World Health Organization. (1946). *Constitution of the World Health Organization*. https://apps.who .int/gb/bd/PDF/bd47/EN/constitution-en.pdf?ua=1

World Health Organization. (2010, January 12). *Violence prevention: The evidence*. https://www.who .int/publications/i/item/violence-prevention-the-evidence

World Health Organization. (2021, March 19). *Injuries and violence*. https://www.who.int/news -room/fact-sheets/detail/injuries-and-violence

Zajacova, A., & Lawrence, E. M. (2018, April 1). The relationship between education and health: Reducing disparities through a contextual approach. *Annual Review of Public Health, 39*, 273–289. https://doi.org/10.1146/annurev-publhealth-031816-044628

CHAPTER 10

TELEHEALTH

Noreen B. Brennan

"Technology may change rapidly, but people change slowly. The principles [of design] come from understanding of people. They remain true forever."

Donald A. Norman (author)

LEARNING OBJECTIVES

- Describe the historical development of telehealth.
- Differentiate between the variety of telehealth technologies.
- Assess implementation components of a telehealth program, from the patient, provider, and organizational perspectives.
- Investigate the legal, ethical, and regulatory issues associated with telehealth programs.

INTRODUCTION

This chapter examines telehealth—an all-encompassing term that has become a significant part of current and future healthcare delivery. Rapid technological advancements have occurred over the last 100 years but have exploded in the past 30 years. As such, a review of the history and the development of the language and naming conventions of telehealth are reviewed in the first sections of this chapter.

Telehealth is a system of electronic communication that has become instrumental in the delivery of healthcare services whether through complex imaging machinery or wearable devices. The possibilities of providing and improving access to care are limitless: Individuals who are in remote areas receive care through telecommunication platforms, intensive care patients are monitored from different global regions, clinicians can collaborate across large geographical regions, patients can transmit real time data to their healthcare provider, and data can be used to inform patient care.

As telehealth continues to expand and morph, nursing leaders must be at the forefront of technological innovation and the commiserate education, research, and ethical challenges that may arise. Additionally, this chapter contains a discussion of nursing leadership competencies and future considerations regarding nursing workflow in light of many technological advancements. Telehealth is an active part of the nurse leader's role and will continue to be an important component in the future, particularly as we incorporate more artificial intelligence and in light of the most recent COVID-19 pandemic. As leaders, the utilization of telehealth technology and the resultant big data will be significant components of new healthcare delivery models.

HISTORY OF TELEHEALTH

Although it may seem as though telehealth is a new concept in healthcare delivery, depending upon how it is classified, the origins of telehealth can be traced as far back as the bubonic plague, when smoke signals were used to communicate information. However, for the purpose of this chapter, we will look at the development of electronic telecommunication as the beginning. As far back as the Civil War, medical supplies and casualty reports were communicated via the telegraph.

The advent of the telephone made an impact on reducing the number of patient visits and improved communication between physicians. Next to arrive on scene was the radio, which allowed treatment to be delivered to remote geographical areas. This was followed very quickly by the advent of closed-circuit television. For example, in 1959, the University of Nebraska School of Medicine tested the use of a closed-circuit television link to provide mental and other health services (Benshoter, 1967). Using biometrical data transmission of animal biometrics data from space, the National Aeronautics and Space Administration (NASA) space program helped pave the way for telehealth monitoring of astronauts while in space.

These systems were extremely costly; during the 1970s, practitioners had difficulty integrating technology with clinical practice (Nickelson, 1998). Some federal funding was provided in the late 1960s and 1970s through demonstration projects. These projects did show that telemedicine was a viable option for providing medical care. By the late 1980s, organizations such as military and correction institutions began to use more technology due to geographical distance or safety concerns related to the transport of certain individuals (Nickelson, 1998). The public began to express interest in the concepts of the expanded internet, and with financial support from the federal government, technology firms increased in number. Rural communities, which did not have a variety of medical specialists, were strong advocates for the development of telehealth programs, seeking political and public support.

During the late 2000s with the growth in internet use and with more affordable and smaller devices, telehealth capabilities expanded at a more rapid pace than any of the prior decades. The internet was a tipping point in the transformation of telemedicine. The speed of communication and the ability to send large amounts of data, combined with the reduction in the cost of care, has pushed telemedicine to the forefront of healthcare. The growth of telehealth has moved from the provider to the recipients of care.

Wearable technology, health apps, virtual reality, and interactive platforms are proving to be effective new modalities for individuals to participate in their well-being. Telehealth expanded particularly during and after the COVID-19 pandemic. Traditional visits to hospitals and physician's offices were changed to telehealth visits that were done through web application technologies, such as Zoom, Microsoft Teams, or Webex, to name a few. Patient monitoring was done through wearable technology; although this was not new, it came to be used with more frequency.

As we progress through 2022 and beyond, additional technologies will be developed that assist in healthcare (Brown et al., 2020). Virtual reality, artificial intelligence, robots, implantable technology, and clinical decision-making applications are just some of the technologies that are on the forefront of healthcare delivery. These new modalities will also redesign how and where healthcare delivery is received, likely shifting from traditional offices or hospitals to patients' homes.

TELEHEALTH TERMINOLOGY

Often when new ideas are introduced there is a development of the language that occurs as the concept develops, so some confusion exists regarding what is truly meant by the topic, with terms being used interchangeably. Such is the case with telehealth and telemedicine. "Telehealth" is an umbrella term that broadly refers to electronic telecommunications technologies and services that are used to distantly provide care and services, specifically using electronic information and telecommunications technologies that support geographically vast healthcare, patient and professional health education, and public and health administration (U.S. Department of Health and Human Services, 2021).

"Telemedicine," on the other hand, is a term coined in the 1970s and refers to the practice of medicine using technology to deliver care at a distance over multiple different sites. The two terms differ in that telehealth refers to a broader scope of remote health services and telemedicine is specific to remote clinical services. Some would also state that telemedicine refers primarily to care delivered by physicians, whereas telehealth is delivered by all other clinicians. Both use cell phones, computers, and the internet to communicate, exchange information, and inform the health of communities. Additionally, both are opening access, equity, and cost-effective quality care to urban and rural communities.

USE OF TELEHEALTH

Telehealth is used in a variety of different ways—clinical care, personal healthcare, videoconferencing, and education. Technology associated with telehealth often includes computers, internet, cell phones, electronic medical records (EMRs), apps, wearable devices, and virtual reality. Telehealth allows for a broad scope of remote healthcare services and nonclinical services such as clinical education, meetings/conferences, and training.

There are currently four different types of telehealth technology: live videoconferencing (synchronous); store and forward (asynchronous); remote patient monitoring (RPM); and mobile health (MHEALTH; Box 10.1). Live videoconferencing is a live interaction between a practitioner and person using an audiovisual telecommunication technology. Some examples are videoconferencing units; peripheral and web cameras from tablets, phones, laptops, and large monitors; or specialized telemedicine carts. Live videoconferencing is a cost-effective method for connecting people with providers, providers with specialists, and holding education or meetings.

BOX 10.1: FOUR TYPES OF TELEHEALTH

- Live videoconferencing
- Store and forward
- Remote patient monitoring
- Mobile health

The next type of telehealth modality is "store and forward" whereby recorded health history is transmitted through an electronic communication system to a practitioner who uses the information to review clinical cases. Some of the common technologies are electrocardiograms, sonograms, and x-rays. Data from these devices is stored locally then transmitted to other locations for consultation or second opinions.

Many acute care facilities and physician practices are investing in RPM. This technology allows for the collection of personal health and medical data from people who are in one location; this data is then transmitted through electronic communication to a provider in a different location. Some examples of internet-connected devices include heart monitors, blood glucose monitors, scales, blood pressure monitors, or oxygen monitors. Vital data is transmitted allowing for healthy aging at home, care of highly infective disease, and care for patients with a high risk for readmission.

The last modality, MHEALTH, is supported by mobile devices such as cell phones, tablets, or wearable personal devices. The technology transmits information to providers or to mobile applications. Typically, MHEALTH is used for setting reminders, notification of emergency news, and tracking exercise/sleep/heart rate/diet.

EVIDENCE-BASED PRACTICE AND APPLICATION

The COVID-19 pandemic thrust the acute care environment from in-person visits to virtual visits overnight. With the shutdown of in-person services, the world of telehealth transformed out of necessity and was supported by waivers and regulatory changes expedited by legislative changes. In relation to telehealth and telemedicine, Totten et al. (2016) conducted an evidence-based report of systematic reviews finding that telehealth interventions have positive outcomes in relation to mortality, quality of life, and readmissions when utilized for

- RPM for chronic cardiovascular or respiratory conditions,
- psychotherapy—behavioral health, and
- communication/counseling for those with chronic conditions.

In one search of published scholarly articles since 2020, over 17,200 articles have been published on telehealth, with only 300 articles published in the previous 3 years. In addition to the patients' groups identified earlier, these articles relate to the fields of oncology, pediatrics, gastroenterology, and occupational therapy. The COVID-19 pandemic resulted in an explosion of research focused on processes for successful telehealth visits, caregiver training, patient outcomes, and expansion of patient care groups. Telehealth is the leading innovation in patient care and interdisciplinary practice and is on point to continue to disrupt traditional healthcare. Important in the discussion is the use of checklists by not only providers, but also ones needed for patients (Table 10.1).

COMMUNICATION

Telehealth has been used as not only a platform for patient health but also as a means of communication between healthcare providers (Mataxen & Webb, 2019). There are several tools currently in use by clinicians: EMR, e-consults, social media platforms, email, secure texting, instant messaging, push notifications, video, and phone calls. Telehealth has also been used in educating individuals and disseminating information to clinicians using computer-based learning management systems, intra/internet websites, and simulation of skills through role-play (Smith et al., 2018).

With this new blend of technology and telecommunications, there has been discussion about "Netiquette," which is basically the blending of the words "network" and "etiquette," which provides a guideline for the communication that occurs between providers and patients. Kumar et al. (2020) suggest during telehealth visits that you be ergonomically comfortable, refrain from multitasking while communicating, and turn off email/text

TABLE 10.1: Provider and Patient Checklists for Telehealth Visits

Providers	Patients
Assess and plan for community needs	Available technology/internet
Plan for language and accessibility	Secure, private environment
Test all equipment	Provide patient education and tip sheet
Quiet, confidential space	Provide patients with troubleshooting information
Identify self, patient, and consent	Provide contact information
Document, follow-up with labs, pharmacy, prescriptions, and appointments	Check in with patient through evaluation

notifications while engaged in communication. Additionally, Kumar et al. (2020) outline 13 key rules of Netiquette:

1. Practice or perform a trial run to prevent audio/visual challenges, having alternative technology available as a standby.
2. Use a neutral background when taking part in video calls (blank wall or screen).
3. Check your internet service and speed.
4. Verify the time management of calls; ensure enough turnaround time exists between calls.
5. Keep the caller appraised of delays/cancellations; establish trust.
6. Ensure the remote setting is safe, secure, and confidential.
7. Have the room well-lit and free of background distractions.
8. Dress professionally.
9. Have the patient call in.
10. Maintain eye contact, set boundaries, acknowledge and respect others' points of view, maintain face-to-face presence, and clarify questions.
11. Listen for tone and be supportive to anxious persons.
12. Be careful with use of chat boxes and emojis.
13. Be empathic and thank the person for the session.

⬡ CASE SCENARIO

CHOOSING TELEHEALTH TECHNOLOGIES

SITUATION

New City Hospital Center is a safety net hospital system that has four acute care facilities, two critical access hospitals, 15 outpatient centers, and two home healthcare agencies. Geographically, the catchment area is about 250 miles. The system is embarking on a comprehensive plan to reduce readmission of patients with congestive heart failure (CHF). Administration believes that the use of telehealth can reduce readmission rates.

APPROACH

As the nursing leader, you have been tasked with forming a committee to choose telehealth devices, review interoperability with the EMR, design the workflow, and develop outcome measures for the program.

OUTCOME

New City Hospital is looking to reduce the cost per case for patients with CHF and to improve patient outcomes in the community. They are looking to reduce recidivism rates by 20% and to reduce readmission within 30 days by 30% over the course of 6 months.

DISCUSSION QUESTIONS

1. In assembling the team to address the initiation of telehealth, develop a project plan that describes the following: Who are the stakeholders, what type of data is needed for device selection, and what outcome measures will you choose to measure the success of the program?
2. Describe the rationale and use of the telehealth devices that you will use to ensure the success of this program. What types of considerations will need to be included?

⬢ **CASE SCENARIO**

SELF-CARE: USING WEARABLE DEVICES

SITUATION

Nurses working in the medical unit have decided to enter a healthcare challenge as inspired by the American Nurses Association (ANA) Healthy Nurse, Healthy Nation Initiative.

APPROACH

Each nurse has a wearable health device which will enable them to track physical activity, nutrition, rest, safety, and quality of life.

OUTCOME

Nurses participating in the challenge have noticed some visible changes in their levels of stress, weight, and overall well-being.

DISCUSSION QUESTIONS

1. What are some of the physical activity, nutrition, rest, safety, and quality of life challenges you would choose for yourself? Why?

2. For 2 weeks, choose one challenge—daily meditation, steps goal, sleep monitoring, journaling, or other activity. What changes did you notice? Would you continue with the challenge? Why or why not? Would you include it in your education plan for your patients? Why or why not?

SPECIAL CONSIDERATIONS IN TELEHEALTH

ETHICAL AND LEGAL CONSIDERATIONS

Prior to COVID-19, the use of telehealth in urban areas truly was behind rural areas in terms of connectivity and utilization. Traditional urban environments were dependent on brick-and-mortar buildings with appointment times. However, a massive shift to telehealth occurred during the pandemic, thereby thrusting telehealth utilization ahead by light years.

There are a few ethical considerations regarding telehealth: erosion of the patient–provider relationship, privacy/confidentiality threats, forcing one-size-fits-all implementations, assuming that new technology must be efficacious, and ensuring use improves equitable access to care. Clinicians need to be aware that all individuals may not have access to mobile technology or internet service. The lack of face-to-face assessment also challenges the nurse to make critical decisions based on patient self-report. The nurse must carefully query patients to provide the visual, tactile, and olfactory information.

In a systematic review, the ethical principle of autonomy and subthemes including consent, individual choice, independence, empowerment, control, and self-determination were main points identified. A balance of a multipronged approach to care is suggested, so that independence is maintained. Beneficence, doing good for others, and nonmaleficence, doing no harm, were also identified (Keenan et al., 2021). Delivering education so that patients can act in their best interest and ensuring patients are protected and safe is suggested. Lastly, justice or fairness was discussed in relation to access, with suggestions that telehealth modality includes equal access to communities. As future technologies develop, the alignment of policy and practice with ethical considerations will need to be incorporated.

According to the American Hospital Association (AHA; 2022), there are many legal and regulatory challenges that exist with establishing a telehealth program, including

- payment or insurance coverage;
- health professional state licensure;

- credentialing and privileging of physicians;
- online prescribing particularly controlled substances;
- medical malpractice and professional liability insurance;
- privacy and security; and
- fraud and abuse.

Another concerning risk is cyberattacks, which threaten patient confidentiality. There have been reported breaches ranging anywhere from 40 to 155.8 million healthcare records impermissibly disclosed during 2020, which include unauthorized disclosures of protected health information (PHI), improper disposal of PHI, cybercriminals or rogue employees stealing private information, and other security or privacy breaches. Cybersecurity has become a predominant part of healthcare budgets. Multiple redundant safety measures, referred to as "cybersecurity," are employed by local informational technology (IT) departments. Some safety measures in place include strong password-protected hardware, two-way authentication, encrypted data, redundancy backed up systems, cybersecurity insurance, use of antimalware solutions, educating employees on the risks associated with using unsecured networks, and limiting the access to nontrusted websites.

FINANCIAL IMPLICATIONS

Telehealth requires outlays of money for hardware, software, programs, personnel, and internet connections. Programs for EMRs can cost organizations millions of dollars. Telehealth can also create a financial impact when patients need to have a device, internet service, a cell data plan, and applications. Additionally, there are significant personnel costs for information technologists and nursing informaticists. However, not having the information systems can be just as costly.

REGULATORY STANDARDS

To further the widespread adoption of telehealth, there are many regulations/questions that need to be addressed at the state level. There are four in particular: state professional licensure, billing, informed patient consent, and malpractice. Currently, healthcare providers are licensed in the state in which they geographically work, but for states that do not have compact licensure, providers cannot technically treat patients outside of their current state. As with licensure, cross state billing is also a concern, as it is a barrier for those who are participating in state networks (Shachar et al., 2020). Changes in payment are also an issue being addressed, so that there is parity in televisits and clinic care. State laws vary on the format of informed patient consent and there is limited precedent for telehealth malpractice cases, as many states do not require malpractice coverage.

An issue that crosses both state and federal regulations is prescribing, with controlled substances falling under federal guidelines. Prescribing includes items such as the practitioner relationship with the patient, whether it involves a controlled substance, and if an emergency situation exists.

Federal level changes to the Health Insurance Portability and Accountability Act of 1996 (HIPAA) may need to be addressed as the Act may be perceived as a potential barrier to a wider adoption of telehealth. HIPAA regulations have built-in violations for not using secure communication that are compliant with HIPAA. For example, platforms like Google Meet, FaceTime, and Zoom are not secure platforms, but during the pandemic regulations were eased to enable the use of these platforms. Another issue that needs to be revisited in the HIPAA regulations is the challenges that come along with partner companies who are unwilling to sign privacy agreements (Shachar et al., 2020).

Lastly, credentialing criteria is used, which verifies information related to the qualifications of a healthcare practitioner. While each hospital has the responsibility for the credentialing process, that information is submitted to the Centers for Medicare & Medicaid Services (CMS) as a condition of participation (CoP) and is a defining part of accrediting bodies such as The Joint Commission (TJC) or Det Norske Veritas (DNV).

NURSING LEADER COMPETENCIES

Nurse leaders are in a pivotal position when the discussion arises about telehealth as they are at the forefront of patient care and safety. Opportunities exist for the nurse leader to be at the forefront of creation of telehealth devices, nursing workflows, legislation, patient care, policy development, and input into device selection. Nurse leaders are poised to make decisions and plans that will change the care of patients. In 2015, the American Organization for Nursing Leadership (AONL) provided seven competencies for information management and technology:

- Use technology to support improvement of clinical and financial performance.
- Collaborate to prioritize for the establishment of information technology resources.
- Participate in evaluation of enabling technology in practice settings.
- Use data management systems for decision-making.
- Identify technological trends, issues, and new developments as they apply to patient care.
- Demonstrate skills in assessing data integrity and quality.
- Provide leadership for the adoption and implementation of information systems.

Nurse informatics is a specialty that has emerged over the last 25 years to assist nurses in fully integrating technology with patient care. The ANA (2014) scope and standards defines "nursing informatics" as managing communications, nursing science, computer technology, data, and information to inform nursing care delivery. They add a specialized knowledge that helps support nurses and nursing leaders through suggestions for electronic documentation and interoperability, nursing workflow-eliminating redundant documentation, assisting with collection and analysis of big data, health education, and incorporation of new patient care devices.

The American Association of Colleges of Nursing (AACN) also identifies 10 points in Domain 8: Informatics and Healthcare Technologies (see www.aacnnursing.org/AACN-Essentials). Lastly, Quality and Safety Education for Nurses (QSEN) describe nursing informatics competency as "Use information and technology to communicate, manage knowledge, mitigate error, and support decision making" (see https://oadn.org/resource/qsen-competency-5-informatics/). Each professional organization describes the importance of communication, advocacy for patients, and data management for patient care.

FUTURE CONSIDERATIONS

There is no question that telehealth will continue to rapidly grow in the future.

Telehealth will continue to redesign healthcare in ways that have not been experienced in generations before. Telehealth has enabled connections to 24-hour care, in the comfort of an individual's home. Vital statistics can be sent via the internet to tele-ICUs, home care monitoring agencies, or primary care providers. The cost of technology is now within the reach of the general population, to the point that individuals can do home sonograms, perform three-dimensional printing, transmit vital statistics, call for help, and receive instant information through a search on the internet. The greatest health promotion activities are connected to wearable devices that track exercise, steps, nutrition, stress reduction, sleep, and heart rhythms.

The future of telehealth will enable increased access to specialists, reduce hospital admissions, and provide improved patient outcomes. Healthcare will move from the traditional brick-and-mortar buildings of hospitals to care delivery at home, avoiding costly ED visits. The availability of telehealth visits will potentially reduce the number of missed or cancelled appointments. Data analytics will assist with addressing social determinants of health (SDOH) concerns as well as inform population health.

There are some barriers that need to be addressed such as federal and state regulations in regard to licensure and payment, as well as access to services. Internet and hardware costs need to be taken into consideration from both a clinician and a patient perspective. The pandemic helped to propel the conversations regarding some of the barriers, but more work needs to be done. Research and development along with dissemination of data analytics related to telehealth need to be widely shared. The consumer voice will be an important component not only to successful outcomes, but also changing outcomes, leading to healthier individuals. As healthcare providers and consumers, one thing we need to remain sensitive to is electronic technology fatigue. While telehealth has opened a whole new chapter in patient care, we need to not lose sight of the personal touch that comes along with caring for human beings.

● | CASE SCENARIO

SETTING UP NURSING WORKFLOW TO ADDRESS TELEHEALTH

SITUATION

NS is a nursing leader in an outpatient clinic. NS has noted that 2 million people in New York State, or 12.3% of the population, have diabetes; and more than 500,000 have diabetes but are unaware of their status. Diabetes rates in New York City vary by neighborhood and borough; for example, the Fordham/Bronx Park (14.6%) neighborhoods where NS works in the ambulatory clinic have the highest rates. The borough of the Bronx has a hospitalization rate of 553.8 per 100,000 for diabetes-related conditions as compared with the statewide average of 386.2 per 100,000. The health system serves more than 50,000 adults with diabetes as well as many adults who are at risk of developing the disease.

APPROACH

NS has decided that they would like to introduce a telehealth program for diabetic patients. This program would incorporate a variety of technology.

OUTCOME

NS is seeking to reduce the complications associated with diabetes and plans to measure the outcomes through glucose control (HgBA1C), diet and exercise, and medication management adherence. NS is looking to reduce complications to the statewide average and will be focusing on the geographical location of the Bronx, New York.

DISCUSSION QUESTIONS

1. What are some of the telehealth options that will assist NS, and what data outcomes would be most effective?

2. As an intervention, telemedicine is an economical and effective way to provide care to many patients. What considerations would you have regarding establishing this program among low- and middle-income patients?

◆ WHAT EVERY NURSE MANAGER NEEDS TO KNOW ABOUT TELEHEALTH

Nurse managers are at a pivotal point when it comes to telehealth. There are a multitude of competencies and need-to-know elements of information on telehealth that should be a component of the work environment (Rutledge et al., 2021). Nurse managers are a conduit between the healthcare leadership, nursing caregivers, and the patients.

WHAT EVERY NURSE MANAGER NEEDS TO KNOW

- Use information and technology to communicate, manage knowledge, mitigate error, and support decision-making.
- Identify best evidence and practices for the application of information and communication technologies to support care.
- Manage and establish communication expectations among the nursing caregivers, patients, and local leadership.
- Recognize and support interoperability.

◆ WHAT EVERY NURSE EXECUTIVE NEEDS TO KNOW ABOUT TELEHEALTH

Nurse executives need to be at the table in any discussion or suggestion of changes, additions, and deletions of telehealth technology. Nurses are extremely innovative, and feedback on their experiences or potential workarounds are essential in improving the process. Nurse executives are instrumental and should focus on four key areas: engagement, communication, financial, and evaluation.

WHAT EVERY NURSE EXECUTIVE NEEDS TO KNOW

Engagement

- Be aware of the importance of nursing engagement in the planning, selection, and evaluation of healthcare technologies.
- Work with technology firms to share innovative nursing ideas for product development.
- Inform local, state, and federal authorities regarding legislation changes and payor changes.

Communication

- Use information and communication technologies in accordance with ethical, legal, professional, and regulatory standards, as well as workplace policies in the delivery of care.
- Provide feedback regarding telehealth processes and workarounds.
- Request technology that will aid in outcomes or improved nursing workflows.

Financial

- Explore the fiscal impact of information and communication technologies on healthcare.
- Create budgets that are inclusive of technology costs (direct and indirect).
- Approximate the cost of not engaging in telehealth solutions.

Evaluation

- Evaluate the use of technology to improve consumer health information literacy.
- Evaluate the unintended consequences of information and communication technologies on care processes, communications, and information flow across care settings.
- Become facile with big data and meaningful reporting.

KEY POINTS

- Telehealth is not a new concept, but it has been readily adapted because of cost-effective technology.
- Four distinct types of telehealth modalities are live videoconferencing, store and forward, RPM, and MHEALTH.
- Nursing professional organizations have established competencies for nurse leaders regarding use of technology, including engagement in process; knowledge regarding terminology and functionality; application of big data; and workflow and security of health information.
- Telehealth is an adjunctive method for engaging people in the care of their health.
- Data obtained from EMRs needs to be utilized to inform nursing care in the future.

SUMMARY

Telehealth has been around in healthcare in a variety of formats for many years, most notably having a particular use in rural geographical regions. The COVID-19 pandemic helped to quickly ignite a wider transition to telehealth. With the mandates of social distancing and healthcare services closed, practitioners and patients established new ways of communicating through televisits. These new communication formats were done via telephone or videoconferencing. The quick switch to this type of care required multiple changes and new challenges for the clinicians. Clinicians had to learn about technology, use new equipment, revisit ways to maintain confidentiality, and depend on internet connectivity. Although movement to telehealth services expands the number of available providers, there remains a concern for access to care for some individuals who may not have internet or devices to participate in a visit.

Telehealth also provided many changes to clinician workflow. Clinicians had to change their skills assessment to be more mindful of different cues, specifically auditory and visual, that may assist with diagnosis, treatment, level of understanding, and overall patient care. Workflow changes may need to be made around scheduling and managing appointments, education of the employees to deliver telehealth services, and supporting patients with disabilities through their visit (Koivunen & Saranto, 2018).

Access to technology and platforms that are well connected are items that need to be addressed prior to and throughout telehealth. With all upgrades, browser changes, and new software programs, testing needs to be completed to ensure no disruption in service.

The availability of technology experts or IT help desks will assist in mitigating challenges faced by both providers and patients. Access to high-speed internet remains a challenge that the federal government is working to address by offering access to low-cost government programs.

Nurse leaders and care providers will need experience with large data sets so that clinical determinants of health and SDOH can be better addressed in the community. EMRs and wearable technology will assist providers, payors, and other stakeholders to support population health initiatives. Some information that can be included in healthcare data sets are medical/surgical information, various measurements, demographics, assessments, financial/insurance data, and community-specific disease management. Using big data and analytics can improve patient care at the local level, serve to inform about detection of disease earlier, and monitor the quality of healthcare institutions.

END-OF-CHAPTER RESOURCES

⬡ DISCUSSION QUESTIONS

1. What is your personal experience with telehealth and wearable technology?
2. To what extent are healthcare services in your area providing telehealth and remote monitoring options and does this benefit the patient population?
3. Describe some of the risks and opportunities that can arise with telehealth and how, as nursing leaders, we can address them.
4. As a nursing leader, what tactics would you use to engage nursing employees to utilize telehealth?

⬡ ADDITIONAL RESOURCES

- American Association of Critical Care Nurses: https://www.aacn.org/nursing-excellence/standards/aacn-teleicu-nursing-consensus-statement
- American Organization of Nursing Leaders: https://www.aonl.org/system/files/media/file/2019/06/nec.pdf
- American Nurses Association: https://www.himss.org/sites/hde/files/File Downloads/ANA%20NI%20Scope%20%26%20Standards%20of%20Practice.pdf

PODCASTS

- See You Now Podcast: https://nursing.jnj.com/see-you-now-podcast
- Telehealth 20 Podcast: https://soundcloud.com/telehealth20/tracks
- Telehealth Talk: https://blog.feedspot.com/telehealth_podcasts/#:~:text=learntelehealth.org/sctrc-po
- My Telehealth Podcasts: https://www.southcarolinapublicradio.org/podcast/my-telehealth-podcasts
- Therapy Tech With Rob and Roy: https://therapytechrobroy.com/episodes-pag
- Healthcare NOW Radio: https://www.audible.com/pd/Healthcare-NOW-Radio-Podcast-Network-Discussions-on-healthcare-including-technology-innovation-policy-data-security-telehealth-and-more-Podcast/B08K58GC2G
- Voices in Healthcare Finance: https://podcasts.apple.com/us/podcast/hfmas-voices-in-healthcare-finance/id1102859089

TED TALKS

- The COVID-19 Telehealth Accelerator: https://www.ted.com/talks/jack_miner_the_covid_19_telehealth_accelerator
- Nurse Innovation: Saving the Future of Healthcare | Rebecca Love: https://www.youtube.com/watch?v=IPBcRW8NQPY&t=6s
- VR and Telehealth Could Transform Diagnosis and Treatment of Concussion: https://www.ted.com/talks/jennifer_reneker_vr_and_telehealth_could_transform_diagnosis_and_treatment_of_concussion

WEBLINKS

- American Telemedicine Association: https://www.americantelemed.org
- National Telehealth Technology Assessment Resource Center: https://telehealthtechnology.org
- Healthcare Informatics: https://www.himss.org/resources/healthcare-informatics
- Online Journal of Nursing Informatics: https://www.himss.org/resources/online-journal-nursing-informatics

◆ LEARNING EXERCISES FOR STUDENTS

1. Download and use a health app and review your data stored on the device after 2 weeks.
2. Participate in an IT committee meeting.
3. Review organizational downtime procedures and make some suggestions for additions.
4. Visit the Healthcare Informatics website (Healthcare Information and Management Systems Society [HIMSS]; American Medical Informatics Association [AMIA]; American Telemedicine Association [ATA]; International Council of Nurses [ICN]; International Society for Telemedicine and eHealth [ISfTeH]) and review the mission and focus of the organization.
5. Visit policy driven sites (Health Resources and Services Administration-Office for the Advancement of Teleheath [HRSA-OAT]; Certified Correctional Health Professional [CCHP]) and review one policy statement about telehealth.
6. Participate in a telehealth visit.
7. Review position statements from nursing professional organizations and compare/contrast to current practices in your work environment.

◆ GLOSSARY OF KEY TERMS

- **Business continuity plan (BCP):** A formal process of instructions and procedures that enable a healthcare setting to respond to internal or external disasters and emergencies that may affect the electronic systems with ongoing continuity of information. Also known as a disaster or recovery plan.
- **Database:** Structured data held in a computer that can be accessed in a variety of ways.
- **Electronic medical record (EMR):** A digital record of any assessments or documents that would be in a paper chart, such as chief complaint, medical/surgical history, medications, consents, immunizations, or patient physical, psychological, or psychosocial health information, in addition to payment information.

- **Firewall:** Part of a computer and network security system that is designed to block unauthorized access while permitting legitimate communication. Firewalls can be hardware, software, or both.

- **Hardware:** Includes physical parts of a computer and related devices; for example, the case, monitor, central processing unit (CPU), mouse, keyboard, and speakers.

- **Informatics:** The science of process data for storage and retrieval; information science on how to use data, information, and knowledge to improve healthcare services.

- **Internet:** Global computer network that provides information and communication through interconnected networks using standardized communication protocols.

- **Telehealth:** Provision of healthcare services remotely by means of a telecommunication strategy.

- **Telemedicine:** Remote diagnosing and treatment of persons by means of a telecommunication technology.

- **Software:** Programs and other operating systems used by a computer.

- **Wearable technology:** Electronic devices that are worn as accessories, embedded in clothing or shoes, implanted in the body, or tattooed on the skin.

A robust set of instructor resources designed to supplement this text is located at http://connect.springerpub.com/content/book/978-0-8261-7795-7. Qualifying instructors may request access by emailing textbook@springerpub.com.

REFERENCES

American Hospital Association. (2022). *Fact sheet: Telehealth.* https://www.aha.org/factsheet/telehealth

American Nurses Association. (2014). *Nursing informatics: Scope and standards for practice* (2nd ed.). Author.

Benshoter, R. (1967). Multipurpose television. *Annals of the New York Academy of Sciences, 142,* 471–477. https://doi.org/10.1111/j.1749-6632.1967.tb14360.x

Brown, P., Oliver, E., & Harrison Dening, K. (2020). Increasing need for telehealth services for families affected by dementia as a result of COVID-19. *Journal of Community Nursing, 34*(5), 59–64. https://www.jcn.co.uk/journals/issue/10-2020/article/increasing-need-for-telehealth-services-for-families-affected-by-dementia-as-a-result-of-covid-19

Keenan, A. J., Tsourtos, G., & Tieman, J. (2021). The value of applying ethical principles in telehealth practices, *Systematic Review Journal Medical Internet Research, 23*(3), e25698. https://doi.org/10.2196/25698

Koivunen, M., & Saranto, K. (2018). Nursing professionals' experiences of the facilitators and barriers to the use of telehealth applications: A systematic review of qualitative studies. *Scandinavian Journal of Caring Sciences, 32*(1), 24–44. https://doi.org/10.1111/scs.12445

Kumar, M. S., Krishnamurthy, S., Dhruve, N., Somashekar, B., & Gowda, M. R. (2020). Telepsychiatry netiquette. Connect, communicate, consult. *Indian Journal of Psychology Medicine, 42*(5 Suppl.), 22S–26S. https://doi.org/10.1177/0253717620958170

Mataxen, P. A., & Webb, L. D. (2019). Telehealth nursing: More than just a phone call. *Nursing2020, 49*(4), 11–13. https://doi.org/10.1097/01.NURSE.0000553272.16933.4b

Nickelson, D. W. (1998). Telehealth and the evolving health care system: Strategic opportunities for professional psychology. *Professional Psychology, Research and Practice, 29*(6), 527–535. https://doi.org/10.1037/0735-7028.29.6.527

Rutledge, C. M., O'Rourke, J., Mason, A. M., Chike-Harris, K., Behnke, L., Melhado, L., Downes, L., & Gustin, T. (2021). Telehealth competencies for nursing education and practice: The four P's of telehealth. *Nurse Educator, 46*(5), 300. https://doi.org/10.1097/NNE.0000000000000988

Shachar, C., Engel, J., & Elwyn, G. (2020). Implications for telehealth in a postpandemic future: Regulatory and privacy issues. *JAMA, 323*(23), 2375–2376. https://doi.org/10.1001/jama.2020.7943

Smith, T. S., Watts, P., & Moss, J. A. (2018). Using simulation to teach telehealth nursing competencies. *Journal of Nursing Education, 57*(10), 624–627. https://doi.org/10.3928/01484834-20180921-10

Totten, A. M., Womack, D. M., Eden, K. B., McDonagh, M. S., Griffin, J. C., Grusing, S., & Hersh, W. R. (2016). *Telehealth: Mapping the evidence for patient outcomes from systematic reviews*. Technical Brief No. 26. (Prepared by the Pacific Northwest Evidence-Based Practice Center Under Contract No. 290-2015-00009-I.) AHRQ Publication No.16-EHC034-EF. Agency for Healthcare Research and Quality.

U.S. Department of Health and Human Services. (2021). *What is telehealth?* Retrieved July 17, 2022, from https://telehealth.hhs.gov/patients/understanding-telehealth/

CHAPTER 11

INNOVATION

Cole Edmonson and Tim Raderstorf

*"You can design and create and build the most wonderful place in the world.
But it takes people to make the dream a reality."*

Walt Disney

LEARNING OBJECTIVES

- Demonstrate an understanding of the innovation continuum and how to develop a culture of innovation.
- Apply the concept of innovation to healthcare and the nursing profession.
- Critique the core competencies of innovation as they relate to the role of nurse leaders and nurse executives.
- Investigate how different leadership styles and system structures influence innovation.

INTRODUCTION

Innovation in nursing has deep historical roots beginning in the 1800s with Florence Nightingale and her leadership in reducing infections among soldiers in the Crimea and influencing health outcomes by addressing causes of infections and creating healing environments in healthcare settings (Sheingold & Hahn, 2014). Innovative practice changes have historically centered around improving patient care quality and health outcomes. As technology burgeons and patient care delivery systems and reimbursement models evolve, innovation continues to broaden in depth, scope, and focus to address efficiency, effectiveness, consumer-centric care partnerships, and value-based economic outcomes.

Emerging global diseases and trends, transformation of care environments, technology advances, health disparities, and population health concerns continue to challenge all healthcare professionals and have specific implications for nurses in all roles and settings. The global coronavirus (COVID-19) pandemic posed challenges for nurses unlike any previously encountered in our lifetimes. Unlike various natural or manmade disasters that, while devastating, are time-limited, this pandemic disease crisis has lasted more than 2 years, testing communities and healthcare professionals across the globe in ways never dreamed possible.

Nurses are well positioned to respond to emerging challenges, lead innovation, and transform care delivery models and environments. As the largest healthcare profession with the greatest direct contact with patients, nurses have substantive big picture knowledge and perspectives about care delivery systems and what patients and caregivers need. Nurses also have tremendous practical understanding of how things work in their settings and are acutely aware of factors that pose challenges or lead to failures. Nurses do not typically view themselves as innovators, yet they constantly employ workarounds and find solutions to the most perplexing patient care problems in their environments. The same is true for frontline nurses, who do not view themselves as leaders despite the reality that they consistently lead at the point of care, often making tough or even unorthodox decisions to implement actions in the best interest of patients and families in their care. Nurse leaders and educators have an enormous responsibility to educate undergraduate and graduate students and nurses at all levels about their roles as innovators, and to help them develop skill sets and empower them with confidence and autonomy to embrace and deploy innovation.

Nurse executives and leaders have a key responsibility to create and support cultures of innovation. First and foremost, these leaders must work collaboratively with interprofessional healthcare leaders to provide the infrastructure to inspire and sustain cultures of innovation. Infrastructures include policies and standards, shared governance, human and financial resources, and an organizational climate that supports risk taking and disruptive innovation, allows failure, facilitates learning communities, and promotes autonomy.

This chapter is devoted to nurse leader and executive roles and responsibilities in innovation and provides case studies as examples of successful, sustainable structures of innovation led by nurse executives in healthcare organizations. The authors also review leaders' roles and responsibilities in fostering and supporting innovation and provide practical implementation strategies, tactics, and actions leaders can apply and adapt to their respective settings and roles.

DEFINING INNOVATION

Nurse leaders and executives must first understand basic definitions of innovation and how innovation can be applied in their roles and settings. Based on the information presented earlier and your personal experience, take a moment to reflect on what innovation means to you. Consider what you know and understand about innovation, its characteristics, and who should be engaged in assuming responsibility for the entire innovation cycle from idea through implementation and outcome.

Moving forward, compare your definition, experience, and understanding of innovation with the following. Innovation is the process of implementing new products, services, or solutions in ways that create new value (Melnyk & Raderstorf, 2021). Simply stated, innovation is creating new value. As we continue through this chapter, we encourage the reader to constantly challenge the assumptions that we make. How do the topics we discuss add new value? Take the initiative to apply these topics to your vast professional experience to determine where innovation applies to your practice and how you can leverage innovation to maximize your impact.

THE *NOVATION DYNAMIC*

As you look to maximize your impact in healthcare, examining the *Novation Dynamic* (Ackerman et al., 2020) will shine light on what changes can be made to create new value. The *Novation Dynamic* (Figure 11.1) showcases how innovation, renovation, and exnovation (or de-implementation) are all related. At the heart of each of these issues is understanding a *gap* that exists. In this dynamic, the "gap" refers to an opportunity that exists. When there is a gap between what is known and what is needed, *innovation-based practice* is the pathway to creating new value. If a gap exists, no current solution is readily available, so some product, service, or solution must be produced to generate value.

Yet there are times when a product is readily available, but that product does not fully address the problem at hand. When the gap occurs within an existing solution that needs improvement, *renovation* is required. Making strategic changes to an existing solution can maximize impact while reducing the cost and time to market compared to innovation and starting from scratch. The challenge for leaders is to determine if the renovation will result in lasting change, or if the renovations will be required regularly to address the issue. If regular renovations are needed, exnovation should be considered as a next step, before proceeding to innovation-based practice.

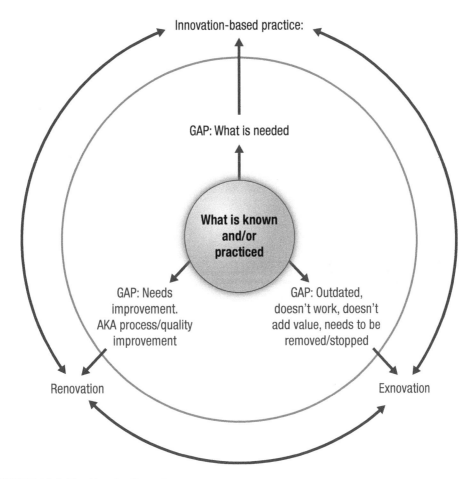

FIGURE 11.1: The *Novation Dynamic.*

Does the gap occur because a product, service, or solution is outdated, or is the solution of choice purely because it maintains the status quo of doing things the way they have always been done; if so, *exnovation* is the path to value. With exnovation, a decision is made to remove a product, service, or solution from practice, thus allowing for a path to innovation, while eliminating unnecessary work. Exnovation may be the most challenging aspect of the *Novation Continuum*, as leaders struggle to remove solutions that may have worked in the past with hope that they will become successful once again. It is imperative for leaders to continually seek opportunities to exnovate to ensure their teams can maximize their potential.

WHAT'S THE DIFFERENCE BETWEEN INNOVATION AND ENTREPRENEURSHIP?

The terms "innovation" and "entrepreneurship" are used so frequently together that sometimes they are used as the acronym I&E. This is not to say that innovation and entrepreneurship are the same thing but rather to showcase their interconnectivity. The key distinction between innovation and entrepreneurship is the intent of the innovator, the person leading innovation. As discussed earlier, innovation is the process of implementing new products, services, or solutions that create new value. Entrepreneurship is the process of implementing new products, services, or solutions that create new value for the intention of generating profits. So head-to-head, innovation is creating new value, and entrepreneurship is creating new value with the intent of profit. It is important to note that it is the *intent of generating profit*, not the act of generating profit itself, as entrepreneurship is extremely challenging and profits are equally as hard to generate. Intrapreneurship is also a salient concept to understand in this description when contrasting innovation to entrepreneurism, since in many organizational settings nurse employees viewed as entrepreneurs are more likely intrapreneurs. Intrapreneurs take risks to solve problems and improve care delivery and health outcomes within organizational structures and without taking personal financial risks. While their actions may generate profit for an organization, their goals are focused on improving patient and work environment outcomes (Wilson et al., 2012), and profitability is not central to their intent or actions.

INNOVATION COMPETENCIES

Before diving into the concepts of leading innovation within organizations, it is imperative for leaders to first understand the innovator within themselves. Pillay and Morris (2016, p. 398) have identified 19 innovation competencies showcasing how innovation is truly a universal language of leadership. These 19 competencies are:

1. Opportunity recognition
2. Conveying a compelling vision/seeing the future
3. Maintain focus/adapt
4. Resilience
5. Interdisciplinary teamwork and collaboration
6. Opportunity assessment
7. Building and using networks
8. Self-efficacy/confidence
9. Tenacity and perseverance
10. Understanding of healthcare systems
11. Ability to leverage resources/bootstrapping
12. Risk management/mitigation
13. Creativity problem-solving/imaginativeness
14. Guerilla skills/unconventional approaches
15. Design thinking
16. Change management
17. Cross-disciplinary knowledge
18. Information management
19. Behavioral economics

While some of these concepts or terms may seem foreign to nurses, once defined, the parallels between these innovation competencies and common nursing terminology become evident. For example, "behavioral economics" is simply defined by Pillay and Morris (2016) as understanding the reasons why people make decisions. As nurses, we regularly place extended effort in understanding why a patient may or may not be able to take a prescribed medication or attend a follow-up appointment—perhaps the drug is too expensive or they do not have transportation to the appointment. And as leaders, we are regularly evaluating ways to motivate our teams to function at their highest potential—and pizza parties will only go so far. Therefore, nurses are regularly engaging in behavioral economics, but often recognize it by other terms (or do not name it at all).

Even more interesting, when these innovation competencies are displayed side-by-side with the nursing process (assessment, diagnose, plan, implement, evaluate [ADPIE]), it is clear to see how these two separate frameworks nearly mirror each other (Figure 11.2). Opportunity recognition, opportunity assessment, understanding systems, and utilizing design thinking are all listed within the innovation concepts. Yet they, too, directly relate to the "assess" paradigm within the nursing process.

Comparing the nursing process to the innovation competencies is depicted graphically in Figure 11.2, but a brief explanation of these relationships provides additional context for the comparison.

- **Assessment:** The assessment provides opportunities for individuals and teams to identify and describe opportunities for innovation; for instance, to solve recurring problems or improve quality outcomes, while gaining an understanding how healthcare system structures and processes may either prevent or support proposed innovations.

- **Diagnose:** The diagnostic phase is a complex process where the team needs to stay focused on specifics and desired outcomes, learning from interprofessional perspectives and adapting to failures along the way. Diagnosis also involves the collective team ability to design uncharted methods and plans that do not use traditional conventional approaches to achieve desired results. Individual and team resilience are key to

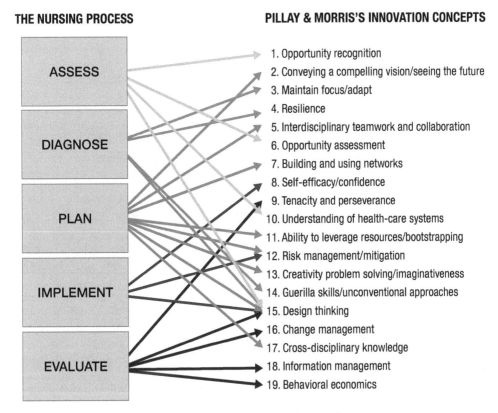

FIGURE 11.2: The nursing process compared and how it relates to the innovation competencies.

Source: © Tim Raderstorf (2021).

this process and the commitment to hear and value diverse perspectives and see the project through to fruition.

■ **Plan:** The key foundational aspect of the innovation planning process is presenting a compelling vision and coming to team consensus about the future of what is possible with the proposed innovation, creating a shared vision. Garnering leadership support, creating a diverse interprofessional collaborative team, while tapping into internal and external resources are necessary building blocks for successful implementation. Understanding the risks and benefits and weighing the risk-to-benefit ratio requires intention, cross-disciplinary understanding, and true collaboration. Team members also need to consider stakeholders' perspectives that are not represented on the team.

■ **Implement:** Each interprofessional team member must possess confidence and a history of self-efficacy for the innovation to be successful, since the implementation phase may be faced with challenges, barriers, pushbacks, and failures. At each step during the process, the team continues to assess risks and benefits and redesign specific elements based on team input, unforeseen problems, and progress toward goals.

■ **Evaluate:** First, team members must possess tenacity and perseverance and commit to the process involved. Sustainable innovation is not a quick fix nor a short-term process. As previously noted, the ability to design and redesign are key to any innovation's success and sustainability. Innovations evolve based on real-world applications and environments. Information management resources are crucial to document, communicate, and objectively evaluate project outcomes, whether the innovation directly involves technology. Part of the evaluation process also relates to behavioral economics, as previously described. Understanding the reasons why those implementing the innovation made decisions not to follow the protocol or plan is important to redesign.

Even with a clear relationship between the nursing process and innovation competencies, the nursing profession has not done enough to prepare nurses to lead innovation within systems. A recent study has shown that while nurse leaders view all 19 of these innovation competencies as vitally important to the advancement of the profession, they only felt that they were proficient in leading one (White et al., 2016). Take a moment to look back at those 19 competencies and make your guess as to which one nurse leaders felt they had mastered. If you guessed "tenacity and perseverance," give yourself a round of applause. Nurses felt extremely competent in demonstrating tenacity and perseverance because in healthcare we operate within complex systems that are often broken. While having tenacity and perseverance are incredibly important characteristics for any professional, having it be the only innovation concept that is widely demonstrated in nursing poses a problem.

MOVING FROM RESILIENCE TO AMBITION

Resilience is one of Pillay and Morris's innovation competencies that nurses surely have become very familiar with, as resilience has been widely promoted as a key determinant to reducing clinician burnout. Resilience is a very important factor for both bedside clinicians and healthcare leaders. Yet it is essential that we do not see resilience as this magic bullet that will solve all our issues.

The key problem with resilience is that while it does acknowledge that the system is inherently flawed, it places the burden on the individual to cope with the system's failures. Instead of addressing the flaws within the system, the individual is asked to change to adapt to the brokenness of the system; in other words, to be resilient and to accept the environment in which they work. With resilience, there is no empowerment for the individual; there is only the option to adapt or be swallowed up by the broken system.

Instead of focusing on resilience as the key approach to working within complex systems, leaders should instead consider pairing resilience with ambition to help both individuals and teams overcome the complexities of the systems in which they work. Just as in resilience, ambition recognizes that the system is broken. The key difference here is that ambition then empowers the individual to change the system instead of changing themselves. Building a culture of ambition combines the best of resilience with the notion that the people on the front lines who understand the problems being faced most frequently should have the power, resources, and autonomy to make the changes our systems so desperately need to succeed.

CULTURES OF INNOVATION

Creating and sustaining innovation cultures in healthcare involves first understanding the innovation continuum and cycle, organizational readiness to value and embrace innovation, and the infrastructures necessary for supporting innovation. Kahan (2021) describes the innovation continuum as ranging from "incremental" to "truly transformational," also known as disruptive. While many organizations readily accept incremental change that addresses problems and improves efficiency and effectiveness, valuing transformative innovation is a far greater leap for organizations. Incremental change is also a rapid cycle process that often involves problem-solving and trial and error on a small scale and may not be duplicatable or sustainable over time. Incremental changes implemented in the moment in response to situations in specific settings or populations also may not be generalizable. On the other end of the innovation continuum, innovators challenge traditional ways of being and doing in organizations to find creative solutions and design new ways forward, questioning policies, practices, and rituals along the way. Leaders are not always comfortable with significant disruption to the status quo.

In addition to understanding the innovation continuum, nurse leaders must have knowledge of their organizations' infrastructures and resources that either support or limit various levels of innovation and the readiness to enable innovation to grow, thrive, and flourish along the continuum in their settings.

Cooperrider's (2012) appreciative inquiry tenets create a foundation for innovation thinking, design, and implementation. Appreciative inquiry is based on the 4-D (discovery, dream, design, destiny) cycle aimed at moving away from "negative, deficit-focused" organizational behaviors to creating "positive, strengths-based" approaches to change. The 4-D cycle encourages individuals and teams to look at their strengths, learn from the past, and carry elements of what works forward into their new designs, while identifying what their ideal would look like. The destiny phase of the cycle "empowers, learns, and improvises" to influence sustainability. These tenets have been applied broadly in high-performing, successful corporations, far beyond healthcare, to create and sustain positive, innovative cultures.

Healthcare settings have traditionally been problem-oriented and deficit-focused. Shifting that paradigm is essential to promoting design thinking, creativity, and innovation. May and colleagues (2011) authored a toolkit and practical guide for healthcare organizations and leaders to use in facilitating strengths-based interprofessional team collaboration in finding creative solutions to challenges in care delivery and quality outcomes. Armstrong and colleagues (2020) describe ways that organizations can integrate appreciative inquiry and an appreciative mindset in the face of emerging challenges such as the COVID pandemic to identify strengths, build and sustain collaborative relationships, inspire curiosity, move toward opportunities, and meet future challenges with realistic optimism.

Naca-Abell (2020) describes positive implications of applying appreciative inquiry principles and strategies in a clinical setting to improve interprofessional team relationships and collaboration and improve performance. The author discusses the use of storytelling and sharing experiences to increase team members' understanding of individual and collective strengths, knowledge, and perspectives and focuses on similarities and shared vision rather than differences,

In 2016, Cianelli and colleagues published a "roadmap" for nurse leaders to drive innovation. They describe the characteristics of innovation that include "divergent thinking, risk taking, failure tolerance, agility and flexibility and autonomy and freedom" (p. 6). The authors go on to say, "Being willing to tolerate and learn from failure is a foundation of the innovative organization" (p. 9). The authors describe events such as infectious disease outbreaks and disasters and system and equipment malfunctions as those that provide ripe opportunities for frontline nurses and nurse leaders to improve their agility and flexibility.

Cianelli and colleagues (2016) outline and describe in depth numerous infrastructure components necessary for building, supporting, and sustaining cultures of innovation in healthcare organizations, including, but not limited to, role modeling, employee feedback and engagement, education, protected time, technological support, rewards, leadership, and financial resources.

Engaging nurses in innovation in all roles and settings is foundational to successful innovation cultures. The American Nurses Association (ANA; 2019) reports that nurses constitute the greatest number of healthcare professionals in clinical environments, are the most frequent end users of clinical technology and systems, and bring practical real-world knowledge, expertise, and perspectives to care delivery needs and systems. While nurses in clinical settings frequently do workarounds and implement creative solutions to problems, educators and nurse leaders need to facilitate frontline nurses to share their experiences and learn to view themselves as the true innovators they are. Organizational leaders also need to provide and support innovation labs that offer opportunities for research and development. Organizational innovation labs and resource allocation promote and support design thinking, allow for failure and learning, and are essential components of innovative cultures. Transforming healthcare requires organizational leaders and interprofessional teams to collaboratively work together and think differently to design, implement, and evaluate innovations, forging new efficient, effective ways forward.

LEADERSHIP IN INNOVATION CULTURES

Leadership in innovation cultures requires many of the same traits necessary for leading evidence-based practice and research cultures. Melnyk and Raderstorf (2021) point out that leaders must make evidence-based decisions in innovative cultures, despite that often evidence is lacking for creative solutions identified to solve the problems organizations face. A basic tenet in evidence-based cultures is curiosity. Leaders need to be curious and reward curiosity and a spirit of inquiry in their team members and employees. These authors address broad areas of current trends filled with opportunities for innovation, including preventable errors, employee burnout, economic returns on investment, mental health and opioid crises, chronic illness epidemics, social determinants of health (SDOH), and the need for "so what outcomes," to name a few. They go on to point out that few healthcare start-ups are initiated by those with clinical knowledge and expertise. No doubt nurse leaders can identify numerous additional areas of opportunity for improvement in their organizations that lend themselves to innovation. All too often, technology, equipment, supply, care delivery models, and other clinical decisions and changes are not driven by end users with the greatest first-hand knowledge of associated problems, workflow effects, and overall effectiveness resulting from the change.

Communication is also a key component of successfully leading innovation with an emphasis on *listening* and adopting less directive and more collaborative leadership styles. Leaders need to be comfortable with risk taking and learning from failures, diverse perspectives and approaches, and autonomous thinking and action, while supporting these behaviors in their team members and employees. For innovation to be successful in organizations, hierarchical and transactional leadership styles must be replaced with transformational, collaborative ones. Leaders in successful innovation cultures are comfortable with role modeling, mentoring, and coaching others. These transformational leaders serve as consultants to individuals and teams. Serving as a consultant, mentor, and coach requires tremendous commitment and a unique skill set, and is far more time consuming than transactional, directive approaches.

The American Organization for Nursing Leadership (AONL) defines competencies for nurse executives (2015a) and nurse managers (2015b). While these competencies do not specifically address their roles in innovation, they do address evidence-based leadership, executives' and managers' roles as change agents, and executives' collaboration with academic partners, to name a few, which all contribute to innovation in healthcare environments. Several additional competencies in the areas of communication, organization and community relationships, professional behaviors, technology implementation, and business acumen are also necessary for leading cultures of innovation.

Partnering with academic organizations can provide opportunities for educating students and clinical nurses about their roles in innovation and can design specific initiatives, programs, and projects that focus on developing skills and abilities as innovators. Interprofessional academic partners and programs in engineering and other clinical and nonclinical disciplines can also offer programs and learning labs where interprofessional teams can work together to study processes, define problems, and identify innovative solutions together.

STRUCTURES OF INNOVATION

Building a culture of innovation is extremely important for the success of an organization. However, it is imperative for any leader to understand that a culture of innovation cannot thrive without a proper and formidable *structure of innovation*. In his book *Loonshots* (2019), Safi Bahcall addresses this concept through a phrase that many of you have probably heard before. There is a famous quote attributed to "the father of modern management," business consultant Peter Drucker, which goes something along the lines of *culture eats strategy for breakfast*. Though Bahcall does not challenge this assumption, he has one important addendum: *If culture eats strategy for breakfast, then structure eats culture for dessert.*

What is he getting at? Well, first is the recognition that no matter how strategic you may be as a leader, the culture you create can be a rate limiting step for your success. For sustainability, structure must come into play. Bahcall asserts that your culture's success is bound by the structure in which it is built upon. Culture can change with people coming and going within an organization. From leaders to those working in the trenches, the culture changes almost directly in line as personnel changes if there is no structure of innovation in place. Foundations that make up the structure of innovation include incentives, educational programs, policies, job descriptions, mentoring and coaching programs, partnerships, and innovation centers. With these foundations in place, your culture is more stable and less likely to be impacted by changes within the organization.

INCENTIVES FOR CLINICIANS, MANAGERS, AND LEADERS

Ask yourself this question: What was the first thing I did when I arrived at work today? With that question answered, now think about this: Why was that the first thing I did? Maybe it was grabbing a coffee for a friend or colleague, and you love the way that teamwork and collaboration make you feel. Or maybe it was to do a dressing change for a patient because you knew that action would improve the patient's outcome. It is more than likely that you engaged in that behavior because in some way you were incentivized to do so. Incentives are the greatest predictor of human behavior. We make decisions and take actions because we know what the outcome most likely will be, and we know how we will be rewarded for that behavior. Whether it be through recognition, friendships, or paychecks, humans take action to receive incentives.

In an effort to incentivize clinicians to engage in innovation behaviors, some organizations host pitch competitions where staff share their ideas, and the winners are provided with funding to advance their innovation. But incentives do not always need to take monetary form. To foster innovation behaviors, incentives could also take the form of introductions to collaborators and content experts who can help with the development of prototypes, or access to 3-D printers, laser cutters, or other pieces of technology that can help one turn ideas into actions.

NURSE MANAGERS AND EXECUTIVE LEADERS

While incentives can certainly motivate clinicians to engage in innovation, incentives are also important for nurse leaders and executives. Leading their teams and organizations to accomplish unit, department, service line, and organization quality, safety, and financial goals and outcomes has intrinsic rewards, but may not only be associated with financial incentives. It also offers personal satisfaction and a sense of pride in such achievements. Nurse leaders are responsible for creating cultures of innovation, removing barriers, accessing internal and external resources, and actively supporting clinicians to innovate. Their roles in clinician innovation shift into those of coach, mentor, advisor, consultant, and champion as they encourage and support failure and celebrate successes along the way. These leaders bring expertise, knowledge of organization structure and processes, and financial and operational acumen that support these clinical innovators and lead to successful outcomes for these teams. Their rewards come with satisfaction and a sense of pride derived from each individual and team success.

EDUCATIONAL PROGRAMS

While incentives can change behavior in the short term, there are arguments that incentives may not result in a lasting change in behavior. Therefore, multiple structural components are necessary for innovation to thrive, and a workforce that has been educated on the concepts of innovation is another key element to a structure of innovation. With healthcare and technology advancing at such a rapid pace, it is imperative for organizations to develop regular educational programming that helps their team stay on the cutting edge. There are many examples of organizations that do this well. Examples of innovative structured programs and education initiatives that drive innovation and entrepreneurship follow. First, Rebecca Love, a nurse innovator and entrepreneur, leads Nurse Hackathons at Northeastern University where nurse innovators have opportunities to collaborate with a host of interprofessional colleagues from engineering, medicine, technology, allied health disciplines, and administrators to develop innovative solutions to current challenges in healthcare environments. In her work, Love (2018) emphasizes the importance of shifting nurses' conversations from describing themselves as "just" nurses to being proud of their identities and the knowledge base, abilities, and impact they bring to healthcare. Additionally, Love stresses the importance of embracing the role of innovator and understanding the business side of healthcare. The Society of Nurse Scientists, Innovators, Entrepreneurs, and Leaders (SONSIEL) has partnered with Microsoft and Johnson & Johnson to host biannual Hackathons, connecting nurses and information technology (IT) specialists committed to developing new IT solutions that improve healthcare.

Two additional examples of structured programs that drive innovation in clinical and academic settings are described in the text that follows. The Cleveland Clinic hosts an Annual Nursing Innovation Summit that helps those at the front lines develop skills for innovation leadership while also showcasing innovation projects that have been initiated within the organization.

The Ohio State University College of Nursing delivers two recurring programs focused on innovation leadership and the entrepreneurial mindset. In the fall, they host the Innovation, Design, and Entrepreneurship Amplified (IDEA) Workshop focused on helping clinicians be more innovative in their practice by teaching them entrepreneurial skills such as developing an elevator pitch, developing a personal brand, and creating a business plan. In the spring, the Interprofessional Innovation Symposium teaches the components of design thinking while highlighting a healthcare business that has been founded by both a clinical and nonclinical entrepreneur. The complementary skill sets of these co-founders are examined by the audience and often viewed as a linchpin to their success.

POLICY

Have you ever engaged in a "workaround" for one of your organization's policies? While policy is often what defines the structural framework for innovation within an organization, it is not uncommon for organizations to overlook the important relationship between innovation and policy. As policy dictates how employees behave, it is imperative for leaders to examine when employees are not aligned with organizational policy; this is not to be diminutive and reprimand them for the behavior, but rather to identify weaknesses within the system. Nurse workarounds have increased exponentially with rapidly advancing health information and patient care technology, evolving documentation requirements, and increased complexity in care delivery systems and environments (Seaman & Erlen, 2015).

You see, when individuals engage in a workaround, they are pointing out a flaw within the system. As nurses implement workarounds, they are frequently identifying workflow problems and inefficiencies associated with technology, practice, and policy implementation and changes, and may not be involved in decision-making with organization leaders in policy changes and technology systems implementation. While some leaders may view such workarounds negatively, these nurses are being disruptive innovators. Many such disruptive innovations are implemented to improve processes and efficiency and may lead to improvements in patient safety and quality outcomes. Organizations that recognize this behavior as a positive disruption that identifies the need for change will have a competitive advantage by adapting quickly to this ever-changing environment and set their employees up for success. Additionally, nurse leaders that seek and value nurses' input reduce frontline clinicians' frustration levels and improve their satisfaction, fostering a spirit of innovation in their organizations. Policies must change when workarounds occur, and policy iteration must be a regularly used gadget in the innovation leader's toolbox.

JOB DESCRIPTIONS

Consider your organization's mission, vision, and values. (If you do not have them committed to memory, take time to do a quick search to refresh your memory.) How many times is the word "innovation" listed? It is a wonderful testament that most healthcare organizations now regard innovation as a core tenet of their missions, but one must ask how deeply are the structures that allow innovation to thrive embedded into these statements? Often innovation is postured as a position statement for the entire organization, yet in reality it does not permeate beyond the organization's mission, vision, and values.

One clear way to address the issue of innovation permeation throughout an organization is to add job responsibilities related to innovation to job descriptions. An argument can be made that every position within an organization should have innovation job responsibilities. Others may protest that if innovation becomes the responsibility for everyone, then innovation will be run by no one. Yet as organizations thrive upon the maximization of value, requiring all employees to *create new value* as part of their job descriptions is a clear path to ownership and empowerment to engage in innovation.

CALL TO ACTION

Ask your human resources (HR) team for a copy of your job description and review it to see if innovation is mentioned. If the term is mentioned, examine how clearly innovation work responsibilities are outlined and make recommendations to your supervisor on how you can be supported to advance innovation within your organization.

If the term "innovation" is not mentioned, examine which job responsibilities could be interpreted as innovative. Also consider the gaps that exist between your job responsibilities and the innovation needs for your organization. Make recommendations to your supervisor for alterations to your job description to maximize your impact in leading innovation.

MENTORING AND COACHING

Navigating the complexity of innovative systems is challenging for even the most accomplished innovation leaders. With such complexity, mentoring and coaching are key to helping transfer institutional knowledge and lead to the development of meaningful peer-to-peer relationships within the organization.

To boot, there is ample evidence that showcases these coaching and mentoring programs have a positive impact on not only the mentee, but the mentor as well. These employees are more likely to stay with their organization and report a higher level of job satisfaction (www.mentoring.org). With such impactful outcomes, mentoring and coaching programs are a must have for any organization looking to be a leader in innovation.

PARTNERSHIPS

Surely no one individual can be responsible for all the innovation within their organization, and the same must be true that no organization can take responsibility for all innovation within its sector. The most innovative organizations in the world thrive on partnerships to achieve success. For example, Texas Instruments, before making the best graphing calculator in the world (that you exclusively used to play video games in calculus class), invented the world's first silicon transistor. This transistor went on to be the leading technology behind transistor radios, Texas Instrument's first commercial success, even before calculators. Yet they also partnered with other manufacturers to license their technology so more radios could be made, and more profits generated.

And as Texas Instruments continues to innovate, a recent evolution of their processing chips has led to the creation of portable ultrasound probes that connect to smartphones. By partnering with organizations that incorporate Texas Instruments's products into new devices like smartphones, Texas Instruments continues to evolve while maintaining a competitive advantage as one of the world's top technology companies.

With examples like that, it is easy to understand how partnerships can improve an organization's value. Just think of all the times at the bedside you partnered with another nurse or clinician to improve a patient's outcome. The more work we do together, the more impact we have. Developing pathways for partnerships, from templates for collaboration, to non-disclosure and licensing agreements, all help partners better understand how to engage with organizations. Strategic partnerships open the doors to new possibilities and are a catalyst to impact.

INNOVATION CENTERS

Innovation centers serve as the physical or virtual epicenter for innovation within an organization. However, it is important to understand that these centers are not the sole location where innovation occurs within an organization. Innovation occurs most frequently at the point of pain, where the problem that needs to be solved surfaces. From the bedside to the operating room, clinicians regularly engage with pain points (problems) and develop solutions to ease the pain. That is the point where innovation centers step in to serve as an innovation structure to help propel these solutions by turning ideas into actions.

Innovation centers come in a variety of shapes, sizes, and locations. Some are moveable, some are virtual, and all seek to accelerate the work of those who truly understand the problem trying to be solved the most. Most are the home to prototyping tools like 3D printers, laser cutters, and CNC (Computer Numerical Control) routers, yet it is the people within these locations that determine the success of the center. And it is the policies of the organization that drive engagement and maximize the center's impact.

A number of interprofessional makerspaces have been opened in academic and community healthcare settings where nurses and their colleagues can develop innovative solutions to common care delivery problems. The Robert Wood Johnson Foundation identified a number of these makerspaces across the country, including providing funding for the partnership between MakerNurse and The University of Texas Medical Branch (UTMB) to open the MakerHealth space on a patient care unit at John Sealy Hospital at UTMB (Robert Wood Johnson Foundation, 2015). These spaces provide frontline nurses with readily accessible tools and resources to test their ideas, instead of piecing together materials from supply and equipment closets. Some of the real-time patient care solutions created by nurses include customized dressings and IV shields and specialized clips and methods for securing catheters and tubing.

● | CASE SCENARIO

THE INNOVATION STUDIO

One of the most recognized healthcare innovation centers of the last 5 years is The Innovation Studio at The Ohio State University. Run by the college of nursing, The Innovation Studio is a university-wide initiative dedicated to democratizing innovation for every student, faculty, and staff member. First launching as a moveable makerspace (Figure 11.3), The Innovation Studio travels across campus taking extended residencies of 7 to 10 weeks at high traffic locations. It may take up a residency in the lobby of the hospital, before making its next stop at the

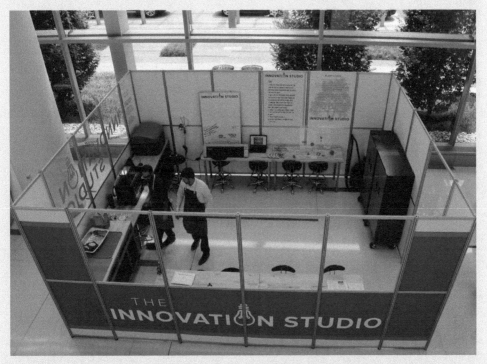

FIGURE 11.3: The Innovation Studio in the lobby of The James Comprehensive Cancer Center.

Source: © Tim Raderstorf (2017).

library. During each stay, The Innovation Studio staff interacts with the students, faculty, and staff that enter the space and encourages them to solve the problems that they run into the most. These innovators then create an interprofessional team to codesign a solution to the problem and consult with The Innovation Studio staff along the way. At the end of The Innovation Studio's extended stay at every location, a pitch day is held for teams to present their ideas and request additional support.

The empowerment to solve the problems that personally impact these teams leads to high levels of buy-in. But the most empowering tool at The Innovation Studio is their policy to *fund each and every team* that pitches their idea on pitch day. As long as teams meet three simple criteria (Figure 11.4), they are guaranteed at least one round of funding from The Innovation Studio. As teams continue to develop their innovation, they are encouraged to return to subsequent pitch days and ask for additional funding and resources to advance their ideas. As long as these teams continue to be good stewards of these resources and achieve the milestones they collectively set with The Innovation Studio staff, they continue to receive support from The Innovation Studio.

This model to fund every team has resulted in over 1,000 students, faculty, and staff submitting ideas to The Innovation Studio in its first 4 years of operating, adding to the evidence that the *ideation rate* is one of the best predictors of return on investment when it comes to innovation (Minor et al., 2017). The success of this program has led to the university investing heavily in The Innovation Studio model, opening a permanent location in central campus named The Innovation Studio—Mirror Lake (Figure 11.5), adding another location in an addition to the college of nursing, and planning a fourth location to open in the near future.

PLANT A SEED

Need funding to mature your idea?
Healthcare solutions created by
(1) a team of two or more OSU students, faculty, or staff
(2) from different disciplines/professions that have
(3) disclosed their invention to TCO (when applicable)
will be eligible for **Seed Funding**
to further incubate their innovation.

Collaborators will present their products, solutions, or services at The Innovation Showcase on April 18th at Newton Hall. Top innovations will be awarded seed funding from the Innovation Studio.

Teams that meet set milestones and demonstrate maturation of their innovation will continue to be eligible for additional, larger grants from the Innovation Studio.

Visit go.osu.edu/innovationstudio for more details.

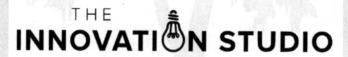

THE
INNOVATION STUDIO

FIGURE 11.4: The investment criteria for The Innovation Studio platform.

Source: © Tim Raderstorf (2017).

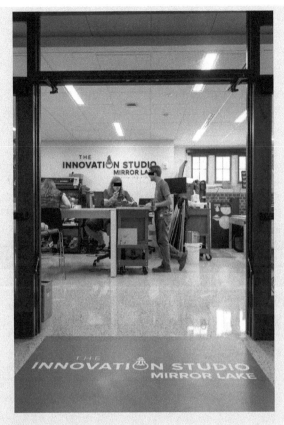

FIGURE 11.5: The Innovation Studio—Mirror Lake.

Source: © Tim Raderstorf (2017).

DISCUSSION QUESTIONS

1. How would you engage internal and external resources to implement "Innovation Studios" in your setting?
2. Which actions can you take to increase the "ideation rate" in your organization?
3. What strategies can you identify to secure funding for implementation of innovation projects?

IDEATION RATE

Ideation rate is an imperative concept for every nurse leader to understand, as it serves as a reminder of two of the biggest hindrances of innovation from nurses: permission and validation. The ideation rate is defined as the number of ideas generated by frontline staff that are approved by management, divided by the total number of employees in that system. Mathematically, there are only three ways to increase your ideation rate. The first is to generate more ideas, and this is where permission comes into play. Leaders need to encourage their team members to solve problems that impact them most. We need to encourage them to come forward with ideas and provide explicit permission to speak up when a problem is identified.

The second way to improve your ideation rate is to approve more ideas that are generated by frontline staff. This can be tricky for nurse leaders to navigate as many do not have access to budgetary resources or have the power to universally approve new initiatives. Yet, nurse leaders must find ways to support the ideas coming from the front lines and provide validation to our colleagues that their ideas are indeed valid and worth pursuing. By validating idea generators, leaders ensure that the pipeline of ideas will continue to flow and the opportunity for impact will increase.

Innovation centers are the most tangible examples of a structure of innovation. When combined with the proper incentives, educational programs, policies, job descriptions, mentoring and coaching programs, and partnerships, innovation centers can raise an organization to new heights and empower clinicians to engage in solving the problems that impact them most. With these structures in place, the organization's culture of innovation will thrive!

⬡ CASE SCENARIO

ROBOTICS AND ARTIFICIAL INTELLIGENCE— INNOVATION SUPPORTS NURSES

Andrea Thomaz and Vivian Chu, social robotics experts, founded Diligent Robotics in 2017 to build robots with ever-evolving mobile manipulation, social intelligence, and human-guided learning capabilities (Figure 11.6).

Moxi is the first robot teammate in healthcare today that works in hospitals to assist care teams with non-patient-facing tasks, freeing up more time for patient care (Figure 11.7).

With up to 30% of nurses' time spent fetching and delivering patient care items, Moxi is designed to complete routine tasks for nurses and hospital staff, providing a valuable time-saving resource to patient care.

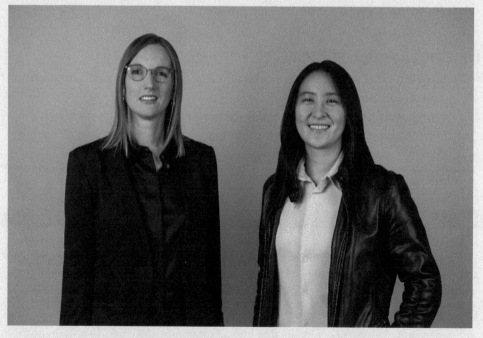

FIGURE 11.6: Meet the founders of Diligent Robotics, Andrea Thomaz and Vivian Chu.

Source: Reproduced with permission from Diligent Robotics, Inc.

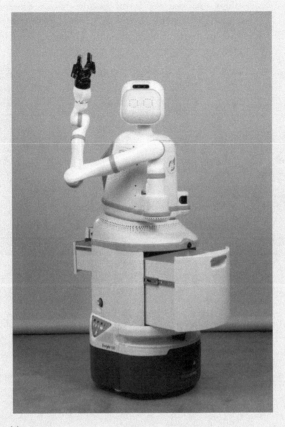

FIGURE 11.7: Meet Moxi.

Source: Reproduced with permission from Diligent Robotics, Inc.

Considering current and predicted nurse shortages, Diligent's core technology enables Moxi to help hospitals provide 24/7 care by assisting clinical staff with non-patient-facing tasks such as

- delivering lab samples that are normally hand-delivered,
- running patient supplies and items left at the front desk for patients,
- fetching items from central supply not normally stocked on patient care units,
- distributing personal protective equipment (PPE) and lightweight equipment just-in-time to make efficient use of limited resources, and
- delivering medications that are normally hand carried.

Nurses are patients' best line of defense, and these examples of many "one-off" tasks are routinely added to their plates, taking time away from crucial patient care delivery, ultimately impacting direct care hours. Moxi enables nurses to spend more quality time with patients.

An important example is Moxi's impact on workflow, such as securing and delivering telemetry devices for patients urgently in need of remote monitoring. For the safety of such patients, monitoring needs to begin as quickly as possible. With one partner hospital, Moxi delivered hundreds of telemetry boxes, averaging less than 16 minutes from receipt of the request.

Moxi's software permits dynamically adding new activities as staff needs change. Moxi's artificial intelligence (AI) properties continuously adapt to changing hospital workflows, learning from human teachers along the way. During the COVID-19 pandemic, Moxi's workflows adapted to evolving hospital and frontline staff needs, delivering PPE, lab samples, and other essential items where and when needed. Moxi's tasks related to staff needs sometimes changed on a weekly basis. Moxi's agility, flexibility, and adaptability played a key role on healthcare teams to support their patient care and contribute to staff resiliency during a difficult and challenging time.

State-of-the-art AI technology enables new levels of automation beyond the kinds of systems implemented in years past (Figure 11.8). Unlike older systems, Moxi contains everything internally needed to work in hospital environments. Diligent's implementation team can

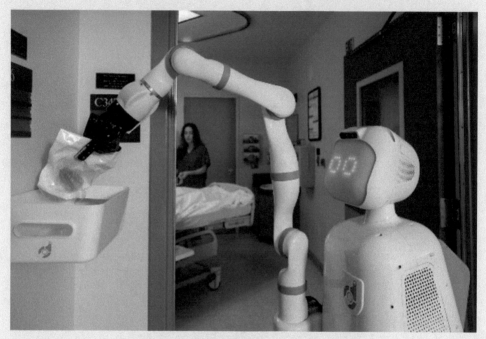

FIGURE 11.8: State-of-the-art AI technology.

Source: Reproduced with permission from Diligent Robotics, Inc.

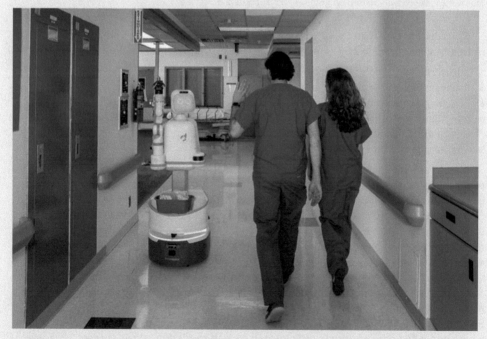

FIGURE 11.9: Robots work in harmony with humans to improve care.

Source: Reproduced with permission from Diligent Robotics, Inc.

add any number of operational workflows customized to specific hospital workspaces, getting Moxi up and running in 2 to 4 weeks.

Moxi's core technical features include:

- Social intelligence: Moxi opens elevators and doors on its own, will not bump into people or objects in hallways, and happily poses for selfies.
- Mobile manipulation: Moxi can grab, pull, open, and guide objects with no human assistance.
- Human-guided learning: The more staff use Moxi, the more Moxi learns and adapts to the specific environment and way of doing things (Figure 11.9).

Moxi testimonials:

- After Moxi delivered three telemetry devices to the unit, a busy charge nurse thanked Moxi saying, "Thanks for the help. You're my hero! I'm your biggest fan!"
- After Moxi retrieved and delivered a 3 L bag of saline to an ICU nurse, the nurse said, "Thank you! I was able to stay here [in the ICU] because of you, Moxi!"

DISCUSSION QUESTIONS

1. How would a nurse-assistive robot benefit frontline team members in your care delivery environment?
2. What characteristics and skill sets do nurses need to implement AI and robotics in patient care settings?
3. Which interprofessional team members would need to be included in a robotics implementation project in a healthcare organization?

SUSTAINING INNOVATION

Sustaining cultures of innovation is a far more difficult and challenging process than creating them. Creating cultures of innovation and infrastructures to support such cultures is certainly complex and cannot be minimized. Innovations are not always successful or effective over time, even if certain innovative solutions implemented may produce desired results initially or are effective in the short term. Implementation of any innovation, no matter how rapid the cycle or long lasting the strategy, requires that data and outcome metrics be established and then gathered at each phase along the way to determine effectiveness. Quantifiable measures of success enable leaders to build business cases for change and sustainability. Innovative solutions to problems are often implemented anecdotally in urgent situations, and data is not gathered nor at times the specifics of the action even documented in such ways that duplication or replication is even possible. In the moment, the innovator may qualitatively measure success, whether the action worked effectively to address the situation or not, but specific actions and outcomes may not be well described and documented.

Organizational infrastructures are the foundation and bedrock of sustainability in innovation cultures. Complex variables either support, serve as barriers to, or limit innovation. Nurse executives and leaders must understand and constantly assess and evaluate the influence these variables exert and related effects on innovation in their cultures. Some of the key infrastructure components to consider include, but are not limited to, history, values, beliefs, rituals, standards, policies and procedures, organizational structure, individual and collective leadership styles, resources (human, financial, community, system, and other), view of risk taking and failure, level and maturity of shared governance structures and functions, and internal and external funding sources and partners. The organization's corporate structure and mission also contribute to infrastructure and sustainability of innovation cultures. For instance, for-profit health systems may not have access to foundation or grant funding in the same way that not-for-profit and academic centers often do. Organizations that seek and retain nursing excellence awards such as Beacon, Magnet®, or Pathway to Excellence, or quality awards such as Baldrige or The Joint Commission Centers of Excellence, generally have infrastructures that prioritize, support, and demonstrate innovation.

Organizations that do not have robust infrastructures also deal with challenging care delivery situations on a daily basis that require rapid cycle problem-solving and call for innovative solutions. Frontline nurses in these settings may not consider their actions as innovative, but those clearly fall on the incremental change end of the innovation continuum.

WHAT EVERY NURSE MANAGER NEEDS TO KNOW ABOUT INNOVATION

During leadership courses for nurse managers, many have been told that they are the chief executive officers (CEOs) of their units (or areas for which they are directly accountable). Given that, nurse managers are charged with responsibilities for complex microsystem operations and clinical, financial, quality, and employee outcomes for the areas they manage. Creating, supporting, and sustaining a culture of innovation in their areas of responsibility requires maturity and creativity and a unique skill set that includes taking risks, letting go, avoiding micromanagement, and capitalizing on individual and team strengths. These managers must also have credibility with their employees, teams, and organization leaders, and establish trust, accept failure, serve as an advocate, and garner necessary resources, while creating learning environments and shared vision and team accountability for achieving unit goals and outcomes. Nurse managers must also identify barriers to innovation and recognize and accept when unit strategies and rituals need to change to accomplish shared goals and desired outcomes. Cianelli and colleagues (2016) recommend that leaders hire employees that can adapt quickly to change and create employee teams that respond to emergent situations.

Nurse managers play crucial roles in microsystem innovation by implementing diverse interprofessional teams, assessing and capitalizing on individuals' and team strengths, and serving as a coach and mentor to teams, individuals, and unit-shared governance leaders. Successful nurse managers have broad knowledge of and can access and garner organization resources to support innovations on their units. Above all, nurse managers need to listen to and value employee and team member perspectives and feedback, foster and facilitate storytelling and sharing of experiences, and learn from innovation failures.

WHAT EVERY NURSE EXECUTIVE NEEDS TO KNOW ABOUT INNOVATION

Nurse executives are responsible and accountable for the microsystems that report to them, the mesosystem that connects microsystems, and the macrosystem that contains them. These executive officers must own innovation for it to grow and flourish in their organizations. For innovation to be successful and sustainable, nurse executives require authority over key infrastructure components, as well as the ability to identify and remove barriers that limit innovation and expand boundaries to enable innovation to flourish and thrive. Nurse executives are charged with creating and supporting organizational design and strategies that reward agility and flexibility, collaboratively developing structures, rules, and procedures that promote agility, flexibility, risk taking, and frontline empowerment.

Nurse executives serve as role models, mentors, consultants, and coaches for interprofessional leaders and team members. They anticipate changes by seeking best evidence, reading current literature, and keeping abreast of internal and external environments and current trends. They have collaborative, transformational leadership styles, abilities, and competencies. These senior executives are skilled advocates and are successful at navigating internal and external boundaries, readily garnering essential resources to support innovation. They create employee teams and empower them to respond to emergent situations with innovative actions and solutions. These executives provide infrastructures and resources to facilitate and support shared governance and learning communities. Nurse executives are accessible, transparent, and listen to diverse stakeholders' perspectives and ideas.

Nurse executives in successful cultures of innovation are risk takers, learn from past failures, and are unafraid of generative design thinking, new ideas, or disruptive change. They are committed to creating shared, rather than individual, vision, evidence-based data-driven decision-making, and using outcome metrics to build business cases for sustaining innovation cultures in the organizations they lead.

These nurse executives are pioneers, trend setters, and possess entrepreneurial spirits that position them to successfully implement, support, and sustain innovation cultures, transforming health for all they serve.

KEY POINTS

- Innovation is created and led by individuals, not organizations or policy.

- Nurses are natural innovators and have a long history of changing the world for the better.

- It is imperative for nurses to stretch their comfort zones in leading innovation. Growth and comfort do not coexist, so to grow in innovation leadership, nurse leaders must become comfortable with being uncomfortable.

- Leaders must build a structure of innovation that allows a culture of innovation to thrive.

SUMMARY

Your challenge as the reader is now to make sense of this chapter content and decide what to take away and how to apply it in the context of your role, work setting, and organization. First and foremost, each nurse is responsible for embracing innovation and understanding that every nurse is an innovator. Understanding innovation and the *Novation Dynamic* and how to practically apply the principles and concepts in each work setting while gaining mastery over the innovation competencies is essential to any innovator's success.

Next, review your organization's mission, vision, and values and your job description to develop your personal plan as an innovator. Identify resources and gaps. Study examples of successful innovation. Learn from mistakes. Welcome mentoring from within and outside nursing, embracing the knowledge and skill sets other disciplines and professions bring to innovative problem-solving and solutions.

And finally, do not let perceived barriers or fear of failure win; even the most brilliant innovators started at the beginning with an idea and a vision, which evolved over time, and along the way they learned from failed attempts before creating the successful products, solutions, or services that dramatically changed the course for all who came after them.

END-OF-CHAPTER RESOURCES

DISCUSSION QUESTIONS

1. What must every innovation create?
2. Examine your own organization and identify the structures of innovation that are currently in place.
3. What changes would you like to make to your organization's structure of innovation that would lead to an improvement in your culture of innovation?
4. What are three workarounds that you have completed as a nurse? How could you turn that workaround into a sustained innovation within your organization?

◼ ADDITIONAL LEADERSHIP RESOURCES

AMERICAN ASSOCIATION OF COLLEGES OF NURSING

- Graduate level education—American Association of Colleges of Nursing. (2021). *The essentials: Core competencies for professional nursing education.* Author. https://www.aacnnursing.org/Portals/42/AcademicNursing/pdf/Essentials-2021.pdf

AMERICAN ORGANIZATION FOR NURSING LEADERSHIP COMPETENCIES

- Chief nurse executive—American Organization of Nurse Executives & American Organization for Nursing Leadership. (2015). *AONL nurse executive competencies.* Author. https://www.aonl.org/system/files/media/file/2019/06/nec.pdf
- Nurse executive: population health—American Organization of Nurse Executives & American Organization for Nursing Leadership. (2015). *AONL nurse manager competencies.* Author. https://www.aonl.org/system/files/media/file/2019/10/population-health-competencies.pdf
- Nurse executive: post-acute care—American Organization of Nurse Executives & American Organization for Nursing Leadership. (2015). *AONL nurse executive competencies: Post-acute care.* Author. https://www.aonl.org/system/files/media/file/2019/06/nec-post-acute_0.pdf
- System chief nurse executive—American Organization of Nurse Executives & American Organization for Nursing Leadership. (2015). *AONL nurse executive competencies: system CNE.* Author. https://www.aonl.org/system/files/media/file/2019/06/nec-system-cne.pdf
- Nurse manager—American Organization of Nurse Executives & American Organization for Nursing Leadership. (2015). *AONL nurse manager competencies.* Author. https://www.aonl.org/system/files/media/file/2019/06/nurse-manager-competencies.pdf

QUALITY AND SAFETY EDUCATION FOR NURSES INSTITUTE

- Quality and Safety Education for Nurses Institute. (2016, January 25). *Leadership in healthcare.* https://qsen.org/leadership-in-healthcare
- Quality and Safety Education for Nurses Institute. (2012, September 24). Graduate-level QSEN competencies. https://qsen.org/competencies/graduate-ksas

◼ LEARNING EXERCISES FOR STUDENTS

1. Identify three common workarounds nurses in your practice area routinely do. Choose one and propose possible innovative solutions. Identify potential risks and benefits. Develop a plan for developing, implementing, and evaluating the innovation.
2. Identify leadership styles, traits, and competencies that support or serve as barriers to innovation in care delivery.

A robust set of instructor resources designed to supplement this text is located at http://connect.springerpub.com/content/book/978-0-8261-7795-7. Qualifying instructors may request access by emailing textbook@springerpub.com.

REFERENCES

Ackerman, M. H., Guilano, K. K., & Malloch, K. (2020, March). The *Novation Dynamic*: Clarifying the work of change, disruption, and innovation. *Nurse Leader, 18*(3), 232–236. https://doi.org/10.1016/j.mnl.2020.01.003

American Nurses Association. (2019, February 20). *How to engage nurses in innovation*. MedTech Boston Features. https://medtechboston.medstro.com/blog/2019/02/22/how-to-engage-nurses-in-innovation/

American Organization of Nurse Executives & American Organization for Nursing Leadership. (2015a). *Nurse executive competencies*. https://www.aonl.org/system/files/media/file/2019/06/nec.pdf

American Organization of Nurse Executives & American Organization for Nursing Leadership. (2015b). *Nurse manager competencies*. https://www.aonl.org/system/files/media/file/2019/06/nurse-manager-competencies.pdf

Armstrong, A. J., Holmes, C. M., & Henning, D. (2020). A changing world, again. How appreciative inquiry can guide our growth. *Social Sciences and Humanities Open, 2(1), Article 100038*. https://doi.org/10.1016/j.ssaho.2020.100038

Bahcall, S. (2019). *Loonshots: How to nurture the crazy ideas that win wars, cure diseases, and transform industries*. St. Martin's Press.

Cianelli, R., Clipper, B., Freeman, R., & Goldstein, J. (2016, June). *The innovation road map: A guide for nurse leaders*. Innovation Works. innovations-roadmap-english.pdf

Cooperrider, D. (2012). *What is appreciative inquiry?* David Cooperrider and Associates. https://www.davidcooperrider.com/ai-process/

Kahan, S. (2021). *The innovation continuum*. The Innovation Continuum - Seth Kahan's Visionary Leadership. https://visionaryleadership.com/the-innovation-continuum-incremental-improvement-to-total-transformation/

Love, R. (2018). *Healthcare's top innovators: Nurses*. Nurse innovator challenges students to redefine nursing. Plenary session at National Student Nurses Association Convention, Nashville, TN. April 18, 2018. https://www.jnj.com/

May, N., Becker, D., Frankel, R., Haizlip, J., Harmon, R., Plews-Ogan, M., Williams, A., & Whitney, D. (2011). *Appreciative inquiry in healthcare*. Crown Publishing.

Melnyk, B. M., & Raderstorf, T. (Eds.). (2021). *Evidence-based leadership, innovation and entrepreneurship in nursing and healthcare: A practical guide for success*. Springer Publishing Company.

Minor, D., Brook, P., & Bernoff, J. (2017). *Data from 3.5 million employees shows how innovation really works*. Harvard Business School Publishing.

Naca-Abell, K. J. (2020, October 19). Appreciative inquiry: Building teamwork and leadership. *My American Nurse*. https://www.myamericannurse.com/appreciative-inquiry-building-teamwork-and-leadership/

Pillay, R., & Morris, M. H. (2016). Changing healthcare by changing the education of its leaders: An innovation competence model. *Journal of Health Administration Education, 33*(3), 393–410.

Robert Wood Johnson Foundation. (2015, September 25). *Nation's first medical makerspace opens in Texas*. https://www.rwjf.org/en/library/articles-and-news/2015/09/nations-first-medical-makerspace-opens.html

Seaman, J. B., & Erlen, J.A. (2015). Workarounds in the workplace: A second look. *Orthopedic Nursing, 34*(4), 235–242. https://doi.org/10.1097/NOR.0000000000000161

Sheingold, B. H., & Hahn, J. A. (2014). The history of healthcare quality: The first 100 years 1860–1960. *International Journal of Africa Nursing Sciences, 1*(1), 18–22. http://dx.doi.org/10.1016/j.ijans.2014.05.002

White, K. R., Pillay, R., & Huang, X. (2016). Nurse leaders and the innovation competence gap. *Nursing Outlook, 64*(3), 255–261. https://doi.org/10.1016/j.outlook.2015.12.007.

Wilson, A., Whitaker, N., & Whitford, D. (2012). Rising to the challenge of health care reform with entrepreneurial and intrapreneurial nursing initiatives. *OJIN: The Online Journal of Issues in Nursing, 17*(2), Manuscript 5. https://doi.org/10.3912/OJIN.Vol17No02Man05.

SECTION IV
ORGANIZATIONAL ANALYSIS

CHAPTER | 12

STRUCTURES, PROCESSES, AND ORGANIZATIONAL GOALS

Deirdre O'Flaherty and Mary Joy Garcia-Dia

"An empowered organization is one in which individuals have the knowledge, skill, desire, and opportunity to personally succeed in a way that leads to collective organizational success."

M. Shawn Covey

LEARNING OBJECTIVES

- Describe the organizational models and theories as they relate to healthcare organizations' structure and performance.
- Differentiate among structures, processes, and goals of an organization.
- Appraise the nurse leaders' role in supporting the organization's overall quality, regulatory, and safety outcomes.
- Formulate a strategy for supporting and/or leading organizational change.

INTRODUCTION

Structure, processes, and organizational goals are the building blocks that provide focus, stability, and direction. The policies, procedures, and organizational standards served as the foundation for nurse leaders and our healthcare systems to quickly respond to meet the challenges encountered during moments of celebration but even more so during moments of crisis. Any disaster situation or global pandemic requires swift, rapid response and purposeful intervention. Lessons learned from previous responses to emergent situations provide an opportunity to reflect, learn, and change existing policies and procedures. Hence, nurse leaders require a formalized process analysis and the situational awareness to precisely strategize, mobilize essential resources, work collaboratively with other disciplines, and determine a positive course of action. As an example, the ongoing global nursing shortage is a challenge for many healthcare organizations (HCOs) and nurse leaders. Competition for human resources (HR) and budget constraints will require nurse leaders to reimagine the organization's reporting structure and governance model without compromising patient safety and quality care.

An overall assessment of structure, process, and goals of existing organizational governance and service line reports or relationships across systems must be conducted to identify vulnerabilities and minimize risks. Creating a workplace environment that incorporates concepts or models rooted in looking at structural components and processes that can support the full potential of nurses in their careers and professional development will set nurse leaders apart in getting ahead with retaining and recruiting an engaged workforce during these challenging times.

This chapter highlights the historical perspective of organizational structures with reference to change and adaptation. Current day scenarios and the expansion of technology as a key player in healthcare, the complexities of delivering care, and the speed of new innovations and mobility in the workforce are discussed, and present-day examples are provided for aspiring nurse leaders as a foundation for evaluating structure and organizational goals.

EVOLUTION OF ORGANIZATIONAL STRUCTURES

Organizational structure refers to the way in which a group is formed, its line of communication, and its means of channeling authority and decision-making processes (Marquis & Huston, 2021). According to *The Encyclopedia of Management* (Gale Research Inc., 2019), the traditional or classical structure of an organization based upon the machinist views of industrial thinkers like Frederick Winslow Taylor (1856–1915) and Henri Fayol (1841–1925) matched German Sociologist Max Weber's (1864–1920) ideas of bureaucracy in which power is ascribed to positions rather than to the individuals holding the position. The scientific management principles of efficiency and productivity based on studied time and motion, unity within the chain of command, and unity of direction through discipline, task specialization, and job separation are characteristics of a formal bureaucratic organizational structure. This hierarchical and vertical structure, which was developed during the Industrial Age, functioned well into the 1970s and early 1980s and focused on positions and formal power while it provided a framework for managerial authority, responsibility, and accountability. The roles and functions are systematically defined with rank and hierarchy as highly visible (Marquis & Huston, 2021) where the chief executive officer (CEO) is the highest rank in a vertical position while there are multiple managers in a horizontal position (Figure 12.1).

However, this formal structure may fail to consider the social context and human needs of workers, particularly in HCOs wherein informal alliances and relationships with peers influence empowerment and shape work behaviors and attitudes (Daft, 2021; Matthews et al., 2006). According to Daft (2021), the Hawthorne studies that began in the 1930s focused on how human behavior and relations affect organizational performance and provided evidence that informal work groups (social relationships) and group pressure have a positive effect on motivation and group productivity.

Globalization and a competitive market between the 1960s to the 1980s led bureaucratic organizations to be flexible, engage with employees, and respond rapidly to customers. This management shift flattened the hierarchical structure, creating distributed teams that engaged with each other and promoted collaborative work, problem-solving, and brainstorming. In this decentralized organizational structure, whereby regional directors manage a team of supervisors and staff, each team is independent and makes autonomous decisions (Figure 12.2). This combination of formal and informal structures ushered its own communication network known as the grapevine wherein conversations occur in the hallway or break rooms and create informal group relationships (Marquis & Huston, 2021). This is true for professional organizations, where formal meetings are accompanied by informal, less structured discussions. Team members can find common ground and create shared intentions that eventually lead to a network of connections and even friendships (Newton et al., 2019).

The internet revolution, beginning in the 1990s, led later to advances in communications and information technology (IT) in the mid-2000s as the use of social media platforms such as Facebook, Twitter, and LinkedIn matured. The use of interactive communication technology extended patient and provider interactions and peer-to-peer dialogues beyond hospital walls as more people adopted electronic communication. Many HCOs have become more interconnected and agile in response to continuous technological change, clinical and scientific advances, and unexpected global health challenges. This collaborative interconnection was manifested during the development and rapid deployment of

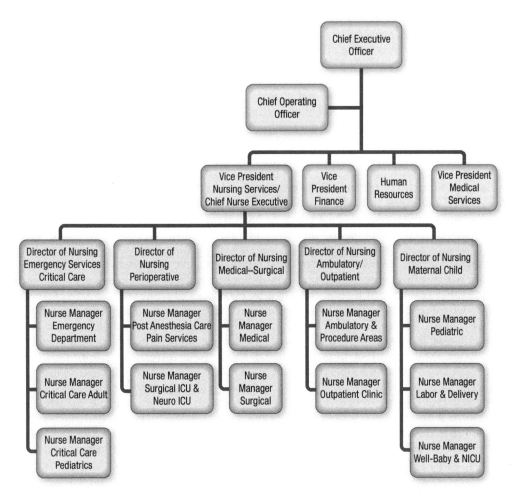

FIGURE 12.1: Traditional hospital organizational structure with a vice president of nursing services and chief nursing executive showing the hierarchical structure with horizontal and vertical lines.

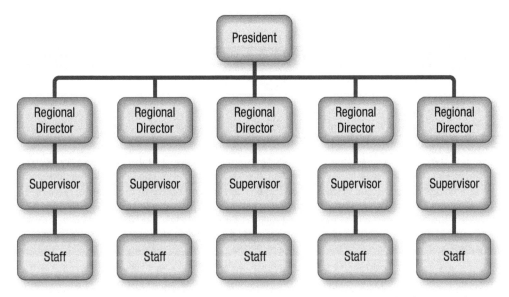

FIGURE 12.2: Decentralized organizational structure. This decentralized hierarchical structure has distributed teams.

the COVID-19 vaccine during the pandemic. Increasing levels of educational and technical skills, diversity, and access to knowledge among the workforce, coupled with a rise in information-driven work in analytics, has created a new mobile workforce. The fast-paced mobility and portability of information allowed for virtual workspaces (i.e., telecommuting) to coexist with formal workspaces. Today, people work side-by-side—often without ever meeting each other—in disparate time zones and geographic locations. This evolution has led to the development of a critical new concern for staff well-being, which may suffer because of information overload, social isolation, and burnout. Consequently, demand among employees for improved work–life balance has increased, and senior leaders in many organizations have implemented wellness and mental health programs to engage and retain staff.

The American Recovery and Reinvestment Act (ARRA) of 2009 provided a stimulus plan for HCO to invest in health information technology (HIT) to promote accountability, security, and quality care. HCOs' journey to meet the HIT components of ARRA entailed looking at clinical and core quality measures, privacy rules, workflow, access, and government reimbursements and penalty fees associated with meeting the meaningful rules of the regulations. The complexity and mix of effectiveness, efficiency, productivity, and quality—together with the high ethical and moral expectations of leaders and care delivery systems in implementing government regulations—require clear lines of authority and accountability (de las Heras-Rosas et al., 2021). Increasing hospital costs and economic pressures led to a shift toward a corporate business model approach wherein hospital administrators must remain flexible and stay competitive. This business model led to program management and necessitated a shift toward an interprofessional, enterprise-level leadership approach. New positions, such as that of the chief nurse executive (CNE), gained more visibility in the hierarchy. The scope of an RN widened to include nurse leaders who held the highest executive positions in HCOs—for example, serving as vice president of patient care in a line structure and assuming operational responsibility for clinical care (Matthews et al., 2006). Nurse leaders who desire to keep abreast and succeed in this ever-changing work environment need to arm themselves with key management and leadership concepts to influence the design and care delivery process in promoting a healthy workplace and quality care environment.

The next section of this chapter will correlate the importance of analyzing management structures and utilizing organizational models in transforming the healthcare system. As a nurse leader, equipping oneself with this organizational knowledge and these skills will amplify the role of the nurse to function at one's full leadership capacity.

● CASE SCENARIO

CLINICAL PRACTICE OUTCOMES

SITUATION

MT is the nurse manager of a 24-bed surgical specialty unit in a large urban HCO with a 600-bed capacity. The average length of stay (ALOS) is 3.5 days for the majority of the post-op patients. Several of the surgeons that admit to the unit have been championing enhanced recovery protocols (ERP) for their patients to reduce the ALOS to 2.5 days or less. The hospital's mission is to utilize innovative approaches to care as well as to remain competitive in the healthcare market. An ERP council was developed, and MT's nursing director, Dr. JS, ensured that they were involved in all the planning meetings. Due to personal health reasons, Dr. JS has been on medical leave and MT's unit has been overseen by another nursing director, EC, temporarily.

At a department head meeting, one of MT's staff nurses shares that there is news that their existing unit will be transitioned to a medicine service and a new, short stay unit will replace the surgical unit. MT is compelled to get an earlier meeting date with EC to clarify if there have been changes that MT has not been privy to. MT has been a nurse manager for 3 years and is worried about their own position, how best to communicate the potential changes to the team, and the overall impact on patient care.

APPROACH

The nature of managing an HCO requires leadership, supervision, and coordination of employees. An organizational chart defines the formal relationship, chains of communication, and a defined line of authority. The added charge of participating in an interprofessional team through the ERP council creates new responsibility and accountability for the nurse manager. The first strategy for strengthening accountability is establishing a line of sight for frontline staff to recognize the connection between their daily work and their institution's larger priorities.

In this scenario, the organizational changes and reporting structure create confusion on the chain of command despite the presence of a formal structure in delineating the line of authority. The large span of control—where too many people are reporting to a single director—can result in a top-heavy, hierarchical structure and lead to ineffective communication and delays in decision-making. MT's approach in pursuing appropriate channels of communication is essential to clarifying roles and structural unit changes. EC can leverage the informal structure of the organization and establish an interpersonal relationship with MT and MT's staff by setting regularly scheduled meetings. This will provide a formal opportunity for staff to share their peer feedback and for MT to listen to their concerns while sharing plans and goals. EC can coach MT as they carry out their expansive responsibility from operations, administrative, and quality management. This will reestablish trust and improve the communication process, allowing MT to share their management style, unit goals, and concerns.

OUTCOME

Research studies show that shared governance and professional practice structures in which staff nurses' involvement in decision-making is encouraged promotes engagement. Clavelle et al. (2016) noted that accountability, professional obligation, collateral relationships, and effective decision-making are the attributes of professional governance. Structure enables behavior and ownership is the underpinning of accountability, which requires a professional practice environment that supports and advances processes for individual empowerment and engagement (Porter-O'Grady & Clavelle, 2020). According to Berkow et al. (2012), staff's knowledge of unit-level quality goals and their awareness of overall clinical excellence are essential to obtaining buy-in and help to foster compliance in supporting organizational goals.

Both MT and EC are appointed to a position of authority in which each must contribute to important decisions that will impact patient and nurse satisfaction, service additions and reductions, and allocation and spending of financial resources. The role of the nursing director is to ensure that the unit, service, division, or organization that they manage and lead achieves high performance against the goals set. Soliciting MT's input on goals, specific targets, and solutions gives MT a greater sense of overall ownership and accountability in their role as nurse manager.

DISCUSSION QUESTIONS

1. How can managers cope with organizational changes, especially in a large, complex, and bureaucratic organization?

2. Describe your current organization according to the structural and contextual dimensions. How would you compare this with other organizations where you have worked in the past?

ORGANIZATIONAL ANALYSIS

Nursing represents the largest group at the structural level of healthcare institutions. Nurse managers are faced with the demands of delivering high-value clinical care according to excellent standards while meeting the clinician's job satisfaction and psychosocial well-being. They need to be familiar with the formal hierarchy (organizational chart) and understand the line of authority, chain of command, and cross-functions that are rooted in various organizational models. Nurse managers serve as an essential link between senior leadership and staff nurses.

Depending on the nurse manager's career trajectory, it is beneficial to conduct an organizational analysis based on models and theories focused on structure, processes, and goals that address job satisfaction, recruitment and retention, and quality indicators by senior nursing management. Table 12.1 presents several models (rational, natural system, sociotechnical, cognitive) from *The Encyclopedia of Management* (Gale Research Inc., 2019). The authors used the model to compare the functional processes and advantages of each model.

TABLE 12.1: Models of Organizational Structure

Model	Description	Functional Roles	Pro	Con
Rational Model	Scientific based on time and motion; Pyramidal—managers are at the apex and employees are at the bottom	Managers have the authority to assign tasks to employees and evaluate performance	Employees complete the tasks to drive efficiency Distribute rewards and punishments based on performance	Repetitive tasks lead to boredom Monetary compensation may not be the primary driver for motivation
Natural System Model	Holistic and strives to balance everyone's needs; members belong to at least one effective work group (department, committee, staff group)	Managers are encouraged to change the organization as a whole	Foster communication and exchange of information across the organization	Changes are difficult as any change in one part of the organization impacts other parts of the organization
Sociotechnical Model	Systems view: Interaction is affected by human, social, technological, and organizational inputs	Managers are engaged with the effective design of tasks through inputs and outputs; tasks are broken down to subtasks	The premise is focused on minimizing conflicts by designing tasks effectively	Gaps with technology (techniques, skills, materials), geographic location, and time (work shifts) can affect the overall performance
Cognitive Model	Focused on cognition, decision-making, and problem-solving	Managers identify areas of specialization that can be broken into and delegated as subtasks	Streamline changes as flow of information is facilitated to and from specialized units	Constant analysis to cope with changes can lead to defensive tactics and burnout

DEVELOPMENT OF ORGANIZATIONAL STRUCTURES

Familiarity with these functional processes guides nurse managers in choosing a model that supports daily operations, promotes a positive workplace environment, and ensures safe quality care. Research studies from Gale Research Inc. (2019) showed that there are four basic decisions that managers need to process in the development of organizational structures:

a. **Division of labor:** Work is divided into specific jobs (e.g., nursing, unit assistant, respiratory therapist). How do staff see the contribution of their work in achieving the overall Magnet® designation?

b. **Departmentalization:** Jobs are grouped based on functions, geographic location, product, and customer/market service. In terms of function, how does the unit interact and communicate updates and manage issues with other departments? Is there a standardized request process for regional hospitals compared to integrated hospital networks from a geographic perspective? Is telehealth offered only in the ED for urgent visits and not for behavioral health?

c. **Span of control:** Refers to the number of people reporting directly and needing to be managed by a single person or a manager. Is the unit efficient based on the number of staff?

d. **Authority:** The power to act and make decisions officially. Is the structure clear for staff to identify who they can reach out to for escalation?

These four decisions, when factored within the organizational models, can lead to various organizational design structures. As an example, the third Case Scenario in this chapter (Disaster Response During COVID-19—Project Organizational Structure) shows how one can use a combination of the sociotechnical and cognitive model while assessing how division of labor and authority can make the structure effective.

ORGANIZATIONAL AWARENESS

Aside from organization models, the nurse manager's awareness that organizations can shape the lives of people is critical in shaping organizations, particularly with promoting engagement, accountability, and workplace satisfaction. This is where the structural and contextual dimensions of the organization come into play. Structural dimension marks the internal characteristics of an organization, allowing the basis to measure and compare one from the other, whereas contextual dimension describes the character of the whole organization based on size, technology, environment, and goals (Daft, 2021; Kottke & Pelletier, 2017). Both structural and contextual dimensions can interact with each other to accomplish a common purpose. Table 12.2 enumerates examples of structural and contextual dimensions identified by these authors.

An example of a formal organization is an academic medical center as it will have volumes of manuals that describe the governance, financial and clinical operations, and clinical specialties. A small family-owned yoga wellness center may not have written rules and would be considered informal, whereas HCOs will have extensive written documentation to which organizational policies and procedures, practices, job descriptions, regulations, and ways of completing tasks are standardized. Regardless of the service or product offered, the nurse manager needs to consider the size (number) of the employees, as well as the technology to facilitate the input and output process of its services and communication. The centralization of power in an organization may be dictated and described in formal rules, policies, and job descriptions. Top level decision-making is centralized while decisions delegated to a lower level is considered decentralized. These decisions can include hiring staff, purchasing clinical systems, and creating quality goals. The unit's staffing level, assignment, and acuity are taken into consideration by first-level

TABLE 12.2: Examples of Structural and Contextual Dimensions

Structural Dimension	Contextual Dimension
Formalization	Size
Differentiation	Innovation or technology
Specialization	Environment
Hierarchy of authority (Management)	Organization's goal and strategy
Centralization	Organization's culture
Professionalism	Interdependence
Personnel ratio	
Complexity	

managers; thus, the hierarchy of authority and personnel ratio needs to be defined. These factors influence productivity and staff satisfaction. Promoting professionalism through education, training, succession planning, and career-ladder development contribute to longevity and retention. Other environmental drivers such as the government, regulatory bodies, and competitors create uncertainty that can either be low or high depending on the tasks, adding a layer of complexity.

The key take-away when performing organizational analysis is to help managers and leadership understand the dynamic structure and interactive dimensions within the organization and equip leaders with a toolkit and roadmap in making better business, clinical, and management decisions (Flynn, 2015; Kottke & Pelletier, 2017).

 CASE SCENARIO

DECENTRALIZATION

SITUATION

Hospital A is a 250-bed regional medical center; it has been providing emergency and acute medical services for over 20 years, and currently has over 1,200 employees on staff. The recent merger with an academic medical center will simplify the organizational structure by merging its existing resources and departments.

APPROACH

Nurse executive leaders have knowledge of the implications and anticipated changes that come with organizational mergers and understand this requires careful thought and planning. Chief nursing officers (CNOs) and system-level CNEs must map out the transition plan by identifying key communication content; outlining checklists or steps to identify structure, process, and resources; and creating a timeline on when to set meetings with targeted audiences. There are several steps in planning the merger that include pre-merger planning, due diligence, regulatory approval, possible litigation, and post-merger organization redesign (Roth Piper & Schneider, 2015). The nurse leaders start by creating an inventory of projects—including their status and priorities. The implementation timeline may last a year or more before the merger is finalized and it is essential that work continues for projects to remain on track. This interval provides an opportunity for nursing leadership in both organizations to establish communication and gain the trust of employees through open forum meetings and workgroups at all levels.

The new merger structure requires proactive guidance from senior leadership. A well-conceived and detailed plan needs to be mapped to clarify new expectations. To promote engagement with staff, leadership hosts a retreat that facilitates feedback and input on what the practice model, support structures, resources, and lines of communication will look like. In planning for integration of processes, management agrees on what model will bring cooperation, trust, and engagement. Facilitating structures that can support professional governance, structural and psychological empowerment, and system recognition such as Magnet and/or achieving Magnet designation are also reassessed. Nursing management from both organizations need to understand their roles and responsibility and articulate the value that they bring.

OUTCOME

A proper plan on the reporting relationships and integration of processes can be developed and shared with stakeholders to promote engagement and adoption. This will minimize resistance and support a shared vision for viability, sustainability, and success. Creating a checklist and inventory will ensure that details are captured and mapped out to ensure a successful endorsement and transition.

DISCUSSION QUESTIONS

1. What activities and considerations would you include in planning for an organizational merger?
2. What are the overarching expectations that you need to anticipate in managing stakeholders before and after the merger?

◻ WHAT EVERY NURSE MANAGER NEEDS TO KNOW ABOUT STRUCTURE, PROCESSES, AND ORGANIZATIONAL GOALS

Healthcare as a complex industry requires standard procedures, a command hierarchy, and decision makers with a high degree of accountability. Levels and roles must be defined clearly as healthcare's business and clinical operations involve many tasks that are interdependent, and oftentimes time-sensitive. Organizational models such as high reliability organizations (HROs) are associated with a culture of safety, increased patient satisfaction, and decreased harm as reported by the Agency for Healthcare Research and Quality and the Consumers Assessment of Healthcare Providers and Systems (CAHPS) hospital survey (Larson, 2012). Nurse managers can utilize organizational models to flex formal and informal structures in promoting a positive workplace environment. The essential component of a HRO is teamwork. The need for immediate feedback because of critical outcomes occurring simultaneously rely on organizational models such as HRO to attain high reliability. Evidence correlates that increased employee engagement positively impacts patient outcomes and the patient experience while reducing costs (Lapaine, 2021). Utilizing models such as HROs that incorporate the goals set forth by the Institute for Healthcare Improvement (IHI) embraces the concepts of the Quadruple Aim. Ultimately, nurse managers serve as advocates toward improving patient health outcomes and patient care experience, as well as reducing cost, while adding joy and meaning to work.

Organizational models are instrumental in the development of organizational structure. Nurse managers need to have a clear understanding of conceptual frameworks as this is an essential step when conducting organizational design decisions. The transformation of organizational structure depends on how people and resources are organized collectively to accomplish the desired goals and outcomes (Aubrey & Lavoie-Tremblay, 2018). According to Rydenfalt et al. (2017), incorporating

294 | IV ORGANIZATIONAL ANALYSIS

organizational design principles in healthcare can promote desirable characteristics of a team such as cohesion, collaboration, communication, conflict resolution, coordination, and leadership. Implementing these principles can lead to good teamwork and success. For example, the IPO (Input-Process-Output) model of teamwork provides structure at three levels: individual, group, and environment (Rydenfalt et al., 2017). The interaction, interdependency, and relationship between the three levels are supported by organizational principles that drive the effectiveness of the teamwork process. One principle is team stability, where trust is central in building communication. The second principle is creating opportunities for communications that promote patient safety through huddles and handoff processes. The third principle is promoting engagement with individuals who can step up and formally lead based on participative and adaptive approaches and leadership training.

The relationships between structure and contextual dimensions with process and goals drive organizational engagement. Contextual dimensions describe the organization and represent its purpose, size, and goals. This serves to influence and shape the structural dimensions which depict the internal features of an organization. In measuring and comparing organizations, responses to engagement surveys can be indicative of the organizational climate and are the employee's perception of the organization. Engaging managers in an initiative that they have contributed to, and/or designed, to increase employee engagement supports the process and the means to achieve organizational goals. As an example, the use of TeamSTEPPS methodology utilizes formal models to enhance performance and patient safety. This initiative nurtures a culture of safety and a shared mental model requiring the nurse leader's engagement and support from the top-down. This teamwork promotes inclusion, mutual respect, and a positive workplace environment leading teams to succeed.

LEADING THROUGH ORGANIZATIONAL CHANGE

The globalization of work and expansion of healthcare systems have triggered changes in traditional organizational structures. Organizations became more vulnerable with downsizing and outsourcing employees that potentially led to diminished job security (Zinn & Brannon, 2014). These changes have sequential implications on the evolution and transformation of the healthcare industry as they affect the ability of management to maintain operational processes while adapting to change. The nurse executive, as the recognized leader, is in a pivotal role to understand the company's culture and spearhead changes in organizational policies and practices. One of these changes is supporting nurse managers' transition and onboarding process. According to the study by Warshawsky et al. (2020), the blueprint in ensuring success for nurse managers depends on the influence of nurse executives in establishing an organizational culture of mentoring and coaching. Empowered nurse leaders who are highly motivated and knowledgeable are committed to achieving organizational goals and delivering patient care effectively. As transformational leaders, nurse executives can support a psychologically safe climate that promotes empowerment and learning (Warshawsky et al., 2020). DiNapoli et al. (2014) illustrated a neo-theoretical model of empowerment where the co-existence of organizational and psychological empowerment influences a healthy environment for nurses and patients to thrive well. Figure 12.3 shows the relationship between organizational empowerment (access to information, resources, support, and opportunities to learn and grow) with psychological empowerment (perception of power, meaning in work, and sense of belonging) in creating a positive healthy workplace environment for nurses and patients. For nurses, the sense of autonomy, decision-making, job satisfaction, and open communication leads to trust, teamwork, respect, and higher retention rate. Patients thrive well as they experience a sense of autonomy in managing their health concerns that can lead to better or improved health outcomes, and satisfaction with their quality care.

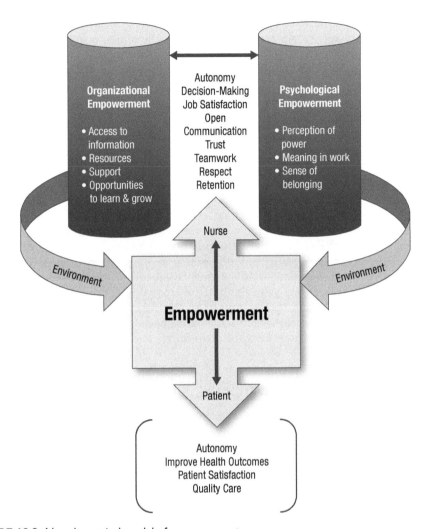

FIGURE 12.3: Neo-theoretical model of empowerment.

Source: Illustration by Mary Joy Garcia-Dia, MA, RN. Copyright © 2013. All rights reserved; from DiNapoli, J. M., O'Flaherty, D., & Garcia-Dia, M. J. (2014). Theory of empowerment. In J. J. Fitzpatrick & G. McCarthy (Eds.), *Theories guiding nursing research and practice: Making nursing knowledge development explicit* (pp. 303–322). Springer Publishing Company, LLC.

STRUCTURAL AND CONTEXTUAL DIMENSIONS OF AN ORGANIZATION

In correlating this neo-theoretical model of empowerment where CNEs are challenged by managing a volatile, uncertain, chaotic, and ambiguous (VUCA) climate, nurse leaders can apply the theory of contingency in tandem with analyzing the structural and contextual dimensions of an organization. In this context, CNEs must consider relevant circumstances before designing and consciously molding the organizational structure to drive and produce high performance. Donaldson (2013) and Gale (2017) noted that organizations need to determine the fit of core structural dimensions with the five contingency factors prior to planning any changes. These contingency factors are:

- **Uncertainty:** A major source of uncertainty is the environment relevant to the decision-making and management of the organization. These external forces include social and cultural norms, governmental regulations, economic conditions, and market competition.

- **Innovation:** This can be in the form of a product or service where cross-functional project teams interact spontaneously and carry out activities to solve new problems.
- **Interdependence:** Tasks vary in their interdependence between pooled, sequential, and reciprocal input and output activities where certain rules may apply. In some instances, further planning or coordination is required. This is frequently seen with clinical-systems projects where resources pool together with designing workflow while dependencies may occur with procurement.
- **Strategy:** Key aspects of organizational strategy are diversification and vertical integration. Diversification refers to the degree of difference among the products or services produced by an organization, whereas in vertical integration, decision-making is centralized.
- **Size:** This is the key aspect relative to the number of members or the number of hospital sites or practice offices, net assets (research and patents), gross reimbursements/payments (insurance, grants, or service industries), or number of units that can be set-up to deliver services or populations who can be served. Large HCOs lead to bureaucratic and structural differentiation. Based on size, larger HCOs have more departments, divisions or departments, job titles and specialization, and a greater number of hierarchy levels that run from the CEO to the chief operating officer (COO), CNE, and to the bottom-level worker compared to smaller ones. Enterprise-wide healthcare systems have more specialization in job types, standardization of rules and formalization of procedures, and often more decentralization with decision-making.

REDESIGNING ORGANIZATIONAL STRUCTURE

Based on evidence, there is no one structure that will best fit an enterprise's integrated healthcare delivery system (Gale, 2017). For example, Table 12.3 provides the most common organizational structures: traditional, hybrid, and matrix. Although this is not an exhaustive list, it provides a baseline for CNEs to apply the contingency theory with multiple existing structures that can be designed as traditional and matrixed. In cases where market changes brought by regulatory, technological, or environmental factors occur at any given point in time, CNEs can redesign the organizational structure or change processes to meet organizational goals.

Within an integrated healthcare system, there could be two or three traditional organizational structures representing multiple hospital campuses that are geographically dispersed but share one functional department such as the HR or quality department. This hybrid

TABLE 12.3: Example and Description of Organizational Structures

Organizational Structure	Description	Use Case Scenario
Traditional	Represented by an organizational chart with vertical and horizontal lines like a pyramid	Enterprise-wide healthcare systems
Hybrid	Combination of two or more types of structure	Transition of two healthcare organizations during merger
Matrix	Combination of two or more different structures (vertical and horizontal) that are working simultaneously	Nursing informatics department reporting to nursing and information technology department

Note: Example and description of organizational structures with corresponding use case scenarios applicable in healthcare.

organizational structure combines different structures to minimize redundant services and consolidate functions (e.g., accounting, education) for efficiency. With the advent of distance and online learning, technology has given HCOs an opportunity to revisit how orientation and onboarding are facilitated cross campus. Nurse executives can adopt these new processes of teaching within a hybrid state.

SUPPORTING ORGANIZATIONAL CHANGE

As a visionary leader, the nurse executive sets the tone for staff to adapt and support change. There are situations where highly specialized teams need to come together and deliver a product, service, or both. In this case, a matrix structure can be created on a project basis where resources are shared, and subject matter experts may need to divide their time between several projects while reporting to two departments. Another example is with market competition wherein CNEs are challenged in maintaining or achieving Centers for Medicare & Medicaid Services (CMS) star rating and Magnet status designation. The scoring, certification, and compliance processes impact quality of care, patient and staff satisfaction, and hospital reimbursement. The nurse executive needs to be creative and transform the current environment fraught with uncertainties by combining structures and processes that can support the shared mission and vision of the organization.

HORIZONTAL AND VERTICAL INTEGRATION

In responding to a VUCA environment, nurse executives must understand horizontal and vertical integration. The interpersonal process aimed at improving relationships, creating positive relationships, and minimizing conflicts are dynamic and can affect anyone within the vertical chain of command and horizontal dependencies that are within multiple departments. For example, the recent COVID-19 pandemic pushed CNEs to implement new structures and support innovative ideas. The unprecedented number of critically ill patients surged beyond the healthcare system's capacity. Spaces were restructured and converted while pop-up units and field tents were built rapidly that required nurse executives to adjust staffing models and implement deployment strategies. Nurse leaders supported staff's creativity in repurposing baby monitors to observe patients in maintaining safety and enhancing communication while they are in isolation. The majority of the nurse executives applied management principles of engagement and blended formal and informal structures to promote staff's empowerment.

ROLE OF TECHNOLOGY IN ORGANIZATIONAL CHANGE

Even prior to the pandemic, the rapid and constant changes brought about by the ubiquitous presence of computerization, the internet, and innovative technologies from wearable devices to mobile communication have a major impact on the overall work environment. However, nursing executive leaders pivoted quickly in staying ahead of the curve of technology. Virtualization and cloud computing offered a new environmental paradigm to meet the communication and interaction of a global and geographically dispersed team through telecommuting. This required coordination to group or cluster jobs within a department either by function or based on skill sets using a team approach pushed HCOs to reimagine and adopt a flexible and mobile workforce. This team approach is the organizational structure of the future where clusters of teams and individuals collaborate, share information, and move from team to team, depending on what issues are at hand. This virtualization expanded care through virtual visits and remote patient monitoring (RPM). RPM allows a team to monitor, observe, and assess patients in a variety of settings such as e-ICUs, telehealth, and remote call centers. Creating this new work environment and care delivery required a three-dimensional structure that combines vertical and horizontal linkages relying on a strong technical infrastructure that can support the virtualization of care services and support project-driven initiatives (Figure 12.4).

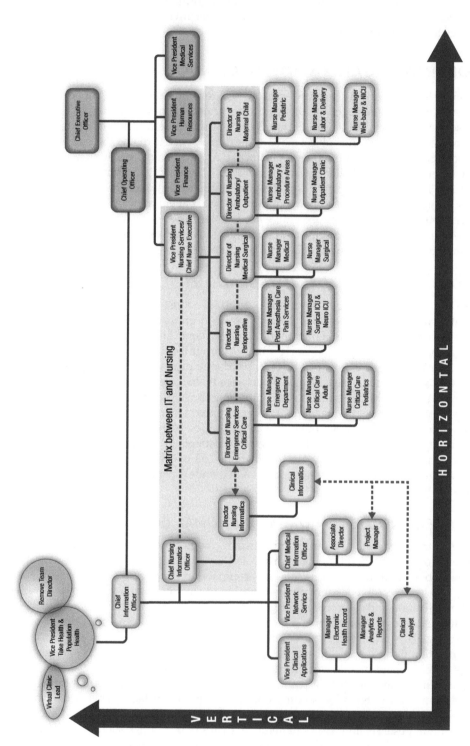

FIGURE 12.4: Vertical and horizontal linkages with defined hierarchical structure.

Note: Vertical and horizontal linkages with defined hierarchical structure that outlines matrix role of chief nursing informatics officer (CNIO) and team between information technology (IT) and nursing in the blue-shaded area. A virtual team portrays a reporting structure to the chief information officer (CIO) that showcases remote monitoring and telehealth practice.

Daft (2021) describes vertical linkages as the process of coordinating activities between the top and bottom of the organization through structural devices, which includes the referral process through the chain of command, rules and plans, and information gathered from written and periodic reports. Horizontal linkages include information systems, direct contact, task forces, and a system integrator. These linkages are supported by a highly centralized and standardized wired environment that relies on technological tools to support communication, coordination, and exchange of information effectively.

ALIGNING ORGANIZATIONAL STRATEGY

The CNE is central in leading change and effectively promoting organizational structures that integrate and blend structural and psychological empowerment with organizational models. There are some practical considerations that CNEs need to weigh when facilitating structural changes to align with the overall organizational strategy. Table 12.4 provides examples of helpful questions that CNEs and/or nurse managers can review in coaching staff and determining the impact of work–life balance (Kottke & Pelletier, 2017).

Creating a balance in being a change-agent, mentor, coach, and executive leader can be challenging and rewarding. The CNE has the sphere of influence, innovative ideas, and collaborative partnerships that they can lean in through sound and flexible structures, and processes that can support HCO's goals while sustaining success.

TABLE 12.4: Practical Considerations in Structuring Organizations

Practical Considerations	Practical Questions
Differentiation versus integration	Does the project require more resources (i.e., staff) where roles need to be defined or can the work be integrated with the same number of resources?
Gaps versus duplication	Were the tasks clarified and is there an outline of staff's scope of responsibility and accountability to address gaps and minimize overlaps?
Underuse versus overload	Is the assignment created by nurse managers fair in relation to staff's capability to promote engagement and prevent burnout?
Lack of clarity versus lack of creativity	Do staff understand the "why"? For example, shared governance structure promotes initiative and creativity. How do directors, nurse managers, and staff align their innovative ideas with the organization's goals in achieving Magnet designation?
Excessive autonomy versus excessive interdependence	Are the staff able to act independently without feeling isolated and disconnected? Do staff rely on layers of approval that can delay decisions? How do points of escalation impact communication relative to safety and care quality?

● CASE SCENARIO

DISASTER RESPONSE DURING COVID-19—PROJECT ORGANIZATIONAL STRUCTURE

SITUATION

During the pandemic, integrated delivery networks had to act swiftly to update the electronic health record (EHR) to capture COVID-19 data close to real-time, coordinate staffing levels, and manage equipment and supplies. There are various departments (e.g., laboratory, infection prevention, IT, nursing providers, respiratory, pharmacy, professional education, registration and admissions, environmental/housekeeping) that need to be part of the workgroup committee as the change process potentially affects workflow, care delivery processes, and optimization. This will affect over 2,000 end-users in seven hospitals and five geographic locations.

APPROACH

Typically, HCOs have a disaster response process to respond to internal and external disasters. In this scenario, the COVID-19 pandemic presents a layer of challenge and complexity in terms of coordination, communication, and control. According to Cristobal et al. (2018), the main factors in Table 12.5 affect the formation of an organizational structure, particularly during crisis situations in the successful execution of a project.

It is an assumption that HCOs have disaster-preparedness policies and procedures. The complexity of any disaster will test the endurance of any organizational structure. Taking these main factors into consideration will keep management and staff focused in formalizing a committee to lead the disaster response. Organizations may need to revamp the old bureaucratic structure to align their purpose and need in meeting the demands in responding and managing crisis situations.

TABLE 12.5: Decentralized Organization Structure

Project Organizational Factors	Description Within the Context of COVID-19 Pandemic
Division of labor	Shifting of labor in specialized areas (ED, critical care, telehealth) divides the throughput of patient, acuity, and staffing needs.
Background and experience	Pooling of subject matter experts to lead specific tasks. For example, information technology, project managers, and service line directors can huddle for a quick analysis of pressing issues and provide recommendations.
Interdependence and interactive management	Coordination of systems communication, interdependence of departments, and schedules in methodological and used case (philosophical) processes to anticipate the risks and unknowns.
Concurrent engineering	Integration of team members through interprofessional collaboration and cross-functional teams.
Authority, leadership, and responsibility	Leading with vision, strategy, and team effort
Unity of command	Activating and establishing lines of commands and understanding obligations
Personnel	Selecting staff with adequate skills and talents to accomplish goals and objectives
Stakeholders	Identifying key project leads and how information will be shared (top-down and bottom-up)
Spans of control	Ensuring adequate levels of control on work processes
Flexibility	Being agile and adapting quickly with change and external environment
Culture values	Commitment and alliance to ensure safety and compliance with quality and regulations
Other factors	Projecting the duration, technology needs, and environment

OUTCOME

An organizational planning structure looks at different units, departments, and teams to maximize efficiency. Setting an organizational structure, particularly during disaster, requires careful planning and considerations such as physical constraints, market conditions, staffing resources, and time needed for procurement of supplies. Roles and responsibilities within the project organizational structure need to look at technical, social, cultural, and administrative reporting lines. Implementing changes (even if temporary) requires communication. Proactive anticipation, flexibility, and early activation of an emergency-disaster organizational structure rooted in project management principles provide an opportunity for senior leadership to explore the best method to meet the challenges and complexities effectively and efficiently.

DISCUSSION QUESTIONS

1. Differentiate ways of conducting analysis from an individual, group, and organizational level.

2. Review your unit/hospital policy for responding to emergency situations and share the communication process with the class. Compare the similarities and differences. Evaluate the following questions based on the most recent emergency experience you participated in: Was the policy effective? What would you suggest changing? Was the leader/organization effective in conveying the necessary change and assuring communication reached the essential team members?

◆ WHAT EVERY NURSE EXECUTIVE NEEDS TO KNOW ABOUT STRUCTURE, PROCESSES, AND ORGANIZATIONAL GOALS

Emerging technologies and virtual workforce are the new normal. The rapid growth of innovation and the ability of early adopters to embrace technology necessitates leaders to be flexible and to foster an environment where creativity can flourish. Communication should be tailored to the needs of a multigenerational workforce. Staff with longevity in the organization might be onsite, remote, and/or virtual. There will be a continued desire for varying work schedules that meet their lifestyles. Nurses desiring more flexibility and the options for travel assignments, reduced work hours, and/or per diem shifts will also influence continuity and creativity. Look to adapt the best practices and tips that have been learned from hospitals where they have had assignments. The need for consistent and clear communication, standardizing practices, evidence-based bundles, and handoff helps ensure safe care. New graduates have less clinical experience, so be prepared to tailor orientation to meet their needs. They may understand the concepts and are adept at accessing information and adapting to electronic medical records, mobile devices and connecting the information.

The other emerging technology to keep at top of mind is artificial intelligence (AI), which has the potential to transform the healthcare industry with not only the advent of applications but the ability to gather data for predictions that can identify at-risk patients and improve outcomes. The ability for analysis of large data sets is also a means to understanding and strategically applying knowledge of the healthcare arena for better resource allocation.

Transactional versus transformational leadership styles will be instrumental in success. The situations that leaders may face will necessitate the ability to possess the skills to be transactional and transformational as needed. Knowledge of different approaches, authentic nurse leadership, appreciative leadership, compassion, an open mind, and critical thinking will serve to guide the appropriate response. With different generations in the workforce, leaders will need to have the age-specific knowledge to manage employees' diverse needs.

Collaborative partnerships to achieve a clear vision and interprofessional collaboration will be essential to success. Nurses, by virtue of their experience in delegating and leading the patient care team, are in roles to further their ability as the interprofessional leaders. Their knowledge of the key roles and disciplines to facilitating wellness and acute patient care is integral to initiatives that impact quality such as efforts to decrease length of stay, facilitate safe discharge, ensure care in the community or at home, and prevent complications and readmissions. Additionally, nurse executives will need to manage diversity in the workforce and work locations, including virtual and nontraditional. They also will need to foster optimism and fairness while providing the opportunity for employees to flourish in all aspects of their lives and to develop the competencies recommended by the American Organization of Nurse Executives (AONE), which are strategic thinking and decision-making, executive presence and communication skills, methods for innovation and change leadership, governance and board relations, executive business skills, and large data sets or big data (Sanford & Janney, 2019).

KEY POINTS

- HCOs rely on structure, process, and goals for success.
- Concepts and models on empowerment, shared governance, and organizational theories are important tools to transform HCOs. Partnership and collaboration are essential in achieving shared purpose and job satisfaction.

SUMMARY

Healthcare's complexity requires an organizational structure that is ideally shaped and implemented for the primary purpose of achieving shared safety goals and quality outcomes in an efficient manner. Nurse leaders must be aware of various organizational structures in business and technology industries that can be adapted in healthcare to set oneself up for success. With the changing global market and VUCA climate, one can design a suitable organizational structure that recognizes and addresses the various human and business realities of HCOs. The advent of innovative technology provides limitless opportunity for CNEs in leading a patient-centered care that is adaptable, flexible, and competitive.

On the other hand, organizational structures share common characteristics in supporting an effective work environment. A traditional organizational chart with a structured reporting process versus a decentralized hybrid structure can thrive by analyzing common characteristics, structure, and dimensions. Nurse leaders can go through this analysis exercise, compare best practices, and go through the following checklist (Gale, 2017):

- What are the strengths and weaknesses of various organizational forms?
- Are there legal advantages and disadvantages of organizational structures?
- Is there a list that identifies the advantages and drawbacks of departmentalization options?
- What are the projected growth patterns of the organization in a 3-, 5-, and 10-years cycle?
- What are the current reporting relationships from a formal/informal chain of command?
- What will be the future state of reporting and authority relationships if structures are changed?
- What is the optimum staffing, that is, ratios of supervisors/managers to subordinates based on regulations?
- What programs are in place to support or develop autonomy/empowerment of staff and promote staff and patient satisfaction?

- What structures are in place that promote joy at work and work–life balance?
- What ongoing structures support optimum operational efficiency and a culture of safety?

Nurse leaders (managers, senior leaders, executives) have a critical and significant role in fostering a climate that is equitable while promoting a shared governance model that is empowering staff to be creative and engaged. Mentoring future nurse leaders to have managerial courage lays the foundation in developing a trusting relationship with staff, influencing individuals' commitment levels while creating an environment that supports the meaning, joy, and value in nurses' work and contributions. Senior management plays an important sponsorship role for facilitating empowering supportive policies that enable organizational members to accomplish their work in meaningful ways.

Nursing is central to the operations of any HCO. Meaningful relationships exist between organizational structure and organizational strategy, performance, and individual attitudes and behaviors (Gale, 2017). A collaborative partnership between cross-departments across the enterprise healthcare system promotes regionalization and virtualization. This collaborative process will reinforce standardized processes through policies that support organizational and professional goals. Sharing success and achieving positive results lay the ground for structural strategies that facilitate successful transitions and leadership transformations in HCO.

END-OF-CHAPTER RESOURCES

◨ DISCUSSION QUESTIONS

1. Conduct an organizational analysis on your current unit. Based on the models, what structure, process, and goals would you improve, retain, or replace?
2. As a leader, how would you prepare your staff in responding to an emergency hospital-wide or statewide crisis? Share with your team any formal communication and planning strategies that your organization has in place.
3. Develop a training module for onboarding new nurse leaders that would encompass organizational structure, process, and outcomes.

◨ ADDITIONAL RESOURCES

Podcast: Today in Nursing Leadership (https://www.aonl.org/nursing-leadership-podcast)

TED Talk: What are you willing to give up to change the way we work? (https://bit.ly/3x2BGSF)

Web Links

- Organizational Health Podcasts: https://player.fm/podcasts/Organizational-Health
- The Kornferry channel—Korn Ferry is a global organizational consulting firm that works with clients to design their organizational structures, roles, and responsibilities. Visit kornferry.com

◨ LEARNING EXERCISES FOR STUDENTS

1. Create an organizational chart that details the structure and relationships of units and departments.
2. Interview a nurse leader and ask about what they consider to be the most challenging aspects of their role and any recommendations for future leaders.
3. Provide an example of effective and ineffective communication through role-playing.

⬤ GLOSSARY OF KEY TERMS

- **Centralization:** The distribution of decision-making authority, information, and power throughout an organization.

- **Contingency theory:** In this context, it refers to the idea that relevant circumstances must be considered before applying a specific organizational design.

- **Departmentalization:** The existence of formal and informal divisions within an organization.

- **Environment:** The total of the factors that occur outside of the organization but are relevant to the decision-making and management of the organization.

- **Formalization:** The extent to which organizational policies, practices, and ways of completing tasks are standardized.

- **Innovation strategies:** Emphasize being the leader in the industry in introducing new products or services.

- **Interdependency:** (also called integration) The integration of tasks and activities across different workers.

- **Mechanistic models of structure:** Denoted by high specialization, rigid departmentalization, strong centralization and formalization, and narrow spans of control with clear authority lines.

- **Organic model of structure:** Has decentralized authority and decision-making, low standardization, and formalization with self-directed teams or work groups as the primary departmentalization strategy.

- **Organizational structure:** The formal and informal way in which people, job tasks, and other organizational resources are configured and coordinated.

- **Physical dispersion:** The extent to which organizational members are physically distinct from one another.

- **Span of control:** The number of subordinates who report to a single manager.

- **Specialization:** The extent to which job tasks require highly specific (i.e., specialized) work skills or, conversely, can be carried out successfully by individuals who possess more universally available knowledge, skills, and abilities.

- **Technology:** Often considered interchangeable with computerization, but technology, in its broadest sense, may be defined as the knowledge necessary to process raw material and represents one aspect of the environment affecting an organization.

 SPRINGER PUBLISHING CONNECT™ | A robust set of instructor resources designed to supplement this text is located at http://connect.springerpub.com/content/book/978-0-8261-7795-7. Qualifying instructors may request access by emailing textbook@springerpub.com.

REFERENCES

Aubrey, M., & Lavoie-Tremblay, M. (2018). Rethinking organizational design for managing multiple projects. *International Journal of Project Management 36*, 12–26. https://doi.org/10.1016/j.ijproman.2017.05.012

Berkow, S., Workman, J., Aronson, S., Stewart, J., Virkstis, K., & Kahn, M. (2012). Strengthening frontline nurse investment in organizational goals. *The Journal of Nursing Administration, 42*(3), 165–169. https://doi.org/10.1097/NNA.0b013e31824809b7

Clavelle, J. T., Porter-O'Grady, T., Weston, M. J., & Verran, J. A. (2016). Evolution of structural empowerment: Moving from shared to professional governance. *Journal of Nursing Administration, 46*(6), 308–312. https://doi.org/10.1097/NNA.0000000000000350

Cristobal, J. R., Fernandez, V., & Diaz, E. (2018). An analysis of the main project organizational structures: Advantages, disadvantages, and factors affecting their selection. *Procedia Computer Science, 138*, 791–798. https://doi.org/10.1016/j.procs.2018.10.103

Daft, R. L. (2021). *Organizational theory and design* (13th ed.). Southwestern, Cengage Learning.

de las Heras-Rosas, C., Herrera, J., & Rodríguez-Fernández, M. (2021). Organisational commitment in healthcare systems: A bibliometric analysis. *International Journal of Environmental Research and Public Health, 18*, 2271. https://doi.org/10.3390/ijerph18052271

DiNapoli, J. M., O'Flaherty, D., & Garcia-Dia, M. J. (2014). Theory of empowerment. In J. J. Fitzpatrick & G. McCarthy (Eds.), *Theories guiding nursing research and practice: Making nursing knowledge development explicit* (pp. 303–322). Springer Publishing Company.

Donaldson, L. (2013). Organizational structure and design. In E. H. Kessler (Ed.), *Encyclopedia of management theory* (Vol. 2, pp. 569–574). Sage.

Flynn, D. N. (2015). Building a better model: A novel approach for mapping organizational and functional structure. *Procedia Computer Science, 44*, 194–203. https://doi.org/10.1016/j.procs.2015.03.003

Gale. (2017). Organizational structure. In V. L. Burton III (Ed.), *Encyclopedia of small business* (5th ed., Vol. 2, pp. 804–805). Gale.

Gale Research Inc. (2019). Organizational analysis and planning. In V. L. Burton III (Ed.), *The encyclopedia of management* (pp. 818–822). Gale.

Kottke, J. L., & Pelletier, K. L. (2017). Organizational structure. In S. G. Rogelberg (Ed.), *The SAGE encyclopedia of industrial and organizational psychology* (2nd ed., Vol. 3, pp. 1142–1146). Sage.

Lapaine, M. (2021). Embracing the Quadruple Aim: One hospital's experience. *Healthcare Management Forum, 34*(1), 26–28. https://doi.org/10.1177/0840470420942791

Larson, J. (2012). *The connection between employee satisfaction and patient satisfaction.* https://www.amnhealthcare.com/amn-insights/news/want-to-boost-your-patient-satisfaction-scores-try-investing-more-resources-and-attention-in-your-clinical-staff

Marquis, B. L., & Huston, C. J. (2021). *Leadership roles and management function in nursing: Theory and application.* Wolters Kluwer Health/Lippincott Williams & Wilkins.

Matthews, S., Laschinger, H. K. S., & Johnstone, L. (2006). Staff nurse empowerment in line and staff organizational structure for chief nurse executives. *The Journal of Nursing Administration, 36*(11), 526–533. https://doi.org/10.1097/00005110-200611000-00008

Newton, J., Wait, A., & Angus, S. D. (2019). Watercooler chat, organizational structure and corporate culture. *Games and Economic Behavior, 118*, 354–365. https://doi.org/10.1016/j.geb.2019.09.004.

Porter-O'Grady, T., & Clavelle, J. T. (2020). The structural framework for nursing professional governance: Foundation for empowerment. *Nurse Leader, 18*(2), 181–189. https://doi.org/10.1016/j.mnl.2019.08.004

Roth Piper, L., & Schneider, M. (2015). Nurse executive leadership during organizational mergers. *Journal of Nursing Administration, 45*(12), 592–594. https://doi.org/10.1097/NNA.0000000000000269

Rydenfalt, C., Odenrick, P., & Larsson, P. A. (2017). Organizing for team in healthcare: An alternative to team training? *Journal of Health Organization and Management, 31*(3), 347–362. https://doi.org/10.1108/JHOM-12-2016-0233

Sanford, K., & Janney, M. (2019). Preparing the nurse executive of the future. *Journal of Nursing Administration, 49*(4), 171–173. https://doi.org/10.1097/NNA.0000000000000732

Warshawsky, N. E., Caramanica, L., & Cramer, E. (2020). Organizational support for nurse manager role transition and onboarding. *The Journal of Nursing Administration, 50*(5), 254–260. https://doi.org/10.1097/NNA.0000000000000880

Zinn, J. S., & Brannon, S. D. (2014). Finding strength in numbers; bringing theoretical pluralism into the analysis of healthcare organizations. In S. S. F. Mick & P. D. Shay (Eds.), *Advances in health care organization theory* (2nd ed., pp. 53–78). John Wiley & Sons.

APPENDIX A: CHECKLIST DURING A PLANNED ORGANIZATIONAL MERGER

Timeline Prior to Merger Date	Checklist
12 Months Prior	Is there a transition plan that identifies mission, vision, and organizational structure?
	What is the new organizational leadership model and structure? Include reporting process, meeting structures, and programs such as Magnet.
	Did you schedule a site visit for a meet and greet session with key leaders? Include regular meetings with staff and leadership to apprise and provide updates.
	What is the baseline data on quality, safety, and performance indicators?
	Do you have an inventory list of the clinical applications, information systems, and services?
	Did you do a gap analysis to identify documentation standards, norms, policies, and procedures? Delegate the work to a system-wide practice council.
	How would you describe the culture, professional practice, and communication? This will drive the composition of a system-wide steering committee to lead the integration process.
	Are there contracts requiring priority for renewal and consolidation of services?
6–9 Months Prior	Did you review nursing systems and structures, organizational goals, and timelines?
	Did you check in with system-wide practice councils with their recommendations on quality improvement/metrics, professional education and practice, staffing, policies and procedures, practice alerts, and patient satisfaction?
	What are the recommendations from human resource, medical staff leaders, and service line structures on nurse–physician processes and programs?
	What is the recommendation from information technology on the current and future state of electronic medical records and other clinical systems?
3 Months Prior	Are you on target with your transition goals?
	Who is monitoring for service disruptions and patient care?
	What is the ongoing feedback from clinical staff with the merger and change?
1 Month Prior	Did you consider stakeholders' feedback on the changes and expected reporting structure? Was this formally communicated to internal (leaders, staff) and external stakeholders (i.e., vendors, schools, community partners)?
	Is there a unified voice with the system-wide council and a unified front with the steering committee in adhering with the schedule and timeline?
Day of Transition	Conduct a town hall meeting to formally welcome stakeholders to the new integrated system; continue to hold huddles and meetings and have a 1-year celebration as a milestone.

CHAPTER 13

STRATEGIC DEVELOPMENT AND PLANNING

Moreen Donahue

*"If your actions inspire others to dream more, learn more,
do more, and become more, you are a leader."*

John Quincy Adams

LEARNING OBJECTIVES

- Describe the nature of strategy formulation, implementation, execution, and evaluation.
- Distinguish among strategic planning, strategic management, and strategy execution.
- Explicate the formulation of corporate level strategy, business level strategy, and functional level strategy.
- Evaluate the strategic plan of the organization in which you work.

INTRODUCTION

The focus of strategic initiatives in healthcare has evolved over the last five decades in response to the ever-changing and challenging healthcare environment. Cost-based reimbursement prevalent during the 1960s through the 1980s encouraged strategies based on growth and expansion of the physical plant. New payment models that emerged from the 1980s through 2010 such as managed care, prospective payment, and the Affordable Care Act (ACA) resulted in a change of focus from expanding brick-and-mortar facilities to offering broader services, extending the geographic footprint, and strengthening relationships with referring physicians. Since 2010, the focus of strategic planning for healthcare delivery has shifted from the volume and profitability of services provided to maximizing value for consumers (Grube & Crnkovich, 2017; Meadows, 2016).

Notable events that significantly changed the strategic direction of the world of business and healthcare delivery include the events of September 11, 2001; the financial crisis of 2008; and the COVID-19 crisis of 2020 to 2022. The events of September 11, 2001, caused world leaders to examine and review safety practices. New York City's healthcare service providers including public health and social services were subjected to unanticipated pressures. Staff and patients experienced high levels of stress, hospital revenues declined, and the proportion of uninsured patients increased. The airline industry was changed overnight, financial markets and institutions needed to respond to the expanding crisis, and healthcare organizations needed to create new ways of leading, such as the establishment of incident command centers. The financial crisis of 2008 to 2009 affected business and healthcare in ways that are still prevalent. Lack of employment and therefore lack of insurance caused a dramatic decline in elective procedures and routine healthcare. The COVID-19 crisis of 2020 to 2021 dramatically changed the future of healthcare and organizations needed to completely redesign their short- and long-term goals (Betts et al., 2020; Morse & Warshawsky, 2021).

As the healthcare industry responded to these life-changing situations, nurse leaders became more central to the strategic planning process. Engaging the nursing workforce in all settings where care was provided in designing and delivering new models of care became critical to the successful attainment of strategic initiatives. In order to be an effective partner on the strategic planning team, nurse leaders needed to be able to translate visionary thinking about improved patient care delivery to actionable outcomes. Nurse leaders were able to obtain guidance from the leading nursing organizations, academic institutions, and other nurse leaders on how to accomplish this (American Nurses Association [ANA], 2018; American Organization of Nurse Executives [AONE], 2016; AONE & American Organization for Nursing Leadership [AONL], 2015).

The strategic plan is often described as a blueprint or roadmap to where the organization is going and directions for how to get there (Broome & Marshall, 2021; Drewniak, n.d.; Lal, 2020; Schaffner, 2009; Spear, 2015). Just as there is no one way to define strategic planning, there is no one way of doing it. Numerous strategic planning and development experts have developed templates and guides to assist healthcare organizations to develop their strategic plan (Broome & Marshall, 2021; Daft, 2021; Drewniak, n.d.; Jeffs et al., 2019; Lal, 2020). Most agree on four key phases for creating a successful plan:

1. The analysis and assessment phase

2. The strategy formulation phase

3. The strategy execution phase

4. The strategy evaluation phase

This chapter addresses the history of strategic development and planning, best practices for addressing the four key phases of successful strategy creation and implementation, different strategy levels, and translating organizational strategy into execution and results at all levels of nursing practice.

HISTORICAL PERSPECTIVE

The concept of strategic planning is not new. Strategic planning has long been a component of the business culture but not historically part of healthcare, and even less so for nursing. A review of the history relevant to strategic planning provides insight into the evolving best practices for strategy formulation, dissemination, and execution (Fisher, n.d.; Horwath, 2006).

Blackerby (1994/n.d.) traced the history of strategic planning from its Greek beginnings through modern practices. According to Blackerby, the word "strategy" is a derivative of the Greek word "strategos" which translates to "general of the army." The strategos elected by the Greek tribes formed a council to advise the political ruler on new ways of managing battles to win wars. As early as 500 BC Sun Tzu, a Chinese military strategist, revolutionized military thinking. He suggested alternatives to waging battles and emphasized the value of making and keeping strategic relationships. Blackerby contends that from these military beginnings the focus on strategic planning has been on the big picture rather than on tactics. Blackerby addresses the evolution of modern strategic planning with a review of various strategic models. The Harvard Business school developed the Harvard policy model in the 1920s. This model was one of the first strategic methodologies for private business. Strategy in this model refers to purposes and policies that define the company. Resources, leadership, market analysis, and social considerations inform strategies that lead to improved financial outcomes. Other models outlined by Blackerby included the portfolio model of the 1950s that incorporated risk management and growth as strategic initiatives, and the industrial economics model of the 1960s that stressed the importance of customers and competition.

Woyzbun (2001) maintained that the process of strategic planning has existed since man needed to "get from point A to point B." Woyzbun highlighted notable pioneers in the theoretical foundations of planning including Igor Ansoff, Peter Drucker, and Michael Porter. Igor Ansoff created the Ansoff Matrix. This matrix model consists of a decision-making guide for corporate or business unit direction. Components of the model include strategies for future growth related to market penetration, market development, product development, and diversification. Peter Drucker contended that management should approach planning as a discipline of science. Drucker defined planning as a continual process of decision-making and evaluating results against expectations. He believed that the purpose of strategy was to enable an organization to achieve its goals in an unforeseeable environment. In the 1980s, Michael Porter proposed that strategy based on external competitive forces would lead to competitive advantage. Porter's Five Forces model provided a framework for business to achieve financial outcomes. These forces are:

1. Internal competition (rivalry)
2. The threat of new entrants
3. The threat of substitutes
4. Supplier bargaining power
5. Customer bargaining power

Woyzbun offered thoughts on the reasons strategic planning lost favor throughout the 1980s. Since most approaches to strategic development and planning contained similar components, common issues emerged as possible causes of the failure of strategic plans to deliver expected outcomes. First, the top-down approach utilized in the planning process did not include input from those who were most knowledgeable about the actual capability of the business to reach the objectives. Also, in many organizations employees were not able to articulate the main objectives of the plan. The complexity of many of the organizations contributed to failures in the implementation of the plan. In addition, the 1980s was a time of increasing globalization and increased economic pressures. Despite these issues that emerged with strategic planning and development, Woyzbun maintained that the foundational work of strategy pioneers such as Ansoff, Drucker, and Porter remained relevant (Fisher, n.d.; Woyzbun, 2001).

Horwath (2006) provided insight into the history of business strategy by describing seven phases of business strategy evolution. The evolution of business strategy as outlined by Horwath is presented in Table 13.1.

TABLE 13.1: Phases of Business Strategy Evolution

Phase	Time Period	Characteristics
Budgetary planning	1950–1960	Financial control was created through operating budgets and investment planning.
Corporate planning	1960–1968	Setting long-term goals and objectives and determining actions and resources needed to meet those goals.
Corporate strategy	1968–1975	The relationship between market share and profitability was stressed.
Industry and competitive analysis	1975–1985	Review of choice of industries, markets, and position were assessed during this phase.
Internal sourcing of competitive advantage	1985–1995	Core competencies that enable a company to provide benefits to customers emerged during this phase.
Strategic innovation and implementation	1995–2001	The application of technology to the business planning process highlighted the importance of strategic innovation during this phase.
Strategic thinking and simplification	2001 and beyond	Utilization of simple frameworks that promote strategic thinking as a daily practice emerged in this phase.

LEVELS OF STRATEGY

Strategy development and execution occurs at the corporate, business, and functional levels within organizations (Business-to-you, 2020). Many larger healthcare organizations create corporate structures that include a board of directors, senior executives, and corporate staff.

The corporate level oversees the strategy for the entire enterprise. The organization's mission and vision as well as the overall strategic direction are defined at this level.

The business level strategy focuses on product line development. Managers at this level develop goals, actions and interventions that will assist their areas of responsibility to achieve the corporate strategic imperatives.

The functional level strategy supports the corporate and business levels. Many healthcare organizations develop service-line driven functional strategies to promote their specialty areas. Managers have the responsibility for assuring that functional strategy initiatives and expected outcomes are understood by all employees and each employee knows how their individual performance contributes to the overall success of the organization.

BEST PRACTICES FOR STRATEGIC DEVELOPMENT AND PLANNING

The Institute for Healthcare Improvement (IHI) created the IHI High-Impact Leadership Framework as a practical way for leaders at all levels of healthcare organizations to improve care, improve the health of populations, and reduce costs. The high-impact leadership behaviors identified by the IHI as essential to improving the health and outcomes of populations served by the organization include

- person-centeredness;
- frontline engagement;
- relentless focus on vision and strategy;
- transparency about results, progress, aims, and defects; and
- systems thinking and collaboration across boundaries.

This framework provides a useful model for strategic development and planning. The six domains of the framework and related leadership actions, behaviors, and efforts were developed based on social science leadership and decades of evidence-based improvement efforts by the IHI. The six domains of the framework are

- driven by persons and community,
- create vision and build will,
- develop capability,
- deliver results,
- shape culture, and
- engage across boundaries.

The recommendations inherent in the IHI High-Impact Leadership Framework are incorporated into the four key phases for developing and executing a successful strategic plan (Swensen et al., 2013).

PHASES OF STRATEGIC DEVELOPMENT AND PLANNING

THE ASSESSMENT AND ANALYSIS PHASE

The assessment and analysis phase assists the organization in examining their present state. The relevance of its mission, vision, values, and goals in relation to the current cultural, financial, and patient care delivery climate is examined in this phase (Drewniak, n.d.).

A mission statement usually describes why an organization exists (Broome & Marshall, 2021; Spear, 2015; Wright, 2020; Zuckerman, 2016). Sample mission statements from industry and healthcare are reflected in Box 13.1.

BOX 13.1: SAMPLE MISSION STATEMENTS

INDUSTRY:

Jet Blue: "To inspire humanity—both in the air and on the ground"
LinkedIn: "To connect the world's professionals to make them more productive and successful"
TED Talks: "Spread ideas"
Tesla: "To accelerate the world's transition to sustainable energy"

HEALTHCARE:

Cleveland Clinic, Cleveland, Ohio: "Caring for life, researching for health, educating those who serve"
Johns Hopkins Medicine, Baltimore, Maryland: "To improve the health of the community and the world by setting the standard of excellence in medical education, research, and clinical care"
Massachusetts General Hospital, Boston, Massachusetts: "Guided by the needs of our patients and their families, we aim to deliver the very best healthcare in a safe, compassionate environment, to advance that care through innovative research and education, and to improve the health and well-being of the diverse communities we serve"
Virginia Mason, Seattle, Washington: "To improve the health and well-being of the patients we serve"

A vision statement is aspirational and reflects the desired future state of the organization (Broome & Marshall, 2021; Crawford et al., 2017; Enochson, 2020; Stichler, 2006; Wright, 2020; Zuckerman, 2016). Sample vision statements from industry and healthcare are reflected in Box 13.2.

BOX 13.2: SAMPLE VISION STATEMENTS

INDUSTRY:

Apple INC.: "To make the best products on earth, and to leave the world better than we found it"
Google: "To provide access to the world's information in one click"
Habitat for Humanity: "A world where everyone has a decent place to live"
Walt Disney Company: "To be one of the world's leading producers and providers of entertainment and information"

HEALTHCARE:

American Academy of Nursing: "Healthy lives for all people"
Fox Chase Cancer Center: "To be a regional, national and international leader in oncology nursing care and services"
Mayo Clinic: "Transforming medicine to connect and cure as the global authority in the care of serious or complex disease"
St. Jude Children's Research Hospital: "To accelerate progress against catastrophic disease at a global level"

Values reflect the organization's principles and expected behaviors necessary for carrying out the mission and vision (Broome & Marshall, 2021; Zuckerman, 2016). Common values that many organizations cite as part of their culture and foundational to the expected code of conduct for all members of the organization are reflected in Box 13.3.

BOX 13.3: SAMPLE VALUES

- Caring
- Compassion
- Diversity
- Equity
- Excellence
- Inclusion
- Integrity
- Quality
- Respect
- Service

Approaches to performing the assessment and analysis of the organization include a SWOT (strengths, weaknesses, opportunities, threats) analysis and/or the SOAR (strengths, opportunities, aspirations, results) analysis. The SWOT methodology typically examines the organization's environment. Strengths and weaknesses reflect internal factors, and opportunities and threats reflect external factors. The SOAR model, based on appreciative inquiry, is gaining favor in healthcare strategic planning as a way to encourage a positive interdisciplinary approach to the formulation of innovative goals and objectives (Broome & Marshall, 2021; Schaffner, 2009; Spear, 2015; Wadsworth et al., 2016; Wright, 2020; Zuckerman, 2016). Common elements of the SWOT or SOAR analysis are listed in Box 13.4.

BOX 13.4: COMMON COMPONENTS OF THE SWOT AND SOAR ASSESSMENT AND ANALYSIS

- Centers of excellence
- Differentiating opportunities
- Financial resources
- Image
- Key staff
- Key relationships
- Market changes
- Market opportunities
- Market recognition
- Organizational culture
- Organizational structure
- Satisfaction survey results
- Technology capability

SOAR, strengths, opportunities, aspirations, results; SWOT, strengths, weaknesses, opportunities, threats.

Engaging key stakeholders in the assessment and analysis of the organization is an important step in obtaining a comprehensive picture of the current state of the organization. This promotes ownership, which will be essential for executing and sustaining the plan (Daft, 2021; Jeffs et al., 2019; Schaffner, 2009). Sample questions for key stakeholders to address are listed in Box 13.5.

BOX 13.5: QUESTIONS FOR KEY STAKEHOLDERS

1. What is the organization's culture?
2. What is the structure of the organization?
3. What is the image of the organization internally and externally?
4. Who are the key staff and are there any gaps or flight risks?
5. What are the financial resources? Is there access to resources?
6. What key relationships exist that need to be cultivated?
7. What differentiates this organization?
8. What new programs should be considered?
9. Are there market opportunities?
10. Should this service area be expanded?
11. What is the technology capability of the organization?
12. What innovative technologies should be explored?
13. How satisfied are various stakeholders with the organization?

The use of data in assessing and analyzing the organization is a critical factor. Data relative to quality, safety, financial performance and stability, human resources (HR), and use of technology must be considered (Morse & Warshawsky, 2021; Sanford & Janney, 2019; Wright, 2020).

THE STRATEGY FORMULATION PHASE

The next phase in strategic development and planning involves the formulation of the strategic plan based on the results of the assessment and analysis phase. Two frequently cited models for strategy formulation are Porter's model of competitive strategies and the Miles and Snow strategy typology. Porter created his model based on his evaluation of a number of businesses that suggested that organizations could become more profitable and less vulnerable by choosing either a differentiation strategy or a low-cost leadership strategy. Apple, Inc. is an example of a company that has successfully embraced differentiation, and Ryanair is a company that has successfully implemented a low-cost leadership strategy (Daft, 2021). The Miles and Snow strategy typology is based on organizational fit with the external environment. This model focuses on four formative strategies. The prospector strategy is based on new growth opportunities. Creativity is emphasized over efficiency. Nike is a company that exemplifies this strategy. The defender strategy is based on efficiency, control, and the retention of valued customers. Paramount Pictures is an example of a company that utilized this approach in making the strategic decision to produce reliable films but few high-risk productions. The analyzer strategy attempts to balance stable environments and customer retention with innovation and new product line development. Amazon is a company that has successfully utilized this strategy. The reactor strategy is employed by companies that respond to immediate opportunities and threats without a defined long-range plan. Blockbuster is an example of a company that failed to adopt a strategy based on changing customer preferences (Daft, 2021; Zuckerman, 2016).

Scenario planning is a technique that may assist healthcare organizations in the formulation of their strategic plan. This technique encourages leaders to be future focused and to consider structures that allow unplanned events and situations to be addressed. Scenario plans should be based on the organization's current state as determined by the assessment and analysis phase and include situations such as capacity surges, loss of communication systems and technology, storm damage, supply chain disruption, loss of key personnel, and new competition. The COVID-19 crisis underscores the importance of scenario planning related to unanticipated healthcare emergencies (Betts et al., 2020; Daft, 2021; Kirkpatrick, 2021; Mohammad, 2020; Zuckerman, 2016).

Once key themes have been identified as a result of the assessment and analysis of the organization's current state, the strategic planning committee determines the strategic imperatives, goals, and objectives that will allow the organization to achieve its mission and vision. Some organizations may choose to engage healthcare consulting firms to assist with this process. Typical plans include short-term and long-term timelines with goals and objectives to be accomplished within a specified time frame, usually ranging from 1 to 5 years. One common challenge during this phase is the failure to determine the critical issues at the corporate level and then failing to develop clear, measurable goals at the business and functional levels. The board of directors in partnership with the executive leadership team is responsible for determining a finite number (usually five to 10) of strategic imperatives among competing priorities and directing resources to support those imperatives. The senior leadership team then translates these imperatives into actionable goals and objectives. Goals are usually broad in focus and state desired outcomes. Objectives are measurable and include actions to be taken by whom and by when. Effective objectives are specific; have a defined time period for completion; and are challenging, achievable, and results oriented. The SMART (specific, measurable, achievable, realistic, time-bound) guide to setting performance goals and objectives is a useful tool for executive leaders to use in assisting managers to set goals and objectives based on strategic imperatives. Once the goals and objectives have been established, the metrics that will be used to monitor progress will need to be determined (Lal, 2020; Smith, 1999; Spear, 2015; Wright, 2020).

THE STRATEGY EXECUTION PHASE

Best practices for strategy execution emphasize the importance of the commitment of the leadership team to the implementation of the plan. Senior leaders communicate the key steps that were taken during the strategy assessment and analysis and formulation phases to ensure that everyone understands the clinical, financial, operational, and workforce benefits of a well-executed plan. The selection of specific execution leaders with the right skills to be able to communicate and direct the essential components of the plan is critical. Each individual's responsibility in achieving specific goals and outcomes should be clearly indicated. Timelines should be established for implementation of the plan's objectives and for reporting of results. Plan implementation progress and results are often included as standing agenda items for executive, management, and staff meetings. Many organizations use scorecards or dashboards to facilitate review of progress (Crawford et al., 2017; Jeffs et al., 2019; Kaplan, 2020; Kaplan & Norton, 1996; Lal, 2020; Schaffner, 2009; Wright, 2020).

The balanced scorecard is a useful tool for managing and tracking operational and financial objectives. Many healthcare organizations use this tool to communicate the organization's initiatives and progress toward goals. Usually, the scorecard is depicted on one page and includes measures such as performance on quality, financial, patient satisfaction, and learning goals (Daft, 2021; Horwath, 2006; Wright, 2020; Zuckerman, 2016). A sample scorecard is depicted in Figure 13.1. Kaplan and Norton (1996), the creators of the balanced scorecard, recommended four steps for managing strategy and suggested rationales for use of the balanced scorecard with each step. These four steps and related rationales are presented in Table 13.2.

Scorecard:				
Goal		Strategic Imperative	Measure	Weight
Quality and Safety				30%
1	Reduce readmissions		CHF, PN, AMI, COPD	
2	Reduce infections		CAUTI	
			CLABSI	
3	Increase patient safety		#SSEs	
Service Excellence				15%
4	Improve patient experience inpatient		HCAHPS – Hospital 1	
			HCAHPS – Hospital 2	
			HCAHPS – Hospital 3	
Skilled and Motivated Workforce				15%
5	Increase employee engagement		Employee Engagement—Transitional Composite	
Growth and Innovation				15%
6	Recognize as innovative, accessible, and comprehensive		Increase clinical services for cancer, ortho, and maternal/child	
			New services are the option of choice	
			Increase clinical research studies	
Financial Strength				25%
7	Increase margin		EBITDA	
8	Increase philanthropy		Development funding	
9	Community benefit investment		Investing equivalent to tax liability	

FIGURE 13.1: Sample scorecard.

AMI, acute myocardial infarction; CAUTI, catheter-associated urinary tract infections; CHF, congestive heart failure; CLABSI, central line-associated bloodstream infection; COPD, chronic obstructive pulmonary disease; EBITDA, earnings before interest, taxes, depreciation, and amortization; HCAHPS, Hospital Consumer Assessment of Healthcare Providers and Systems; PN, pneumonia; #SSE, number of serious safety events.

TABLE 13.2: Four Steps for Managing Strategy and Rationale for Using the Balanced Scorecard

Step		Rationale
1	Translating the vision	The balanced scorecard can serve as a useful tool to translate the mission and vision into understandable performance expectations.
2	Communicating and linking	The balanced scorecard can be used as a communication tool that links individual performance to organization objectives.
3	Organizational planning	Development of the balanced scorecard assists organizations to link strategy with operations and implementation.
4	Feedback and learning	The balanced scorecard approach to strategic management provides a framework for setting goals, monitoring progress toward goals, and a mechanism to alert management if a plan needs revision.

THE STRATEGY EVALUATION PHASE

According to the Agency for Healthcare Research and Quality (AHRQ; 2018), determining when and how to measure success is one of the most important decisions to be made during the planning process. Questions to be answered during this phase include:

- What worked?
- What did not work?
- What could be done differently to create a better process and a better outcome?

The evaluation phase allows management to determine whether goals were achieved on time and on budget. It is important to consider time, resources, and funding that will be needed as part of the evaluation process during the initial planning phases. Common criteria include relevance, compliance, effectiveness, efficiency, impact, and sustainability. Questions to be asked in this phase include:

- Were objectives met?
- Were key steps omitted?
- Was there enough money in the budget?
- Was enough time allotted?
- Were conflicts addressed?
- Were the right partners selected?

STRATEGIC DEVELOPMENT AND PLANNING—A NURSE LEADER COMPETENCY

Leading nursing organizations identified strategic planning and development as a core competency nursing leaders must master to be successful in meeting the challenges of the rapidly changing healthcare environment. In 2005 the AONE, renamed the AONL in 2019, published the AONE nurse executive competencies (NECs). These competencies were deemed essential for impactful executive nurse leadership. The NECs include leadership, professionalism, business skills and principles, knowledge of the healthcare environment, and communication and relationship management. Included in the leadership competency is the expectation that nurse executives provide visionary thinking on issues that affect the healthcare organization and take into account the importance of nursing decisions on the organization (Morse & Warshawsky, 2021; Waxman et al., 2017).

Beginning in 2010, AONE focused on the establishment of core competencies for system chief nurse executives (CNEs). In 2016, AONE published the *System CNE White Paper: The Effective System Nurse Executive in Contemporary Health Systems: Emerging Competencies.* Meadows (2016) provided an overview of this document and the competencies that system CNEs must embrace and exhibit in the ever changing, more complex healthcare environment. "System CNEs must be competent in improving population health, increasing quality, expanding provider coverage, and managing increasingly complex health information technology systems" (Meadows, 2016, p. 235).

Nurse manager competencies were published by AONE in 2015. These competencies were based on three domains:

1. The Science: Managing the business
2. The Art: Leading the people
3. The Leader Within: Creating the leader in yourself

THE LEADER WITHIN: CREATING THE LEADER WITHIN YOURSELF

The ANA published the ANA Leadership Competency Model in 2018. This model includes three domains:

1. Leading yourself

2. Leading others

3. Leading the organization

Vision and strategy are included in the leading organization competency. Behaviors of nurse leaders exhibiting competencies in vision and strategy include the ability to translate vision into realistic long-term objectives and business strategies, and the development of plans that are flexible enough to account for future challenges (ANA, 2018).

THE NURSING STRATEGIC PLAN—TRANSLATING STRATEGY INTO EXECUTION

The first phase in the development of an organization's strategic plan usually occurs at the corporate level and includes the board of directors, senior administrators, and clinical leadership. The CNE is a member of the executive team that prepares an executive summary of the plan for the strategic planning committee of the board of directors. This document typically includes an environmental analysis, strategic imperatives identified by the analysis, and outcome indicators. If the executive summary is approved by the committee, the complete strategic plan is presented to the full board of directors for approval. A sample table of contents for an executive summary of a strategic plan is depicted in Box 13.6. The CNE can use this summary as a guide for preparing documents to translate and communicate the content of the plan for all nursing staff when the complete strategic plan has been approved by the board of directors.

BOX 13.6: SAMPLE EXECUTIVE SUMMARY TABLE OF CONTENTS

1. Introduction
   Overview of system/organization
   Purpose of the strategic plan
   Plan development process

2. Environmental analysis
   Key issues affecting healthcare delivery
   Competencies to proceed
   Primary and secondary markets

3. Strategic plan
   Mission
   Values
   Future vision
   Strategic imperatives

4. Monitoring and evaluation
   Outcome indicators

Nurse leaders in practice and academia have provided guidance and resources for developing the nursing strategic plan and integrating it into the overall system/organizational strategy (Broome & Marshall, 2021; Schaffner, 2009). In 2009, Schaffner proposed a 10-step process that could assist new nurse leaders as well as seasoned nurse executives to design a nursing strategic plan:

STEP 1: Appoint a Nursing Strategic Planning Committee

- The CNE usually chairs the committee and is responsible for determining its membership. The committee members usually include nurse representatives from practice, education, shared governance councils, nursing research committees, and advanced practice. Other members who are often included on this committee include colleagues from finance, HR, information technology (IT), and public relations (PR) departments. Issues determined by this committee include roles, responsibilities, and level of authority. Committee goals, objectives, and available resources should be made clear.

STEP 2: Use strategic analysis to guide the planning, using key nursing indicators

- Data analysis is a critical step in determining the nursing strategic plan. Nursing sensitive indicators, quality data, and HR data such as nursing turnover, vacancy rates, and level of staff engagement should be collected. Patient acuity and satisfaction data also provide important information.

STEP 3: Conduct key stakeholder interviews to assess perceptions regarding the nursing enterprise

- Interviews with key members of the organization are an important source of information. Common issues and themes can emerge and can assist the planning team to formulate strategic initiatives. Standard survey tools should be used, and responses can be further analyzed to enhance appropriate targeting goal formation.

STEP 4: Share key stakeholder interviews and analytical data

- Results of the stakeholder interviews should be shared with stakeholders who participated in the interviews and with other colleagues and departments. Integral to nursing are groups such as physician leadership, educational partners, and the IT department.

STEP 5: Use a SWOT analysis

- As previously stated, a SWOT analysis is a technique that encourages the strategic planning team to take a look at the current state of the nursing enterprise. Information obtained through the SWOT analysis combined with the data analysis and the stakeholder interviews help inform and effect strategic plans.

STEP 6: Brainstorm potential strategies

- Brainstorming is a technique that can help the nursing strategic planning team to identify the main strategies that relate to the overall strategic direction of the organization and are key to the impactful contribution of nursing in attaining the organization's mission and vision.

STEP 7: Complete a gap analysis around the strategies

- Once the strategies have been established, it is important to engage staff at all levels to identify gaps that have not been addressed in the proposed initiatives.

STEP 8: Develop a tactical plan for selected strategies

- The tactical plan should include targeted objectives relative to each strategy. Timeline, metrics, and responsibility for proposed outcomes should be established.

STEP 9: Develop metrics for this strategic plan

- Determining the metrics that will be used to evaluate the success of the plan is a critical step. Responsibility for data collection and reporting results should be clearly outlined for each objective.

STEP 10: Communicate the strategic plan

- Multiple communication techniques and methods should be used to communicate the nursing strategic plan. One of the reasons the plan could fail would be inadequate communication to key stakeholders (Schaffner, 2009).

In addition to the 10 steps recommended for the creation of a nursing strategic plan, Schaffner (2009) outlined benefits and barriers associated with effective planning. In addition to providing a roadmap for the future, benefits include

- establishment of a clearly defined strategy for nursing,
- provision of a sense of ownership,
- nursing resources that are focused on priorities,
- promotion of the value of nursing services, and
- progress that is communicated to the nursing enterprise on established timelines and in multiple ways.

Barriers to effective planning outlined by Schaffner (2009) include

- lack of time,
- lack of strategic planning skills,
- perceived lack of value, and
- lack of organizational support.

If these barriers are not addressed, frustration and disengagement will result.

Broome and Marshall (2021) expanded on Schaffner's 10-step nursing strategic plan to include guidance for healthcare systems strategic planning. Recommendations for steering committee membership were to include visionary thinkers and realists from across the organizations as part of the team. Broome and Marshall stressed the importance of communicating the strategic plan broadly and proposed the assignment of champions to monitor progress of the plan. The use of a specific evaluation plan was recommended to document achievement of goals.

Wright (2020) emphasized the importance of a multidisciplinary approach to the construct of the strategic plan. The interdisciplinary team should be involved in all phases of strategic planning and development including the review of the organization's purpose, the assessment of the organization's internal and external position, the establishment of strategic initiatives, and the evaluation of the achievement of outcomes.

Assessment and analysis skills are fundamental to the creation of a nursing strategy that supports the strategic imperatives of the organization. The nursing process provides a useful framework for determining actions that will result in the achievement of strategic priorities. As a result of the assessment and diagnosis of the current state of nursing care delivery, plans can be implemented, and results evaluated to ensure the attainment of desired outcomes. Nursing sensitive quality indicators, benchmark information, and input from nurses across the enterprise need to be considered in the assessment and planning phase.

The IHI (Swensen et al., 2013) recommendations for improving the safety and quality of patient care provide a guide for the formulation of the nursing strategic plan. Based on these recommendations, the following steps should be included:

STEP 1: Be sure to include frontline nurses as well as nursing leaders on the multidisciplinary nursing strategic planning team.

STEP 2: Set nursing goals that include the delivery of safe, effective, timely, patient-centered, equitable, and efficient care.

STEP 3: Define areas of concern and establish desired outcomes that could result from a change in practice.

STEP 4: Provide staff time, funding, and technological support for delivering results.

STEP 5: Establish monitoring and evaluation teams to evaluate progress and challenges.

STEP 6: Create a learning system that increases the likelihood that the nursing strategic plan will achieve the intended results.

Nurse leaders in executive and management roles are key to the successful execution of the nursing strategic plan. Implementation of the strategic initiatives selected to meet the objectives that have been set is a joint responsibility. Executive nurse leaders communicate the content and intent of the plan and translate the goals to be achieved into actionable objectives (Burke & Erickson, 2020; Crawford et al., 2017; Stichler, 2006).

◻ WHAT EVERY NURSE EXECUTIVE NEEDS TO KNOW ABOUT STRATEGIC DEVELOPMENT AND PLANNING

Executive nurse leaders across healthcare systems, organizations, and agencies are prepared by education and practice to lead strategic planning and development. Key competencies including collaboration, coordination, and communication position executive nurse leaders as essential to achieving stakeholder consensus on key priority issues. Nurse executives communicate the content and intent of the plan and translate the goals to be achieved into actionable objectives. Executive nurse leaders must advocate for a future state that is more diverse, equitable, and inclusive.

WHAT EVERY NURSE EXECUTIVE NEEDS TO KNOW

- Executive nurse leaders should be part of the corporate level strategy development and planning team.

- The executive nurse leader should translate the vision into actionable strategies and interventions that are understood at all levels of the nursing enterprise.

- The nurse executive should conduct regular meetings to determine current progress toward goals, to remove barriers, and to hold crucial conversations with middle and low performers.

⬡ CASE SCENARIO

DEVELOPING A STRATEGIC PLAN FOR IMPROVED CARE ACROSS THE CONTINUUM

SITUATION

Facilitating a safe transition from acute care to the most appropriate post-acute care setting is an important aspect of high-quality comprehensive patient care. One healthcare system in the northeast part of the United States recognized that their transition processes needed to be improved. The senior executive team proposed "improved care across the continuum" as one of their strategic imperatives. The board of directors of the system endorsed the strategic plan, and the system CNE was appointed as the lead executive for developing and planning the goals, objectives, and metrics for the improved care across the continuum strategy.

Other strategic priorities that were part of the system strategic plan included "improving the health of populations" and "maintaining system financial stability." The CNE held a meeting with the lead executives assigned to each of these strategic imperatives. These executives quickly reached consensus on the key objectives to be met. Unnecessary hospital admissions, readmissions, and utilization of hospital emergency services were major contributors to the high cost of care. Finding ways to partner with community agencies to reduce unnecessary hospitalizations and emergency department visits could improve the overall quality, efficiency, and outcomes for high-risk populations.

APPROACH

The system CNE convened a multidisciplinary steering committee to assess the care provided to patients who were frequent utilizers of care. Team members included system physician and nurse clinical leaders, community MDs, and APRNs; members of the palliative care team; post-acute care providers from skilled nursing facilities and homecare agencies; and representatives from the state Area Agency on Aging. Steering committee team members were asked to conduct an audit of the medical records of their current patients/clients who were frequent utilizers of care. Once these patients were identified, the members obtained permission from the patients/clients to allow the steering committee to review their records and conduct a pilot project. The team identified patients/clients who were known to both acute and post-acute providers and determined common themes. As a result of the audit, the pilot program was designed with the overall goal to reduce unnecessary hospital readmissions.

Communication among providers was identified as a major problem. The pilot program was designed to improve communication and support patients at high risk for readmission with an enhanced care plan of services to allow them to safely transition to the community. The pilot project interventions included the placement of community agency coaches in the acute care hospitals, primary care offices, skilled nursing facilities, and homecare agencies. High-risk patients and their caregivers were educated about medication management, their personal health record, keeping appointments, and disease self-management. The enhanced care plan included additional support from community providers such as post-discharge phone calls, home visits, and additional home health services when appropriate.

OUTCOME

The pilot's success was measured by tracking readmissions to the hospital for the identified high-risk patients. Comprehensive audits were conducted to determine the effects of the interventions. Prior to the interventions, the pilot group received an average of 5.3 hospital or emergency care visits per quarter post-interventions; one visit was required for the same high-risk population during the same quarter. Post-intervention, one visit as required for the same high-risk population per quarter.

The success of the pilot project to improve care across the continuum by reducing unnecessary hospital admissions served as a model for continued collaboration. Funding for expansion of this initiative was obtained from the state Area Agency on Aging, and the interventions and outcomes were shared with other healthcare systems across the state.

DISCUSSION QUESTIONS

1. What system CNE competencies were instrumental in achieving the successful outcomes for this strategic initiative?
2. What best practices were utilized in creating the pilot program to accomplish the strategic objectives?
3. What lessons can be learned from this scenario?

WHAT EVERY NURSE MANAGER NEEDS TO KNOW ABOUT STRATEGIC DEVELOPMENT AND PLANNING

Nurse managers engage frontline staff in the execution of strategic initiatives and actions. Communication to all nursing staff about expectations and responsibilities is essential. Appointing champions who are able to articulately communicate the goals, actions, responsibilities, accountability, and timelines is one strategy for assuring that each nurse understands the plan and their role in it.

A best practice for communicating the plan consistently and clearly is the use of a one-page document that succinctly maps out the key components of the plan. This strategy map can be adapted for executives, key stakeholders, and all employees. Figure 13.2 shows a sample strategy map.

The key to successful execution of the plan is to create clear linkages between each individual and the strategy. Nurse leaders can help make these connections for their team by demonstrating to frontline staff how their work contributes to departmental goals, and how their department contributes to the organization and system strategy. Keeping staff aware of progress toward goals through updated metric reports presented at staff meetings and in written communication can encourage engagement and buy-in

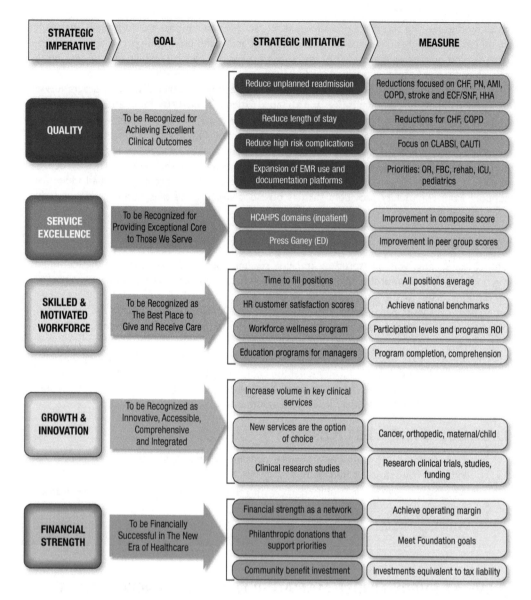

FIGURE 13.2: Sample strategy map.

AMI, acute myocardial infarction; CAUTI, catheter-associated urinary tract infections; CHF, congestive heart failure; CLABSI, central line-associated bloodstream infection; COPD, chronic obstructive pulmonary disease; ECF, extended care facility; EMR, electronic medical record; FBG, fasting blood glucose; HCAHPS, Hospital Consumer Assessment of Healthcare Providers and Systems; HHA, home health agency; HR, human resources; OR, operating room; PN, pneumonia; ROI, return on investment; SNF, skilled nursing facility.

(Broome & Marshall, 2021; Jeffs et al., 2019; Stichler, 2006). One strategy for linking individual performance to the major strategic initiatives of the organization is to tie annual performance evaluation and compensation to targeted outcomes. For example, if the strategic imperative is to provide exceptional quality care and the critical objective is to reduce high-risk complications, the functional level nursing metrics could include the number of hospital-acquired infections, falls with injury, and hospital-acquired pressure ulcers. Each metric is assigned a target goal and value, and performance ratings range from below target to exceeds target.

⬡ CASE SCENARIO

STRATEGIC DEVELOPMENT AND PLANNING FOR PALLIATIVE CARE

SITUATION

Providing palliative care to patients who would benefit from this specialized service was identified as an important aspect of improving the overall quality of care at an acute care facility located in the eastern part of the United States. The board of directors and senior executive leaders of the hospital determined that increased utilization of palliative care would be a strategic initiative of the plan to "improve the health of populations" for patients with a serious or end-stage illness. The chief nursing officer (CNO) of the hospital was appointed as the leader with responsibility for this initiative.

The CNO convened a meeting with the nursing directors and nurse managers of the medical, surgical, and oncology units to determine the best ways to approach increasing appropriate and timely utilization of palliative care services. The nurse managers identified team members who should be included on the committee to improve palliative care. The director of the hospitalist service who was also the director of palliative care and three APRNs were members of the palliative care team. They all agreed to participate on the committee. The nurse managers also identified physicians, social workers, and chaplains who should be included.

One of the first issues identified by the committee was the lack of identified patients appropriate for palliative care consults. Patients were only being identified after multiple hospital admissions despite having a serious life-limiting illness. The committee recognized that patients who could benefit from a palliative care consult were being missed or not seen in a timely manner. This was leading to increased readmissions and longer lengths of stay. The nurse managers from the medical and surgical units expressed the need for frontline nursing staff to have greater knowledge about patients who would be appropriate for a palliative care consult. The nurse managers decided to include the successful completion of an educational program on palliative care as part of the frontline nurses' performance evaluation expectations. Inservice education classes and online PowerPoint presentations were prepared by the APRN directing the palliative care team.

APPROACH

A palliative care screening tool was developed and added to the nursing automated admission assessment. The screening tool included criteria such as end-stage cancer, heart failure, chronic pulmonary disorders, and renal disease. Other criteria included functional status of the patient, concomitant disease processes, not being a candidate for curative therapy, and prolonged ICU stay. Points were assigned to the criteria and scoring guidelines were implemented. Patients who scored 8 points or higher were identified as appropriate for a palliative care consultation. Nurse managers voiced concern about adding more steps to the nursing admission process and the reaction of frontline nurses to the addition to their workload. The nurse managers collaborated with the nursing informatics team to create an automatic notification to the palliative care department if a patient scored 8 or higher on the palliative care screening assessment. The nurse managers conducted additional educational sessions on the new palliative care assessment and tool for all nurses during their staff meetings.

OUTCOME

The palliative care committee measured the number of palliative care consult referrals, time to consult, length of stay, and readmissions. Since implementation of the screening tool, the palliative care service has seen a 40% increase in consults, a decrease in days to consults, and a decrease in readmissions. Patient and family satisfaction has increased as a result of early consultation and the creation of a patient-centered plan of care.

DISCUSSION QUESTIONS

1. What leadership competencies were displayed by the nurse managers who were part of the committee to improve palliative care?
2. What strategies did the nurse managers use to achieve the objective to improve palliative care?
3. What other approaches could the nurse managers have utilized to increase the successful outcome of this strategic imperative?

FORECASTING THE FUTURE

As a result of the COVID-19 global pandemic, strategic planning has become even more essential and complicated. Emphasis on personal safety precautions such as telehealth visits and remote work have impacted traditional healthcare delivery. Healthcare organizations will need to adapt and revise strategic plans to respond to increased consumer demand for more accessible, affordable, and equitable care (Blackman, 2020; Morse & Warshawsky, 2021).

Healthcare consulting firms responded to the global pandemic by adjusting their own strategic plans to address the need to assist healthcare organizations through the crisis. The OnStrategy firm conducted a strategic plan stress test to determine the response of organizations to the pandemic. A total of 551 respondents representing healthcare, professional services, and financial organizations completed the survey. Results indicated that organizations that had an agile, adaptable strategy were able to change their approach to achieving their objectives. They cited a strong culture and commitment to core values as integral to team engagement and motivation. Recommendations for survival to the new normal included contingency planning and creating an infrastructure that supports real-time communication with employees. Healthcare organizations should embrace technology expansion, remote visits, and work from home as a means to improve quality and efficiency (Enochson, 2020).

Other recommendations provided by healthcare consulting firms to assist healthcare organizations to respond to the pandemic new normal included increased focus on care delivery at home and decreased service utilization (Kirkpatrick, 2021).

Healthcare organizations evaluated where and how care can be delivered and focused on the positive aspects of virtual care. Many organizations adapted strategic imperatives and objectives to include an enterprise-wide virtual health strategy. Health systems provided education for clinicians on best practices for conducting virtual visits, and changed scheduling and pre-registration procedures (Betts et al., 2020; Mohammad, 2020).

A new era of collaboration and cooperation has emerged as a result of the COVID-19 crisis. Healthcare systems needed to partner with community service providers, technology experts, and supply chain companies. Within health systems, collaboration and cooperation among the workforce became a differentiator for organizations that were successful in meeting surge capacity demands. Cross training and redeployment strategies were quickly implemented. In many instances, these strategies helped fill gaps in care delivery and prevented workforce shortages (Blackman, 2020; Enochson, 2020; Mohammad, 2020).

The American Hospital Association (AHA) Center for Health Innovation forecasted shifts in strategic priorities that could occur as a result of the COVID-19 pandemic. The AHA predicted widening socioeconomic disparities and stressed the need for organizations to increase focus on social determinants of health (SDOH). Other predictions included greater demand for value, expanded crisis preparation, and strategic plans adjusted to prioritize technology and data as strategic imperatives (AHA, 2020).

Sanford and Janney (2019) outlined the general principles and competencies nurse leaders must master to be successful in meeting the challenges ahead. These include "strategic thinking and decision-making; executive presence (EP) and C-Suite communication skills; methods for innovation and change leadership; governance and board relations; and executive business skills as well as how to leverage big data" (Sanford & Janney, 2019, p. 172).

KEY POINTS

- Strategic planning is the organization's process for examining its future state. Strategic planning is an ongoing process that requires continuous monitoring and evaluation to determine if the organization is meeting its strategic imperatives.

- If goals are not achieved, reasons for the variance need to be examined. Actions that need to take place include changing the goal, changing or adding key personnel, changing key timelines for expected outcomes, and adding additional resources.

- Strategic planning and development are based on the organization's mission, vision, and values. Based on the organization's philosophy, strategic planning provides staff with a sense of direction, guidance for decision-making, and setting standards of performance.

- As a result of the COVID-19 pandemic, strategic planning has become more essential and complicated. Strategic plans will need to respond to the demand for more accessible, affordable, and equitable care. Increased focus needs to be placed on SDOH.

SUMMARY

Nurse leaders at all levels of healthcare organizations are uniquely prepared by education and professional practice to assume key roles in strategic development and planning. Competencies including collaboration, coordination, and communication position nurses as skilled leaders in the preparation, implementation, and evaluation of strategic imperatives and initiatives that will assist the organization in achieving its vision and mission.

Senior nurse leaders who exhibit a transformational leadership style are equipped to envision a future state that is more diverse, equitable, and inclusive. As part of the corporate team, senior nurse leaders in executive roles address critical issues based on science. They assist in achieving stakeholder consensus on key priority initiatives. They serve as champions for change, identify potential roadblocks, and find solutions to overcome them. They analyze data, evaluate outcomes, and adjust the plan as necessary. Nurse leaders in management roles are prepared to operationalize the plan. Nurse managers plan, organize, direct, and control the use of staff, supplies, money, and space to meet goals and objectives. They support the business level of the strategy plan. Nurse leaders at the point of care perform assessments, plan actions, and facilitate interdisciplinary teams. They educate, motivate, and empower patients and families. Nurse leaders on the frontline of care support the corporate and business level strategic initiatives through the provision of care that is safe, equitable, patient centered, effective, efficient, and timely (Beauvais, 2018; Swensen et al., 2013; Wright, 2020).

This chapter reviewed the history of strategic planning, levels of strategy within organizations, and best practices for strategy development, execution, and evaluation. Business, healthcare, and nursing perspectives were presented. Competencies that demonstrate the contributions of nurse leaders at all levels of the organization's strategic planning processes were highlighted. See Box 13.7 for a list of recommendations for successful strategic development and planning that were discussed in this chapter. The main reasons why strategic plans fail are listed in Box 13.8. The challenges of forecasting the future of healthcare delivery in uncertain times was stressed. Nurse leaders who are visionary, strategic thinkers, innovative, and able to adapt to unanticipated events are fundamental to successful healthcare delivery in the future.

BOX 13.7: KEY ACTIONS FOR SUCCESSFUL STRATEGIC PLAN DEVELOPMENT AND IMPLEMENTATION

- Include team members and stakeholders on the planning team who represent diverse cultures and points of view.
- Address critical issues.
- Achieve stakeholder consensus on key priority initiatives.
- Include a financial plan.
- Assess and analyze key data.
- Communicate the plan to all stakeholders.
- Implement the plan on time and on budget.
- Address resistance to change.
- Evaluate outcomes and adjust the plan as necessary.
- Continue to monitor the plan and communicate results.

BOX 13.8: WHY STRATEGIC PLANS FAIL

- The purpose is not clear.
- The process is misunderstood.
- The plan is not linked to the mission, vision, and goals.
- The plan is based on opinion, not research.
- The goals are not objective or achievable.
- There is lack of engagement and buy-in.
- There is no action plan for implementation.
- The plan is not aligned with resources.

(continued)

BOX 13.8: WHY STRATEGIC PLANS FAIL *(continued)*

- There is no follow-up evaluation.
- Failure to include the right people.
- Failure to incorporate a financial plan.
- Failure to address critical issues.
- Failure to achieve stakeholder consensus.
- Failure to be flexible.
- Failure to address resistance to change.

END-OF-CHAPTER RESOURCES

DISCUSSION QUESTIONS

1. What are four key phases for developing a successful strategic plan?
2. What are some best practices for strategic planning and development?
3. What nurse leader strengths and competencies position nurse executives and nurse managers as essential to strategic planning and development?

 A robust set of instructor resources designed to supplement this text is located at http://connect.springerpub.com/content/book/978-0-8261-7795-7. Qualifying instructors may request access by emailing textbook@springerpub.com.

REFERENCES

Agency for Healthcare Research and Quality. (2018, November). *Evaluating the process of creating and promoting a quality report.* https://www.ahrq.gov/talkingquality/assess/what-you-evaluate/process.html

American Hospital Association. (2020, August). *Forecasting shifts in strategic priorities amid COVID-19.* https://www.aha.org/aha-center-health-innovation-market-scan/2020-08-25-forecasting-shifts-strategic-priorities-amid

American Nurses Association. (2018, July). *ANA leadership: Competency model.* https://www.nursingworld.org/~4a0a2e/globalassets/docs/ce/177626-ana-leadership-booklet-new-final.pdf

American Organization of Nurse Executives. (2016). *System CNE white paper: The effective system nurse executive in contemporary health systems: Emerging competencies.* https://www.aonl.org/system/files/media/file/2019/04/system-cne-white-paper.pdf

American Organization of Nurse Executives & American Organization for Nursing Leadership. (2015). *Nurse executive competencies.* https://www.aonl.org/system/files/media/file/2019/06/nec.pdf

Beauvais, A. M. (Ed.). (2018). *Leadership and management competence in nursing practice: Competencies, skills, decision-making.* Springer Publishing Company.

Betts, S., Burrill, S., Kroll, A., Sowar, J., & Wheeler, T. (2020). *Implications of the COVID-19 crisis for the health care ecosystem.* https://www2.deloitte.com/content/dam/Deloitte/us/Documents/life-sciences-health-care/us-implications-of-the-covid-19-crisis-for-the-health-care-ecosystem.pdf

Blackerby, P. (n.d.). *History of strategic planning*. Blackerby Associates. http://www.blackerbyassoc
.com/history.html (Original work published in *Armed Forces Comptroller, 39*(1), 23–24, (Winter
1994).)

Blackman, M. (2020, December 10). *Guide your hospital successfully through the COVID-19 crisis: 4
strategies*. https://www.healthleadersmedia.com/strategy/guide-your-hospital-successfully
-through-covid-19-crisis-4-strategies

Broome, M. E., & Marshall, E. S. (2021). Transformational leadership. In M. E. Broome & E. S. Marshall
(Eds.), *Transformational leadership in nursing: From expert clinician to influential leader* (3rd ed., pp.
35–66). Springer Publishing Company.

Burke, D., & Erickson, J. I. (2020). Passing the chief nursing officer baton: The importance of succession planning and transformational leadership. *JONA: The Journal of Nursing Administration,
50*(7/8), 369–371. https://doi.org/10.1097/nna.0000000000000901

Business-to-you. (2020, August 29). *Three levels of strategy: Corporate strategy, business strategy and functional
strategy*. https://www.business-to-you.com/levels-of-strategy-corporate-business-functional

Crawford, C. L., Omery, A., & Spicer, J. (2017). An integrative review of 21st-century roles, responsibilities, characteristics, and competencies of chief nurse executives. *Nursing Administration Quarterly,
41*(4), 297–309. https://doi.org/10.1097/naq.0000000000000245

Daft, R. L. (2021). *Organization theory and design* (13th ed.). Cengage Canada.

Drewniak, R. (n.d.). *7 Steps to healthcare strategic planning [White paper]*. Hayes Management Consulting. https://cdn2.hubspot.net/hub/19712/file-13392848-pdf/docs/hayes_white_paper_7_steps
_to_healthcare_strategic_planning.pdf

Enochson, H. (2020, August 14). *What 551 organizations are doing to thrive in the next normal*. OnStrategy.
https://onstrategyhq.com/resources/what-551-organizations-are-doing-to-thrive-in-the-next-normal

Fisher, A. (n.d.). *The evolution of strategic planning*. Sutori. https://www.sutori.com/story/the-evolution
-of-strategic-planning--XtqXoff4X933J7bz1GCLVGD2

Grube, M. G., & Crnkovich, P. (2017, November 1). *Giving a consumer focus to strategic planning in health
care*. HFMA. https://www.hfma.org/topics/article/56575.html

Horwath, R. (2006). *The evolution of business strategy*. Strategic Thinking Institute. https://www
.strategyskills.com/Articles/Documents/evolution.pdf

Jeffs, L., Merkley, J., Sinno, M., Thomson, N., Peladeau, N., & Richardson, S. (2019). Engaging stakeholders to co-design an academic practice strategic plan in an integrated health system. *Nursing
Administration Quarterly, 43*(2), 186–192. https://doi.org/10.1097/naq.0000000000000340

Kaplan, R. (2020, May). *Using the balanced scorecard for successful health care M&A integration*. NEJM
Catalyst. https://catalyst.nejm.org/doi/full/10.1056/CAT.20.0286

Kaplan, R., & Norton, D. (1996). Using the balanced scorecard as a strategic management system.
Harvard Business Review, 75(I), 75–85. https://hbr.org/2007/07/using-the-balanced-scorecard
-as-a-strategic-management-system

Kirkpatrick, K. (2021, March 23). Strategic outlook for hospitals post-COVID. *Becker's Hospital Review*.
https://www.beckershospitalreview.com/strategy/strategic-outlook-for-hospitals-post-covid
.html

Lal, M. M. (2020). Why you need a nursing strategic plan. *JONA: The Journal of Nursing Administration,
50*(4), 183–184. https://doi.org/10.1097/nna.0000000000000863

Meadows, M. T. (2016). New competencies for system chief nurse executives. *JONA: The Journal of
Nursing Administration, 46*(5), 235–237. https://doi.org/10.1097/nna.0000000000000336

Mohammad, N. (2020, November 27). *Strategic planning during a pandemic*. Hospital News.
https://hospitalnews.com/strategic-planning-during-a-pandemic

Morse, V., & Warshawsky, N. E. (2021). Nurse leader competencies. *Nursing Administration Quarterly,
45*(1), 65–70. https://doi.org/10.1097/naq.0000000000000453

Sanford, K., & Janney, M. (2019). Preparing the nurse executive of the future. *JONA: The Journal of
Nursing Administration, 49*(4), 171–173. https://doi.org/10.1097/nna.0000000000000732

Schaffner, J. (2009). Roadmap for success: The 10-step nursing strategic plan. *JONA: The Journal of
Nursing Administration, 39*(4), 152–155. https://doi.org/10.1097/nna.0b013e31819c9d28

Smith, D. K. (1999). *Make success measurable!: A minbook-workbook for setting goals and taking action*. John
Wiley & Sons.

Spear, M. (2015). Strategic planning: Building for the future. *Plastic Surgical Nursing, 35*(4), 152–153.
https://doi.org/10.1097/psn.0000000000000115

Stichler, J. F. (2006). The emerging nurse executive. *AWHONN Lifelines, 10*(1), 71–73. https://doi
.org/10.1111/j.1552-6356.2006.00014.x

Swensen, S., Pugh, M., McMullan, C., & Kabcenell, A. (2013). *High-impact leadership: Improve care,
improve the health of populations, and reduce costs.* IHI White Paper. Institute for Healthcare
Improvement.

Wadsworth, B., Felton, F., & Linus, R. (2016). SOARing into strategic planning. *Nursing Administration
Quarterly, 40*(4), 299–306. https://doi.org/10.1097/naq.0000000000000182

Waxman, K. T., Roussel, L., Herrin-Griffith, D., & D'Alfonso, J. (2017). The AONE nurse executive
competencies: 12 Years later. *Nurse Leader, 15*(2), 120–126. https://doi.org/10.1016/j.mnl.2016
.11.012

Woyzbun, R. P. (2001). *The evolution of strategic* planning. www.the-marketing-works.com/pdf/
planning.pdf

Wright, P. (2020). Strategic planning: A collaborative process. *Nursing Management (Springhouse), 51*(4),
40–47. https://doi.org/10.1097/01.NUMA.0000654860.02889.d3

Zuckerman, A. M. (2016). *Healthcare strategic planning.* Health Administration Press.

CHAPTER 14

SYSTEM PERSPECTIVES FOR ORGANIZATIONS

Michele P. Holskey and Reynaldo R. Rivera

"Yet we act as if simple cause and effect is at work. We push to find the one simple reason things have gone wrong. We look for the one action, or the one person, that created this mess. As soon as we find someone to blame, we act as if we've solved the problem."

Margaret J. Wheatley

LEARNING OBJECTIVES

- Identify the value of system perspectives for organizations.
- Delineate competencies needed for a system perspective.
- Examine organizations from a system perspective through real-world examples.
- Evaluate an organization for its system perspective.

INTRODUCTION

A "system" is defined as several components that function with a common goal. Merriam-Webster (n.d.) described a system as interacting or interdependent groups, known as subsystems, that act as a unified whole. The term "system" is inherent when referencing healthcare organizations. Healthcare systems are made up of departments, numerous disciplines, and individuals—including patients—which act as subsystems or interrelated parts. Systems have boundaries that separate them from other systems. In healthcare, organizations promote their mission, vision, and values as distinct from other systems and the business of healthcare as a whole. Success for an organization is dependent on the synergy between the different subsystems.

Systems have three essential components: input, process, and output. A feedback mechanism links these three components to ensure the effective functioning of the system. When we manage a system, we usually regulate the inputs and processes to produce our desired output. Temperature control serves as an effective example. The inputs are the current room temperature and the target temperature. The process is the heater or air conditioning unit. The output is either hot air to warm the room if it is below the desired temperature or cool air to cool the room if it is above the desired temperature. The negative feedback is the delta between the current room temperature and the ideal.

Organizational systems follow the same model. Changes in one subsystem or part of a system influence other subsystems and the entire organization. For example, if the supply chain is interrupted for a single component, the entire manufacturing process can come to a screeching halt, resulting in loss of revenue, temporary layoffs, the inability to meet financial obligations, and a loss of customer loyalty. To prevent this, processes must be put in place that can compensate for the supply chain interruptions. These processes could include alternate suppliers, inventory management of critical components, or an alternate design that does not require that exact component. Whether it is a small community hospital or a major academic medical center, integrated system dynamics apply.

A system perspective—called systems thinking—takes into account the interconnections and interrelationships within the subsystems and how they interact with their environments through a holistic lens. The Institute of Medicine's *The Future of Nursing: Leading Change, Advancing Health* (IOM, 2010) report provides key messages for the profession of nursing, including the importance of committing to lifelong learning and strengthening competencies. The report highlights the need for nurses to gain new competencies in systems thinking to lead change within healthcare systems, including quality improvement, system redesign, and improving patient safety. When nurse leaders and nurse managers engage in systems thinking, they can identify patterns, interactions, and interdependencies among people, processes, products, and services (Dolansky et al., 2020). Systems thinking enhances nurse leaders' and nurse managers' ability to gain insight into how actions can strengthen or undermine the whole system and the importance of these considerations when making improvements.

For nurse leaders and nurse managers to succeed in healthcare organizations and systems, they need to understand how organizational structures, relationships, and the environment interact and influence nurse, patient, organization, and community outcomes. This chapter examines real-world examples of the interdependences within healthcare organizations and the role of nurse leaders and nurse managers.

GAINING SYSTEM PERSPECTIVES

Nurse leaders and nurse managers need a broad skill set to gain system perspectives due to the dynamic nature of change and the complexities inherent in healthcare organizations. Professional organizations have developed core competencies, with specific competencies for each domain, that can be used to self-appraise your strengths and opportunities for growth, plan professional development and nursing curriculum, and set expectations for evaluating job performance. Although the path to competency may be complex, several key competencies set the foundation for nurses to lead others through a system perspective.

Some of the competencies for systems thinking include the American Organization for Nursing Leadership (AONL) nurse executive (nurse leader) and nurse manager competencies (NECs and NMCs, respectively). Key competencies associated with gaining a system perspective for a nurse manager relate to the domain of science, and for a nurse leader key competencies relate to the domains of communication and relationship building and leadership (Table 14.1). The specific competencies include foundational thinking skills for nurse managers (AONL, 2015) and identifies systems thinking as an approach to analyzing and solving problems. The foundational thinking skills scaffold with advanced knowledge, skills, and attitudes expectations for nurse executives (American Organization of Nurse Executives [AONE], 2015) and combine with visionary thinking on issues that impact the organization. Additional competencies such as effective communication and collaboration, relationship management, and diversity are essential for nurse leaders to achieve a system perspective.

TABLE 14.1: Key Competencies for Gaining System Perspectives

Competency Type	Competency Domain	Competencies
Nurse leader	Communication and relationship building	• Effective communication and collaboration • Relationship management • Diversity
	Leadership	• Systems thinking
Nurse manager	The science	• Foundational thinking skills, systems thinking knowledge as an approach to analysis and decision-making

In addition to the AONL competencies, the Quality and Safety Education for Nurses (QSEN) competencies in patient-centered care, teamwork and collaboration, quality improvement, evidence-based practice (EBP), informatics, and safety assist in system perspectives. The Interprofessional Education Collaborative, embraced by more than 60 professions, including nursing, developed core competencies in 2011 for interprofessional collaborative practice, and expanded the scope in 2016 (Interprofessional Education Collaborative, 2016). These competencies reinforce the fundamental need for disciplines to reach beyond their profession-specific point of view to gain a global perspective of different professions and to collaborate effectively to improve health outcomes.

The key competencies for gaining a system perspective enlighten nurse leaders and nurse managers to develop professional development plans for integrating knowledge, skills, values, judgments, and attitudes into their daily practice. As part of the AONL competencies, tenets were developed to guide reflective nursing practice. One of the tenets is expanding awareness, respecting, and appreciating race, gender, religion, sexual orientation, and generational diversity to fully achieve a holistic systems view (AONL, 2015). When used for self-assessment of competency, these tenets help nurses better understand their leadership behaviors. The professional development plans for nurse leaders and nurse managers can mirror the five stages of proficiency, novice to expert, described by Benner (1982). As competencies are achieved, refined, and applied to the practice environment, nurse managers and leaders strengthen their capacities for gaining system perspectives. Mentoring is key to advancing competencies and promoting professional growth, as well as building culture (Beauvais, 2019). When nurse leaders and nurse managers establish mentoring relationships, leaders help develop succession planning activities to prepare future nurse leaders. Many of the competencies associated with mentoring align with AONL and QSEN competencies, including communicating, receiving feedback, and creating a culture of safety.

Nurses at all levels have opportunities for demonstrating competencies by obtaining national board certification, such as via the American Nurses Credentialing Center (ANCC), to validate expert knowledge in specialty fields, including nurse leaders and advanced nurse executives. Evidence suggests that certification may affect patient care outcomes, specifically related to nurses making decisions about fall prevention strategies (Aydin et al., 2015) and reducing fall rates (Boyle et al., 2015).

KEY COMPETENCIES FOR NURSE LEADERS

COMMUNICATING AND BUILDING RELATIONSHIPS

An effective nurse leader achieves strategic goals by developing and applying key competencies that take into account all the moving parts within the environment and system, including competencies for effective communication, collaboration, and relationships management with a global or system perspective. Most importantly, nurse leaders understand the inputs, processes, and outputs of communication and collaboration which contribute to systems thinking. Examples of the inputs, processes, and outputs of communication and collaboration are listed in Table 14.2.

SYSTEM COMPONENTS

System components include inputs which are characteristics that impact the system. Processes are the interactions that occur related to the inputs. Another attribute, outputs, are the results of the effectiveness and efficiencies of the system. When nurses apply evidence-based knowledge using a holistic system thinking approach, the outputs are more likely to reflect effectiveness, efficiencies, affordability, and excellent patient outcomes.

TABLE 14.2: Inputs, Processes, and Outputs of Communication and Collaboration Examples

Inputs	Processes	Outputs
• Individual people characteristics: perspective of their profession, personal perspective, skill set, personality, experiences, education, knowledge, strengths, weaknesses, communication style, communication preferences, and include patient and family characteristics • Unit/hospital/organization characteristics: staffing, resources (such as internal and external experts), information technology and equipment, policies, procedures, communication style • Team/council characteristics: diversity, relationship status, leadership, history of working together, synergy (individual and team dynamics), education, communication style as a group (meetings, between meetings), handoffs • Environment characteristics: leadership support for innovation, culture, facilities and sites for interactions (rooms, hallways), dedicated time for communication and collaboration • Overall inputs: Formal vs. informal communication, language (choice of words), communication style (electronic, virtual, paper, verbal, nonverbal, newsletter), preferences for communication (visual, auditory, tactile)	• Sending or transmitting information and/ or messages: cyclical processes • Interferences, disruptions, or failure in sending messages: technology, language, and cultural barriers • Distractions: environmental (noise), team/council discourse • Incongruence of messages (verbal, nonverbal) • Assurance for respect and diversity • Processes for speaking up and voicing opinions and concerns • Reporting processes for errors and concerns • Decision-making processes • Performance reporting	• Overall outputs: interpretation of messages (visual, auditory, tactile) • Feedback: response of the receiver to the sender's message • Patient-centered care outcomes, patient experiences • Adverse events • Missed care • Effective vs. ineffective teams/councils • Improved communication • Innovations • Efficiencies • Employee satisfaction, retention, turnover • Recognitions and rewards

Effective communication is critical for true collaboration to occur. Collaboration is built and optimized with strong inputs and processes that change one's perspective from me, my patient, my unit, to encompass diverse perspectives and consideration to the web of inter-dependence among all parts of the organization. Fundamental to communication and collaboration is the accurate transfer of information interpreted the way nurse leaders intended it to be. However, this can be challenging within complex healthcare systems with many concurrent interactions. Interferences, distractions, and incongruent messages may result in tunnel vision. Understanding how communication and collaboration contribute to systems thinking is important for nurse leaders so messages and information are not misconstrued or dropped and teams produce the planned results. The characteristics of all individuals, units, teams, and environments involved in the interactions (inputs), such as their knowledge, preferences, and experiences, contribute to the processes and outputs. When nurse leaders create a trusting environment that encourages safe, open engaging processes for communicating and building relationships, individual preferences, team preferences, cultures, and diverse perspectives combine to create synergy for system perspectives to grow. This environment is conducive to collaboration and collaborative problem-solving using a holistic approach resulting in buy-in and creative solutions. Ultimately, nurse leaders consider outputs of communication and collaboration such as performance outcomes and feedback mechanisms to evaluate and inform ongoing leadership decisions and advance patient-centered care. Outputs such as decreased satisfaction may indicate inefficient processes, fragmented care, and a siloed approach to solving problems. As a leader of a learning organization, nurse leaders continually apply critical analysis and evidence when re-designing structures and processes to improve outcomes. Honing skills in giving and receiving feedback, negotiating, and advocating for others sustain the gains in achieving system perspectives.

LEADING THROUGH SYSTEMS THINKING

The ANCC Magnet Recognition Program® is a national recognition program that designates organizations for achieving and sustaining nursing excellence. Magnet® organizations demonstrate transformational leadership, structural empowerment, exemplary professional practice, new knowledge, innovations, and improvements, with empirical outcomes, which are components of the Magnet Model (ANCC, n.d.). Nurse leaders and organizations seeking Magnet designation follow the Magnet Model as a framework, often referred to as a roadmap, for creating a culture of excellence and includes global nursing and healthcare issues. The journey to Magnet designation and nursing excellence begins with a shared mental model for transforming the culture and achieving excellence. The shared vision includes structural empowerment and a healthy work environment which serve as catalysts for systems thinking.

Empowerment is authority or power given to someone who uses that power to become stronger and achieve more autonomy or control. Structural empowerment in nursing refers to nurses' perceptions that nurse leaders provide nurses with access to organizational resources, education, policies, people, supplies, and equipment and that they leverage that access to make autonomous decisions, positive change, and achieve goals. When this synergy exists, a healthy work environment develops. Examples of empowering structures include

- access and incentives for formal education and continuous professional development,
- promotion and support for engagement in professional organizations,
- recognition programs for nurses who contribute to strategic initiatives,
- involvement of nurses in organizational interprofessional decision-making groups,
- promotion of programs that ensure the effective transition of nurses into practice environments, and
- recognition and support for nurse involvement in community population health initiatives.

Research supports a positive correlation between nurse leaders who exhibit transformational leadership behaviors and nurse managers' perceptions of structural empowerment (Asif et al., 2019; Khan et al., 2018). In addition, a positive relationship was shown among staff nurses' perception of their manager's transactional and transformational leadership behaviors and staff nurses' perceptions of their empowerment (Khan et al., 2018). There is an abundance of literature suggesting that nurse leaders within Magnet organizations contribute to positive professional practice environments. Nurse leaders were found to positively influence professional practice environments, including the structures necessary to empower nurses and support quality patient outcomes (Ducharme et al., 2017). The findings suggest that a nurse leader's understanding of their influence was essential for excellent professional practice environments, particularly related to providing access to resources. Raso et al. (2020) found a positive relationship between authentic nurse leadership and healthy work environment. In a healthy work environment, honest relationships emerge, and sharing opinions is valued and leveraged to achieve nurse and organizational goals and outcomes (AONE, 2015).

Nurse leaders apply competencies for systems thinking when asserting views, building consensus, and inspiring a culture that includes a positive, healthy work environment. A nurse leader's role, as incorporated in the AONL nurse executive competencies, is to establish an environment conducive to systems thinking and promote systems thinking as an expectation of nurse managers and staff. Nurse leaders who transform nursing practice environments with structures that strengthen nurses' voices spark innovative and systems thinking at all levels. These structures will likely result in improved nurse satisfaction and the quality of care provided to patients. When challenges are presented in the future, nurses are more resilient with effective structures to assist in dealing with economic and complex problems. When nurses are empowered, professional nursing practice flourishes, and nursing excellence thrives.

KEY COMPETENCIES FOR NURSE MANAGERS

MANAGING THROUGH SYSTEMS THINKING

Addressing the complexities of healthcare delivery at a department or unit level requires foundational thinking skills. Nurse managers also create and sustain empowering structures for effective communication and collaboration. Most importantly, nurse managers' critical contributions occur at the unit level where they apply systems thinking as an approach to analysis and decision-making. Nursing management roles and responsibilities for gaining a system perspective include activities for planning, organizing, staffing, directing, and controlling.

PLANNING

Nurse managers provide valuable input as strong advocates for nurses and patients. They help frontline staff to understand a system perspective by planning for and providing effective unit-based structures that support unit, hospital, and organizational outcomes, such as supporting shared governance. When planning for unit-based quality improvement activities, nurse managers maintain trust among staff and prioritize a communication plan for facilitating diverse and system perspectives during change.

ORGANIZING

At the unit level, nurse managers ensure nurses have access to resources for autonomous, evidence-based decision-making, such as an academic librarian, safe space, and allocated time. When resources are available, frontline nurses are more likely to deliver safe patient care despite competing priorities.

STAFFING

Nurse managers understand the complexities of balancing a unit-budget while meeting patient care needs, and the relationship to how their decisions impact the system budget. They predict staffing needs by scheduling and re-allocating resources with consideration of the concomitant variables such as patient, nurse, unit, and organizational needs.

DIRECTING

In addition to creating and sustaining a healthy work environment where diverse opinions are welcomed and valued, a nurse manager facilitates change through clear communication and anticipation of resistance to change. When nurse managers consistently message to the team how unit-level decisions are related to the organization's goals, they eliminate barriers and accelerate opportunities for collaboration.

CONTROLLING

Nurse managers ensure that staff have access to data and assist nurses to evaluate nurse- and patient-centered outcomes for trends and opportunities for improvement. When nurse managers consistently recognize nurses for their contributions to the profession, unit, and organization, they create a positive practice environment.

ASSESSING SYSTEMS THINKING IN A TEAM

How do you know if you and your team are systems thinkers? Dolansky et al. (2020) developed the Systems Thinking Scale (STS), a 20-item user-friendly tool, deemed to be valid and reliable for assessing systems thinking in the clinical and educational settings. The STS tool helps to inform leaders about the relationship between systems thinking and important outputs and outcomes, such as safety. Nurses who reported a high perception of systems thinking reported high safety knowledge and skill (Dillon-Bleich, 2018) and systems thinking was found to be a strong predictor of safe nursing care (Moazez et al., 2020). In a study investigating medication administration practices, nurses' perceptions of safety culture were more positive after receiving systems thinking education (Tetuan et al., 2017). These findings support that systems thinking nurses considered impacts beyond their individual patients and units and recognized the influence of their actions on systems. Therefore, nurse leaders can use the STS to assess systems thinking in their organizations. Based on the findings, nurse leaders can promote systems thinking with activities such as quality improvement projects, interprofessional education, and risk management reviews and plans.

Systems thinking can be developed over time and help people shift perspectives from a discipline-specific and unit-specific view to a more holistic global view of the interconnectedness of systems. When nurses are engaged in expanding their views, they can be creative problem-solvers who consider diverse perspectives to optimize outcomes.

◆ CASE SCENARIO

A SYSTEM APPROACH TO IMPROVE PATIENT SAFETY

SITUATION

One example to illustrate the interdependences and interrelationships in a healthcare organization involves the organization's structures, processes, and outcomes, also known as outputs, related to patient safety. Clinical nurses across a multihospital healthcare system implemented a fall prevention program known as Tailored Interventions for Patient Safety (TIPS; Dykes et al., 2010). The Fall TIPS program is an evidence-based fall prevention toolkit in which clinical nurses perform a falls risk assessment using the Morse Fall Scale, a valid risk assessment scale, and then utilize electronic decision support that generates fall prevention interventions tailored for each patient based on the patient's fall risks. The tailored interventions are incorporated into an individualized Fall TIPS poster for each patient. The poster is intended to facilitate communication among patients, nurses, and the interprofessional care team about the patient's recommended evidence-based fall prevention interventions, such as the use of assistive devices and the patient's individual out-of-bed assistance needs. TIPS supported the systems' strategic initiative for standardization across the system and goals to sustain the high reliability organization.

To monitor the effectiveness of the newly implemented fall prevention program, unit-based clinical nurses throughout the system reviewed monthly unit-level patient fall rates (falls per 1,000 patient days). During unit-based shared governance council meetings, clinical nurses discussed, planned, and evaluated nursing practices and quality performance outcomes, such as fall prevention strategies and patient fall rates. In addition to unit-based evaluation of the effectiveness of the fall prevention program, clinical nurses actively participated in fall prevention councils and quality and safety councils, which have a reporting structure at the hospital level and the system level. The hospital and system-wide councils have interprofessional members and may include representation from medicine, rehabilitation services, pharmacy, information technology (IT), safety, environmental services, and quality departments, in addition to nurses at all levels—clinical nurses, advanced-practice nurses, nurse managers, and nurse leaders. Following the implementation of the TIPS program, nurses noted improved patient safety at the unit level with a reduction in patient fall rates.

Over time, clinical nurses on several units within the system began to notice an increase in patient falls and an increase in unit-level patient fall rates. During unit council meetings, clinical nurses discussed the findings and questioned if the evidence-based strategies which were fully adopted upon the initial launch of the TIPS program were still being implemented. They reflected upon the challenges of sustaining EBP changes as supported in the literature. The clinical nurses agreed that professional development in the form of continuing education focused on the Fall TIPS program was indicated. Because of the reporting structure within the organization, which optimized nurses' voices to be heard, clinical nurses communicated their concerns to nurse managers and nurse leaders and advocated for improved patient safety at the hospital and system level.

APPROACH

The system's nurse leaders listened carefully to the clinical nurses' concerns and supported the nurses' request for education related to the Fall TIPS program. The leaders acknowledged and applauded the clinical nurses' utilization of unit councils to champion patient safety, understanding that shared governance has been associated with nurse empowerment. The experienced nurse leaders synthesized that one critical approach to leading change is the dissemination and translation of research findings into daily practice (Graystone, 2018). Who would be better to assist the organization with hard-wiring adoption and best practices for reducing patient falls than the researchers involved in the Fall TIPS program? Nurse leaders of the professional development department arranged for Patricia Dykes, PhD, MA, RN, senior nurse scientist, Center for Nursing Excellence, Brigham and Women's Hospital, to provide a continuing education program for all system stakeholders invested in improving patient safety. Dr. Dykes is considered an external expert in inpatient falls research and was an investigator in the randomized controlled trial that showed a statistically significant improvement in patient fall rates with TIPS program utilization (Dykes et al., 2010). Throughout the system, nurse leaders and nurse managers partnered to plan the education program and strategize about nurse schedules to ensure that key clinical nurses could attend. They shared the program with all stakeholders, including the interdisciplinary teams, who engaged in interprofessional collaborative practice with nurses to create shared plans of care for fall prevention. Clinical nurses, and attendees from rehabilitation services, quality, and other clinical departments throughout the system, attended the program and disseminated the education to their colleagues, including unit-based and hospital-level councils.

The following are sample initiatives from different hospitals within the system that describe how clinical nurses, in partnership with their interprofessional colleagues and nursing leadership, assumed ownership and leveraged organizational structures, which empowered them to gain a system perspective for improving patient safety.

HOSPITAL A

The clinical nurses listened to Dr. Dykes's teaching points about fall prevention practices and compared the evidence from a literature search and the education to current nursing practices. The nurses noted that current practice included nursing interventions such as yellow "fall risk" alert wristbands and yellow no-skid socks for patients to communicate to care team members about the patients' risk for falls. The clinical nurses recalled that not only were these practices not supported by the most current evidence, but that their implementation may hinder the implementation of other EBPs included in the Falls TIPS program. Since alternative practices such as the alert wristbands and yellow socks could prevent the standardized communication of risk status that was already incorporated into the TIPS bedside poster, the clinical nurses agreed to change nursing practice and discontinue the interventions of "fall risk" alert wristbands and yellow socks for fall risk patients. Nurse managers collaborated with supply chain managers to advocate for removing the alert wristbands and yellow socks from stock.

In addition, clinical nurses identified that a critical component of the TIPS program included the importance of engaging patients as active partners in their tailored fall prevention care plan. However, nurses reported that they were not consistently prioritizing fall prevention patient education for patients to become fully engaged in their risk reduction plans. The clinical nurses agreed to prioritize educating and engaging patients as an essential part of implementing the Falls TIPS program. By gaining a system perspective that extended beyond their unit, the clinical nurses aligned nursing practice with the evidence-based TIPS program.

HOSPITAL B

Clinical nurses reported to the interprofessional quality and safety council that a barrier to full implementation of the Fall TIPS program was the nurses' lack of easy access to the patient's historical fall risk factors and fall interventions documented in the electronic health record (EHR). The nurses explained that a new Fall TIPS page was added to the EHR when documenting their assessment of the patient's fall risk and fall risk factors. However, when a patient's fall risk status matched the prior assessment, the EHR generated documentation that noted that the patient's fall risk remained unchanged. The unchanged status page hid important details, which meant the clinical nurses could not visualize the patient's previous fall risk factors and fall interventions. The nurses proposed streamlining Fall TIPS documentation in the EHR. The interprofessional colleagues agreed that streamlining documentation for ease of access to important patient information for monitoring and implementing patient safety measures was essential, especially for reducing falls.

The quality director and director of nursing championed the clinical nurses' idea by taking the innovative solution to the IT team, who agreed to a change in the EHR. Clinical nurses collaborated with IT specialists to design and test the new streamlined Fall TIPS documentation. After the EHR revisions were implemented, the clinical nurses reported that the new Fall TIPS documentation processes were efficient. Also, the nurses were able to visualize the patients' comprehensive fall risk history, risk factors, and tailored fall interventions and utilize the essential data to complete fall risk assessments and keep patients safe.

OUTCOME

Because of the dynamic nature and inherent challenges associated with patient falls, the organization's leaders had established unit, hospital, and system-wide structures to optimize quick identification and resolution of problems. The clinical nurses leveraged their access to structures within the organization such as shared governance councils and external experts to identify potential root causes for the increased patient falls and possible variation in practices that deviated from the evidence. Following education and implementation of the changes in nursing practice that strengthened alignment to evidence-based strategies found to effectively reduce patient falls, both hospitals had a decrease in patient falls (falls per 1,000 patient days) at the unit and hospital levels. In addition, the councils continued to evaluate performance by comparing their performance to national benchmarks, which was an ongoing action step of the organization's quality and safety strategic plan. The synergy achieved among clinical nurses, nurse managers, nurse leaders, and interprofessionals resulted in a system perspective and improved patient safety. The success of prioritizing patient safety was realized because the clinical nurses communicated their concerns, the nurse managers listened, and they advocated on behalf of patients and nurses. Later, they planned strategies to sustain best practices and hard-wired checks and balances to ensure ongoing implementation of the evidence-based Fall TIPS program.

DISCUSSION QUESTIONS

1. Discuss factors that changed over time to create interdependencies across the system.
2. List five empowering structures for nurses that contributed to perspective sharing and systems thinking.

⬡ **CASE SCENARIO**

JOURNEY TOWARD AMERICAN NURSES CREDENTIALING CENTER'S MAGNET RECOGNITION PROGRAM®

SITUATION

One organization's journey to achieve ANCC's Magnet Recognition Program included a strategic plan for nurse leaders to engage nurses at all levels in establishing one nursing professional practice model (PPM) across a seven-hospital system (Holskey & Rivera, 2020). A PPM "describes how nurses practice, collaborate, communicate, and develop professionally to provide high quality care" (Holskey & Rivera, 2020, p. 468). With over 7,000 nurses across multiple hospitals that comprised the organization, nurse leaders needed to be transformational. Although there are tools available to help nurses identify and make complex decisions on the road to formulating a system perspective for a PPM, many tools and processes are not effective in achieving goals and are less efficient, potentially wasting financial and people resources.

APPROACH

As defined by ANCC (2017), transformational leaders motivate and inspire others to achieve outcomes and simultaneously build their own leadership capacity. In this initiative, nurse leaders transformed the structures and processes for learning and practicing nursing by breaking down siloes and incorporating effective strategies for engaging nurses that were inclusive and empowering. Nurse leaders examined the evidence and identified liberating structures (LSs) by Lipmanowicz and McCandless (2014) as innovative engagement strategies. LSs are creative activities that can be used with large groups to share individual perspectives on the road to identifying system perspectives. Initially, nurse experts educated nurses about the value and expectations for a system PPM that represented all levels of nurses in all practice settings. They disseminated examples of PPMs from other organizations, introduced PPM definitions and language, and discussed evidence about the relationship of PPM for driving exemplary professional practice. After providing nurses with knowledge and evidence, the nurse experts inspired nurses to share their ideas, as they were exposed to diverse perspectives of their colleagues working in different units, specialties, and hospitals. The visionary nurse leaders reinforced the shared goals of everyone—achieving excellence for patient-centered care. As LSs were leveraged to assist in identifying and prioritizing elements of a PPM, nurse leaders collaborated with clinical nurses as they considered best practices for communicating and coordinating feedback from nurses who were members of interprofessional teams.

OUTCOME

The structures and processes for learning and decision-making empowered nurses to share their voice and energized collaboration. Clinical nurses advocated for patients, themselves, and their profession as they were coached by nurse leaders to achieve a system perspective and consensus in an efficient manner. The organization's nurses designed a PPM which was adopted across the system as a guide for excellence in patient-centered care. Overall, nurses at all levels established a successful environment conducive to systems thinking and stimulating new knowledge, innovations, and improvements for achieving organizational goals and outcomes.

DISCUSSION QUESTIONS

1. After reviewing the AONL competencies, identify two nurse executive competencies demonstrated in this case scenario and give an example of their actions that demonstrate each competency.
2. What role would nurse managers have in this case scenario?

SYSTEM PERSPECTIVE AS AN APPROACH TO ACHIEVING GOALS

System perspective is a holistic approach to achieve its goals. This initiative aims to build a culture of inquiry across a large health system with multiple hospitals resulting in advancing nursing science and improving patient-centered care, which are strategic initiatives of the organization.

The culture of inquiry is an environment designed to solve clinical questions through research when existing literature is insufficient and embark on improvement projects to support practice change when data are sufficient. Additionally, nurses are supported, valued, and understood to recognize, implement, and generate best practices to advance the nurse practice environment, patient-centered care, and patient outcomes (Carter et al., 2018).

◆ CASE SCENARIO

A SYSTEM APPROACH IN BUILDING A CULTURE OF INQUIRY AT A LARGE SYSTEM WITH MULTIPLE HOSPITALS

SITUATION

In 2014, the organization started the Nursing Research and Innovation office to build a culture of inquiry across New York-Presbyterian Hospital (NYP). Nurse leaders assessed the current state of EBP and research and found: (a) knowledge deficits among EBP and research committee members and nurse leaders in the similarities and differences between EBP, research, and quality improvement; (b) a lack of understanding of how and why research studies were conducted; (c) a lack of EBP and research mentors, while EBP and research team members were incredibly enthusiastic about EBP and research; (d) few were doctorally prepared or had participated in a research study, and had limited exposure to conducting a research study or seeking Institutional Review Board (IRB) approval; (e) a lack of awareness around completed ongoing and pending research studies; (f) a lack of opportunity to share the work done by each hospital with the remaining hospitals; and (g) most importantly, a lack of awareness of the PEACE model developed by NYP clinical nurses. The PEACE model is a mnemonic simplifying the EBP process for clinical nurses (Rivera & Fitzpatrick, 2021).

Nurse leaders considered the many studies that identified barriers to nurses' participation in EBP, including lack of EBP and research education, lack of time, heavy workload, staffing issues, feeling intimidated by research, lack of institutional support, lack of access to scholarly support, low prioritization among chief nurse executives, and lack of institutional research infrastructure (Melnyk et al., 2012, 2016).

INPUTS AND OUTPUTS

In building a culture of inquiry, the inputs are the knowledge deficits. The process is reviewing related literature to determine if the answer is readily available and, if it is not, to find novel solutions. The output will be the available information or the innovative solutions.

APPROACH

The system's visionary nurse leaders created and implemented changes through a series of structural interventions to increase research capacity, increase information dissemination, and improve patient-centered care (Table 14.3).

REINVIGORATE EVIDENCE-BASED PRACTICE AND RESEARCH COMMITTEE

The organization had existing EBP and research committees across the different hospitals. The committees were part of the existing system's shared governance structure. Standing monthly meetings were reinvigorated to engage more participation among members. Journal clubs were

TABLE 14.3: Systems View Changes for Building a Culture of Inquiry

Inputs	Process	Output
Knowledge deficits regarding research and EBP	To support the process, the following structures were developed to increase research capacity, increase information dissemination, and improve patient-centered care: • Reinvigorate EBP and research committee • Hiring of nurse scientists, which are joint faculty appointments between Columbia University School of Nursing and New York-Presbyterian • Academic-Practice Research Fellowship program • Partnership with nurse residency program coordinator • Provide educational programs such as monthly grand rounds, the PEACE model deep dive, annual research, EBP, innovation symposium, and journal clubs • Mentoring program through nurse residency program, Academic-Practice Research Fellowship program, and EBP and research committee	Knowledge gained to reduce deficits with the use of the newly developed structures

EBP, evidence-based practice.

added to assist nurses in critically appraising articles for quality and evaluating studies for clinical relevance. Nurses were provided a dedicated time to discuss and brainstorm questions identified in their clinical work.

HIRING OF NURSE SCIENTISTS

The AONL nurse executive competencies include academic relationships as a nurse executive competency. Nurse scientists were hired as an integral part of building a culture of inquiry and scholarship. They are PhD-prepared nurses with a joint appointment between Columbia University School of Nursing (CUSON) and NYP. Nurse scientists served as experts who shared their expertise in EBP and research to transform the system by providing nurses with related education and guidance. They strengthened the EBP and research competencies of nurses by providing support and one-on-one mentoring in addition to the monthly committee meetings.

ACADEMIC-PRACTICE RESEARCH FELLOWSHIP PROGRAM

The Academic-Practice Research Fellowship program is a competitive 2-year program. Fellows are given: (a) didactic time on research methods; (b) dedicated time to complete their research studies; (c) one:one mentorship from faculty affiliate; (d) statistical consultations; (e) hands-on guidance in disseminating study results; (f) ongoing continuing education credits; and (g) access to library services.

PARTNERSHIP WITH NURSE RESIDENCY PROGRAM

NYP has an accredited-with-distinction nurse residency program that supports new graduates transitioning to their first professional nursing role. Nurse residents are introduced to the importance of EBP and the use of the PEACE model. Nurse residents are required to complete an EBP project as part of their residency program to demonstrate competencies.

EDUCATIONAL PROGRAMS

Nurse leaders designed and implemented professional development programs that included engaging nurses in system perspectives for a culture on inquiry, such as

- research and EBP teaching and learning through monthly grand rounds;
- the PEACE model deep dive (offered three times a year to all nurses to discuss EBP, research, and the use of the PEACE model);
- annual research, EBP, and innovation symposium; and
- journal clubs (hospital specific).

MENTORING PROGRAM

Nurse leaders and nurse scientists provided mentoring and coaching through EBP and research committees, the Academic-Practice Research Fellowship program, and the nurse residency program.

OUTCOME

Nurse leaders gained knowledge to reduce deficits with the newly developed structures. As a result, the system's leaders found that these structures to building a culture of inquiry and scholarship were associated with the following:

- increased research capacities and research projects
- increased publications and podium presentations
- improved outcomes and patient-centered care

DISCUSSION QUESTIONS

1. Reflect on a system change you have participated in lately. What were the processes you implemented or optimized to achieve your goals? What were the lessons learned in terms of system perspectives?
2. If you failed to achieve your goal on the first iteration of the system change, what would be your next steps?

◻ WHAT EVERY NURSE MANAGER NEEDS TO KNOW ABOUT SYSTEM PERSPECTIVES FOR ORGANIZATIONS

Key points for success for nurse managers begin with recommendations for polishing their skills for engaging others to achieve unit and/or department goals, repeating often how individuals, teams, and units contribute to the strategic initiatives for the organization. When employees understand how their contributions fit into the big picture, they are more likely to conceptualize a system perspective. Creating a safe and healthy practice culture is paramount to achieving improved nurse, patient, organization, and community outcomes.

Nurse managers are leaders, followers, and partners to improve patient-centered care. To achieve these goals, nurse managers plan strategies, such as a communication plan for sharing knowledge and collaborating with nurses and interprofessionals. In their commitment to lifelong learning, nurse managers seek opportunities for professional growth of self and others, validating core competencies and incorporating peer feedback. These actions allow them to identify emerging nurse leaders for succession planning and mentoring relationships.

Nurse managers challenge the status quo by creating and strengthening a culture of inquiry where nurses' voices are diversified, valued, and respected. Careful listening and providing resources empower nurses to identify problems and make data-driven decisions about the root causes of problems. A nurse manager collaborates with nurses to justify projects based on accurately identified issues that align with the organizational priorities and advocates for funding as required resources. These key points support system perspectives for organizations and prepare nurse managers to be frontline leaders in patient-centered care.

WHAT EVERY NURSE MANAGER NEEDS TO KNOW

- Recognize your influence for system change by communicating, sharing knowledge, collaborating, and challenging the status quo.

- Utilize core competencies defined by professional organizations for professional growth and development, succession planning, mentorship, and peer feedback.

- Confirm the root cause of system issues is accurately identified.

- Advocate for system perspectives to ensure alignment with strategic initiatives and full adoption of system changes.

WHAT EVERY NURSE EXECUTIVE NEEDS TO KNOW ABOUT SYSTEM PERSPECTIVES FOR ORGANIZATIONS

What are key points for nurse executives? Nurse executives set the stage for empowering others to be their best selves, coworkers, nurses, managers, and community members. To role model a system perspective, nurse executives need fine-tuned system thinking competencies that start with developing self-awareness and understanding of how their own words and actions influence others. Executives focus on big-picture concerns and plans, and are effective delegators. Critical to success is skill in establishing a shared vision that incorporates a system perspective. This requires nurse executives to know the subsystems and understand the interdependencies and interrelationships of the organization.

A key point for nurse executives is communicating strategic initiatives and partnering with other executives to reward and recognize others who significantly impact the strategic goals. At the same time, working with interprofessionals, a nurse executive advocates for nurses and the profession helps others gain a nursing perspective for informing their holistic view. Since nurse executives are committed to lifelong learning, they co-create structures and processes for professional growth of self and others, succession planning, and mentoring programs. Top priorities for nursing executives relate to patient-centered care and ensuring exemplary professional practice thrives. Nurse executives apply evidence-based leadership practices and ensure that clinical nurses and interprofessional teams translate and adopt EBPs, even when it involves change. When nurse executives role model effective skills for system change, others follow. The identification of problems and errors is encouraged, and teams are reassured that projects are supported independently of the outcome. Effective nurse executives integrate systems thinking when making decisions and transform organizations to achieve excellence.

WHAT EVERY NURSE EXECUTIVE NEEDS TO KNOW

- Establish a shared vision that incorporates a system perspective, an interprofessional approach, and a funding source.

- Utilize core competencies defined by professional organizations for professional growth and development, succession planning, mentorship, and peer feedback.

- Collaborate with nurses to design empowering structures as an evidence-based strategy for improving outcomes.

- Promote and demonstrate reassurance to the team that projects are supported independently of the outcome.

KEY POINTS

- Nurse managers and nurse leaders role model the necessity for a system perspective through everyday actions.
- Strategic planning for excellent nursing organizations requires system perspectives.
- System perspectives take into account the interdependencies and interrelationships of the subsystems to achieve a holistic view.
- A culture of inquiry promotes system perspectives for organizations.

SUMMARY

The system perspectives for organizations are based on the concept that an organization has a number of interdependent parts functioning as a whole for some shared purpose. Changes in one part or subsystem influence other parts and the entire organization. Within healthcare organizations, the interdependencies among the subsystems are sensitive to the complexities, unpredictable changes (patient load, staffing, and structural barriers), and competing priorities (regulatory, community, and organizational) that occur daily and may trigger barriers to systems thinking. When this occurs, individuals, departments, and organizations may assume tunnel vision, focusing on a single area in isolation or a cause-and-effect relationship, rather than understanding the interrelationships and interdependences of the system. This results in unintended consequences or improvements in a single area, rather than improvements across the entire system.

The integration of systems thinking is considered a critical competency of nurse managers and nurse leaders. Nursing leaders demonstrate these competencies by facilitating change with a shared vision of the big picture, thinking beyond immediate responsibilities and problems. This often includes consideration of how things are interconnected and interrelated. For example, nursing leaders are influential in building and sustaining a healthy work environment, a culture of inquiry, EBP, and structures for empowering nurses—all of which influence patient care outcomes. When nursing leaders identify and understand these relationships, they recognize that solving problems in one area can greatly impact another area. Therefore, to achieve and sustain the best patient experiences, nurse outcomes, and organizational goals, nurse leaders take a systems approach to improvements. In everyday practice, nurse leaders model effective communication skills so true collaboration occurs and the culture thrives.

Although patient-centered care and safety performance serve as beacons across healthcare organizations to guide teams in their improvement efforts, a nurse leader contributes to the organization's success by engaging all stakeholders beyond their department, sharing knowledge about the importance of systems thinking and providing support independently of the outcomes. As key strategic members of the organization, nurse managers partner with interprofessional counterparts closest to the patient for a holistic view. System perspectives emerge when all stakeholders recognize how the interdependencies and interrelationships among subsystems (patients, people, departments, resources, and communities) are interconnected and that any change results in a ripple effect, effecting change throughout the system. These events are tied to the interrelationships between system components of inputs, processes, and outputs. Synergy among the different subsystems promotes a holistic view, which is necessary for excellent organizations.

As competent system thinkers, nurse leaders welcome opportunities for new knowledge, innovations, and improvements. Problems are identified, validated, and resolved using a systems approach and strategic initiatives are planned to align with the organization's mission, vision, and values. In an organization where nurses are leading change using a system perspective, nurse, patient, organization, and community outcomes are improved.

END-OF-CHAPTER RESOURCES

⬡ DISCUSSION QUESTIONS

1. Select a nurse leader whose leadership skills you admire. What are the competencies that you observe?

2. Reflect on your experience on how you created a better work environment by applying systems concepts and strategies/tools to your circumstances and issues.

3. Explain the essential components (inputs, processes, and outputs) for gaining a system perspective within your organization (hospital, place of employment, college, etc.).

4. Reflect on a real-world problem that you solved using a systems approach. What were the lessons learned?

⬡ ADDITIONAL RESOURCES

PODCASTS

Gagel, G. (Host). (2020, September 14), Taking a systems approach to complex change [Audio podcast episode 27]. *Greatness Podcast.* https://www.conversant.com/greatness-podcast-anne-murray-allen-complex-change

TED TALKS

Pilkington, K. (2018, January). *It all started in the garden: A systems thinking approach to community-based urban agriculture* [Video]. TEDxMacEwanU. https://www.ted.com/talks/kalen_pilkington_it_all_started_in_the_garden_a_systems_thinking_approach_to_community_based_urban_agriculture

WEB LINKS

Magnin, A. (2014, May). *System thinking: A cautionary tale (cats in Borneo)* [Video]. YouTube. https://www.youtube.com/watch?v=17BP9n6g1F0&t=188s

Plack, M. M., Goldman, E. F., Scott, A. R., & Brundage, S. B. (2019). *Systems thinking in the healthcare professions: A guide for educators and clinicians.* The George Washington University. https://hsrc.himmelfarb.gwu.edu/cgi/viewcontent.cgi?article=1000&context=educational_resources_teaching

⬡ LEARNING EXERCISES FOR STUDENTS

1. Circles Are Us Exercise: Create a Venn diagram to illustrate the dynamic interrelationships and interdependencies for systems thinking within a hospital. The Venn diagram has three overlapping circles, as depicted in Figure 14.1. One circle represents your perspective, another circle represents your unit and coworkers' perspectives, and the third circle represents other department perspectives within a hospital setting (medicine, finance, environmental services, pharmacy, quality, etc.). The fourth component of the Venn diagram is the connected section among the three circles which implies a system perspective. Consider the complexities of nurse staffing within an organization. Illustrate the similarities and differences of the perspectives of all stakeholders. The key to completing the overlapping inner circle for a system perspective is finding common themes or characteristics (strategies, goals, outcomes, etc.) among you, your coworkers, your unit, and your departments. Reflect on all stakeholders' unique perspectives and shared perspectives and discuss the importance of a system perspective. Tip: Be sure that a patient's perspective is considered and included in the center of the overlapping perspectives.

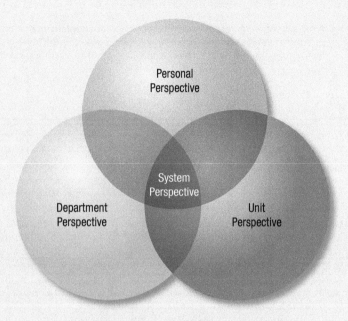

FIGURE 14.1: Circles Are Us exercise.

2. Balls of Fire Exercise: Toss a ball with your classmates as a way to share your professional development plans for growing competencies for system thinking, using the AONL competencies for nurse managers and nurse executives. Form a circle and take turns tossing the ball around to other students. As students receive a ball, they share one competency that they are "fired up about" and committed to improving. The activity can be repeated. The next time the student catches the ball, they share one strategy or goal for how they plan to strengthen a competency, such as through specific professional development activities, mentoring relationships, and so on.

3. High Hopes Exercise: As a nurse manager or nurse leader, write a step-by-step plan for making a system change. Using a highlighter, mark or highlight specific steps that you consider are reflective of a system perspective. Share your plan with a peer and exchange feedback about other opportunities and views you may have missed. Review Case Scenario: A System Approach in Building a Culture of Inquiry at a Large System With Multiple Hospitals to ensure you covered the important considerations for a system perspective.

⬤ GLOSSARY OF KEY TERMS

■ **Interdependencies:** When each subsystem or part contributes to the greater good but falls short of achieving system goals.

■ **Interprofessional collaborative practice:** "When multiple health workers from different professional backgrounds work together with patients, families, [careers], and communities to deliver the highest quality of care" (World Health Organization, 2010, p. 7).

■ **Interrelationships:** Occur when every subsystem or part depends on the behavior of subsystem(s) and that navigating the interrelationships is critical to the organization's mission.

■ **Synergy:** When the whole is greater than the sum of its parts.

■ **System:** An entity with several components that function with a common goal.

A robust set of instructor resources designed to supplement this text is located at http://connect.springerpub.com/content/book/978-0-8261-7795-7. Qualifying instructors may request access by emailing textbook@springerpub.com.

REFERENCES

American Nurses Credentialing Center. (n.d.). *ANCC Magnet recognition program*. Retrieved June 30, 2021, from https://www.nursingworld.org/organizational-programs/magnet/magnet-model

American Nurses Credentialing Center. (2017). *2019 Magnet® application manual*. American Nurses Association.

American Organization of Nurse Executives. (2015). *AONE nurse executive competencies*. American Nurses Association. https://www.aonl.org/sites/default/files/aone/nec.pdf

American Organization for Nursing Leadership. (2015). *AONL nurse manager competencies*. American Nurses Association. https://www.aonl.org/system/files/media/file/2019/06/nurse-manager-competencies.pdf

Asif, M., Jameel, A., Hussain, A., Hwang, J., & Sahito, N. (2019). Linking transformational leadership with nurse-assessed adverse patient outcomes and the quality of care: Assessing the role of job satisfaction and structural empowerment. *International Journal of Environmental Research and Public Health, 16*(13), Article 2381. https://doi.org/10.3390/ijerph16132381

Aydin, C., Donaldson, N., Aronow, H. U., Fridman, M., & Brown, D. S. (2015). Improving hospital patient falls: Leveraging staffing characteristics and processes of care. *Journal of Nursing Administration, 45*(5), 254–262. https://doi.org/10.1097/NNA.0000000000000195

Beauvais, A. M. (Ed.). (2019). *Leadership and management competence in nursing practice: Competencies, skills, decision-making*. Springer Publishing Company.

Benner, P. (1982). From novice to expert. *The American Journal of Nursing, 82*(3), 402–407. https://journals.lww.com/ajnonline/citation/1982/82030/from_novice_to_expert.4.aspx

Boyle, D. K., Cramer, E., Potter, C., & Staggs, V. S. (2015). Longitudinal association of registered nurse national nursing specialty certification and patient falls in acute care hospitals. *Nursing Research, 64*(4), 291–299. https://doi.org/10.1097/NNR.0000000000000107

Carter, E. J., Rivera, R. R., Gallagher, K. A., & Cato, K. D. (2018). Targeted interventions to advance a culture of inquiry at a large, multicampus hospital among nurses. *The Journal of Nursing Administration, 48*(1), 18–24. https://doi.org/10.1097/NNA.0000000000000565

Dillon-Bleich, K. (2018). *Keeping patients safe: The relationships among structural empowerment, systems thinking, level of education, certification and safety competency*. Case-Western Reserve School of Graduate Studies.

Dolansky, M. A., Moore, S. M., Palmieri, P. A., & Singh, M. K. (2020). Development and validation of the Systems Thinking Scale. *Journal of General Internal Medicine, 35*(8), 2314–2320. https://doi.org/10.1007/s11606-020-05830-1

Ducharme, M. P., Bernhardt, J. M., Padula, C. A., & Adams, J. M. (2017). Leader influence, the professional practice environment, and nurse engagement in essential nursing practice. *The Journal of Nursing Administration, 47*(7–8), 367–375. https://doi.org/10.1097/NNA.0000000000000497

Dykes, P. C., Carroll, D. L., Hurley, A., Lipsitz, S., Benoit, A., Chang, F., Meltzer, S., Tsurikova, R., Zuyov, L., & Middleton, B. (2010). Fall prevention in acute care hospitals: A randomized trial. *The Journal of the American Medical Association, 304*(17), 1912–1918. https://doi.org/10.1001/jama.2010.1567

Graystone, R. (2018). Disseminating knowledge through publication: Magnet® nurses changing practice. *The Journal of Nursing Administration, 48*(1), 3–4. https://doi.org/10.1097/NNA.0000000000000571

Holskey, M., & Rivera, R. (2020). Optimizing nurse engagement: Using liberating structures for nursing professional practice model development. *Journal of Nursing Administration, 50*(9), 468–473. https://doi.org/10.1097/NNA.0000000000000918

Institute of Medicine. (2010). *The future of nursing: Leading change, advancing health*. National Academies Press.

Interprofessional Education Collaborative. (2016). *Core competencies for interprofessional collaborative practice: 2016 update*. https://hsc.unm.edu/ipe/resources/ipec-2016-core-competencies.pdf

Khan, B. P., Quinn Griffin, M. T., & Fitzpatrick, J. J. (2018). Staff nurses' perceptions of their nurse managers' transformational leadership behaviors and their own structural empowerment. *The Journal of Nursing Administration, 48*(12), 609–614. https://doi.org/10.1097/NNA .0000000000000690

Lipmanowicz, H., & McCandless, K. (2014). *The surprising power of liberating structures: Simple rules to unleash a culture of innovation*. Liberating Structures Press.

Melnyk, B. M., Fineout-Overholt, E., Gallagher-Ford, L., & Kaplan, L. (2012). The state of evidence-based practice in US nurses: Critical implications for nurse leaders and educators. *The Journal of Nursing Administration, 42*(9), 410–417. https://doi.org/10.1097/NNA .0b013e3182664e0a

Melnyk, B. M., Gallagher-Ford, L., Thomas, B. K., Troseth, M., Wyngarden, K., & Szalacha, L. (2016). A study of chief nurse executives indicates low prioritization of evidence-based practice and short-comings in hospital performance metrics across the United States. *Worldviews on Evidence-Based Nursing, 13*(1), 6–14. https://doi.org/10.1111/wvn.12133

Merriam-Webster. (n.d.). *Systems*. Merriam-Webster.com dictionary. Retrieved June 30, 2021, from https://www.merriam-webster.com/dictionary/system

Moazez, M., Miri, S., Foroughameri, G., & Farokhzadian, J. (2020). Nurses' perceptions of systems thinking and safe nursing care: A cross-sectional study. *Journal of Nursing Management, 28*, 822–828. https://doi.org/10.1111/jonm.13000

Plack, M. M., Goldman, E. F., Scott, A. R., & Brundage, S. B. (2019). *Systems thinking in the healthcare professions: A guide for educators and clinicians*. The George Washington University. https://hsrc .himmelfarb.gwu.edu/cgi/viewcontent.cgi?article=1000&context =educational_resources_teaching

Raso, R., Fitzpatrick, J. J., & Masick, K. (2020). Clinical nurses' perceptions of authentic nurse leadership and healthy work environment. *The Journal of Nursing Administration, 50*(9), 489–494. https://doi.org/10.1097/NNA.0000000000000921

Rivera, R., & Fitzpatrick, J. (2021). *The PEACE model evidence-based practice guide for clinical nurses*. Sigma Theta Tau International.

Tetuan, T., Ohm, R., Kinzie, L., McMaster, S., Moffitt, B., & Mosier, M. (2017). Does systems thinking improve the perception of safety culture and patient safety? *Journal of Nursing Regulation, 8*(2), 31–39. https://doi.org/10.1016/S2155-8256(17)30096-0

World Health Organization. (2010). *Framework for action on interprofessional education & collaborative practice*. WHO Press. http://apps.who.int/iris/bitstream/handle/10665/70185/WHO_HRH_HPN_10.3_eng .pdf;jsessionid=F30B239A28D1E1CF85FEA95F7002021A?sequence=1

SECTION V
ESSENTIAL MANAGEMENT ISSUES

CHAPTER 15

QUALITY AND SAFETY

Mary Cathryn Sitterding and Amy Dee Wilson

"Transformational leadership means moving a profession, an institution, or some aspect of healthcare down a new path with different expectations, structures, and ways of conceptualizing how the mission can be achieved in light of changing conditions."

Angela Barron McBride (2020, p. 199)

LEARNING OBJECTIVES

- Contrast various cultural influences on safety and quality within healthcare.
- Appraise high reliability principles within one's existing work environment and/or clinical setting.
- Differentiate between various levels of situation awareness and types of situation awareness demons influencing quality and safety in healthcare.
- Design a leadership development strategy integrating complexity leadership as a framework driving innovation that results in quality and safety within healthcare.
- Compose a quality strategy integrating evidence-based spread, sustain, and scale lessons.

INTRODUCTION

The basis of all patient care should revolve around the delivery of safe care to patients, families, healthcare workers, organizations, communities, and the nation. Failure to do this places an incredible economic and emotional burden on the people and organizations affected. While progress has been made in patient safety, the pace must be accelerated. Nurse leaders have a tremendous opportunity to join and accelerate patient safety improvement. However, change will only occur if leaders are intentional about making a difference with patient safety (Kerfoot, 2016). The past decade of nursing excellence has yielded a bevy of tools and methodologies for safety and quality care, many of which have been borrowed from other industries with a similarly obsessive, mission-critical focus on safety, like air travel. What we have not focused on as much is how leadership plays a key role in the adoption of these tools. The tools that exist are only as useful as the organizations with the motivation and ability to put them into use. How are nursing leaders creating—or not creating—an environment in which a culture of safety can be seeded, then grow and develop?

The COVID-19 pandemic highlighted shortcomings in our safety culture. Nurses' situation awareness was understandably diminished. While caring for a patient with a fast-changing disease with limited resources and data, not to mention concerns over their own safety and that of their colleagues and family, it is no wonder we have seen safety incidents skyrocket over the last year (Weiner-Lastinger et al., 2022). There are many lessons to be learned from this, and much is being studied and observed about how nursing and healthcare can adapt and adjust post-pandemic. One of those lessons relates to a culture of safety vis a vis nursing leadership. This public health crisis revealed that our leaders were not as agile as they needed to be. "Just use the tool" did not get us very far. We are not nearly as close to being highly reliable organizations as we previously believed (Vogus et al., 2022). We have had a lot of safety tools working in a lot of organizations for a long time. But what are the leadership competencies that really drive quality and safety results?

CREATING A CULTURE OF QUALITY AND SAFETY

WHY QUALITY AND SAFETY MATTER

Quality and safety in healthcare matter. Approximately 400,000 patients experience some type of preventable harm each year. Studies suggest iatrogenic deaths are the third leading cause of death in the United States with estimates ranging from 210,000 to 440,000 deaths per year (James, 2013; Makary & Daniel, 2016), though Rodwin et al. (2020) maintain that the number of deaths due to medical error is lower than has been reported and that most inpatient deaths are caused by underlying disease rather than differences in quality of care. Carver et al. (2021) suggest the number of deaths due to medical error can only be estimated as medical records are often inaccurate, and providers may be reluctant to disclose error-related illness. Medical errors cost approximately $20 billion annually (Rodziewicz et al., 2021). As caregivers committed to serving our patients, we know that any healthcare-related harm or death is unacceptable.

Two decades after the publication of the Institute of Medicine's (IOM's) seminal report, *To Err Is Human* (Corrigan et al., 1999), it is more and more evident that safety issues have been persistent and that patients are frequently injured as a result of the care they receive (Bates & Singh, 2018). Common causes of hospital-related harm include medication errors, surgical injuries, error during handoff between units, failure to recognize and rescue, misidentification of patients, pressure ulcers, and falls. Significant reductions in harm have been gained by partnering with and learning from other disciplines (human factors engineering, psychology, social sciences); incentives built into payment structures (the Centers for Medicare & Medicaid Services [CMS] stopped reimbursing hospitals for hospital-acquired conditions such as pressure ulcers, falls, and infections); and national policy and practice initiatives such as the Patient Safety and Quality Improvement Act of 2005, authorizing the creation of patient safety organizations (PSOs). The PSOs bring groups together to share data about patient harm from voluntary reporting with privacy and confidentiality safeguards. Most noteworthy in spurring national efforts in harm reduction have been the impact of the Institute for Healthcare Improvement (IHI), which galvanized the patient safety movement with its 100,000 Lives Campaign (Berwick et al., 2006) and the National Patient Safety Foundation (NPSF).

Care delivery work in the best of circumstances can be emotionally, physically, and cognitively demanding. Emotional exhaustion among the healthcare delivery team has been well documented (Barello et al., 2021; Caldas et al., 2021; Portoghese et al., 2017). We are approaching a nursing shortage—again. The retirement of the baby boomers combined with less-than-optimal enrollment in nursing programs (as a result of faculty retirements) have had a dramatic impact on the nursing workforce. The result is missed nursing care and an array of negative outcomes: less/poorer quality of patient care, lower patient satisfaction, a decline in job satisfaction among nurses, more patient adverse events, and increases in hospital length of stay and hospital readmission (Chaboyer et al., 2021). Categories of missed care include

- communication and information sharing;
- self-management, autonomy, and education, including care planning, discharge planning, and decision-making;
- fundamental physical care; and
- emotional and psychological care, including spiritual support.

Missed care is related to factors such as staffing levels and skill mix, lack of availability of material resources, patient acuity, and teamwork/communication (Chaboyer et al., 2021). The conceptual definition, antecedents, and consequences of missed nursing care were introduced by Kalisch and colleagues (2009). What followed was a seminal program of research still relevant today describing, explaining, and predicting errors of omission (missed nursing care) including, but not limited to, the development and psychometric testing of tools to measure missed nursing care. Evidence demonstrating the impact of staffing levels, teamwork, and non-Magnets® on missed nursing care and the influence on patient harm and patient experience is well documented (Hessels et al., 2019; Kalisch & Lee, 2010; Kalisch & Williams, 2009; Kalisch et al., 2011, 2014).

Quality and safety competencies and contributions matter. Nurse leaders have a moral imperative to understand and improve factors affecting quality and safety, for those we serve and those we serve beside. In this section, we will look at the endeavor of creating a culture of quality and safety through several lenses. First, we explore the tenets of the high reliability organization (HRO) by taking a close look at the principles of high reliability as well as key concepts that are essential for the creation of a culture where high reliability behaviors and the caregivers who practice them can thrive: mindfulness, situation awareness, psychological safety, and growth mindset. Next, we consider the role of governance in creating the vision, structure, and process accountability necessary to prioritize quality and safety in an organization. Finally, we return to the fundamentals of culture to describe the importance of organizational coherence and transformational leadership in aligning teams around common goals and higher purpose and in inspiring them to work together to achieve measurable improvements in quality and safety.

HIGH RELIABILITY ORGANIZATIONS

HROs have been described as "organizations in industries like commercial aviation and nuclear power that operate under hazardous conditions while maintaining safety levels that are better than in healthcare" (Chassin & Loeb, 2013, p. 459). Individuals and teams are trained to proactively recognize and speak up about abnormalities or subtle weaknesses in the system and to use robust improvement strategies to address them. Within HROs, reward systems are designed to incentivize these behaviors that reflect continuous learning for individuals, teams, and organizations (Chassin & Loeb, 2013). Healthcare delivery, and particularly the work of nurses, is high-hazard work involving complex and continuous information flow. The work requires constant cognitive and relational processing. In short, nursing work is emotionally, physically, and cognitively demanding. High reliability behaviors absent a work environment enabling high reliability practices results in emotional exhaustion, impaired situation awareness, and high risk for harm (Vogus et al., 2014). It is up to nursing leaders to build a work environment that supports their teams in adopting and embracing the behaviors and attitudes that are integral to a culture of high reliability.

THE PRINCIPLES OF HIGH RELIABILITY

In the first edition of *Managing the Unexpected*, Weick and Sutcliffe (2001) introduced five principles or hallmarks of HROs, describing how organizations detect problems (hazard anticipation) and manage them (hazard containment): preoccupation with failure, reluctance to simplify, sensitivity to operations, commitment to resilience, and deference to expertise (Table 15.1). In the years since, these principles have informed the understanding of high reliability in healthcare and other industries.

TABLE 15.1: Applying the Hallmarks/Principles of High Reliability Organizations (HROs)

High Reliability Principle	Definition	Example of Application in Healthcare	Consider and Describe Your Real-World Examples
		Hazard Anticipation Principles	
Preoccupation with failure	Alertness to failures, especially as indicated by weak signals. Prepares for and prevents failure where feasible and responds and recovers from failures when they do occur.	Daily operations brief where all units report on staffing, acuity, operations status, and/or challenges. Safety officer of the day and nurse administrator of the day notice one unit describes less-than-optimal staffing numbers, including >50% nurses with <2 years' experience combined with higher-than-expected acuity. Decision made to consider the unit *at-risk* for error/harm with resources reallocated accordingly.	
Reluctance to simplify	Does not overlook subtle aspects of complex problems and avoids classifications of conditions into convenient categories.	Medical–surgical unit. Healthy 18-year-old, non-English speaking male admitted post appendectomy. Day of surgery postoperative blood pressure drops noted by float nurse, who communicates to charge nurse, "likely just dehydrated and needs fluids." Expert nurse notices drop in pressure combined with low-grade fever and decides to call a team huddle to ensure the team is not over-simplifying the clinical picture.	
Sensitivity to operations	HROs understand that potential problems can lie in a little-recognized location in a process or system. Sensitivity to operations underscores that failures are usually the result of processes or systems and the result of more than one cause.	Central line-associated bloodstream infections dramatically reduced by two-person line change practices. High-risk medications policy often requires two-person verification. The airline industry practice of preflight checklists has been adopted in surgical suites.	
		Hazard Containment Principles	
Commitment to resilience	Some problem events may be unavoidable, but an HRO will identify, plan for, and execute recovery measures to ensure continued service.	Many pediatric hospitals have a code word (e.g., "watcher") to signal that a child is at-risk for physiological decline. The signal alerts the entire team, enabling the team to plan for and execute recovery immediately should that child deteriorate clinically.	
Deference to expertise	HROs ensure that those with the specific problem-solving knowledge, skills, and abilities are engaged in providing solutions and avoid restrictions caused by hierarchy and chain-of-command.	Before a case, it is standard for surgical teams to introduce themselves where the surgeon will humbly ask the entire team to let her know if there is any concern. This is evidence in other teams on other units in other settings where teaming is required.	

Source: Data from Weick, K. E., & Sutcliffe, K. M. (2007). *Managing the unexpected: Assuring high performance in an age of complexity* (2nd ed.). Jossey-Bass.

INDIVIDUAL AND ORGANIZATIONAL MINDFULNESS

Cantu et al. (2020) proposed that a culture of mindfulness is the fundamental difference between reliable and highly reliable operations. They conducted a systematic literature review that revealed five foundational characteristics of a culture of reliability: (a) leadership, (b) individual accountability, (c) learning organization, (d) training and competence, and (e) communication. Mindfulness is the sixth principle that elevates and connects these five characteristics to create a culture of high reliability.

The five principles of high reliability reflect mindful organizing behaviors or reliability-enhanced leader work practices (Vogus & Iacobucci, 2016). Mindful or reliability-enhanced organizing is beneficial to nurses in multiple ways, especially on nursing units with high levels of adverse events over time.

SITUATION AWARENESS

The current work environment in healthcare requires a constant state of attention to the unexpected, with the capacity to perceive multiple points of data, conditions, and disparate decision-making. Nursing work environments are considered high-hazard and require interdependent and effective stacking of priorities and focused attention, with little margin for human error (Ebright, 2010; Ebright et al., 2003, 2009; Sitterding et al., 2012). Multitasking is required! The average inpatient nurse completes 100 tasks per shift, spending about 3 minutes on each task before being interrupted by other tasks or priorities. One nurse who was observed displayed cognitive shifts or interweaving among five patients 74 times in 8 hours (Tucker & Spear, 2006). The relationship between human factors, situation awareness, and harm is well documented (Brady et al., 2013; Goldenhar et al., 2013; Sitterding et al., 2014).

Understanding situation awareness in acute care nursing and the identification of factors that influence situation awareness can lead to the design and implementation of interventions maximizing nurse and team attention. As defined by Endsley and Garland (2000), situation awareness exists in three levels:

- Situation Awareness 1: Perception of environmental elements with respect to time or space
- Situation Awareness 2: Comprehension of their meaning
- Situation Awareness 3: Projection of their future status

Differences in stacking and situation awareness between newly licensed nurses, experienced non-expert nurses, and expert nurses are noteworthy and have been described (Ebright et al., 2003; Patterson et al., 2011; Sitterding et al., 2014). Situation awareness in nursing has been defined as "a dynamic process in which a nurse perceives each clinical cue relevant to the patient and his or her environment; comprehends and assigns meaning to those cues resulting in a patient-centric sense of salience; and projects or anticipates required interventions based on those cues" (Sitterding et al., 2012, p. 89).

Endsley (1995) describes "demons" that interfere with situation awareness: attentional tunneling, errant mental models, requisite memory trap, out-of-the-loop (overreliance on automation), WAFOS (workload, anxiety, fatigue, and other stressors), misplaced salience, and complexity creep. Sosa et al. (2021) demonstrated a 70% reduction in emergency transfers per 10,000 patient days as a direct result of individual and team situation awareness improvements targeting situation awareness demons or corrupters and psychological safety. Table 15.2 illustrates how situation awareness demons can block a nurse's capacity to provide highly reliable care.

PSYCHOLOGICAL SAFETY

Psychological safety is defined as the belief that the work environment is safe for interpersonal risk-taking. Psychological safety is a feeling that one is comfortable expressing themselves, speaking up, sharing concerns, or making mistakes without fear of embarrassment, ridicule, shame, or retribution (Edmondson, 2019). Edmondson writes that psychological safety is not simply a perk but essential to producing high performance in a volatile,

TABLE 15.2: Situation Awareness Demons in Action

Situation Awareness Demon	Conceptual Definition	Voice and Experience of a Registered Nurse
Attentional tunneling	Tunnel vision: The person drops their scanning behavior. Attentional tunneling occurs when the nurse fixates on one set of information to the exclusion of others. The problem is not physical interference but attentional distraction— switching attention.	*"The clinician was so focused on tasks in front of them, they completely missed this child's subtle and continuous change in LOC."*
Errant mental models	I think I see; I think I see, but it's actually the wrong mental model. People tend to explain away conflicting cues to fit the mental model they already selected— results in poor situation awareness.	*"The resident and I talked early in the shift. We just knew all along, this child was fine. It was simple gastroenteritis. We were wrong."*
Requisite memory trap	The memory bank is limited. We can hold 7 ± 2 chunks of new information in working memory. Short-term or working memory— where features of the current situation come together and are processed as a meaningful picture— is fed by knowledge stored in long-term memory as well as current information taken in.	*"Wait! What? What's the MRT criteria for this patient? Hey, did anyone see and call MJ's critical labs? What are our numbers for tonight? Is someone handling staffing?"*
Out-of-the-loop	Out-of-the-loop occurs when there is a cognitive overreliance on automation and less attention on the person/patient right within the nurse view.	*"The patient's rhythm was fine. I just couldn't see beyond the monitor. I just missed they were decompensating right in front of me."*
WAFOS	Workload, anxiety, fatigue, and other stressors (WAFOS). Stressors significantly strain situation awareness by reducing an already limited working memory. The stressors exacerbate the reliance on working memory and people are less able to gather information under stress.	*"It's a crazy shift. We have a number of watchers and 50% of our nurses are less than 2 years out. We're exhausted given the past several months working beside travelers with very different benefits packages. We've been in the red for staffing, flow, and census for months!"*
Misplaced salience	Notice or perception is alerted— for example—with the color red, movement, and flashing lights (consider the typical healthcare unit). Some information content such as hearing a particular alarm or one's name also share similar salience characteristics. These salience characteristics can promote or hinder situation awareness.	*"Overhead pages all the time. Making sense of the overhead page and if I need to respond in the midst of the alarms. It's constant. It's really hard to pay attention to all the alarms all the time—especially since some of the alarms are absolutely worthless."*

(continued)

TABLE 15.2: Situation Awareness Demons in Action (*continued*)

Situation Awareness Demon	Conceptual Definition	Voice and Experience of a Registered Nurse
Complexity creep	Technology-enabled nursing practice is great, unless the technology becomes a work burden and impedes the nurse's ability to be situationally aware.	*"Wait! I can't find the admission assessment. What did this woman look like when she came in? How do we know we've established watcher criteria? Where's that at in the EHR? Where's the early warning system note? Who saw this woman last? She's non-English speaking. Where in the EHR can I quickly locate her family? Where can I find all of this in the EHR—quickly!"*

EHR, electronic health record; WAFOS, workload, anxiety, fatigue, and other stressors.

Source: Data from Endsley, M. R. (1995). Measurement of situation awareness in dynamic systems. *Human Factors,* *37*(1), 65–84. https://doi.org/10.1518/001872095779049499; Sosa, T., Sitterding, M., Dewan, M., Segar, B., Bedinghaus, K., Hawkins, D., Maddock, B. H., Hausfeld, J., Falcone, R., Brady, P., Simmons, J., & White, C. (2021). Optimizing situation awareness to reduce emergency transfers in hospitalized children. *Pediatrics, 148*(4), e2020034603. https://doi.org/10.1542/peds.2020-034603.

uncertain, complex, and ambiguous world and work environment like that found in healthcare. Leaders who welcome only good news create fear that blocks them from hearing the truth. When the team fails to speak up with their concerns or questions, the physical safety of patients and of the care delivery team itself is compromised and the result may be harm that could have been prevented (Edmondson, 2019).

The science describing the relationship between psychological safety, fear, and behavior is well documented. Edmondson (2019) describes why it is hard for people to do their best work when they are afraid. Quite simply, fear inhibits learning. Research demonstrates that fear consumes physiological resources, diverting them from the part of the brain that manages working memory and processes new information. Subsequently, this impairs analytical thinking, creative insight, and problem-solving (Edmondson, 2019). The impact of psychological safety on situation awareness, learning, and safety, and, ultimately, the potential for harm to both patients and providers when psychological safety is absent have been described (Edmondson, 2019; Gilmartin et al., 2018; Greene et al., 2020; Hirak et al., 2012; Leroy et al., 2012; Sosa et al., 2021; Torralba et al., 2016).

Psychological safety and fear of repercussions is further explored by White and Delacroix (2020) in an integrative review of second victims' perceptions of the healthcare culture and opportunities for improvement. Second victims are healthcare providers who are involved in a patient-harm event and suffer trauma as a result, often feeling responsible for the harm and losing confidence in their clinical abilities (Scott et al., 2009). Opportunities for improvement described by second victims included: (a) eliminating fear of repercussions associated with reporting medical errors; (b) supporting safety leadership in reducing fear of error reporting; (c) improving education on adverse event reporting, offering positive feedback when adverse events are reported, and developing nonpunitive error guidelines for healthcare professionals; and (d) developing standard operating procedures for healthcare facility peer-support teams (White & Delacroix, 2020).

Edmondson offers a leader's toolkit for building psychological safety, detailing how one might set the stage (frame the work, emphasize the purpose), invite participation (demonstrate situational humility, practice inquiry, set up structures and processes that create forums for input), and respond productively by expressing appreciation and destigmatizing failure (Edmondson, 2019). The impact of psychological safety on teams and teaming is particularly relevant. Edmondson's research demonstrates that teaming requires situational humility, curiosity, and a willingness to take risks to learn quickly. Learning does not happen when you feel you know all there is to know. However, leader situational humility combined with curiosity creates psychological safety, bolstering the confidence of individuals and the team to take risks where they may fail at first, but learn and eventually succeed, as a team. Creating a culture of high reliability that enables excellence in safety and quality demands psychological safety and teaming.

GROWTH MINDSET

The construct of mindset originated from the field of psychology and has become increasingly relevant to academics, healthcare learners and leaders, and organizations (Dweck & Yeager, 2019). Mindset research originated in the study of student motivation in response to difficulty. The question the research addressed was, "What makes some students respond to difficulty or failure with helplessness, while others respond with engagement and come to develop mastery?" The study of motivation shifted the field toward how learners or team members viewed and interpreted situations and sought to understand the cognitive processes that ultimately informed their behavior as a result of how they interpreted the situation (Dweck, 1986). To grapple with the global pandemic of 2020, employees and leaders were oriented toward continuous learning in the face of challenge—even extreme challenge. A growth mindset is defined as "the belief that human capacities are not fixed but can be developed over time" (Dweck & Yeager, 2019, p. 481). Table 15.3 outlines the contrasting behaviors of those with a growth mindset versus those with a fixed mindset.

Canning et al. (2020) examined the impact of mindset on organizational culture and found that employees who perceived their organization as endorsing a fixed (versus growth) mindset reported that their organizational culture was characterized by less collaboration, innovation, and integrity and that they felt less organizational trust and commitment. Klein et al. (2017) applied the construct of mindset to the response of medical doctors in training to medical error. Young doctors with developed fixed mindset, regularly praised for their intelligence and abilities, often feel a loss of confidence and identity following a medical error. Praising students for their intelligence and abilities resulted in poorer performance and less willingness to take on challenges. Lewis et al. (2020) found the construct of mindset to be particularly relevant and promising when applied as a learning strategy for registered nursing students.

Drivers of safety within HROs include but are not limited to human factors, communication, teamwork, and collaboration (Sherwood & Armstrong, 2016). Growth-mindset units or

TABLE 15.3: Differentiating Fixed and Growth Mindsets

How Individuals Respond to . . .	Fixed Mindset: Intelligence Is Static. Leads to a Desire to Look Smart and Therefore a Tendency to . . .	Growth Mindset: Intelligence Can Be Developed. Leads to a Desire to Learn, and Therefore a Tendency to . . .
Challenges	Avoid challenges	Embrace challenges
Obstacles	Get defensive or give up easily	Persist in the face of obstacles
Effort	See effort as fruitless or worse	See effort as the path to mastery
Criticism	Ignore useful negative feedback	Learn from criticism
Success of others	Feel threatened by the success of others	Find lessons and inspiration in the success of others

Source: Data from Dweck, C. S. (2006). *The new psychology of success* (p. 263). Random House.

organizations see positive effects on both teamwork and innovation (Dweck, 2017). Employees in growth-mindset organizations, Dweck (2017) writes, report that their organization supports reasonable risk-taking, innovation, and creativity. Lee et al. (2021) describe how engaging nursing teams and leaders in the development of growth-mindset characteristics, enabled by design thinking and agile methodologies, nurtures joy among clinical nurses, positively influencing professional development, aspiration, and retention. As a result of this growth mindset mediation, the authors report 100% retention at 2 years post-intervention, whereas 65% of nurses expressed an intent to leave the organization prior to participating in the mediation. Growth mindset nurses experienced improvement in leader support in developing skills and careers and in empowerment to try new things and grow from mistakes (Lee et al., 2021).

GOVERNANCE

In order to consistently provide safe, high-quality care, a strong organizational governance structure and process must be in place and permeate the organization. For purposes of this discussion, governance is defined as vision, structure, and process accountability that starts at the highest level in the organization, the board of directors. Historically, boards of directors in healthcare organizations have been hyper-focused on finances (Jones et al., 2017). Some may even argue that this type of governance has been counterproductive to quality outcomes (Jones et al., 2017). However, the call for the achievement of the Triple Aim from the IHI (improving the patient experience of care, improving the health of populations, reducing the per capita cost of healthcare) makes it clear that finances, quality outcomes, and patient experience are not mutually exclusive but rather interdependent and must coexist in order to achieve high-quality, patient-centered outcomes (IHI, n.d.). As a result, the board of directors will need to provide oversight and leadership in the area of quality and safety in order for the organization to demonstrate sustainable results in these areas.

Numerous studies over the years have examined the differences in governance structures of organizations that achieve higher quality and safety outcomes from those of their peers. This literature demonstrates that organizations with boards of directors who take an active role with clinical leadership in establishing long-term and short-term quality and safety priorities achieve better outcomes (Jones et al., 2017; Vaughn et al., 2014). Board of director involvement in quality and safety results in improved engagement from the chief executive officer (CEO) of the organization, and this level of leadership engagement affects organizational resource use, structures, rewards, communication, culture, and accountability at all levels of the organization. In other words, where the organization spends time and resources, results occur, and how the organizational top leaders spend their time, culture follows. This was clearly demonstrated in a study by Vaughn et al. (2006) of 413 hospitals from eight states that completed the executive quality improvement survey, which examined leadership governance and quality performance outcomes. In this study, 25% of the board of directors' time was spent on driving quality and safety in the facilities that demonstrated the most improvement in quality performance indicators (Vaughn et al., 2006).

The literature examining the relationship between governance, leadership, and quality and safety results is not new. This leaves one to question why there has not been more improvement across the country in decreasing medical errors, eliminating patient harm, and sustaining better quality and safety outcomes. It appears that there is often more institutional rhetoric regarding support for quality and safety than actual leadership support from the board, which permeates the organization at all levels (Levey et al., 2007). This may mean that CEOs and board chairs need to choose different skill sets for the board members and ensure there is a complement of skill sets represented that can set the vision and accountability for all aspects of the Triple Aim. Ultimately, quality and safety performance only improves when there is a clear vision from the top of the organization and the organizational structures, resources, incentives, and accountabilities are set up in a manner to reinforce that quality and safety are organizational priorities.

DESIGNING AND DRIVING CULTURE

Organizational culture is a set of shared values and beliefs that drive performance and outcomes. Literature exploring the topic of organizational culture demonstrates that, while the definition of culture might sound simple, creating, shifting, and sustaining culture in healthcare is anything but simple. This is in large part due to the complexity of healthcare delivery and the complexity of the rapidly changing digital environment. This complexity has resulted in immense variation in practices and beliefs, even within a single organization, despite all the work that has been done on evidence-based practice and standardization (Mannion & Davies, 2018). The variation plays out in departments, specialties, service lines, and hierarchy within the organization, resulting in many subcultures, often competing against each other instead of all rowing in the same direction toward a common goal (2018).

Despite multiple subcultures within single organizations, culture remains the most important driver of sustainable, high-quality performance outcomes (Ingelsson et al., 2018; Mannion & Davies, 2018; O'Hagan & Persaud, 2009). As a result, leaders must have intentional plans for designing and creating a culture of quality and safety. Without this intentionality, the organization will have a culture, but it may not be a culture that leads to sustained high-quality and safety performance outcomes, as we see all too often in many healthcare organizations. Two important aspects to consider when creating intentional plans to design and create a quality and safety culture are organizational coherence and transformational leadership.

Coherence is the ability to be consistent and aligned. Organizational coherence is the ability of the organization to be well-aligned and consistent in its values, beliefs, goals, direction, rewards, and measurement at all levels of the organization. McAlearney et al. (2013) designed a conceptual model for organizational coherence that encompasses three components: social system coherence, intraorganizational coherence, and coherent processes (see Figure 15.1). Social system coherence references the need for all individuals within groups and teams to

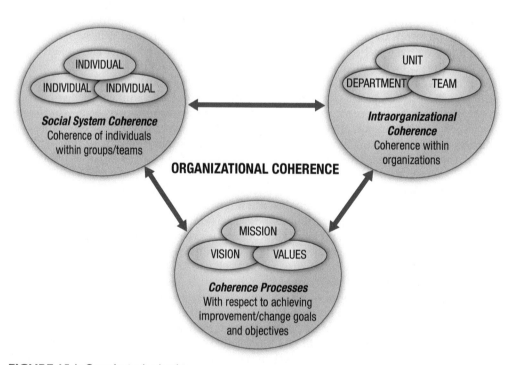

FIGURE 15.1: Complexity leadership.

Source: Adapted from Uhl-Bien, M., & Arena, M. (2017). *Complexity leadership: Enabling people and organizations for adaptability.* Organizational Dynamics.

be aligned around a common set of values, beliefs, goals, and outcomes. Intraorganizational coherence represents the need for this alignment to occur across departments, teams, units, disparate groups, disciplines, and hierarchies. Coherent processes are ways of working in the organization that are aligned around a common set of goals, measurements, incentives, accountability, and rewards, all in turn aligned with the organization's mission, vision, and values. These three dimensions of organizational coherence then must work seamlessly in concert together, which will reduce the confusion and resistance that is often experienced in organizations around quality and safety efforts as a result of competing priorities or values.

ORGANIZATIONAL COHERENCE CONCEPTUAL MODEL

As the leaders in the organization focus on ensuring organizational coherence related to quality and safety culture and performance outcomes, it is also important for them to examine their leadership style and its impact on the culture. A systematic review conducted by Sfantou et al. (2017) demonstrated the strong correlation between leadership, quality and safety culture, quality and safety outcomes, and provision of care. The specific leadership style of transformational leadership has been strongly connected and associated with a safety culture that leads to high-quality, patient-centered outcomes (Moneke & Umeh, 2013).

Transformational leadership is a formal leadership style that encourages and expects both the leader and the leader's followers to work toward a higher purpose and focus on the good of the team and the organization (Bromley & Kirschner-Bromley, 2007). Transformational leaders have the ability to transcend the current situation; paint a vibrant picture of future possibilities, goals, and steps to get there; and influence team members to see how each individual and the team as a whole can have impact on the greater good and share a meaningful purpose. Creating a sense of higher order grounded in meaning, purpose, and inspiring good proves very motivational for clinicians who already likely have an innate calling. This leadership style enables development of a quality and safety culture where performance measurement is an essential element, where reporting errors is encouraged and not punished, and where collaboration between all levels of the organization and across all disciplines is expected (O'Hagan & Persaud, 2009). All of these attributes lead to a culture of safety where everything centers around improvement for the patient, thereby leading to high-quality, patient-centered outcomes.

Transformational leaders fundamentally focus on inspiration as opposed to being authoritarian. A transformational leader understands that their purpose as a leader is to be an "agent" or a coordinator or facilitator of all the factors, intersections, forces, and complexity in the organization in order to create conditions for the success of the team and, ultimately, the organization (Porter-O'Grady, 2020). This facilitation supports and promotes creativity, ideological vision, and high-performing teams. Ultimately, the leader is cultivating a growth mindset in the team, encouraging them to constantly ask questions, push the limits of what might seem possible, expect excellence from themselves and others, and view failure as an opportunity to learn, all in an effort to improve, achieve goals, and create an environment in which patients and families receive the highest quality outcomes.

Some may question what role accountability plays when everything is focused on inspiration and higher moral purpose. Accountability is a key part of any successful organization; however, how accountability is defined is often where the problem lies. Many perceive accountability as punitive or negative, with a focus on what did not go "right." However, healthy accountability in quality and safety cultures focuses on what is possible through continual learning, transparency, and positive motivation. In other words, accountability flows from inspiring a growth mindset in the team, all focused on a common set of team and organizational goals, thereby creating a culture with tools for measuring what success looks like and centered on serving patients. O'Hagan and Persaud (2009) define "accountability" as "encompassing the procedures and processes by which one party justifies and takes responsibility for its activities such as achieving organizational goals" (p. 124), suggesting that accountability is not punitive but rather inspirational and aligned with transformational leadership.

PRACTICING COMPLEXITY LEADERSHIP TO DRIVE INNOVATION AND RESULTS

COMPLEXITY: A FRAMEWORK OR MODEL FOR LEADERSHIP IN QUALITY AND SAFETY

Twenty-first century leadership of complex initiatives and environments requires a different mode of understanding healthcare networks and healthcare delivery models as they unfold into the future. Complexity leadership is a model for enabling people and organizations to adapt to rapid and continuous change. In this model, the leader is seen not as a managerial implementer of top-down directives but as a collaborator who works with others to enhance the overall adaptability and fitness of the system (Figure 15.1; Uhl-Bien et al., 2020). Porter-O'Grady (2020) differentiates situational and servant leadership from what is necessary and available through a leadership framework where the "leader is an agent of forces, factors, and intersection, which create conditions for success" (p. 92). Complexity leadership, in contrast to historical hierarchical models based on control and efficiency, requires skills of assessment, prediction, adaptation, and influence. Complexity leaders create an environment for decisions and action that aligns effort and action in a manner that achieves the desired impact, influenced most by those who own the work (Porter-O'Grady, 2020). The complexity leadership model depicts how networked interactions enable idea generation by entrepreneurial leaders, flowing through an adaptive space into the operating system, captured by operational leaders, generating new order, and resulting in healthcare innovations and improved health outcomes including, but not limited to, improved quality and safety (Uhl-Bien et al., 2020).

THE ADAPTIVE SPACE AND PROCESS

The basic premise of the complexity model is that the core dynamic is tension—tension between the need to innovate and the need to control or produce. The adaptive process engages tension; traditional hierarchical models work to eliminate the tension. The fact that you are reading this text means you are near the adaptive space—you are willing to engage to think differently. The tension dynamic is necessary and simply suggests "conflicting"— conflicting worldviews, conflicting preferences. Instead of trying to manage the conflict or make the conflict go away (command, control, and hierarchy), we need to engage the conflict or tension. It is the engagement between the need to produce or solve and the need to innovate that creates the adaptive space and process. Uhl-Bien asserts that what is necessary is the space—in our minds—for conflicting. Opening up to conflicting creates adaptability that occurs on the individual level, within groups, between groups, in organizations, between organizations. Conflicting only generates adaptability if it is combined with connecting. Innovation is important in that it leads to adaptability, which in turn leads to sustainability. Through effective conflicting and connecting, no one individual or agent owns the idea—the ideas are shared (Uhl-Bien & Arena, 2017).

⬣ | **CASE SCENARIO**

A HIGH-RISK PATIENT LEAVES WITHOUT BEING SEEN

Last week, TS presented themselves at the hospital ED, worried about thoughts of self-harm. As TS had a history of behavioral complaints and suicidality, they were placed in the designated high-risk behavior zone. However, security was not informed that TS was there. Several minutes after TS's arrival, SS, BSN, RN, clinical nurse, ED, entered TS's room to begin triage and noted the patient was gone. The security officer recalled seeing the patient walk to the bathroom but did not see them return. CCTV footage showed TS walking down the street, away from the hospital. This is not the first time a patient at high risk for self-harm left without being seen.

The nurse leader has been asked to solve for this issue. How might you engage a team and think differently about a sustainable solution? Imagine how you would apply complexity leadership, adaptive processes, and adaptive space. How might you enable practices that engage the tension between productivity and innovation, resulting in adaptation? How might you facilitate an adaptive process by creating an adaptive space that enables the combination of conflicting and connecting?

Within a complexity leadership model, enabling leadership practices include brokerage, leveraging adaptive tension, linking up, tags and attractors, simple rules, and network closure (see Table 15.4). Choose either of the following scenarios and apply enabling leadership practices.

TABLE 15.4: Enabling Leadership Practices of the Complexity Leadership Model

Enabling Leadership Practices	Practice Description	Scenario Application
Brokerage	Ideas are triggered at the intersection of networks. Brokerage allows for ideas to be generated and creates bridges for information to flow and agents to link up.	
Leveraging adaptive tension	Increasing and decreasing tension to manage levels of conflicting. Too much conflicting distresses a system, reducing its ability to create; too little conflicting keeps a system and agents in status quo. Conflicting is good—play in the pressure that motivates agents to change or do better.	
Linking up	Creating or energizing network connections that enable information flows, or amplify movements, to feed and fuel emergence.	
Tags and attractors	Listening for language (messages, stories) and symbols (pictures, objects) that "stick" in a system and attract energy and using them to create tags to amplify and channel emergence.	
Simple rules	Creating simple guidelines for behavior that enable network and complexity dynamics (e.g., brokering, cohesion, energizing, conflicting, linking up, network closure) without requiring agents to have an understanding of complexity.	
Network closure	Network closure lets the others make the sale for you. It uses reputation and gossip to get attention and support of sponsors.	

Source: Uhl-Bien, M., & Arena, M. (2017). *Complexity leadership: Enabling people and organizations for adaptability* (p. 17). Organizational Dynamics.

SITUATION #1

Sepsis screening was implemented in the ED, medical–surgical units, and intensive care unit (ICU) in 2018 to promote better patient outcomes by identifying and treating sepsis earlier. However, the mother–baby unit (MBU) was excluded from the implementation of sepsis screening due to physiological changes of pregnancy that can produce a false-positive systemic inflammatory response syndrome (SIRS) screen result. Late in 2018, an antepartum patient was admitted with pyelonephritis symptoms and was receiving routine treatment on the MBU. During the stay, the patient's condition deteriorated and the clinical nurse caring for the patient requested the unit charge nurse and nurse manager assess the patient's changing condition.

APPROACH

Due to prior involvement with hospital-wide sepsis discussions, the nurse manager recognized that the patient was experiencing signs of sepsis and instructed team members to call a sepsis alert.

OUTCOME

Consequently, the sepsis alert was called, and the patient was transferred to the ICU where they received aggressive treatment and made a full recovery.

SITUATION #2

What nurses experienced in 2020 and their heroic response to COVID-19 changed everything. Newly licensed pediatric nurses were holding the hands of dying adult patients while FaceTiming with their families who were not permitted to be present because of COVID restrictions. Protocols and guidelines that were communicated during the morning brief might change by 1 p.m. the same day. Few things tax a person's resilience more than navigating uncertainty, but the team was required to perform demanding work within an atmosphere of extreme uncertainty. Professional nurses rely on evidence, protocols, and procedures to guide practice every minute during the workday. The anxiety and threat around what they were dealing with, how they would deal with it, and the unpredictability of how long they would need to mount a response to this pandemic was disturbing and draining.

APPROACH

Complexity leadership and enabling leadership practices is the approach that best equips the nurse leader to embrace the uncertainty and gather key operators and innovators (representing all levels of nursing) to an adaptive space that enables nurses to practice best evidence while simultaneously innovating to meet the needs of the patient, family, nurse, and team. Consider which team members (within and outside of nursing) who represent the network will energize and fuel emergence of an adaptive solution. Consider opening and revisiting simple rules within the adaptive network you have gathered. Simple rules might include, but not be limited to, the solution is patient-centric, the solution is derived from those closest to the point of care delivery, or the solution represents our very best connecting and conflicting.

OUTCOME

The outcome is a statistically significant decrease in your patient-harm outcome. The outcome is you have a 98% retention rate of clinical nurses otherwise incomparable to your nurse leader colleagues.

DISCUSSION QUESTIONS

1. Describe the differences when comparing the traditional approach to ignore or tame the tension as opposed to the approach taken to embrace the tension and create a network of innovators and operators that generated solutions through an adaptive space.

2. Discuss how enabling connection and conflict within and beyond the network results in innovative and sustained solutions.

3. Name and recognize the ideas generated and tested within the adaptive space. What stories or images were amplified and stuck influencing the emergence of innovation?

INNOVATION THROUGH DESIGN THINKING AND AGILE METHODOLOGY

WHAT IS DESIGN THINKING?

Lorusso et al. (2021) provide one of the most comprehensive definitions of design thinking. Design thinking is a collaborative method of inquiry that fosters innovative, team-generated solutions to complex scenarios that are extraordinarily complicated and difficult to solve. "It is a practical tool in the toolbox of the codesign team, which includes client and design professionals as primary stakeholders" (Lorusso et al., 2021, p. 16). It is an open-sourced framework customizable for each unique application and is reused and revised involving a creative problem-solving (CPS) process (Lorusso et al., 2021). Using an iterative process to understand the problem, generate ideas, and develop a plan for action is foundational for successful design thinking, as well as creative brainstorming, prototyping, and human-centered design (Lorusso et al., 2021; Micheli et al., 2019; Seidel & Fixson, 2013; Treffinger, 1994). The design must be rooted in a deep understanding of users (those closest to the work), their tasks, and their environment. The users themselves must be involved throughout the codesign process, and the design is evaluated by user-focused criteria (Ku & Lupton, 2020).

Critical to the process is ensuring that despite whatever activities are utilized, the design team establishes a methodical way to collect and record narrative feedback during these phases, to document decision-making progression and design validation. Given that design thinking and design teams are new to healthcare, a place to start is by translating the idea of a checklist (common in healthcare) into a healthcare design team codesign checklist, which might include items such as: "(a) create organizational chart displaying codesign team; (b) write "how might we?" statements to frame the kickoff; (c) recruit department champions (superusers); (d) establish calendar holds for the team to conduct initial workshops and recurring touch-base sessions; (e) create template for ongoing summary of findings (print or digital); and (f) establish key performance indicators that will influence design drivers" (Lorusso et al., 2021, p. 25).

An integrative review of design thinking in healthcare summarized facilitators and barriers with this approach. Facilitators of design thinking were categorized into four subthemes: existing literature eased transition, participant enthusiasm, detailed understanding of barriers, and streamlining of goals. In contrast, barriers included limitations in existing literature, extensive time to implementation, social pressure influence, and poor concept definition (Rahemi et al., 2018).

Resources for learning more about design thinking are emerging. For example, Health Design by Us through the University of Michigan is a collaborative of patients and caregivers, healthcare providers and researchers, designers and artists, engineers and technologists, and public health professionals "who are passionate about patient-centered participatory design and applying the model of the maker movement to healthcare" (HealthDesignbyUs, n.d., para 1). To learn more, visit www.healthdesignby.us.

WHAT IS AGILE METHODOLOGY?

The agile process is one that accepts the complexity of a problem and addresses it through frequent inspection, responding with a customer-centric flexible approach to adaptation. Agile methodology values the results of human interactions over traditional approaches.

The traditional process of detailed task definitions, development of flow charts, and defining assignments are less common in agile methodology. The highest priority of agile methodology is to satisfy the customer through rapid and continuous delivery of value (Kitzmiller et al., 2006). It is, however, a lean approach, and some recommend the lean and agile methodology hybrid approach (Tolf et al., 2015).

Agile methodology values communication and harnesses change to an advantage, facilitating the natural evolution of an adaptable implementation process. An agile approach enhances traditional implementation techniques to meet the demands of today's complex healthcare environments. Agile innovation focuses on customer needs, collecting and nimbly responding to customer feedback in sprint cycles and empowering teams to autonomously adjust to demands in contrast to the traditional top-down constraints associated with solution-generation (Holden et al., 2021).

Holden et al. (2021) describe eight steps necessary for agile innovation—four steps for planning and four steps for execution. The eight steps are: (a) confirm demand, (b) study the problem, (c) scan for solutions, (d) plan for evaluation, (e) ideate and select, (f) run innovation development sprints, (g) validate solution, and (h) package for launch. Improvement in dementia care and behavioral healthcare, as well as improved decision-support tools, have been directly attributed to the agile innovation (Holden et al., 2021). Factors enabling the development and sustainability of an agile organization include: (a) transparent and transient interorganizational links at all levels within the organization, (b) market sensitivity and customer focus, (c) management by support for self-organizing employees, (d) organic structures that are elastic and responsive, and (e) flexible human and resource capacity for timely delivery (Tolf et al., 2015). Lee et al. (2021) describe the impact of design thinking and agile methodology on growth mindset and joy in nursing. More work is needed to test and develop the application of agile methodology and design thinking in healthcare, patient care delivery models, and nursing.

USING TOOLS TO DRIVE RESULTS

Work to improve quality and safety is often associated with the use of tools to view systems and processes, gather information, organize information, understand variations, understand relationships, and manage projects (Langley et al., 2009). As important as understanding tools and tactics is, the role of the nurse leader and nurse executive is to drive results. The six aims of improvement in healthcare quality described in the IOM report *Crossing the Quality Chasm* (2001) are no less significant today than when the report was first published. A more recent report expands upon the original six aims to include value, equity, effectiveness, safety, timeliness, patient-centeredness, access, efficiency, care coordination, and capabilities of health system infrastructures (IOM, 2010). The nurse leader or nurse executive of the future must be equipped with the knowledge and experience to drive quality and safety across systems—at scale.

That said, tools can facilitate very helpful diagnostic tactics for quality and safety improvement initiatives. However, it is critical to understand the expected competency and contribution of your particular role as it relates to quality and improvement and the utilization of tools. Your role may be to project manage a particular initiative, and, in that case, you must have expertise in understanding and facilitating the use of improvement tools. Your role may be to serve as a team leader for various quality and safety initiatives where you would be required to understand the tool and ensure that the team is accurately matching the diagnostic of interest with the right tool. You may serve as an executive sponsor, in which case you must ensure your project manager or coordinator, team members, and team leader are adequately resourced with the tools and talent necessary to solve for the quality or safety problem or opportunity they have been challenged to improve.

STRATEGIC EXECUTION

THE IMPORTANCE OF INFLUENCE

Safety and quality outcomes are dependent upon nurse leader capability to drive results through influence. This is not a new idea. Nurses have always been well-prepared academically and experientially to influence quality and safety associated with clinical practice. Beyond clinical practice, it is time for nurses to influence quality and safety in the boardroom and through policy (Adams et al., 2019; American Organization for Nursing Leadership, n.d.; Sundean et al., 2017, 2020). A case study of the experience of a nurse who served as chair of a statewide hospital board's quality and patient safety committee demonstrates the impact of a nurse leader at the system level dramatically influencing quality and safety across a large healthcare system in the Midwest (McBride, 2017).

How is nursing leadership influence described or defined? We have been limited in part by a lack of understanding of influence in the context of nursing leadership. Sundean et al. (2021) answered this question through a concept analysis resulting in proposed attributes, antecedents, and consequences of influence in nursing leadership. Attributes of influence in nursing leadership include advocacy, communication skills, competency, confidence, credibility, and engagement. Antecedents enabling and/or existing prior to the incidence of influence in nursing leadership include authority, collaboration, integrity, and mentorship. Consequences or outcomes as a result of influence in nursing leadership include action, change, commitment, compliance, decision-making, motivation, and resistance (Sundean et al., 2021).

How might you know your capacity to influence? Shillam et al. (2018) developed the Leadership Influence Self-Assessment instrument, building on the Adams Influence Model (Adams & Natarajan, 2016). The model describes influence factors such as "knowledge-based competence (well-qualified intellectually), authority (the right to take actions), status (having high standing or prestige), communication traits (proficiency or dexterity with which one person relates and interacts with other people), and use of time (the understanding of both the interval in which the action is available to be taken and the optional judgment and delivery of when an action is taken)" (Shillam et al., 2018, p. 132).

What can we learn about influence from others outside of healthcare? Sinek asserts that influence is attained when one leads from the position of *why*. He describes why some leaders and organizations influence and others do not. The *why* he describes is your purpose, your belief; inspired leaders lead with the *why* as opposed to the *what*. Stories—the *why*—are a well-known catalyst for improvement in quality and safety (Grissinger, 2014; Siegal & Ruoff, 2015). Consider how the why is integral to the attributes and antecedents (Sundean et al., 2021) associated with influence. The goal is not to sell the idea of improvement; the goal is to positively influence the desire to improve because those you are attempting to influence believe what you believe about healthcare safety and quality.

SPREAD, SUSTAIN, AND SCALE

Knowledge and capability to spread, sustain, and scale are core attributes necessary to accelerate the safety and quality improvement pace, demonstrating our commitment to those we serve and serve beside. Rogers's seminal work demonstrated that it was not only the properties of the innovation (i.e., the care delivery model your team designed, relative advantage, compatibility, complexity, trialabilit, and observability) that made it successful but also a set of factors associated with communication across networks (McGrath & Zell, 2001). Definitions matter. A scoping review of the literature on spreading, sustaining, and scaling healthcare innovations conducted a thematic analysis to arrive at definitions of these terms (Côté-Boileau et al., 2019). The authors define spread as "both passive and deliberate efforts to communicate and implement an innovation and usually involves adapting an innovation to a new setting" (p. 4). Sustainability is defined as "what happens when an innovation becomes routinized within an organization or other setting" (p. 4). Scale-up is "the process in which the coverage and impact of an innovation are expanded to reach all potential beneficiaries" (p. 4). Five lessons that emerged from the scoping review are: (a) focus on the why; (b) focus on perceived-value and feasibility; (c) focus on what people do, rather than what they should be doing; (d) focus on creating a dialogue between policy and delivery; and (e) focus on inclusivity and capability building (2019).

◆ CASE SCENARIO

INFLUENCING BEYOND YOUR TEAM

You have been inspired by the call for next generation care delivery innovation and impact. You believe you have a compelling narrative, signaling a radical call to redesign care delivery. To broaden your perspective, you decide to gather a small group of thought leaders representing interdisciplinary key stakeholders with very diverse backgrounds and perspectives. You have led a collaborative expansion of a most compelling narrative that reflects the unique attributes, meaning, and functional value of each of the diverse team members you have gathered. The product of the team's collaborative narrative was energy, enthusiasm, ingenuity, innovation, and a next generation care delivery model of the future (CMOF) prototype. Your next step was to expand upon feedback through geographic and key stakeholder boundary spanning including the team of physicians, nurses, and therapists closest to the point of care. Through each interaction, you were intentional about listening to what was most salient to your thought partner at the time and integrating that voice in the prototype or testing plan. You applied agile methods as a framework to test, iterate, and evaluate informed by outcome measures most significant to the population and team members serving that population. This approach was reflected in bi-weekly retrospection reviews with those closest to the prototype implementation with three meeting objectives informed by customer feedback: (a) What have we learned that is working? (b) What have we learned that is not working? (c) What is the plan to iterate and how will we measure impact? Six months into what has become a demonstration project with significantly positive outcomes in hospital-acquired harm reduction, patient experience, mortality, length of stay (LOS), and team turnover have emerged. The executive team has noticed. You have now been given the opportunity to spread and scale, influencing where you do not have direct line management authority.

Ponder the following personal reflection questions as an exercise in evaluating how you may approach the challenge to influence those beyond your direct team.

REFLECTION AND DISCUSSION QUESTIONS

1. The compelling narrative: Describe the narrative you would tell outlining the need for change and how the narrative is embedded with what you have learned; this is most meaningful to those with whom you wish to influence.

2. Framing the narrative: How do you tap the intrinsic motivation of the collective resulting in an expanded narrative that reflects diversity in personality and expertise among your thought partners?

3. Empirical outcomes within the evolving narrative: What empirical outcomes complement the narrative you have facilitated? What empirical outcomes are necessary to accelerate and expand upon the intrinsic motivation you have catalyzed?

4. Teaming: You have learned about how you as a leader can facilitate an adaptive space through connecting and conflicting. Describe how you create an environment that promotes positive and productive teaming. How will you promote team autonomy to inform, iterate, fail, and learn?

5. Leader emotional presence: Your emotional presence through design iteration, testing, failing, and learning influences team performance. How will you praise the team through

success? How will you demonstrate empathy with iteration failures? How will you model a growth mindset versus victimhood that embraces failures as learning?

6. Leader emotional intelligence: Your emotional intelligence influences whether to stay the course and/or redirect to call it quits. As a leader, how are you constantly scanning, with a laser-sharp focus on impact on the problem? How do you avoid becoming blinded by the solution that you and the team created, losing sight of the problem? Describe a time when a team was so convinced the intervention was going to solve the problem and there was recognition following implementation that the intervention failed. How did you move the team emotionally, intellectually, and in the most psychologically safe manner from being committed to what they created as a solution to the problem to seeing what they need to impact and influence?

◼ WHAT EVERY NURSE MANAGER NEEDS TO KNOW ABOUT QUALITY AND SAFETY

What every nurse manager needs to know about quality and safety begins with the nurse manager knowing thyself and demonstrating the capacity to lead oneself—enabled by a growth mindset. The nurse manager who embraces a growth mindset embraces uncertainty and the possibility of failure with a sense of optimism, knowing that their application of a complexity leadership model will explain, describe, and/or predict their ability to positively influence quality and safety within their unit, their clinic, and the community they serve. A basic understanding of quality improvement tools is helpful; however, far more important than memorizing quality improvement tools is the need for the nurse manager to understand their moral and ethical responsibility to positively influence the team reporting up through them, ultimately making a difference in quality and safety among the patients we all are privileged to serve.

WHAT EVERY NURSE MANAGER NEEDS TO KNOW

- How nurse manager leadership attributes contribute to a culture of excellence in quality and safety
- How to enable growth mindset within yourself and among your team
- How to ensure psychological safety among your interprofessional and intraprofessional team
- How design thinking and agile methodology can empower your team and help you drive results
- The difference between quality and safety tools and driving results

◼ WHAT EVERY NURSE EXECUTIVE NEEDS TO KNOW ABOUT QUALITY AND SAFETY

Leadership at all levels and especially at the executive level always begins with understanding yourself first and the recognition that as a leader you must be consumed with introspection, retrospection, and growth—representing a true growth mindset. Leadership is a skill set and an art that must be constantly cultivated and viewed as a journey. Each of us as leaders learn and adapt every day.

Leadership is fundamentally about creating and cultivating culture, a culture that is rooted in the mission and vision of the organization. In order for leaders to be able to communicate the why with conviction and purpose, it is always helpful for a leader's own personal mission to be in alignment with the mission and vision of the organization, thereby creating true authenticity when the leader leads. This authenticity provides the leader with the ability to influence others through connecting to the why and purpose—inspiration. This inspiration is in many cases what explains the variation in results between highly competent leaders.

WHAT EVERY NURSE EXECUTIVE NEEDS TO KNOW

- Culture drives quality and safety outcomes both for the good and unfortunately for the bad. The following outlines what every nurse executive should know about driving a culture of quality and safety:
  - Recognizing the number one priority must always be quality and safety.
  - Finance, quality, safety, and patient experience all must coexist in order to have a healthy organization and healthy culture.
  - Healthcare leadership can no longer focus on control and hierarchy. Rather, the nurse executive must recognize that healthcare, today, is a highly complex series of multiple networks which are full of knowledge workers interacting with each other in multidimensional ways in order to deliver care to individuals, families, and communities.
  - Nurse executive leadership which embraces the networks requires strong cross discipline and cross collaborative relationships at all levels of the organization.
  - Nurse executives must embrace these networks of caregivers and other leaders by creating the environment that allows them to foster and grow, individually and collectively, in alignment with the organizational goals.
  - Nurse executives can accomplish this by driving a culture that embraces complexity and tension by ensuring those closest to the work drive most of the decisions.
  - Those closest to the work will always make the best decisions about the work.
  - In turn, this behavior also creates the space and trust necessary for psychological safety. Psychological safety is a key component and input in order to be a highly reliable organization that achieves high-quality results.
  - The nurse executive's primary role is to harness this ability by balancing the need to control and produce and the need to innovate, thereby allowing the adaptive space to form which will lead to sustainability of results. Nurse executives should lean into their inherent ability to cultivate relationships and inspire others in all they do as a leader.

KEY POINTS

- Growth mindset is a required frame for the nurse expecting to dramatically influence sustained excellence in quality and safety. The nurse leader must never, ever underestimate the power of influence regardless of line authority.
- Psychological safety explains a nurse leader's capacity to influence the speed at which the team develops, innovates, fails, learns quickly, and impacts excellence in quality and safety.
- Nurse leaders' understanding of individual, team, and organizational situation awareness informs the nurse leaders' capacity to recognize and mitigate situation awareness demons that are negatively influencing safety.

■ The moral and ethical imperative for the nurse leader to impact quality and safety revealed itself during the COVID-19 pandemic. It was a brutal audit explained by complexity leadership and our decision to stamp out the tension and/or embrace the tension and uncertainty, and innovate—for good.

SUMMARY

The basis of all patient care should revolve around the delivery of safe care to patients, families, healthcare workers, organizations, communities, and the nation. Failure to do so creates an incredible economic and emotional burden on the people and organizations affected. While progress has been made in patient safety, the pace must be accelerated. Nurse leaders have a tremendous opportunity to join and accelerate patient safety improvement. However, change will only happen if leaders are intentional about making a difference with patient safety (Kerfoot, 2016).

The challenges faced by the nursing profession are perhaps unprecedented, and include emotional exhaustion, post-pandemic burnout, worker shortages, a declining workforce, and frustration with on-the-job technologies like EHR which may lack usability. Only 9% of nurses are prepared to practice upon graduation (Kavanagh & Sharpnack, 2021). More than a tool is needed. Nursing leaders must face these challenges with new ways of problem-solving.

Tools are useful, and important, but nursing leaders absolutely must step into a new, more active role in creating a culture of safety. Leaders must drive psychological safety. Leaders must adopt a growth mindset. Leaders must shed hierarchical structures and adopt more collaboration. Leaders must bring agile methodology and design thinking to their challenges.

END-OF-CHAPTER RESOURCES

◆ DISCUSSION QUESTIONS

1. Describe cultural influences on safety and quality within healthcare.
2. Discuss evidence of high reliability principles of quality and safety application within your clinical setting and contrast it to high reliability principles applied in other organizations, such as aviation.
3. Describe your experience and observations of situation awareness within interprofessional teams as well as within organizational cultures.
4. Discuss application of complexity leadership and the contributing influence on quality and safety.
5. Describe what factors most influence spread, sustain, and scale and how you might modify those factors as they relate to quality and safety.

◆ ADDITIONAL RESOURCES

■ TED. (2018, June 4). *How to turn a group of strangers into a team* | *Amy Edmondson* [Video]. YouTube. https://www.youtube.com/watch?v=3boKz0Exros
■ Stanford Alumni. (2014, October 9). *Developing a growth mindset with Carol Dweck* [Video]. YouTube. https://www.youtube.com/watch?v=hiiEeMN7vbQ
■ The Q community. (2019, December 6). *Prof Mary Uhl-Bien: How to master the art of creating 'Adaptive Spaces'* [Video]. YouTube. https://www.youtube.com/watch?v=OBINjMSq9yY

- Beck, K., Beedle, M., van Bennekum, A., Cockburn, A., Cunningham, W., Fowler, M., Martin, R. C., Mellor, S., Thomas, D., Grenning, J., Highsmith, J., Hunt, A., Jeffries, R., Kern, J., Marick, B., Schwaber, K., Sutherland, J. (2001). *The agile manifesto*. https://www.agilealliance.org/agile101/the-agile-manifesto

- A widely used, evidence-based, collaborative resource for those of us who are always students of quality and safety science is the IHI Open School: https://www.ihi.org/education/ihiopenschool/Pages/default.aspx

- For more on the impact of *why*, visit Simon Sinek's TED Talk at https://www.youtube.com/watch?v=u4ZoJKF_VuA

◖ LEARNING EXERCISES FOR STUDENTS

1. You have been asked to interview nurses caring for a child who coded last week. You are interviewing Olive, one of the clinical nurses with just over 2 years of experience. She shares the story of Charles, a 5-year-old patient hospitalized with gastroenteritis. Overnight, she noticed he had worsening diarrhea. She also noticed an elevated heart rate; he wasn't drinking too much, and his parents told her that he wasn't acting right. She reported to the charge nurse, who was busy that night. The charge nurse told her to contact the resident and let him know. Olive and the resident discussed and agreed that they should "keep an eye on him." Olive reported everything—or so she thought—to Caroline during shift change, but they were interrupted several times with alarms, staffing issues, and lab. The family contacted Caroline, who was very busy with a new admit. Lucy, the patient care tech, shared with Caroline that the family felt Charles was much worse than when he came into the ED. Caroline told the patient care tech that she was very busy and that she should assure the family they could share their concerns during rounds a little later in the morning. Lucy felt as though the family concerns and her concerns for the family were dismissed. Lucy noticed Charles's heart rate was higher than when originally reported on nights. Lucy did not say anything to Caroline about the heart rate. During mid-morning rounds, Charles was difficult to arouse. His pulses were difficult to palpate and code was called. Consider the three levels of situation awareness and any psychological safety elements within the scenario.

2. Imagine that you are the nurse leader in charge of the MBU. You are charged with the imperative of ensuring that this situation is not repeated since it could have led to devastating outcomes. How might you engage a team and think differently about a sustainable solution? Use Table 15.4 as a guide to how you might apply enabling leadership practices to address the issue raised in this scenario.

3. Self-care programs can no longer be looked upon as value-added niceties to help sustain your team. You now need a comprehensive program that targets caregiver well-being so that they can maintain a healthy body, mind, and spirit during persistent, uncertain times. How might you engage a team and think differently about a sustainable solution? Use Table 15.4 as a guide to how you might apply enabling leadership practices to address the issue raised in this scenario.

REFERENCES

Adams, J. M., Glassman, K., McCausland, M., Pappas, S., & Manges, K. (2019). A purposeful approach to articulate and enhance nursing influence across policy, research, education, practice, theory, media, and industry. *The Journal of Nursing Administration, 49*(9), 397–399. https://doi.org/10.1097/NNA.0000000000000774

Adams, J. M., & Natarajan, S. (2016). Understanding influence within the context of nursing: Development of the Adams Influence Model using practice, research, and theory. *ANS. Advances in Nursing Science, 39*(3), E40–E56. https://doi.org/10.1097/ANS.0000000000000134

American Organization for Nursing Leadership. (n.d.). *2019–2021 strategic priorities and objectives.* Retrieved June 30, 2021, from https://www.aonl.org/system/files/media/file/2019/07/AONL%20Strategic%20Plan%202019-2021.pdf

Barello, S., Caruso, R., Palamenghi, L., Nania, T., Dellafiore, F., Bonetti, L., Silenzi, A., Marotta, C., & Graffigna, G. (2021). Factors associated with emotional exhaustion in healthcare professionals involved in the COVID-19 pandemic: An application of the job demands-resources model. *International Archives of Occupational and Environmental Health, 94*(8), 1751–1761. https://doi.org/10.1007/s00420-021-01669-z

Bates, D. W., & Singh, H. (2018). Two decades since *To Err Is Human*: An assessment of progress and emerging priorities in patient safety. *Health Affairs, 37*(11), 1736-1743. https://doi.org/10.1377/hlthaff.2018.0738

Berwick, D. M., Calkins, D. R., McCannon, C. J., & Hackbarth, A. D. (2006). The 100 000 lives campaign: Setting a goal and a deadline for improving health care quality. *JAMA, 295*(3), 324–327. https://doi.org/10.1001/jama.295.3.324

Brady, P. W., Muething, S., Kotagal, U., Ashby, M., Gallagher, R., Hall, D., Goodfriend, M., White, C., Bracke, T. M., DeCastro, V., Geiser, M., Simon, J., Tucker, K. M., Olivea, J., Conway, P. H., & Wheeler, D. S. (2013). Improving situation awareness to reduce unrecognized clinical deterioration and serious safety events. *Pediatrics, 131*(1), e298–e308. https://doi.org/10.1542/peds.2012-1364

Bromley, H. R., & Kirschner-Bromley, V. A. (2007, November–Decemebr). Are you a transformational leader? *The Physician Executive, 33*(6), 54–57.

Caldas, M. P., Ostermeier, K., & Cooper, D. (2021). When helping hurts: COVID-19 critical incident involvement and resource depletion in health care workers. *Journal of Applied Psychology, 106*(1), 29–47. https://doi.org/10.1037/apl0000850

Canning, E. A., Murphy, M. C., Emerson, K. T. U., Chatman, J. A., Dweck, C. S., & Kray, L. J. (2020). Cultures of genius at work: Organizational mindsets predict cultural norms, trust, and commitment. *Personality and Social Psychology Bulletin, 46*(4), 626–642. https://doi.org/10.1177/0146167219872473

Cantu, J., Tolk, J., Fritts, S., & Gharehyakheh, A. (2020). High reliability organization (HRO) systematic literature review: Discovery of culture as a foundational hallmark. *Journal of Contingencies and Crisis Management, 28*(4), 399–410. https://doi.org/10.1111/1468-5973.12293

Carver, N., Gupta, V., & Hipskind, J.E. (2021). Medical error. In *StatPearls*. StatPearls Publishing. https://www.ncbi.nlm.nih.gov/books/NBK430763

Chaboyer, W., Harbeck, E., Lee, B. O., & Grealish, L. (2021). Missed nursing care: An overview of reviews. *The Kaohsiung Journal of Medical Sciences, 37*(2), 82–91. https://doi.org/10.1002/kjm2.12308

Chassin, M. R., & Loeb, J. M. (2013). High-reliability health care: Getting there from here. *The Milbank Quarterly, 91*(3), 459–490. https://doi.org/10.1111/1468-0009.12023

Corrigan, J. M., Kohn, L. T., & Donaldson, M. S. (Eds.). (1999). *To err is human: Building a safer health system.* National Academies Press.

Côté-Boileau, É., Denis, J. L., Callery, B., & Sabean, M. (2019). The unpredictable journeys of spreading, sustaining and scaling healthcare innovations: A scoping review. *Health Research Policy and Systems, 17*(1), 84. https://doi.org/10.1186/s12961-019-0482-6

Dweck, C. S. (1986). Motivational processes affecting learning. *The American Psychologist, 41*(10), 1040–1048. https://doi.org/10.1037/0003-066X.41.10.1040

Dweck, C. S. (2017). *Mindset-updated edition: Changing the way you think to fulfil your potential.* Hachette UK.

Dweck, C. S., & Yeager, D. S. (2019). Mindsets: A view from two eras. *Perspectives on Psychological Science, 14*(3), 481–496. https://doi.org/10.1177/1745691618804166

Ebright, P. (2010, January 31). The complex work of RNs: Implications for healthy work environments. *OJIN: The Online Journal of Issues in Nursing, 15*(1), Manuscript 4. https://doi.org/10.3912/OJIN .Vol15No01Man04

Ebright, P., Patterson, E., Chalko, B., & Render, M. (2003). Understanding the complexity of registered nurse work in acute care settings. *Journal of Nursing Administration, 33*(12), 630–638. https://doi .org/10.1097/00005110-200312000-00004

Ebright, P., Patterson, E., & Saleem, J. (2009, January). *Nursing work: Impact of patient safety initiatives on nursing workflow and productivity* [Presentation]. AHRQ Funded Grant Workshop, San Diego, CA.

Edmondson, A. C. (2019). *The fearless organization: Creating psychological safety in the workplace for learning, innovation, and growth.* John Wiley & Sons.

Endsley, M. R. (1995). Measurement of situation awareness in dynamic systems. *Human Factors, 37*(1), 65–84. https://doi.org/10.1518/001872095779049499

Endsley, M. R., & Garland, D. J. (Eds.). (2000). *Situation awareness analysis and measurement.* CRC Press.

Gilmartin, H. M., Langner, P., Gokhale, M., Osatuke, K., Hasselbeck, R., Maddox, T. M., & Battaglia, C. (2018). Relationship between psychological safety and reporting nonadherence to a safety checklist. *Journal of Nursing Care Quality, 33*(1), 53–60. https://doi.org/10.1097/NCQ.0000000000000265

Goldenhar, L. M., Brady, P. W., Sutcliffe, K. M., & Muething, S. E. (2013). Huddling for high reliability and situation awareness. *BMJ Quality & Safety, 22*(11), 899–906. https://doi.org/10.1136/ bmjqs-2012-001467

Greene, M. T., Gilmartin, H. M., & Saint, S. (2020). Psychological safety and infection prevention practices: Results from a national survey. *American Journal of Infection Control, 48*(1), 2–6. https://doi .org/10.1016/j.ajic.2019.09.027

Grissinger M. (2014). Telling true stories is an ISMP hallmark: Here's why you should tell stories, too . . . . *P & T: A Peer-Reviewed Journal for Formulary Management, 39*(10), 658–659. https://www .ncbi.nlm.nih.gov/pmc/articles/PMC4189689/

HealthDesignbyUs. (n.d.), Who we are. https://www.healthdesignby.us

Hessels, A., Paliwal, M., Weaver, S. H., Siddiqui, D., & Wurmser, T. A. (2019). Impact of patient safety culture on missed nursing care and adverse patient events. *Journal of Nursing Care Quality, 34*(4), 287–294. https://doi.org/10.1097/NCQ.0000000000000378

Hirak, R., Peng, A. C., Carmeli, A., & Schaubroeck, J. M. (2012). Linking leader inclusiveness to work unit performance: The importance of psychological safety and learning from failures. *The Leadership Quarterly, 23*(1), 107–117. https://doi.org/10.1016/j.leaqua.2011.11.009

Holden, R. J., Boustani, M. A., & Azar, J. (2021). Agile Innovation to transform healthcare: Innovating in complex adaptive systems is an everyday process, not a light bulb event. *BMJ Innovations, 7*(2), 499–505. https://doi.org/10.1136/bmjinnov-2020-000574

Ingelsson, P., Bäckström, I., & Snyder, K. (2018). Strengthening quality culture in private sector and health care. *Leadership in Health Services, 31*(3), 276–292. https://doi.org/10.1108/ LHS-02-2018-0012

Institute for Healthcare Improvement. (n.d.). *IHI Triple Aim initiative.* Retrieved May 24, 2021, from http://www.ihi.org/Engage/Initiatives/TripleAim/Pages/default.aspx

Institute of Medicine. (2001). *Crossing the quality chasm: A new health system for the 21st century.* The National Academies Press.

Institute of Medicine. (2010). *Future directions for the national healthcare quality and disparities reports.* The National Academies Press. https://doi.org/10.17226/12846

James J. T. (2013). A new, evidence-based estimate of patient harms associated with hospital care. *Journal of Patient Safety, 9*(3), 122–128. https://doi.org/10.1097/PTS.0b013e3182948a69

Jones, L., Pomeroy, L., Robert, G., Burnett, S., Anderson, J. E., & Fulop, N. J. (2017). How do hospital boards govern for quality improvement? A mixed methods study of 15 organizations in England. *BMJ Quality & Safety, 26*, 978–986. https://doi.org/10.1136/bmjqs-2016-006433

Kalisch, B. J., Landstrom, G. L., & Hinshaw, A. S. (2009). Missed nursing care: A concept analysis. *Journal of Advanced Nursing, 65*(7), 1509–1517. doi: 10.1111/j.1365-2648.2009.05027.x

Kalisch, B. J., & Lee, K. H. (2010). The impact of teamwork on missed nursing care. *Nursing Outlook, 58*(5), 233-241. https://doi.org/10.1016/j.outlook.2010.06.004

Kalisch, B. J., Tschannen, D., & Lee, K. H. (2011). Do staffing levels predict missed nursing care? *International Journal for Quality in Health Care, 23*(3), 302–308. https://doi.org/10.1093/intqhc/mzr009

Kalisch, B. J., & Williams, R. A. (2009). Development and psychometric testing of a tool to measure missed nursing care. *JONA: The Journal of Nursing Administration, 39*(5), 211–219. https://doi.org/10.1097/NNA.0b013e3181a23cf5

Kalisch, B. J., Xie, B., & Dabney, B. W. (2014). Patient-reported missed nursing care correlated with adverse events. *American Journal of Medical Quality, 29*(5), 415-422. https://doi.org/10.1177/1062860613501715

Kavanagh, J. M., & Sharpnack, P. A. (2021, January 31). Crisis in competency: A defining moment in nursing education. *OJIN: The Online Journal of Issues in Nursing, 26*(1), Manuscript 2. https://doi.org/10.3912/OJIN.Vol26No01Man02

Kerfoot, K. M. (2016). Patient safety and leadership intentions: Is there a match? *Nursing Economic$, 34*(1), 44.

Kitzmiller, R., Hunt, E., & Sproat, S. B. (2006). Adopting best practices: "Agility" moves from software development to healthcare project management. *CIN: Computers, Informatics, Nursing, 24*(2), 75–82. https://doi.org/10.1097/00024665-200603000-00005

Klein, J., Delany, C., Fischer, M. D., Smallwood, D., & Trumble, S. (2017). A growth mindset approach to preparing trainees for medical error. *BMJ Quality & Safety, 26*(9), 771–774. https://doi.org/10.1136/bmjqs-2016-006416

Ku, B., & Lupton, E. (2020). *Health design thinking: Creating products and services for better health.* MIT Press.

Langley, G. J., Moen, R. D., Nolan, K. M., Nolan, T. W., Norman, C. L., & Provost, L. P. (2009). *The improvement guide: A practical approach to enhancing organizational performance* (2nd ed.). Jossey-Bass.

Lee, S. H. G., Reed, S., & Wilson, A. (2021). *Leading with growth mindsets enabled by design thinking and agile principles among clinical nurses.* Manuscript submitted for publication. Ascension.

Leroy, H., Dierynck, B., Anseel, F., Simons, T., Halbesleben, J. R. B., McCaughey, D., Savage, G. T., & Sels, L. (2012). Behavioral integrity for safety, priority of safety, psychological safety, and patient safety: A team-level study. *Journal of Applied Psychology, 97*(6), 1273–1281. https://doi.org/10.1037/a0030076

Levey, S., Vaughn, T., Koepke, J. D., Moore, D., Lehrman, W., & Sinha S. (2007). Hospital leadership and quality improvement: Rhetoric versus reality. *Journal of Patient Safety, 3*(1), 9–15. https://doi.org/10.1097/PTS.0b013e3180311256

Lewis, L. S., Williams, C. A., & Dawson, S. D. (2020). Growth mindset training and effective learning strategies in community college registered nursing students. *Teaching and Learning in Nursing, 15*(2), 123–127. https://doi.org/10.1016/j.teln.2020.01.006

Lorusso, L., Lee, J. H., & Worden, E. A. (2021). Design thinking for healthcare: Transliterating the creative problem-solving method into architectural practice. *HERD, 14*(2), 16–29. https://doi.org/10.1177/1937586721994228

Makary, M. A., & Daniel, M. (2016). Medical error—the third leading cause of death in the US. *BMJ, 353*, i2139. https://doi.org/10.1136/bmj.i2139

Mannion, R., & Davies, H. (2018). Understanding organisational culture for healthcare quality improvement. *BMJ (Clinical research ed.), 363*, k4907. https://doi.org/10.1136/bmj.k4907

McAlearney, A. S., Terris, D., Hardacre, J., Spurgeon, P., Brown, C., Baumgart, A., & Nyström, M. E. (2013). Organizational coherence in health care organizations: Conceptual guidance to facilitate quality improvement and organizational change. *Quality Management in Health Care, 22*(2), 86–99. https://doi.org/10.1097/QMH.0b013e31828bc37d

McBride, A. B. (2017). Serving on a hospital board: A case study. *Nursing Outlook, 65*, 372–379. https://doi.org/10.1016/j.outlook.2016.12.006

McBride, A. B. (2020). *The growth and development of nurse leaders* (2nd ed.). Springer Publishing Company.

McGrath, C., & Zell, D. (2001). The future of innovation diffusion research and its implications for management: A conversation with Everett Rogers. *Journal of Management Inquiry, 10*(4), 386–391. https://doi.org/10.1177/1056492601104012

Micheli, P., Wilner, S. J., Bhatti, S. H., Mura, M., & Beverland, M. B. (2019). Doing design thinking: Conceptual review, synthesis, and research agenda. *Journal of Product Innovation Management, 36*(2), 124–148. https://doi.org/10.1111/jpim.12466

Moneke, N., & Umeh, O. (2013). Factors influencing critical care nurses' perception of their overall job satisfaction: An empirical study. *Journal of Nursing Administration, 43*, 201–207. https://doi.org/10.1097/NNA.0b013e31828958af

O'Hagan, J., & Persaud, D. (2009). Creating a culture of accountability in healthcare. *The Health Care Manager, 28*(2), 124–133. https://doi.org/10.1097/HCM.0b013e3181a2eb2b

Patterson, E. S., Ebright, P. R., & Saleem, J. J. (2011). Investigating stacking: How do registered nurses prioritize their activities in real-time? *International Journal of Industrial Ergonomics, 41*(4), 389–393. https://doi.org/10.1016/J.ERGON.2011.01.012

Perla, R. J., Bradbury, E., & Gunther-Murphy, C. (2013). Large-scale improvement initiatives in healthcare: A scan of the literature. *Journal for Healthcare Quality, 35*(1), 30-40. https://doi.org/10.1111/j.1945-1474.2011.00164.x

Porter-O'Grady, T. (2020). Complexity leadership: Constructing 21st century health. *Nursing Administration Quarterly, 44*(2), 92–100. https://doi.org/10.1097/NAQ.0000000000000405

Portoghese, I., Galletta, M., Burdorf, A., Cocco, P., D'Aloja, E., & Campagna, M. (2017). Role stress and emotional exhaustion among health care workers: The buffering effect of supportive coworker climate in a multilevel perspective. *Journal of Occupational and Environmental Medicine, 59*(10), e187–e193. doi: 10.1097/JOM.0000000000001122

Rahemi, Z., D'Avolio, D., Dunphy, L. M., & Rivera, A. (2018). Shifting management in healthcare: An integrative review of design thinking. *Nursing Management, 49*(12), 30–37. https://doi.org/10.1097/01.NUMA.0000547834.95083.e9

Rodwin, B. A., Bilan, V. P., Merchant, N. B., Steffens, C. G., Grimshaw, A. A., Bastian, L. A., & Gunderson, C. G. (2020). Rate of preventable mortality in hospitalized patients: A systematic review and meta-analysis. *Journal of General Internal Medicine, 35*(7), 2099–2106. https://doi.org/10.1007/s11606-019-05592-5

Rodziewicz, T. L., Houseman, B., & Hipskind, J. E. (2021). Medical error reduction and prevention. In *StatPearls* [Internet]. StatPearls Publishing.

Scott, S. D., Hirschinger, L. E., Cox, K. R., McCoig, M., Brandt, J., & Hall, L. W. (2009). The natural history of recovery for the healthcare provider "second victim" after adverse patient events. *Quality & Safety in Health Care, 18*(5), 325–330. https://doi.org/10.1136/qshc.2009.032870

Seidel, V. P., & Fixson, S. K. (2013). Adopting design thinking in novice multidisciplinary teams: The application and limits of design methods and reflexive practices. *Journal of Product Innovation Management, 30*, 19–33. https://doi.org/10.1111/jpim.12061

Sfantou, D. F., Laliotis, A., Patelarou, A. E., Sifaki-Pistolla, D., Matalliotakis, M., & Patelarou, E. (2017, December). Importance of leadership style towards quality of care measures in healthcare settings: A systematic review. *Healthcare, 5*(4), 73. https://doi.org/10.3390/healthcare5040073

Sherwood, G., & Armstrong, G. (2016). Current patient safety drivers. In C. Oster & J. Braaten (Eds.), *High reliability organizations: A healthcare handbook for patient safety & quality* (pp. 25–48). Sigma Theta Tau International.

Shillam, C. R., Adams, J. M., Bryant, D. C., Deupree, J. P., Miyamoto, S., & Gregas, M. (2018). Development of the Leadership Influence Self-Assessment (LISA©) instrument. *Nursing Outlook, 66*(2), 130–137. https://doi.org/10.1016/j.outlook.2017.10.009

Siegal, D., & Ruoff, G. (2015). Data as a catalyst for change: Stories from the frontlines. *Journal of Healthcare Risk Management, 34*(3), 18–25. https://doi.org/10.1002/jhrm.21161

Sitterding, M. C., Broome, M. E., Everett, L. Q., & Ebright, P. (2012). Understanding situation awareness in nursing work: A hybrid concept analysis. *ANS. Advances in Nursing Science, 35*(1), 77–92. https://doi.org/10.1097/ANS.0b013e3182450158

Sitterding, M. C., Ebright, P., Broome, M., Patterson, E. S., & Wuchner, S. (2014). Situation awareness and interruption handling during medication administration. *Western Journal of Nursing Research, 36*(7), 891–916. https://doi.org/10.1177/0193945914533426

Sosa, T., Sitterding, M., Dewan, M., Segar, B., Bedinghaus, K., Hawkins, D., Maddock, B. H., Hausfeld, J., Falcone, R., Brady, P., Simmons, J., & White, C. (2021). Optimizing situation awareness to reduce emergency transfers in hospitalized children. *Pediatrics, 148*(4), e2020034603. https://doi.org/10.1542/peds.2020-034603

Sundean, L. J., Han, H. P., Waddell, A., & Adams, J. M. (2021). A concept analysis of influence for nurse leaders. *Nursing Outlook, 69*(3), 286–292. https://doi.org/10.1016/j.outlook.2020.11.006

Sundean, L. J., Polifroni, E. C., Libal, K., & McGrath, J. M. (2017). Nurses on health care governing boards: An integrative review. *Nursing Outlook, 65*(4), 361–371. https://doi.org/10.1016/j.outlook.2017.01.009

Sundean, L. J., Waddell, A., Bryant, D. C., & Adams, J. M. (2020). Amplifying nurses' influence through governance: Responding to a call to action. *Journal for Nurses in Professional Development, 36*(3), 117–120. https://doi.org/10.1097/NND.0000000000000641

Tolf, S., Nyström, M. E., Tishelman, C., Brommels, M., & Hansson, J. (2015). Agile, a guiding principle for health care improvement? *International Journal of Health Care Quality Assurance, 28*(5), 468–493. https://doi.org/10.1108/IJHCQA-04-2014-0044.

Torralba, K. D., Loo, L. K., Byrne, J. M., Baz, S., Cannon, G. W., Keitz, S. A., Wicker, A. B., Henley, S. S., & Kashner, T. M. (2016). Does psychological safety impact the clinical learning environment for resident physicians? Results from the VA's learners' perceptions survey. *Journal of Graduate Medical Education, 8*(5), 699–707. doi: 10.4300/JGME-D-15-00719.1

Treffinger, D. J. (1994). Productive thinking: Toward authentic instruction and assessment. *Journal of Secondary Gifted Education, 6*(1), 30–37.

Tucker, A. L., & Spear, S. J. (2006). Operational failures and interruptions in hospital nursing. *Health Services Research, 41*(3p1), 643–662. https://doi.org/10.1111/j.1475-6773.2006.00502.x

Uhl-Bien, M., & Arena, M. (2017). *Complexity leadership: Enabling people and organizations for adaptability.* Organizational Dynamics.

Uhl-Bien, M., Meyer, D., & Smith, J. (2020). Complexity leadership in the nursing context. *Nursing Administration Quarterly, 44*(2), 109–116. https://doi.org/10.1097/NAQ.0000000000000407

Vaughn, T., Koepke, M., Kroch, E., Lehrman, W., Sinha, S., & Levey, S. (2006). Engagement of leadership in quality and improvement initiatives: Executive quality improvement survey results. *Journal of Patient Safety, 2*(1), 2–9. https://journals.lww.com/journalpatientsafety/Abstract/2006/03000/Engagement_of_Leadership_in_Quality_Improvement.2.aspx

Vaughn, T., Koepke, M., Levey, S., Kroch, E., Hatcher, C., Tompkins, C., & Baloh, J. (2014). Governing board, c-suite and clinical management perceptions of quality and safety structures, process, and priorities in US hospitals. *Journal of Healthcare Management, 59*(2), 111–128. https://journals.lww.com/jhmonline/Abstract/2014/03000/Governing_Board,_C_suite,_and_Clinical_Management.6.aspx

Vogus, T. J., Cooil, B., Sitterding, M., & Everett, L. Q. (2014). Safety organizing, emotional exhaustion, and turnover in hospital nursing units. *Medical Care, 52*(10), 870–876. https://doi.org/10.1097/MLR.0000000000000169

Vogus, T. J., & Iacobucci, D. (2016). Creating highly reliable health care: How reliability-enhancing work practices affect patient safety in hospitals. *ILR Review, 69*(4), 911–938. https://doi.org/10.1177/0019793916642759

Vogus, T. J., Wilson, A. D., Randall, K., & Sitterding, M. C. (2022). We're all in this together: How COVID-19 revealed the co-construction of mindful organising and organisational reliability. *BMJ Quality & Safety, 31*(3), 230–233. https://doi.org/10.1136/bmjqs-2021-014068

Weick, K. E., & Sutcliffe, K. M. (2001). *Managing the unexpected: Assuring high performance in an age of complexity.* Jossey-Bass.

Weiner-Lastinger, L. M., Pattabiraman, V., Konnor, R. Y., Patel, P. R., Wong, E., Xu, S. Y., Smith, B., Edwards, J. R., & Dudeck, M. A. (2022). The impact of coronavirus disease 2019 (COVID-19) on healthcare-associated infections in 2020: A summary of data reported to the National Healthcare Safety Network. *Infection Control & Hospital Epidemiology, 43*(1), 12–25. https://doi.org/10.1017/ice.2021.362

White, R. M., & Delacroix, R. (2020). Second victim phenomenon: Is 'just culture' a reality? An integrative review. *Applied Nursing Research, 56*, 151319. https://doi.org/10.1016/j.apnr.2020.151319

CHAPTER 16

INFORMATION MANAGEMENT AND BIG DATA

Andrew P. Reimer

"What gets measured, gets managed."

Peter Drucker

LEARNING OBJECTIVES

- Demonstrate understanding of how clinical data is generated, stored, and then accessed for secondary use.
- Analyze outcomes of data transfer and storage considerations.
- Evaluate approaches to preprocessing and analyzing clinical data to support clinical practice through quality improvement or research.
- Design a data dashboard that will support nursing management in clinical practice.

INTRODUCTION

The release of the seminal report *To Err Is Human* (Kohn et al., 2000) in 2000 shifted the focus of healthcare delivery to concentrate on patient safety. The passing of the American Recovery and Reinvestment Act of 2009 included the Health Information Technology for Economic and Clinical Health (HITECH) Act, which ushered in the current era of digital healthcare. The primary goal of the HITECH Act was to promote the adoption and meaningful use of health information technology (HIT) to improve the administration of healthcare (Office of the National Coordinator for Health Information Technology, n.d.). The widespread need to adequately capture and make usable all of the clinical information that is generated in the course of patient care was recognized. The HITECH Act provided both the regulatory requirements and financial incentives to employ electronic health record (EHR) systems in clinical care and to then use that electronically captured information to guide care. The resulting explosion of available clinical data in the form of EHR data has led to the pursuit of a learning health system. Charles Friedman and colleagues (2017), one of the original conceivers of the learning health system concept, provides the following description:

> *Learning* refers to the capability for continuous improvement through the collection and analysis of data, creating new knowledge, and the application of the new knowledge to influence practice. *Health* is both an end-goal of universally recognized benefit to humanity and a domain of human endeavor seeking to achieve that end. A *system* consists of component parts acting in unison to achieve goals not attainable by any subset of the components. Integrating these terms, health systems become *learning* health systems when they acquire the ability to continuously, routinely, and efficiently study and improve themselves. (para. 5)

Fully achieving the vision of a learning health system now requires that those engaged in healthcare administration be proficient in understanding all aspects of data generation, storage, and use. This chapter is divided into two sections. The first section is a nuts-and-bolts approach to information management that begins with exploring how clinical data is generated, types of clinical data, and how data is stored and then accessed to be reused for secondary purposes such as clinical dashboards or clinical decision support. The second section focuses on the concept of big data and the steps involved in receiving the data, preprocessing, and making the data work in the intended application, which may include anything from a forward-facing dashboard to support frontline clinical operations of a nursing unit, to quality improvement initiatives and metric tracking, or to executive level management of a hospital. The goal of this chapter is not to provide a comprehensive "how to" guide but, rather, to expose the reader to the important concepts and steps involved in using clinical data so that nurse leaders—from management to the executive level—can develop the requisite knowledge to create and support the teams that are necessary to achieve a learning health system.

INFORMATION MANAGEMENT

A primary challenge for those in healthcare leadership is that they often transition into roles that require additional knowledge beyond that for which they were formally prepared. Information management is the latest example of an emerging domain that has taken hold in essentially every aspect of the healthcare delivery infrastructure. Information management is a broad term that encompasses the range of activities relating to the use of clinically generated data in support of all activities related to patient care and healthcare administration. The following sections present the background information one requires to understand each step of the process.

SOURCES OF DATA

There are three main categories of data to consider when identifying which data sources you will need to access in order to accomplish the goal of your project: data that is clinically generated (i.e., data generated in care of the patient during an encounter), data that is hospital generated (i.e., administrative data generated to support care of the patient or hospital operations), and data that is nonclinical (i.e., data that is not generated in a hospital setting or for administrative support that nonetheless provides additional information to inform care of the patient). Table 16.1 presents an overview of the data categories and data sources typically encountered in each data source.

CLINICAL DATA

The most common source of data that we think about is that which is clinically generated during patient care through EHRs or, in the past, from a patient's chart. Clinical data includes patient demographics, vital signs, clinical notes, diagnoses, orders, lab results, procedures, medications, radiology, and genetic data. Recent applications of technology to monitor patients both in clinical and home settings provide new sources of clinical data as well. Telemonitoring of patient rooms has been applied in many settings, the most notable in ICUs (Udeh et al., 2018). Telemonitoring generates digital recordings that can be analyzed to assess facial cues for nonverbal signs of pain, or for signs that a patient is attempting to get out of bed. Clinical monitoring of the patient in the home is another major area of growth, and is accomplished via phone consults, patient-completed surveys via phone or computer login to their online medical record portal, or monitoring equipment such as pulse oximetry, heart rate, and blood pressure (Mayo Clinic Health System, 2021). Each data source can contain different types of data, which are covered in the next section.

TABLE 16.1: Data Sources and Types

Category	Source	Name
Clinical	Electronic health record	Patient demographics
		Vital signs
		Clinical notes
		Diagnoses—problem lists • past medical history • admitting diagnosis • discharge diagnosis
		Orders
		Lab results
		Procedures
		Medications
		Radiology-digital images
		Genetic testing
Hospital	Administrative data	Billing or claims
		Admission/discharge/transfer
		Patient/provider surveys
	Business intelligence	Quality improvement tracking
		Census—staffing • patients
		Clinical dashboards
Nonclinical	Wearables	Fitness trackers
	Cell phone	Location/movement
	Online applications	Twitter
		Facebook
		patientslikeme
	Home testing	23andMe
		Ancestry
		Cologuard

HOSPITAL DATA

There are multiple disparate sources of data that are generated in the course of a patient encounter that support clinical care and administrative processes. Examples of hospital data, sometimes referred to as administrative data, include billing or claims data, admission/discharge/transfer systems, patient/provider surveys, and business intelligence (i.e., data generated to support administration or operations such as quality metric tracking).

NONCLINICAL DATA

Sources of nonclinical data are too many to include in a comprehensive list, so we will cover several of the major sources. The primary source of interest is wearables (e.g., fitness trackers, cell phone data that includes movement and location tracking capability, and online activity). Wearables provide a robust source of data on exercising habits, help patients with chronic disease monitor their health, or gather data for research activities (Cadmus-Bertram, 2017).

Cell phone data can be used to track an individual's location and movement—recent applications can be used to track and warn of COVID-19 cases and hot spots (Grantz et al., 2020). The natural extension of cell phone data is use of the phone itself to access other sources of data or generate new data. Common social media applications can be used as additional data sources. For example, researchers will analyze social media posts and feeds to identify trending health topics or to analyze the sentiment of individuals' posts for clues that may aid in identifying depression (Reece et al., 2017). Lastly, online support groups such as patientslikeme (www.patientslikeme.com) provide an online resource for patients with chronic conditions to share their experiences. Patientslikeme provides researchers with access to the website to analyze the data and make new discoveries such as how patients are using medications to ameliorate symptoms based on beneficial side effects of medications that others have identified and reported in the discussions.

Another source of data gaining popularity relates to home testing. This source of data does not fit neatly into any of the sources of data already described but can be used to guide care in primary care or hospital settings. Home testing options continue to increase and range from general family ancestry and risk profiles for developing medical conditions such as high blood pressure or cancer to specific tests for the presence of colon cancer. Awareness of these nontraditional testing sources is necessary to consider options of incorporating these data and results into EHRs and patient portals as more care and testing continues to shift to out-of-hospital settings.

DATA TYPES

After identifying all applicable sources of data, we shift to identifying which types of data are contained within each source. There are two main data types to consider when working with EHR data, each requiring different data management and analytic techniques, those being unstructured and structured.

UNSTRUCTURED DATA

Unstructured data, also referred to as free text data, composes a majority of the recorded data/information in the EHR. Even with wide scale EHR implementation, estimates state that around 80% of the data in EHRs are free text, or unstructured (Murdoch & Detsky, 2013). Unstructured data is usually generated in clinical notes that include the history of present illness, clinical consults, nursing care narratives, and pathology and radiology reports. Unstructured data presents multiple challenges to reuse for secondary purposes. For example, clinical notes such as the history of present illness or nursing care narratives provide rich patient-specific data that can be leveraged to inform care models such as early warning alerts for clinical deterioration (Rossetti et al., 2021), but abstracting useful data from free text requires advanced analytics to abstract useful information. A primary approach, natural language processing, identifies word combinations that provide useful information for the specified task at hand. Assale et al. (2019) provides a concise overview of the application of natural language processing to unstructured data from EHRs. Current efforts are focused on reducing the amount of unstructured text by developing and using structured templates for clinical encounters to standardize provider note entry. The goal is to provide as much structure as possible, such as drop-down categorical selections and discrete data entry boxes for observations such as vital signs, that enables data abstraction for secondary use and minimizes the amount of unstructured text entry.

TABLE 16.2: Diagnosis Code Storage Data Table

ID	Encounter ID	Patient ID	Date Created	Code	Code Source	Description	Display As
1	4658970	58902387	04/15/20 00:01.15	J96.00	ICD-10-CM	Acute respiratory failure, unspecified whether with hypoxia or hypercapnia	Acute respiratory failure
2	4658970	58902387	04/15/20 00:02.10	J15.0	ICD-10-CM	Pneumonia due to *Klebsiella pneumoniae*	Pneumonia
3	4658970	58902387	04/15/20 00:03.54	31500	CPT	Intubation	Intubation

CPT, current procedural terminology; ICD-10-CM, *International Classification of Diseases*, 10th Revision, Clinical Modification.

STRUCTURED DATA

Structured data is data that is formally represented in a standardized format. The most common standardized formats we use include diagnosis codes such as the *International Classification of Diseases* (ICD), Current Procedural Terminology (CPT), Logical Identifiers Observations and Codes (LOINC), and Digital Imaging and Communications in Medicine (DICOM), as well as health system specific codes that are generated for specific applications within the hospital such as provider names or unit names and numbers. Coded data facilitates standardized application and use of data both within the same EHR system or in other applications. While not always visible during use of the EHR, structured data is used in many aspects of the EHR. For example, problem lists may only display the diagnosis "acute respiratory failure" that is represented formally by *ICD-10-CM* code J96.00. The code J96.00 serves as a unique identifier, making the discovery of that particular data easier than searching unstructured text for a specific word or word combination. Table 16.2 provides an example of how diagnosis codes can be stored in a diagnosis table. We will cover in more detail how data is stored and retrieved for secondary purposes in "Accessing and Using Data."

LIFE CYCLE OF DATA

One of the least familiar areas for nurse leaders and executives is the behind-the-scenes operation of data generation, storage, and use, often referred to as the life cycle of data. We are most familiar with data entry through interfacing with the EHR. Once the data is entered, however, is when—for most—the black box begins. Developing an understanding of the beginning-to-end data generation pipeline is crucial for today's nurse leaders and executives as more administrative and managerial activities involve using data that originates from the clinical setting.

Primary sources of data are generated during patient encounters. Figure 16.1 displays several primary sources of data that originate from clinical processes and associated data types. For example, the top of the figure depicts nurse charting, in which the front-end clinical nurse will enter data in the EHR that can include both structured data (e.g., vital signs, chart by exception selections) and unstructured data (e.g., beginning of shift assessment, narrative notes). Typically, EHR data is stored in its own database, and in multiple tables (i.e., spreadsheets). Also depicted in Figure 16.1, each source of data, such as laboratory values and radiology images, is stored in their own unique databases and data coding standards. Each of these unique databases can then be fed into the EHR via an application program interface (API) or programs that enable the exchange of data from one unique database to another in a standardized format (Sixicki, 2019). The primary standard employed is Fast Healthcare Interoperability Resources (FHIR), with recent reports indicating that 84% of

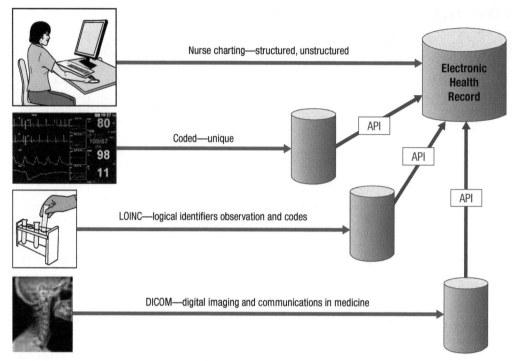

FIGURE 16.1: Primary sources of data from clinical processes and their associated data types.

API, application program interface.

hospitals and 61% of clinicians have adopted and implemented this standard (Nelson, 2021). FHIR provides all of the resources necessary to support connecting one database, regardless of the data formatting, to another using a standardized approach (HL7 International, n.d.). The primary role of FHIR is to facilitate interoperability—the exchange and use of information within the healthcare ecosystem, whether that be within a single hospital or health system or by connecting an entire community of hospitals and community healthcare providers.

PUTTING DATA TO WORK

There are several ways information management projects begin. The first is the end-user identifying a clinical or managerial need and requesting new services such as a clinical dashboard that tracks nursing unit operations or performance metrics for quality improvement. Another is the top-down approach where leadership has identified a need and asks that the new system be developed, whether that involves applying artificial intelligence (AI) to identify at-risk patients as discussed in Chapter 8, "Value-Based Contracting," or developing key performance indicators and associated tracking and reporting. Further considerations on data management reporting needs are provided in the Chapter 8 section on "Infrastructure, Information Technology Platforms, System Structure, and Data Reporting."

Regardless of the initiating source, the crucial next step in beginning any new project is identifying the resources that are available. Resources for information technology (IT) projects include personnel and technological capabilities. Available resources vary at each institution. For example, within a large academic medical center or health system, one will probably have access to a business intelligence or IT department whose primary role is developing new IT projects. However, in a critical access or independent hospital not associated with a large health system, EHR functions such as patient engagement and data analytics will be less common (Apathy et al., 2021), or staff may not have access to IT services that are capable of executing the project. In these situations, engaging a third-party developer or consultant to develop and complete the project may be necessary. Similarly, depending on the scope of the project, health systems will partner with external third-party developers to jointly develop and implement a new IT project such as the teleICU monitoring system with the goal of scaling and providing the new technology as a service to other institutions.

Many projects are handled internally, and, depending on the size and scope, may consist of a small team of only one or two data analysts and programmers working with a unit manager to create a quality metric tracking dashboard to develop a new clinical decision support system for a large interdisciplinary team working across multiple units and departments. Chapter 11, "Innovation," presents useful information on embracing a culture of innovation in interdisciplinary teams and the associated competencies that can be used to facilitate conceptualizing, developing, and deploying new information management systems.

ACCESSING AND USING DATA

Establishing the ability to access, and then use, data for your intended project is a critical step. As mentioned, some hospitals—particularly large academic health systems—have entire departments focused on business intelligence, analytics, and research. Whether positioned within a hospital that has or does not have data support services, a beginning task is to identify the contacts, sometimes referred to as gatekeepers, who are process literate and can provide the necessary access to the system or systems necessary to support your project. To simplify our approach to the process of developing a data use project from start to finish, the following material will refer to developing a metric dashboard (Figure 16.2) to monitor the discharge disposition and readmission tracking for patients in a value-based care program. However, the following information is applicable to any project that uses clinical data.

Depending on the project goals, there are generally two ways to access and use data. The first, and easiest, is accessing already established secondary data sources. For example, one approach is to develop a secondary server that extracts, transforms, and loads (ETL) clinical data from the EHR on a daily basis into a data repository. The data contained in this data repository is easily accessible and, as depicted in Figure 16.3, separated from the clinical

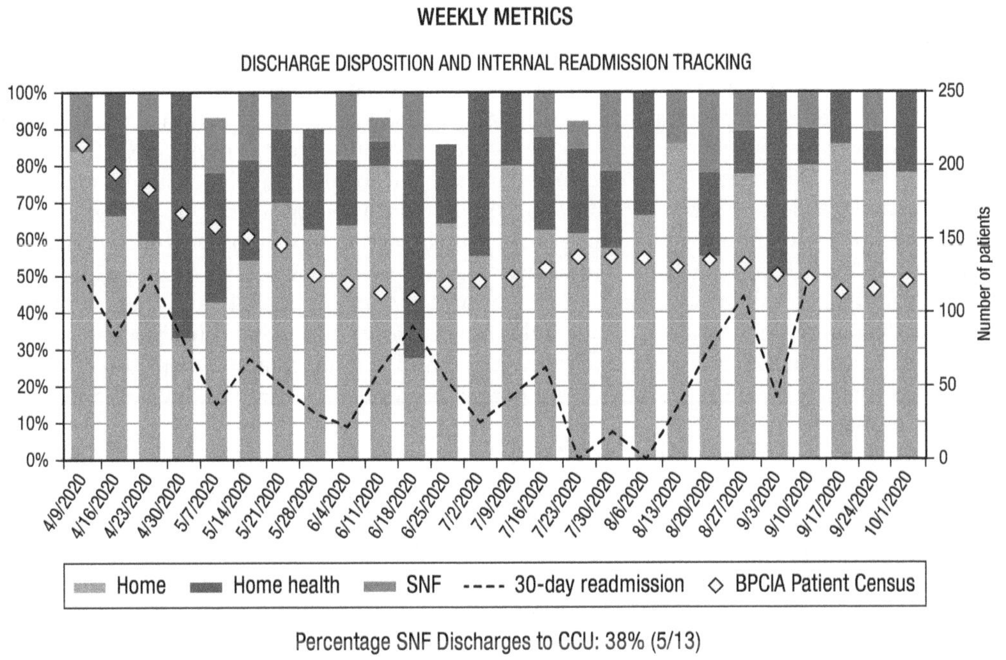

FIGURE 16.2: Example of metric dashboard.

BPCIA, Bundle Payments for Care Improvement–Advanced; CCU, critical care unit; SNF, skilled nursing facility.

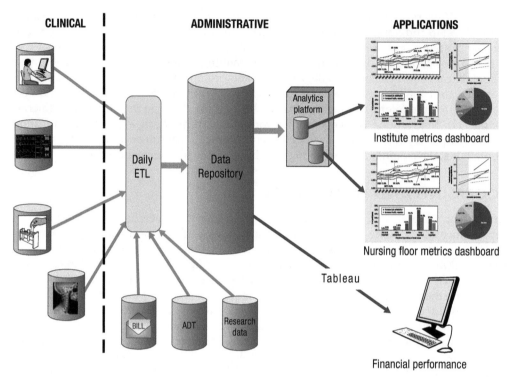

FIGURE 16.3: A secondary server extracts, transforms, and loads (ETL) clinical data from the EHR on a daily basis into a data repository.

ADT, admission/discharge/transfer; EHR, electronic health record.

information systems. This separation is important to support preserving the computing capacity of the clinical programs that are used real-time and to also maintain the security and integrity of the data as originally generated and stored for clinical operations. Developing the secondary data ETL process and data repository is necessary because the way many clinical programs generate and save data in their individual databases are not immediately usable for secondary purposes, thus requiring additional steps of transforming the raw data into usable formats. The benefit of developing a data repository that contains post-ETL data is that the data is easily accessible and in a standardized format that can easily be incorporated into any application. For example, an individual with Microsoft Excel or Tableau skills can connect to the data repository and generate their own data dashboards and visualizations. Without the data repository, an end-user would have to connect to each original data server, identify and pull the data needed to support the new application, and then complete data transformation to normalize all the data into one format to make it usable. Secondary data repositories such as this are usually developed and supported at the institute or hospital level as this work requires large investments in personnel and time to develop and then manage long-term.

Of particular importance is to note that secondary abstraction is time-delayed and will not support applications that require "real-time" data feeds (Figure 16.4). Systems requiring real-time data feeds include sepsis early warning alerts and programs embedded in telemonitoring applications that generate alerts for clinical deterioration based on changing vital signs and laboratory values. Using real-time data to support real-time systems requires different data access and analytics that is typically more labor-intensive due to the need to develop a custom platform that performs a majority of the functions that would otherwise already have been performed in the daily ETL in the secondary data repository. For example, if you wanted to develop a clinical deterioration early warning system, you need to identify each source of vital sign data from the EHR, and each source of laboratory results

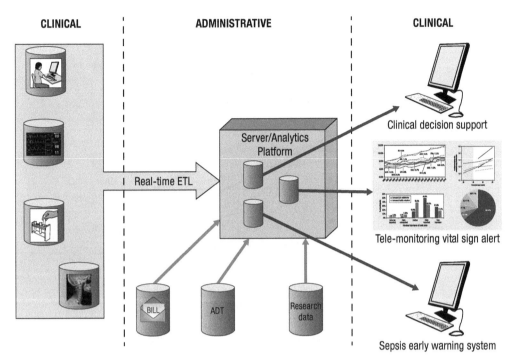

FIGURE 16.4: Real-time data feeds require that each data element be incorporated into a server with an analytics platform.

ADT, admission/discharge/transfer; ETL, extract, transform, load.

from that server to incorporate into the predictive model. Each data element needs to be mapped, extracted, transformed, and loaded, and then incorporated into a server with an analytics platform that can run the predictive model and produce the results to the end user via an EHR alert or dashboard. Lastly, the IT infrastructure available to you may not fit in either of these categories, presenting a hybrid option or blend of the two. Identifying the type of data access and functions you need and support available to you to develop your project is a critical first step.

THINKING ABOUT DATA QUALITY

Once the necessary sources of data and types of data access to support the discharge disposition dashboard are identified, each data element required must be identified. Identifying the correct data elements to abstract from the EHR can be a challenging task in and of itself. For example, EHRs within tertiary and quaternary hospitals contain many entries for blood pressure. Within our health system there are seven discrete places (e.g., intraoperative, floor) that include 20 different measurement types across 89 different tables and patient ID combinations. There are also multiple nondiscrete procedure report types that include 17 different measurement types with 41 different ways the types are represented within the report. Some are recorded as systolic/diastolic and some are recorded as individual measures. It is necessary to also specify the measurement location (e.g., left/right, arm, wrist, calf, umbilical artery, central venous), method (e.g., manual, automated, arterial), body position (e.g., sitting, standing, supine, orthostatic), and pre/post intervention or testing. A continuous monitor feed is another source that has its own considerations. Thus, if you are including vital signs, you must identify each vital sign specifically. Sometimes, identifying the exact blood pressure data to extract is accomplished by taking screenshots of the EHR page that displays the vital sign entries that you want to use and working with your data analyst to identify that exact source within the data repository.

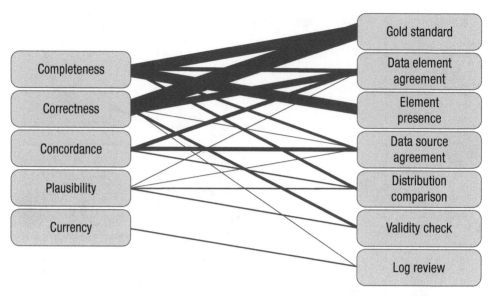

FIGURE 16.5: Weiskopf and Weng's data quality assessment framework.

Source: Reproduced with permission from Weiskopf, N. G., & Weng, C. (2013). Methods and dimensions of electronic health record data quality assessment: Enabling reuse for clinical research. *Journal of the American Medical Informatics Association, 20*(1), 144–151. https://doi.org/10.1136/amiajnl-2011-000681.

Once all of the data has been identified, the quality of that data must be assessed. There are formalized data quality assessment frameworks that can be useful in thinking through the different aspects to consider when assessing data quality. Weiskopf and Weng's (2013) framework presents five dimensions and associated methods of assessment to guide assessing data quality for reusing EHR data for a secondary use such as research (Figure 16.5). There are several schools of thought regarding the integrity of reusing EHR data for secondary purposes and a more in-depth discussion can be found here (Reimer & Madigan, 2018). Whether it be reuse of data in the clinical setting to support weekly reporting of discharge disposition and readmission tracking for patients in a value-based care program, or to conduct clinical research, the intended application will dictate the level of scrutiny and data quality assessment necessary to develop a valid and reliable product.

A first general assessment is to confirm *is this the right data*? Confirming that the data supplied from the data repository or real-time feed matches the original source data is necessary because as we previously identified, there can be multiple sources of the same data. Next steps include assessing if the data feed *will be reliable* or, stated differently, does it provide the necessary data in the appropriate time intervals? For example, depending on the unit, vital sign data may not be entered on a regular schedule, as patients on the same floor can have different frequencies of vital sign monitoring (e.g., every 2, 4, or 6 hours). Do differences in vital sign collection intervals impact the intended implementation such as a prognostic model that requires updating continuously as teleICU applications require, or will the most current vital signs, whether recorded 2 or 8 hours ago, provide the necessary data to support an application such as the daily skin breakdown risk calculator? Refer to Box 16.1 for key questions to consider for data quality assessment.

DATABASE STRUCTURE

Database structure is another one of those black box topics for nurse leaders. Developing a basic understanding of how databases are structured and function will enable you to understand data requirements for connecting requirements for the front-end user doing data entry in the clinical setting and how the data of interest can be collected through to ensuring that

BOX 16.1: KEY QUESTIONS FOR DATA QUALITY ASSESSMENT

- Is the data valid—does it provide the right data (e.g., vital sign recording)?
- Is the data feed reliable?
  - What is the necessary frequency of data required?
    - Continuous feed such as ICU vital sign monitoring
    - A recording once daily
    - The worst or best value
    - Establish when the data is supplied:
      - Only once daily representing previous day's values
      - Updated with each new entry
- Does the data meet quality assessment requirements?

you have the right type of data to perform the statistical analyses. There are several ways to structure databases; we will review the most commonly used, relational databases.

Relational databases are a simple design that consists of multiple tables—think Excel spreadsheets—that have at least one common variable on a table that can be joined or matched to that same variable on another table. For example, a common joining variable can be the medical record number (MRN), date of service, or other variable that can be matched between tables. Figure 16.6 presents several tables and examples of variable matching between tables. For example, when a patient is admitted, an admission is generated on the Admission/Discharge/ Transfer (ADT) table, which will generate an admission ID. When creating the admission, if the patient already exists in the system, the existing MRN can be pulled and attached to the new admission as signified by the top two boxed items in Figure 16.6, or a new MRN can be

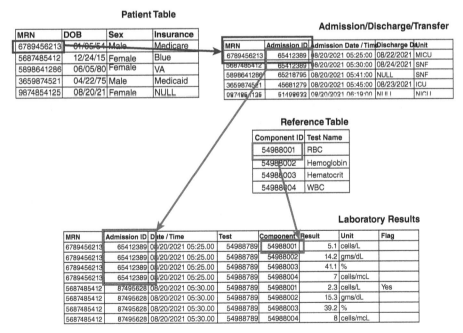

FIGURE 16.6: Variable matching between tables.

generated and added to the patient table—with the MRN acting as the matching variable between the ADT table and the patient table. Then, to query data from a particular admission, you can use the admission ID to pull results from the laboratory results table as signified by the ADT box connected to the laboratory results box in Figure 16.6—specifically using the admission ID and not the MRN alone as a patient can have more than one admission. Note that the same variable may not be used to match between different tables. Lastly, multiple reference tables are created and used to provide additional information, such as the name of an individual test as signified by the two component ID boxes in the center of Figure 16.6. Often data is recorded and stored as indicated in the laboratory table using codes such as ICD-10 (*International Classification of Diseases*, 10th Revision) or CPT and require additional mapping to add in the display name or actual name of the variable such as "RBC" versus the standardized code (e.g., 54988001).

STORING AND TRANSFERRING DATA

The next consideration is how data will be stored, and if data will need to be transferred to another institution. Most projects will be internal to the institution and data storage options are the only consideration; as indicated in Figures 16.3 and 16.4, available options are either already established or you may need to create a new data repository. A data analyst will be the lead personnel to guide this process.

Alternatively, if engaging in a joint project between institutions, requiring that data either be received from one institution or delivered to another, several additional steps are necessary. First, the Institutional Review Board (IRB) will need to be engaged as early as possible. In order to receive or transfer data, most institutions require both IRB approval as well as an executed data use agreement (DUA). The IRB application will outline the project, specify data to be accessed and used, and identify those involved in the project. A DUA, separate from the IRB application, is a specific legal contract between parties that specifies the exact data being transferred and its specifications (e.g., fully identified, limited, or de-identified), as well as how the data will be transferred, stored, and terms of use. For more information on data set types and considerations, see Figure 16.7. DUAs are usually administratively handled by a legal or technology transfer office that will usually provide a template to guide the application process. If lacking experience with preparing IRB and DUA applications, a colleague versed in research and data management practices will be a valuable addition to the team. One important aspect that requires specific attention throughout the IRB and DUA application process and can become quite dubious is the requirement from the IRB that one submit a fully executed DUA with the IRB application, and vice versa (i.e., that the IRB approval to conduct the work be submitted with the DUA application). While this is impossible to achieve, a common remedy is to make each office aware that the other is requesting an approved application. One can then supply the application numbers to the other office and come to an agreement of which one can be approved contingent on the other being approved thereafter.

Once administrative approvals are obtained, data can be extracted and stored. Storage options such as internal institutional drives or cloud-based options will depend on your institutional policies or DUA requirements. Upon establishing that you have the correct data and data quality assessment has demonstrated that it is accurate and adequate, the next consideration is how you will analyze and operationalize the data. The intended application will dictate the level of analysis that is necessary. Data analysis can range from simple tabulations and descriptive statistics that are typically presented in quarterly updates or metric tracking dashboards, or the development of a predictive algorithm that is implemented via a clinical nomogram risk calculator implemented via a webpage, through to the application of AI that is capable of reading digital imaging more accurately than humans. There is a tendency to apply more sophisticated methods of data analytics than is necessary, so maintaining the engineering principle of "keep it simple" is important.

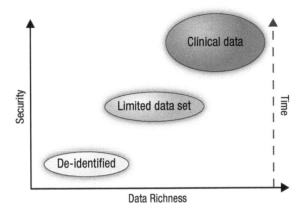

Dataset type	Data richness	Storage/security	Time
Clinical	• Contains all identifiers	• Must meet all HIPAA standards for storage and transfer • Requires IRB and DUA	• Longer approval time, may require full IRB review
Limited Data Set	• Does not contain individual identifiers. • Can contain dates such as admission, discharge, service, DOB, DOD, city, state, five digit or more zip code; ages in years, months, or days or hours	• Must meet all HIPAA standards for storage and transfer • Requires IRB and DUA	• Shorter approval time, usually expedited IRB review • Requires unique patient identifiers to link data across sources
De-Identified	• Does not contain any identifier	• Technically does not require oversight—but institutional policy varies	• Shorter approval time, usually expedited or exempt IRB review

FIGURE 16.7: Data set types and considerations.

DOB, date of birth; DOD, date of death; DUA, data use agreement; HIPAA, Health Insurance Portability and Accountability Act of 1996; IRB, Institutional Review Board.

◆ **CASE SCENARIO**

PRIORITIZING DATA MANAGEMENT PROJECTS

SITUATION

A nurse executive is asked to join the newly formed technology management council. The council is charged with reviewing all applications of technology in the hospital (e.g., smart pumps, EHR, bar code scanning), identify new needs as they arise such as an integrated bed management platform or quality metric tracking dashboard, and review and approve requests for new technology or data management projects. While charged with these three primary tasks, the council is inundated with more requests for new projects or revisions to current applications than the business intelligence department has capacity to complete. Currently, there are five requests to customize charting templates for various specialties to chart their encounter notes, one request to build a new module that will enable the hospital's transport team to move from paper charting to the EHR, one request to build a new computerized provider order entry (CPOE) module to eliminate paper orders and tracking, one request to fully integrate bar code scanning with pharmacy medication orders, and 10 requests to build nursing unit dashboards that track unit-specific metrics that differ based on the requests made by each unit.

DISCUSSION QUESTIONS

1. The council is currently reviewing each project request and needs to prioritize each request from highest priority to lowest. How would you rank order the requests?
2. The council is currently considering the 10 individual requests from the nursing units. What are several ways that these requests could be handled?

OUTCOME

The council triaged the CPOE and bar code medication administration system as the top priority due to high priority for patient safety and requested that the two projects be integrated into one initiative. The second highest priority project was building one dashboard for the 10 nursing units as it covered a wide swath of care providers and institutional needs. The transport EHR was returned back to the requestor to begin initial needs assessment and project scope identification, and that once initial mockups and a concrete project timeline was completed, the project would be slated for initial build the following year. The customized charting requests were triaged to the waiting list.

 CASE SCENARIO

LEVERAGING INFORMATION TECHNOLOGY TO SUPPORT STRATEGY ON THE NURSING FLOOR

You are a nurse manager of a regular nursing floor that cares for post-cardiac surgery patients. The recent focus on tracking and reducing readmissions directly impacts your unit and the administration has tasked you with putting together a comprehensive strategy to track and reduce readmissions. This has been identified as a top priority for the institution and your unit will be the proof-of-concept pilot project to establish a new approach, then test and refine it for eventual rollout to other units within your hospital and then the other hospitals within your health system. You were told that you will have access to all of the necessary resources to complete this project. Working with your unit's shared governance committee and nurse educator, you have identified a multipronged approach to addressing this problem. You have identified the potential of leveraging IT and clinical data as a major component of this new initiative.

1. In what ways can you use clinical data to support this project?
2. What personnel and resources would you need to develop and implement a new clinical decision support system based on in-house clinical data?

DATA ANALYTICS

The analytics phase should entail the involvement of at least one data analyst, and for more intensive applications at least one statistician to plan and complete the data analyses. Of note, there are significant differences between data analysts and statisticians. Data analysts typically have computer coding backgrounds and data wrangling skills—the ability to access and use data from many sources in various ways—but may be limited in their statistical analysis knowledge. Statisticians, on the other hand, can perform the complicated statistical analyses but may be limited in their data wrangling capabilities.

Nurse leaders, and particularly nurse informaticians, play a critical role during all phases of IT projects, particularly those that involve using clinical data. Nurse leaders, especially those with a background or understanding of information management, are able to bridge the different disciplines involved in the project that enable developing a shared vision and understanding between the team members. For example, having an understanding of how data is entered by the clinical facing nurses enables working with the statistician and/or data analyst to assess the practicality of adding or removing new data elements. Conversely, it is not uncommon for statisticians to perform initial data analyses and remove variables that do not meet a certain level of completeness—or, stated differently, because a certain provider type was only listed 40% of the time, the variable was removed from the model. However, the variable indicated when a provider was engaged in the clinical care of the patient, which does not take place for every patient encounter, thus indicating a significant event in the care of the patient and requiring continued inclusion in the model. Including this variable in the model can be handled several ways. Working with the statistician will enable identifying the best way to handle the data. This is only one example of the interplay between the clinicians, statisticians, data analysts, and IT personnel that commonly takes place throughout an IT project.

PREPROCESSING

A common misconception of working with clinical data, or other data that already exists, is that because the data already exists, the work will be easy and proceed quickly. In fact, a majority of time in these projects is dedicated to accessing, extracting, and transforming the data into a usable or analyzable format—or preprocessing the data. Depending on the scope of the project, estimates range anywhere from 40% to 90% of total project time is dedicated to preprocessing data, particularly if preprocessed data does not exist. Data preprocessing is a critical phase in any information management project and will dictate the value of the results generated.

The extent of data preprocessing work is determined by the scope of the project. For example, if we are building our weekly metrics discharge disposition and internal readmission dashboard, the amount of preprocessing will be minimal as we are simply pulling data from the Admission/Discharge/Transfers database and reporting the frequencies of each category to a dashboard.

Alternatively, if developing an active real-time patient status dashboard that will be used to monitor ICU patient status or predict patient instability, such as an early warning system, the amount of preprocessing will increase depending on the types and number of variables you will be abstracting and including. For example, many real-time patient tracking dashboards include vital sign data extracted from the flowsheets section of the EHR. Raw EHR data can be sparsely populated when first abstracted. Depending on the storage structure, several rows of data may be populated for one vital sign entry. Alternatively, if one assessment finding is entered 15 minutes after a regular vital sign assessment, most of the row will be empty except for the new information—leading to a significant amount of missing data (described further in the next section), or all of the data from the previous vital sign entry will be repeated with the only difference being the newly added assessment. These differences in data representation and storage contribute to the amount of preprocessing time that is required to transform data into usable and analyzable formats.

Another frequently encountered problem relates to the granularity of the raw data. For example, diagnosis codes may need to be mapped to or combined into a broader category such as medical or trauma, instead of any one of the many *ICD-10* codes for arm fracture. In this case, identifying the type of patients and creating an indicator for those patients is the goal. Thus, identifying all eligible diagnosis codes that can be mapped to the broader category is the preprocessing work that is required. This is where using one of the standardized terminologies such as SNOMED CT is useful as this mapping work has already been completed and can be used to move up or down levels of abstraction to classify patient groups.

Another example of preprocessing data is creating indicator variables of certain clinical activity or interventions of interest. For example, if we are developing a prognostic model to predict hospital mortality, we may need to indicate if a patient is receiving supplemental oxygen. There are many ways oxygen is delivered and represented in the EHR. But oftentimes, it may not be important to differentiate between simple mask delivery versus nasal cannula, just that the patient is receiving supplemental oxygen. Simple indicator variables can be created that indicate the presence or absence of supplemental oxygen, or in the case of intubation and ventilation that the patient is on a ventilator—with the specific ventilator settings not necessary to account for.

Another consideration for working with vital sign data or flowsheet data is the potential to create new indicator variables that account for clinical changes not explicitly charted. For example, an increased frequency in vital sign charting and observations or nursing assessment notes can indicate a clinical concern for change in patient status that is not explicitly documented as an extractable variable labeled "concern for change in patient status." While some applications will use natural language processing (NLP) or other forms of text analysis to identify the concern via the text notes, one can also simply create a new indicator variable that represents the increased charting frequency anytime the regularly ordered vital sign monitoring (e.g., q 4 hours) is replaced with more frequent recordings. This indicator variable can then be used in prognostic models or calculators. While this is only a basic review of several examples of the different ways in which raw data requires preprocessing, there are many more ways to work with and preprocess data to support the intended goals of the project. There can be a tendency to preprocess or continually explore the data as this work can be exciting and insight generating—in essence, going down the proverbial rabbit hole, ultimately distracting from the original project goals and timeline. This work is both time consuming and expensive; thus, it is imperative for every project leader to start with clear goals and revisit those goals throughout the project to stay on task.

HANDLING MISSING DATA

Missing data is a key concept when working with data in any project, but particularly more important when using EHR data secondarily. As previously mentioned, clinical data is often sparsely represented, presenting significant challenges to use in any statistical analysis as most analyses are sensitive to missing data. There are multiple approaches to handling missing data that can be considered in consultation with your statistician.

However, there is another dimension of missing data that is specific to big data and using clinical data secondarily, that being the discernment of whether data should be present or not. A major difference in secondary data use is that, in contrast to a prospective research study in which one identifies the data needed to answer the research question and then collects that data, in big data approaches (described in the text that follows) and secondary use cases, the opposite is true. One must identify if the data available will be sufficient to answer the research question at hand. In prospective data collection, missing data is minimized and more easily addressed, whereas in secondary use cases, one must discern if the data should be present and is missing (e.g., age, sex) or simply did not happen (e.g., medication administration or procedure). For example, including medication data or procedure data is complicated by the fact that not every patient receives medication or a specific procedure, such as intubation and ventilation, but when they do it is significant. However, it can be difficult to discern if no medication was given for a patient during a specified period of time or clinical encounter, or if the medication data is actually missing and did not complete the ETL process properly. Therefore, attention should be given during the development stage when identifying what data is needed for the project to identify data that is expected to be present, data that by its mere presence is informative and should be included, or data that might be considered missing but did not take place and is not missing.

BIG DATA AND PREDICTIVE ANALYTICS

Big data is considered to be the new frontier in healthcare and particularly for using clinical information to support clinical practice and administrative activities. While attention to big data has increased intensely since the beginning of the 21st century, evidence of humans struggling with large amounts of data date back to 1663 when John Graunt, considered the first to develop and use statistics, stated that he was dealing with "overwhelming amounts of information" while studying the bubonic plague (Foote, 2017). Then, in the 1860s, the seminal work of Florence Nightingale included the coxcomb, which presented complicated statistics and data in an easy to understand visualization (Small, 1998). Fast forward to today, when we grapple with similar problems of having too much data and continually strive to make complicated information easier to understand.

The term "big data" has had an evolving meaning over time. Not too long ago, big data used to refer to data sets that were too large to be analyzed on a personal computer. But now—due to Moore's Law and the doubling of computing power approximately every 2 years (Gregersen, 2011)—big data is considered via the 7 Vs (Table 16.3) as the computing power contained in a smartphone far surpasses that of a desktop computer from only several years prior (Big Data Path, n.d.).

In working through the 7 Vs of big data, one can begin to understand the complicated nature of working with big data. Working with large amounts of data is not new. For example, commonly available administrative data sets such as the Centers for Medicare & Medicaid Services (CMS) billing data can contain millions of rows of data, yet these data would not be considered big data; rather, it is just large data as the data is from one source and is provided in standard formats and easy to analyze. Traditional statistical approaches such as linear regression are capable of analyzing these data without the need for large capacity computing, otherwise referred to as high-performance computing that consists of a cluster that uses 100s to 1,000s of processors working in tandem. The key differentiating factor between large data and big data is not just the amount but, as the Vs present, varying types of data from multiple sources that must be combined into an analytical data set to support the project. For example, if we were to develop a state-of-the-art patient mortality prediction tool for each hospital admission, we could include every data element available for that patient, which would include all the data types presented in Table 16.1 into a predictive model. In this case, prolonged ICU stays can generate thousands of vital sign entries, far surpassing the ability of traditional statistical approaches to incorporate all that data for one patient, creating a situation referred to as high-dimensional data, or more predictor variables than subjects. Thus, different ways of handling the large amounts of data are necessary and have developed into the current focus of big data and data analytics now being applied in healthcare.

TABLE 16.3: The 7 Vs of Big Data

	Definition	Example
Volume	The amount of data being processed	The world produces 2.5 million terabytes/day The average person generates 1.7 mb/hour
Velocity	Speed at which data is generated	90% of data has been generated in the last 2 years
Variety	Types of data	Tweets, genomic, geospatial, text, images
Variability	Meaning depends on context	Single word can have multiple meanings
Veracity	Accuracy or trustworthiness of data	Data can come from multiple sources in multiple formats; data processing may enter noise
Value	How using data improves operation	Using EHR data to predict readmission and target discharge education interventions
Visualization	Presenting data in a readable and understandable format	Clinical dashboards, heat maps

EHR, electronic health record.

ARTIFICIAL INTELLIGENCE

AI is an umbrella term that is commonly applied to many different approaches in data analytics. AI is defined as "the science and engineering of making intelligent machines, especially intelligent computer programs . . . to mimic the problem-solving and decision-making capabilities of the human mind" (IBM Cloud Education, 2020, paras. 1–2). Thus, AI can refer to any of the newer statistical approaches that are typically employed to handle high-dimensional data, particularly in the prognostic model building space. Examples of AI in everyday life include speech recognition such as speech-to-text, which relies on natural language processing that many EHRs support for dictation, online virtual support agents or chat bots, recommendation engines employed in online shopping websites, and automated stock trading. Subfields within AI include machine learning and deep learning (Figure 16.8). Machine learning is "a method of data analysis that automates analytical model building . . . based on the idea that systems can learn from data, identify patterns and make decisions with minimal human intervention" (SAS Institute, n.d., para. 1). A subfield within machine learning is deep learning, which is a specific approach that employs a layered neural network, designed to mimic the neural structure of our brains, and is primarily an automated process that extracts features from labeled data to make a prediction or classification.

MACHINE LEARNING

Machine learning, previously defined as a method of data analysis that automates analytical model building, is becoming more common when analyzing large amounts of data. As opposed to traditional approaches of statistical analysis that include hypothesis generation and testing, big data and machine learning approaches can either be used for hypothesis testing or be employed as a data-driven discovery approach. Considered a primary strength of machine learning, data-driven discovery, sometimes referred to as "letting the data speak," is employed to identify patterns or correlations in the data that might not have been conceptualized or hypothesized prior to analysis. The primary advantage that machine learning provides is the ability to analyze significantly large data sets with many

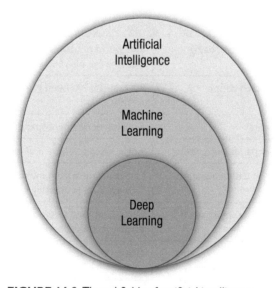

FIGURE 16.8: The subfields of artificial intelligence.

more variables—100s to sometimes 1,000s, with limited to no supervision. "Supervision" is the term used when the analyst or statistician directs the analysis via certain rules that are entered into the equation prior to analysis. Thus, machine learning approaches can be classified into supervised and unsupervised methods. Supervised methods infer function from data that is labeled or having the outcome of interest already identified such as a patient receiving a particular diagnosis or outcome and includes approaches such as classification and regression. In contrast, unsupervised approaches infer function from hidden structures within the data and can use unlabeled data where the outcome may not be specified, and typically consist of clustering and association analyses. Each of these approaches are further described in the text that follows.

Additional data modeling steps are included when working with big data that you may not be familiar with. Big data analyses are powerful statistical tools that are capable of maximally leveraging the data that is being analyzed. While this enables building models that are extremely accurate, it tends to lead to what is called overfitting the data. While not unique to big data approaches, overfitting the data means that the prediction or model that was developed is so specific to the data that was used that if that model were to be applied in a different clinic or hospital the odds of that model predicting the outcome are lower. There are several ways to address this. The first is partitioning the data into training and testing data sets. For example, if the complete data set consists of 10,000 patients, 7,000 would be used to run the initial statistical modeling, and then the remaining 3,000 would be used to test that model with an "independent" sample. It is not uncommon for the model performance to reduce from the training set to the testing set, but it provides valuable insight into how well a model might perform overall and in other populations. Another approach is cross validation that leverages random sampling during model building—the specifics are beyond the goal of this chapter, but it is something to be aware of and discuss with a statistical team.

MODELING OBJECTIVES

The primary consideration during the analytics phase is identifying the type of analysis or modeling that is required to achieve your project goals. The main categories of modeling include descriptive—how many patients had x condition or treatment; predictive—probabilistic forecast of what may happen; association—probability of two or more items co-occurring at the same time; or clustering—similar patients that group around certain characteristics. Once the type of modeling is determined, consideration can be given to employing one or more of the supervised or unsupervised machine learning approaches.

SUPERVISED MACHINE LEARNING

Supervised approaches require labeled data, that is, data where the outcome of interest is already known and is identified and labeled through expert review—trained data reviewers that review the data and label it with the diagnosis or outcome of interest such as patients that have confirmed diabetes via clinical findings and laboratory results. The labeled data can then be analyzed via one of the supervised machine learning methods such as Random Forest or classification and regression trees (CART).

CART identifies combinations of predictors associated with the outcome of interest that involves a tree-building technique in which the choice of "splitting" variables is based on an exhaustive search of all possibilities. The tree-building process leads to terminal nodes (or leaves), at which point the nodes cannot be divided anymore. Figure 16.9 displays one side of a tree with the terminal nodes at the bottom, with the bar graph indicating the mortality rate for that particular group (farthest right indicating a 30% mortality rate). The result is mutually exclusive groups that are the most different with respect to the outcome. CART is a semi-supervised approach because you are able to set criteria such as how deep—or how

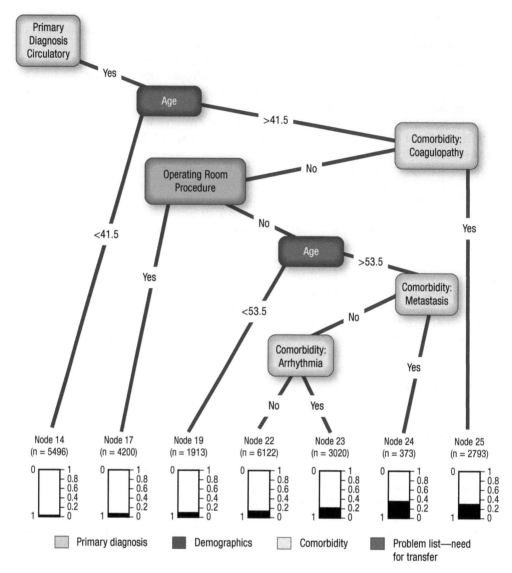

FIGURE 16.9: Classification and regression trees (CARTs) identify combinations of predictors associated with the outcome of interest that involves a tree-building technique in which the choice of "splitting" variables is based on an exhaustive search of all possibilities.

Source: Adapted from Reimer, A. P., Schiltz, N. K., Ho, V. P., Madigan, E. A., & Koroukian, S. M. (2019). Applying supervised machine learning to identify which patient characteristics identify the highest rates of mortality post-interhospital transfer. *Biomedical Informatics Insights.* https://doi.org/10.1177/1178222619835548.

many levels the tree contains (this tree contains eight levels), the criteria to identify when a variable should be split between two groups so that it contributes significantly to the model prediction (age is split at 41.5 years), and the minimum number of patients that are required to be in each final group—terminal node (number of patients is signified by $n =$, which is the terminal node).

Random Forest is an extension of CART and is simply the generation and analysis of many individual CART trees by randomly selecting input variables during each tree building, improving overall prediction. Random Forest generates a list that ranks variable importance from high to low that consist of the overall ranked importance of

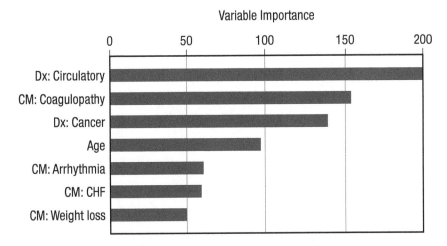

FIGURE 16.10: Overall ranked importance of significant variables.

CHF, congestive heart failure; CM, clinical modification; Dx, diagnosis.

significant variables that predict the outcome of interest by taking the results from each individual tree and averaging them into a final variable importance score for each variable (Figure 16.10). Random Forest is also considered a supervised approach as it too uses labeled data and you can specify the model building criteria such as the maximum number of variables to be included in a tree and how many trees (i.e., 100–10,000) to build.

UNSUPERVISED MACHINE LEARNING

Unsupervised machine learning infers function from hidden structure within the data and can use unlabeled data where the outcome may not be specified. It typically consists of clustering and association analyses. Association rules mining is an unsupervised machine learning approach that identifies items that most frequently occur together, similar to how stores identify items most frequently purchased together (e.g., formula and diapers). Association rules can be used to identify diagnoses or other conditions that co-occur, with the significance of the results being that the co-occurrence of the identified conditions—for example, hypertension, diabetes, and history of smoking—is more significant than any one of the conditions individually or added together—indicating a nonlinear relationship equaling more than the sum of the parts.

Other unsupervised machine learning methods include clustering analysis, a powerful approach to identify patients who may be similar or, more importantly, different on individual factors or multiple variables simultaneously. Clustering analysis is useful to identify new ways to classify patients as it is an unsupervised approach to data analysis that does not require labeled data or prespecified relationships. Clustering analysis is complex and can include using visualizations to assess the results. Clustering methods used include k-means clustering that clusters values on the nearest mean of the value of interest, and expectation-maximization clustering that is an iterative method that finds maximum likelihood estimates based on modeling latent variables—variables that are not explicitly identified or observed.

DEEP LEARNING

Deep learning is a subfield within machine learning and is a supervised approach. The power of this approach is the ability to analyze large and complex data due to the neural network structure that is designed to mimic the structure of our brains (see Figure 16.11). By

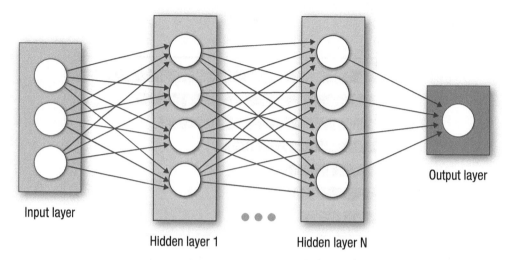

Output layer

Input layer

Hidden layer 1   Hidden layer N

FIGURE 16.11: The power of deep learning is the ability to analyze large and complex data due to the neural network structure that is designed to mimic the structure of our brain.

leveraging high-performance computing clusters, neural network models are able to generate classification models in a matter of days, whereas previously it may have taken several years to identify all of the rules and program one image classification model. A common application of deep learning is radiology image reading. For example, deep learning neural networks are able to analyze digital imaging and diagnose medical conditions such as COVID-19 on chest imaging (Wang et al., 2020). For this type of application, the input layer is the image which is analyzed pixel by pixel or voxel by voxel. The hidden layers consist of individual neurons that store an individual numeric value and a connection to another neuron represents the weight or strength of the connection between the two neurons. Developing neural networks includes determining how many layers or how deep the model is and how many neurons or how wide each layer is. The output layer contains each of the final desired outcomes such as classifying between the presence or absence of a particular condition in the image. Neural networks are developed with labeled images that enable the network to set the model parameters. Then, images not used in training and held out for testing are used to assess the accuracy of the model (Zaharchuk et al., 2018). This is a basic overview to provide an understanding of deep learning as there are many other model building considerations and parameters to set.

An important aspect of deep learning to be aware of is the limited application of the results—typically a model is only accurate in the classification application in which it was originally designed and used, with limited to no ability to extend the model to other applications. Stated differently, deep learning applications are so specific that if you train a model to detect images that display dogs or cats, it will achieve that accurately, but it probably will not be able to distinguish between different types of cats or dogs. Thus, expectations should be that a given deep learning project will only be applicable to the original application and another project will be necessary to apply the approach to a different classification task.

SUSTAINING NEW SYSTEMS

Once the project is complete and operational, there are still several aspects that require continued attention. The first is performing frequent quality reviews of the data that is being used. It is not uncommon for changes to be made to the underlying data that is being used in your dashboard or prognostic tool. For example, a different project may have identified that the data variable for discharge disposition that currently only includes a category for "other nursing facility" would be better served by differentiating between skilled nursing facility, short-term care, or long-term care. While this change is easy to make on the backend, unless you are aware of the change, it may lead to a complete failure of your dashboard to pull and display your discharge disposition categories—an easy problem to identify and remedy. Alternatively, and more pernicious to detect, depending on how the new categories were developed, a new category may contain the same coding as an old category (old category "nursing facility" = 1, new category "short-term care facility" = 1). In this case, data will continue to populate your dashboard with the same label that was already programed in the dashboard of "nursing facility," but in reality, the results being displayed actually reflect only the "short-term care facility" discharges. One may notice a sudden decrease in nursing facility discharges compared to past results as you would now only be indicating "short-term care facility," which is only a fraction of the previous "nursing facility" discharges.

Another similarly related activity is the necessity of regularly scheduled reviews and revision. Once you are using your new system, it is fairly common to identify multiple aspects that could be improved upon. Or like any data-related project, answering questions begets new questions. The desire to make changes needs to be balanced with the ability to make additional changes while also considering the impact on the end-user who can easily be overburdened with increasing charting requirements. Depending on the workflow for your project and the institution generally, the ability to make changes or add additional features can be so restrictive that it does not allow additional modifications as the project is considered complete, through to the ability to make requests on an on-demand basis. A typical approach can include conducting quarterly scheduled meetings to review the performance of the dashboard and solicit feedback on usability and end-user experience and any requests for modifications or additions. Often, necessary changes to the information collected or in user interface are not apparent until it has been in use for some time. By working with your team, you can establish an approach to modifying the project that aligns with the resources and project timeline capabilities of the team and your organizational processes.

If a project entails developing and deploying a prognostic model to support clinical care, which is often the case for decision support applications, an additional, more technical aspect to monitor is calibration drift. Calibration drift is the tendency of predication model calibration, or predictive performance, to deteriorate over time in response to change in clinical environments such as new treatment protocols or changing patient populations (Davis et al., 2020). Calibration drift is a statistical analysis problem, and your statistician will be able to handle this required recalibration of the prognostic model. Calibration drift is a significant patient safety problem and thus must be attended to in any prognostic application. Reviewing this potential problem should be identified during initial project development so that a realistic total project cost and timeline can be developed to ensure proper allocation of time and resources both during the project and after the project is deployed.

◼ WHAT EVERY NURSE MANAGER NEEDS TO KNOW ABOUT INFORMATION MANAGEMENT AND BIG DATA

Nurse managers are uniquely positioned to be the leader of information management projects. Overseeing day-to-day operations of your respective units provides insight into the clinical and administrative needs of the unit that can be improved via the appropriate application of IT. From developing unit facing dashboards that display patient census and staffing through to implementing fully connected smart pumps and vital sign monitoring that interfaces with the EHR, there are numerous opportunities to leverage clinical data and technology resources to improve clinical care and quality management.

Once a need or potential project is identified, the nurse manager must engage their next level management to assess administrative support to move a project forward—and most importantly to get the project on the schedule of the associated departments such as business intelligence to conduct an initial project scope and feasibility meeting. The result of the meeting should be identifying an achievable project with the available resources and a general idea and establish a general project timeline.

While each of us thinks that our projects are important and should be prioritized, most every IT department has more project requests than can be completed in a year. Thus, most departments have review committees that prioritize the order of projects to be completed, and your project may get triaged to a later start date, sometimes months or even years later. Persistent evaluation of the project status is necessary; when able, making the case for increasing the triage priority can expedite project initiation and competition.

Nurse managers, or frontline nurses with direct clinical experience, provide the ideal individual to lead these projects. Identifying an individual who has informatics knowledge or has expressed interest in improving the clinical environment will provide the necessary project champion to move the project forward and will be critical in recruiting other staff involvement and staff buy in if the scope of the project is significant and may entail practice change. Quality committees or practice improvement committees can be ideal groups to oversee these projects, and if neither of these groups exists, now is the time to establish them.

Having an established group is critical to both the short- and long-term success of any IT project. This group will be able to fulfill the necessary steps from front-end user input in design, initial testing, rollout training, and then frequent reassessments for redesign or functional improvements over time. As with most projects, once implemented and the state of practice is improved, other opportunities for improvement will be identified, necessitating a committee to guide project development. This committee should meet regularly and have agenda items to review each project on a regularly scheduled basis as these projects often require revision.

In addition to unit level organization and management of the project, you need to ensure that you have necessary team members to complete the project. While this can be straightforward and usually handled by your collaborating IT department, there are a few items to pay particular attention to. Many projects such as creating clinical facing dashboards can be achieved with just a data analyst who can identify and pull the needed data. Data analysts are typically not statisticians; if your project contains analyses beyond simple tabulations, then a statistician should be engaged—some places offer both master's-prepared and PhD-prepared statisticians and will guide you to the appropriate level of support. Lastly, it is not uncommon for new projects to get off track, the primary reason being project creep or the tendency to stray far beyond the initial scope once those involved discover the endless range of possibilities. Frequent check-ins to get the project started and then frequent assessment of project progress from both your committee or project leader as well as from the IT department are crucial to keep these projects on time.

WHAT EVERY NURSE MANAGER NEEDS TO KNOW

- Nurse managers must engage their next level management to establish administrative support to begin a new IT project that originates from unit management or the frontline staff.

- Nurse managers and nurses who will be using the new technology must be involved in the project design, testing, and implementation phases to ensure user-centered design and usability.

- Strict project management from the initial needs assessment through to testing and implementation is essential to prevent project creep and keep the project on time and on budget.

- Established committees, such as shared governance or a quality committee, present ideal groups to manage IT projects both during development and over time to identify needs for revision and improvement.

WHAT EVERY NURSE EXECUTIVE NEEDS TO KNOW ABOUT INFORMATION MANAGEMENT AND BIG DATA

Nurse executives are in a key position to advocate for IT projects that will improve the ability of the nursing staff to care for patients and improve the clinical care that is provided. Nurses are uniquely positioned to be strong leaders in IT-related projects, especially those with informatics and/or data management knowledge due to the ability to understand both the front clinical use and applications and back-end administrative and technical aspects of the project, allowing them to bridge the approach and language differences between the multiple disciplines engaged in these projects (e.g., data coding, statisticians, staff nurses). The common path for nurse informatician development is to engage in formal education or training after entering a role that requires those skills, or more simply the classic on-the-job training. Thus, specific attention should be given to cultivating a culture of data-savvy nursing personnel and identify key individuals within nursing administration and below to cultivate into nursing informatics and data management experts who are capable of leading these projects and teams.

Another primary challenge related to IT projects generally is the front-end investment in personnel and financial resources required to complete projects. Establishing the business case for any new IT project can be particularly challenging as the ability to establish a return on investment (ROI) for some projects is not always obvious or easy to calculate. Focusing on realized work efficiency, the earlier recognition of problems such as staffing shortages, patient deterioration, or preventing readmissions can have a downstream financial impact on the institution. Other tangible factors to explore can include the influence on staff attrition and burnout that can serve as objective measures to assess the impact of IT projects post-implementation. It is critical to provide the ability for nurse managers to allocate nonclinical time to project personnel to encourage involvement at the staff level. Lastly, you must recognize that IT projects are never really completed. Once implemented, frequent review is necessary and contingencies for updating or establishing updates or upgrades to the project should be included in initial planning and for the life of the project.

WHAT EVERY NURSE EXECUTIVE NEEDS TO KNOW

- Nurses are uniquely positioned to be strong leaders in IT-related projects due to the ability to understand both the front-end clinical use and application and back-end administrative and technical aspects of the project.
- Establishing the business case for any new IT project is challenging as the need to determine an ROI is not always obvious; thus, particular attention should be given to establishing ROI, whether direct or indirect.
- Specific attention should be given to cultivating a culture of data-savvy nursing personnel within nursing administration to develop nursing informatics and data management experts who are capable of leading IT projects and teams at the unit and health system.

TOWARD ACHIEVING A LEARNING HEALTH SYSTEM

Whether your data information management project is developing a clinical dashboard to track unit discharge disposition and readmissions or develop a complex clinical decision support system that reads radiology images with neural network analysis to identify patients with a lung disorder, each project moves us closer to realizing a learning health system. Five observable characteristics of a learning health system outlined by Freidman et al. (2017) are:

- Every patient's characteristics and experiences are securely available as data to *learn* from.
- Best practice knowledge derived from these data is immediately available to support health-related decisions by individual members of society, care providers, and managers and planners of health services.
- Improvement is continuous through ongoing study addressing multiple health improvement and related goals.
- A socio-technical infrastructure enables this to happen routinely, with a significant level of automation, and with economy of scale.
- Stakeholders within the system view the previously noted activities as part of their culture. (pp. 1–2)

This last bullet is the guiding point that can serve as the overarching guiding principle for every information data management project that we engage in. Developing and implementing new information management projects is a time consuming and resource intensive activity that requires nurse leaders with an understanding of all aspects who can contribute to the successful competition and long-term durability of a project. Nurse leaders with clinical care experience and knowledge in information management practices and big data analytics are uniquely positioned as the ideal team leaders to manage the diverse project teams and are critical if we are going to maximize our rich information resources to truly achieve a learning health system.

KEY POINTS

- Data to support patient care comes from a variety of sources that contain differing data types. Key activities to use clinical data include identifying the sources of data, understanding the data types and associated methods to work with the data, and identifying the necessary resources to complete your IT project.
- The scope of your IT project will determine the level of data access required and the associated data storage needs. Data used in multisite projects will require IRB oversight and often require the execution of a DUA if transferring data outside of the institution or receiving data from another institution.
- Identifying and assembling an adequate project team is based on the needs of the project. At a minimum, you will need to include frontline staff that will use the product, a data analyst capable of completing the ETL process on the data, and potentially statisticians to conduct appropriate model building and outcomes analyses.
- There are multiple approaches to analyzing data. AI is the latest advance with machine learning approaches that include supervised, in which data is labeled and the algorithm is guided with statistical considerations, and unsupervised, in which unlabeled data is used to infer meaning. While robust, machine learning approaches require interdisciplinary teams and large resource dedication to complete.
- All projects require review and potential revision over time. Follow-up and review of implemented programs should be included in the initial planning stages and resource allocation decisions at project inception.

SUMMARY

The large-scale availability of electronic health data enables unlimited ways to describe the current state of clinical practice and, more importantly, improve practice by using the data in innovative ways. Data to support patient care comes from a variety of sources that contain differing data types. Key activities to use clinical data include identifying the sources of data, understanding the data types and associated methods to work with the data, and identifying the necessary resources to complete your IT project. Resources required to successfully complete a project include identifying and including the appropriate personnel from those who provide access to the data, data analysts who can extract and make the data usable, and those who can design the user interface or dashboard, through to statisticians and doctorally prepared researchers if data modeling and statistical analyses are required. There are multiple approaches to analyzing data. AI is the latest advance with machine learning approaches that include supervised machine learning, which requires labeled data and enables input to guide the algorithm in developing the statistical model outputs, and unsupervised machine learning, which can use unlabeled data to infer meaning from the data. Nurse leaders are in the ideal position to identify opportunities to use clinical information to improve practice, to provide administrative support at all levels of the organization to facilitate these projects, and to cultivate the current and next generation of data-savvy nurse clinicians and leaders needed to navigate the healthcare data landscape.

END-OF-CHAPTER RESOURCES

◆ DISCUSSION QUESTIONS

1. Identify several IT projects that a nurse manager of a nursing unit could develop to support the operations of the nursing floor.
2. Why is it important for nurse leaders to develop health data literacy?
3. While forming your team to develop a new IT project, who are the various team members to consider adding to the team? Identify their roles and contributions to the project.

◆ ADDITIONAL RESOURCES

- American Medical Informatics Association: https://amia.org
- Nursing Informatics Working Group: https://amia.org/communities/nursing-informatics
- Healthcare Information and Management Systems Society: https://www.himss.org
- *How APIs streamline patient access to health information*: https://ehrintelligence.com/news/how-apis-streamline-patient-access-to-health-information
- *Predictive modeling in healthcare: how to adopt it painlessly*: https://www.itransition.com/blog/predictive-modeling-in-healthcare
- DataCamp: https://www.datacamp.com

◆ GLOSSARY OF KEY TERMS

- **Application program interface (API):** Software program that enables one application to communicate with another in a standardized format.
- **Artificial intelligence (AI):** "The science and engineering of making intelligent machines, especially intelligent computer programs . . . to mimic the problem-solving and decision-making capabilities of the human mind" (IBM Cloud Education, 2020, paras. 1–2).
- **Big data:** Data that exceeds the capacity of standard approaches for analysis (refer to the 7 Vs table).
- **Deep learning:** Employs layered neural network, designed to mimic the neural structure of our brains, and is primarily an automated process that extracts features from data to make a prediction or classification.

- **DUA**: Data use agreement; contract used to regulate the transfer and use of data between individuals or institutions.

- **ETL:** Common acronym that refers to extract, transform, and load data.

- **Fast Healthcare Interoperability Resources (FHIR):** A standard describing data formats and elements and an application programming interface for exchanging electronic health record data.

- **Interoperability:** The ability to exchange and use information between systems.

- **Machine learning:** "A method of data analysis that automates analytical model building . . . based on the idea that systems can learn from data, identify patterns, and make decisions with minimal human intervention" (SAS Institute, n.d., para. 1).

A robust set of instructor resources designed to supplement this text is located at http://connect.springerpub.com/content/book/978-0-8261-7795-7. Qualifying instructors may request access by emailing textbook@springerpub.com.

REFERENCES

Apathy, N. C., Holmgren, A. J., & Adler-Milstein, J. (2021). A decade post-HITECH: Critical access hospitals have electronic health records but struggle to keep up with other advanced functions. *Journal of the American Medical Informatics Association, 28*(9), 1947–1954. https://doi.org/10.1093/jamia/ocab102

Assale, M., Dui, L. G., Cina, A., Seveso, A., & Cabitza, F. (2019). The revival of the notes field: Leveraging the unstructured content in electronic health records. *Frontiers in Medicine (Lausanne), 6,* 66. https://doi.org/10.3389/fmed.2019.00066

Big Data Path. (n.d.). *Understanding the 7 V's of big data.* Retrieved August 30, 2019, from https://bigdatapath.wordpress.com/2019/11/13/understanding-the-7-vs-of-big-data

Cadmus-Bertram, L. (2017). Using fitness trackers in clinical research: What nurse practitioners need to know. *The Journal for Nurse Practitioners, 13*(1), 34–40. https://doi.org/10.1016/j.nurpra.2016.10.012

Davis, S. E., Greevy, R. A., Jr., Lasko, T. A., Walsh, C. G., & Matheny, M. E. (2020). Detection of calibration drift in clinical prediction models to inform model updating. *Journal of Biomedical Informatics, 112,* 103611. https://doi.org/10.1016/j.jbi.2020.103611

Foote, K. D. (2017, December 14). *A brief history of big data.* Dataversity. https://www.dataversity.net/brief-history-big-data

Friedman, C. P., Allee, N. J., Delaney, B. C., Flynn, A. J., Silverstein, J. C., Sullivan, K., & Young, K. A. (2017). The science of Learning Health Systems: Foundations for a new journal. *Learning Health Systems, 1*(1), e10020. https://doi.org/10.1002/lrh2.10020

Grantz, K. H., Meredith, H. R., Cummings, D. A. T., Metcalf, C., Grenfell, B. T., Giles, J. R., Mehta, S., Solomon, S., Labrique, A., Kishore, N., Buckee, C. O., & Wesolowski, A. (2020). The use of mobile phone data to inform analysis of COVID-19 pandemic epidemiology. *Nature Communications, 11,* Article 4961. https://doi.org/https://doi.org/10.1038/s41467-020-18190-5

Gregersen, E. (Ed.). (2011). *Moore's law.* In *Encyclopedia Britannica online.* https://www.britannica.com/technology/Moores-law

HL7 International. (n.d.). *Welcome to FHIR®.* Retrieved July 27, 2021, from https://www.hl7.org/fhir/index.html

IBM Cloud Education. (2020, June 3). *Artificial intelligence (AI).* https://www.ibm.com/cloud/learn/what-is-artificial-intelligence

Mayo Clinic Health System. (2021, February 17). *Remote patient monitoring: Comprehensive care at home.* https://www.mayoclinichealthsystem.org/hometown-health/speaking-of-health/remote-patient-monitoring-comprehensive-care-at-home

Murdoch, T. B., & Detsky, A. S. (2013). The inevitable application of big data to health care. *JAMA, 309*(13), 1351–1352. https://doi.org/10.1001/jama.2013.393

Nelson, H. (2021). *Market leaders drive certified health IT FHIR-enabled API adoption*. EHR INTELLI-GENCE. https://ehrintelligence.com/news/market-leaders-drive-certified-health-it-fhir-enabled-api-adoption

Office of the National Coordinator for Health Information Technology, (n.d.). *Health IT legislation*. Retrieved July 12, 2021, from https://www.healthit.gov/topic/laws-regulation-and-policy/health-it-legislation

Reece, A. G., Reagan, A. J., Lix, K. L. M., Dodds, P. S., Danforth, C. M., & Langer, E. J. (2017). Forecasting the onset and course of mental illness with Twitter data. *Scientific Reports, 7*(1), 13006. https://doi.org/10.1038/s41598-017-12961-9

Reimer, A. P., & Madigan, E. A. (2018). Veracity in big data: How good is good enough. *Health Informatics Journal, 1290–1298*. https://doi.org/10.1177/1460458217744369

Rossetti, S. C., Knaplund, C., Albers, D., Dykes, P. C., Kang, M. J., Korach, T. Z., Zhou, L., Schnock, K., Garcia, J., Schwartz, J., Fu, L.-H., Klann, J. G., Lowenthal, G., & Cato, K. (2021). Healthcare process modeling to phenotype clinician behaviors for exploiting the signal gain of clinical expertise (HPM-ExpertSignals): Development and evaluation of a conceptual framework. *Journal of the American Medical Informatics Association, 28*(6), 1242–1251. https://doi.org/10.1093/jamia/ocab006

SAS Institute. (n.d.). *Machine learning: What it is and why it matters*. Retrieved September 3, 2021, from https://www.sas.com/en_us/insights/analytics/machine-learning.html

Sixicki, B. (2019, April 11). *What you need to know about healthcare APIs and interoperability*. Healthcare IT News. https://www.healthcareitnews.com/news/what-you-need-know-about-healthcare-apis-and-interoperability

Small, H. (1998). *Florence Nightingale's statistical diagrams*. Florence Nightingale Museum. https://www.york.ac.uk/depts/maths/histstat/small.htm

Udeh, C., Udeh, B., Rahman, N., Canfield, C., Campbell, J., & Hata, J. S. (2018). Telemedicine/virtual ICU: Where are we and where are we going? *The Methodist DeBakey Cardiovascular Journal, 14*(2), 126–133. https://doi.org/10.14797/mdcj-14-2-126

Wang, L., Lin, Z. Q., & Wong, A. (2020). COVID-Net: A tailored deep convolutional neural network design for detection of COVID-19 cases from chest X-ray images. *Scientific Reports, 10*(1), 19549. https://doi.org/10.1038/s41598-020-76550-z

Weiskopf, N. G., & Weng, C. (2013). Methods and dimensions of electronic health record data quality assessment: Enabling reuse for clinical research. *Journal of the American Medical Informatics Association, 20*(1), 144–151. https://doi.org/10.1136/amiajnl-2011-000681

Zaharchuk, G., Gong, E., Wintermark, M., Rubin, D., & Langlotz, C. P. (2018). Deep learning in neuroradiology. *American Journal of Neuroradiology, 39*(10), 1776–1784. https://doi.org/10.3174/ajnr.A5543

CHAPTER 17

HUMAN RESOURCE MANAGEMENT

MariLou Prado-Inzerillo and Bertha Ku

"Before you are a leader, success is all about growing yourself. When you become a leader, success is all about growing others."

Jack Welch

LEARNING OBJECTIVES

- Describe four human resource management (HRM) practices that contribute to the organization's overall positive value.
- Analyze key components of HRM and how they affect the daily operations of a nursing unit.
- Calculate the number of full-time equivalents (FTEs) required to care for patients on a nursing unit.
- Evaluate the importance of establishing a strategic nursing plan in order to achieve organizational goals.
- Compare two varying styles of conflict management which could be utilized by a nurse manager to facilitate conflict resolution.

INTRODUCTION

Human resources are valuable capital in healthcare organizations, in which nurses represent the biggest human capital. Nurses are considered the main type of human resources among healthcare professionals who provide direct care to patients. Proper management of human resources can facilitate the achievement of organizational, operational goals and ensure quality patient care. It is therefore necessary that nurse leaders have the required competency to create a healthy, professional nursing environment where nurses are satisfied, engaged, and are delivering safe and quality patient care.

Nurse leaders play a vital role in the creation and maintenance of a professional nursing practice environment that promotes a culture of excellence. Although there are few research studies on nurse leader engagement, it is believed that nurse leaders play a pivotal role in creating a work environment that promotes employee engagement, leading to a high-performing unit and high-quality patient care (Prado-Inzerillo et al., 2018). In addition, the leader's behaviors play an important role in the health and well-being of employees (Arnold, 2017). Leadership is behavior composed of an observable set of skills and abilities (Kouzes & Posner, 2012). Thus, understanding the skills and abilities that need to be cultivated and enculturated in the development of current and future nurse leaders is critical to the nursing profession. As an example, during the 2020 pandemic, a large healthcare system observed that nurse executives who displayed calm, positive, and inspirational characteristics enabled clinical nurses to experience less dissatisfaction in working with reduced staffing and longer hours per staff members. These clinical nurses also expressed less burnout and were better able to deal with rapidly evolving infection control mandates and guidelines.

The competencies that guide the discussion in this chapter are based on the American Organization for Nursing Leadership (AONL) nurse executive competencies (NECs; American Organization of Nurse Executives [AONE] & AONL, 2015a) and nurse manager competencies (NMCs; AONE & AONL, 2015b). These competencies were developed in 2004 by the Healthcare Leadership Alliance to guide the nurse executive and nurse manager practices.

Described in this chapter are real-life scenarios and examples of competencies that nurse executives and nurse managers should possess and exhibit in all practice settings. The following competencies were selected for discussion in this chapter:

- NECs: Communication and relationship building: creating academic partnerships; professionalism; knowledge of the healthcare environment; leadership: systems thinking.
- NMCs: Human resource management: staffing needs, scope of practice; strategic management: facilitate change; relationship management and influencing behaviors: manage conflict; personal and professional accountability: personal growth and development.

LITERATURE REVIEW

Human resource management (HRM) is a strategic approach that helps bridge the gap between employees' performance and achievement of the organization's goals. It is designed to maximize employees' performance to execute their roles and functions safely and effectively.

Professional competency is a fundamental concept in nursing. The World Health Organization (WHO) requires that nurses are equipped with the competency required to deliver quality patient care. Regulatory agencies also require that nurses demonstrate ongoing professional and clinical competency in order to perform certain roles in the organization. It is reported that a nurse's poor competency may lead to job dissatisfaction, turnover, and burnout (Heydari et al., 2016).

The chief nurse executive (CNE) provides strategic direction and leadership to professional nurses and other disciplines within the table of organization. The CNE needs to master the necessary leadership competencies to ensure the value of nursing is integrated into the overall organizational strategic plan and solutions. With rapidly evolving healthcare challenges that organizations are facing, the CNE plays a critical role in monitoring disruptors and responding quickly to innovations that are vital to the organization's success (Boston-Fleischhauer, 2020).

It is essential for healthcare systems to have a sound health resource management. It can improve healthcare models and is critical in providing high-quality care. Effective HRM strategies are needed to achieve better healthcare outcomes (Kabene et al., 2006).

HUMAN RESOURCE MANAGEMENT: STAFFING NEEDS, SCOPE OF PRACTICE

Nurses account for much of the workforce in most, if not all, healthcare organizations. As such, they can be considered the main type of human resources among healthcare professionals who provide direct care to patients. Proper management of these human resources can facilitate the achievement of organizational, operational goals and ensure quality patient care. Hence, HRM is an essential skill for all nurse managers to acquire and hone.

Relative to nursing, HRM is the process by which employees such as RNs and ancillary staff (e.g., nursing assistants, patient care associates, and unit assistants) are managed in alliance with an organization's strategic goals to provide a proficient healthcare delivery system and improve patient health (International Council of Nurses [ICN], 2009). Key components of HRM include recruitment and retention of nursing staff, training and development, performance appraisal, reward and recognition, and career planning. Prudent nurse managers realize the importance of selecting employees with the right skills, knowledge, and attitudes to perform the right tasks in the right place at the right time to achieve the right predetermined health targets (Gunawan et al., 2019; ICN, 2009).

To provide optimal patient care, adequate staffing of a nursing unit is paramount and ensures an effective match between the actual or projected needs of patients and their families with the knowledge, skills, and abilities of the nursing team (Halm, 2019). Comprehending the basic elements of a staffing budget is fundamental when determining the number of employees needed to appropriately staff a specified nursing unit. A significant value is the number of full-time equivalents (FTEs) within a staffing budget; FTEs represent the combined hours worked by full-time and part-time employees. To calculate how much of the allocated budget any one employee consumes, the following equation can be utilized:

$$\frac{\text{Hours worked by employee per day} \times \text{Days per pay period worked by employee}}{\text{80 hours (typical pay period 14 days)}}$$

Example: *If an employee works 12 hours a day and six shifts per 2-week pay period, the calculation would be as follows: 12 hours per day × 6 shifts/80 hours = 0.9 FTE (Hunt 2018a).*

An understanding of other salient, budget-related components such as hours per patient day (HPPD) and the average daily census (ADC) of a nursing unit is also required when calculating how many FTEs a nursing unit needs to adequately care for its patients. Nursing care hours or HPPD is the number of direct patient care hours needed to care for a patient. HPPD can vary from unit to unit as various factors are considered including the number of patients on a unit, patient acuity, staffing skill mix/roles, and organizational support services (Hunt, 2018a). The ADC is typically the average of the unit's daily, midnight census within a given reporting period. To determine the number of staffing hours and FTEs required to meet the patient needs of the unit per day, the following equation can be utilized:

$$\frac{\text{ADC} \times \text{Budgeted HPPD divided by}}{\text{Shift hours}}$$

Example: *If the unit ADC is 25, the budgeted HPPD is 9.2, and the hours per shift are 12, the calculation would be as follows: 25 ADC × 9.2 HPPD = 230 staff hours needed per 24-hour period, then 230/12 hours per shift = 19.2 FTEs within 24 hours (Hunt, 2018a).*

Once the number of FTEs needed within 24 hours has been determined, the nurse manager must carefully consider aspects of the unit environment such as patient acuity or severity of illness, types and frequency of procedures performed, and the average length of stay of patients. Knowledge of these aspects will assist the nurse manager in allocating the correct skill mix of staff to care for patients during each 12-hour shift. Additionally, the staffing plan should reflect a balanced combination of staff members and allow each staff member to practice at their highest potential in order to provide quality patient care while maintaining fiscal responsibility (Hunt, 2018a).

Within the realm of HRM, nurse managers must be able to proficiently develop and train team members according to their scope of practice. Promoting nurses to practice at full scope of practice has been shown to increase job satisfaction, decrease costs, and improve the quality of patient care (Ganz et al., 2016). Scope of practice can be described as the services a healthcare professional is competent in and permitted to perform in keeping with the terms of their professional license (American Nurses Association [ANA], n.d.). Scope of practice is also based on a nurse's educational preparation, training, and experience. Moreover, these services, actions, or interventions within the nursing scope of practice are influenced and bound by regulatory state boards of nursing, and the policies and procedures of a healthcare organization (Van Wicklin, 2021).

Guided by regulatory state boards of nursing and a hospital's nursing policies and procedures, nurse managers should have a clear understanding of each nursing team member's roles and responsibilities. Job descriptions outlining said roles and responsibilities should be developed, consistently reassessed, and updated accordingly to meet the changing health-care needs of society (Feringa et al., 2018). Nursing team member roles and responsibilities should be embedded in the orientation process for newly hired employees and subsequently reviewed for competency during the orientation period. The training and development of employees remain crucial in building nurse competencies to deliver high performance in their practice (Gunawan et al., 2019).

 CASE SCENARIO

A NEW NURSE MANAGER SEEKING HUMAN RESOURCES SUPPORT

SITUATION

KM has been the assistant nurse manager of a 28-bed, medical–surgical unit for approximately 2 years. During this time, the nurse employee turnover rate has increased, and several days a week, the team complains of being short-staffed. After initiating a maternity leave of absence at the beginning of KM's second year as assistant manager, the nurse manager has decided to resign. Consequently, KM is offered the role and promoted to nurse manager. KM has fostered good relationships with the team while in the assistant position. Even so, KM has had limited involvement in HRM. KM is uncertain as to what steps to take first to ensure team members are qualified, as well as sufficient in number, to consistently provide quality care to the patients on the unit.

APPROACH

As a newly promoted nurse manager, KM may not yet fully understand the complexities of HRM. To help build upon this knowledge, KM should first seek out organizational resources already available. These resources may include employee files maintained for each staff member, administrative manuals that contain hospital policies/procedures, and job descriptions outlining employee-specific responsibilities and required credentials. KM may also want to consider connecting with hospital colleagues to supplement any knowledge gaps. KM could learn the basic tenets of unit budgeting by speaking to a member of the finance team. To better understand the qualifications required for each employee, KM could reach out to the human resources department. KM could also garner advice from more experienced nurse managers on how to manage a team. Moreover, KM may find external resources helpful, such as the state's board of nursing when determining employee scope of practice.

OUTCOME

Recognizing the nurse managers of neighboring units have had several years of experience as nurse leaders, KM decides to approach them for advice. The seasoned nurse managers openly shared their experiences with KM. They advised KM to meet with representatives from the finance and human resources teams to gain a better understanding of employee-required qualifications and factors that influence unit staffing. They did this at the beginning of their nurse manager careers and found it beneficial. KM also meets with their managing director. Together they review the foundations of unit staffing, as well as how to calculate daily unit staffing needs. To reinforce budgetary teaching, the managing director arranges an appointment between KM and the nursing finance manager. In addition, KM and the managing director develop a learning plan with set goals to address KM's learning needs. With an established learning plan in place, KM feels more assured about accurately assessing the team's qualifications and the staffing needs for patient care.

DISCUSSION QUESTIONS

1. Name three factors that can impact a nurse manager's unit budgeted HPPD.
2. What two data measurements does a nurse manager need to consider in order to appropriately calculate the number of staff needed to care for the patients on the unit?
3. What entities should nurse managers check to ensure unit nurses and ancillary staff are practicing within their scope of practice?

PERSONAL AND PROFESSIONAL ACCOUNTABILITY: PERSONAL GROWTH AND DEVELOPMENT

According to a 2020 Gallup poll, nursing was voted the most trusted profession by Americans (Johns Hopkins Nursing, 2021). To maintain this level of trust in our profession, it is imperative nursing remains highly accountable for our practice, work environment, and patient safety. In order to do so, nurses must continually seek professional growth and development opportunities to keep current in the ever-evolving realm of healthcare (Davis, 2017). As the cornerstone of healthcare organizations, it is particularly vital for nurse managers to be educationally prepared and competent in their role.

Demanding healthcare settings make it necessary for nurse managers to become proficient in various leadership competencies such as financial and HRM, strategic planning, performance improvement, influencing behaviors, and cultural diversity. As per the American Association of Colleges of Nurses (AACN), nurse managers seeking to broaden their span of knowledge, advance expertise, and impact healthcare delivery at a higher level should engage in graduate studies (AACN, 2019; Fennimore & Warshawsky, 2019). The coursework for advanced nursing degrees, such as a master of science in nursing (MSN), focuses on cultivating leadership competencies and provides nurse managers, especially novice ones, the knowledge and skills required to successfully navigate and improve healthcare systems (Schlaak, 2019). Graduate-educated nurse leaders can critically review current literature and apply evidence-based practice to real-world situations, demonstrate scholarly writing, apply principles of financial management to improve the financial health of an organization, and are more adept at facilitating change and managing relationships (Fennimore & Warshawsky, 2019). Additionally, for nurse managers who are already master's degree prepared though needing reinforced learning in a specific area such as financial acumen, several educational institutions offer an array of graduate courses available via online or in-person training.

Mentorship can also provide the education, advice, and support necessary for nurse managers to achieve the foundational leadership skills required for their positions. Mentoring is considered a long-term relationship that focuses on the overall professional growth of the nurse (Goodyear & Goodyear, 2018). A well-matched mentor can offer a protégé psychosocial support in terms of encouragement, counseling, and a different perspective regarding complex health situations (Dewald & Reddy, 2020). Other functions a mentor can provide include career assistance such as coaching related to setting goals, exposure/visibility to organizational opportunities, as well as helping the mentee create collaborative interprofessional relationships to build on communication and collaboration skills (Goodyear & Goodyear, 2018). Moreover, finding a mentor does not have to entail an elaborate process. The mentor can be the mentee's managing director, a director in another discipline, a fellow nurse manager who may be more seasoned, and/or even someone outside of the organization with whom a professional relationship has been established (Fennimore & Warshawsky, 2019).

Enhancing nurse engagement can be viewed as another leadership skill nurse managers should develop. Healthcare organizations have a vested interest in promoting a culture of engagement among nurses as they comprise the largest share of the workforce (Kutney-Lee et al., 2016). One strategy nurse leaders can use to increase nurse engagement is participation in professional governance. Evolving from shared governance, which has supported the involvement of frontline nurses in organizational decision-making (Kutney-Lee et al., 2016), professional nursing governance implies membership in a professional community and assurance that the decisions and actions derived represent the standards of the profession and positively impact intended outcomes (O'Grady & Clavelle, 2021). Nurse managers who succeed at increasing nurse engagement in professional governance may also see improved patient and nurse outcomes.

A variety of modalities exist to help nurse managers enhance leadership proficiencies. A review of the organizational job description for the nurse manager role can help prepare oneself for the expected responsibilities, as well as identify knowledge and educational gaps for which an action plan can be devised to achieve set learning goals. Nurse managers should familiarize themselves with the organizational policies and procedures utilized most frequently on their unit; they provide guidance with daily operational activities and delineate the specific roles of different disciplines (Dewald & Reddy, 2020). Annual self-assessment and performance evaluation serves as another method for nurse managers to improve leadership competencies. Periodic reflection of one's strengths, weaknesses, and accomplishments can assist nurse leaders to prioritize their learning needs and set future goals for completion. Effective nurse managers also actively seek out feedback to better understand areas of needed improvement (Sherman, 2017). Lastly, nurse managers may find career planning a helpful exercise to discover main interests and define career goals to ensure upward mobility in the nursing profession (Dewald & Reddy, 2020).

Nurse managers can further develop leadership competencies by engaging in professional development activities outside the work environment. Achieving specialty certification in leadership increases nurse manager knowledge and builds confidence. Nurse leaders should also leverage opportunities to attend local and/or national nursing conferences. Networking with and learning from top nursing leaders around the country can be invaluable as they have tried innovative ideas and proven success (Hunt, 2018b). Other professional development activities include membership to local and/or national nursing organizations, subscribing to a professional nursing publication, earning continuing nursing education credits via class participation, listening to nurse leader podcasts, and partaking in leadership book clubs. As the frontline nursing leaders in healthcare organizations, nurse managers must maintain their commitment to the nursing profession, and this requires continuous learning and professional development in order to remain competent in rapidly changing healthcare environments (ANA, 2018).

⬡ | CASE SCENARIO

A NOVICE NURSE MANAGER SEEKING LEADERSHIP SKILLS

SITUATION

Throughout their nursing career, TF has always been an engaged member of the team. As a graduate nurse, TF joined the unit council. After 2 years of frontline clinical experience, TF assumed the role of charge nurse and became one of the team's best preceptors. As TF represented their unit on several nursing and professional governance committees in the hospital, TF naturally became interested in pursuing a nursing leadership position. When the assistant nurse manager position became available on the unit, TF applied and succeeded. Subsequently, TF decided to further their education and enrolled in a graduate program to obtain an MSN degree. Currently, TF is within 6 months of completing their graduate studies and has now been offered the nurse manager position for another unit. TF considers this a great opportunity, though is apprehensive about accepting the role. TF is concerned with being overwhelmed by the position and has low confidence in their leadership abilities. What steps should TF take to attain greater knowledge, enhance nursing leadership skills, and boost their confidence?

APPROACH

As a novice nurse manager, trying to grasp all the responsibilities of the position may feel daunting at first; nonetheless, several opportunities and resources exist for new managers to utilize and help them acclimate to the role, many already available to them within their organization. For overall guidance, new nurse leaders should rely on their direct managers who can review with them the leadership competencies required for the role, assess strengths and weaknesses, and assist them with setting learning goals to offset competency deficiencies. New managers should also seek advice and mentorship from other, more seasoned nurse managers. Shared discussions with experienced colleagues provide new managers with invaluable insight on ideal staffing plans and best practices to optimize unit finances and improve quality and patient experience outcomes. Developing collegial relationships with experienced colleagues can be extremely meaningful for the new nurse manager. It increases team camaraderie, and the new manager benefits from learning from other's perspectives and previous experiences.

OUTCOME

Before making a final decision, TF decides to garner further information about the position. TF schedules ad hoc meetings with the managing director, as well as nurse managers from other units. During the meeting with the managing director, they review the organization's job description of the role. Upon doing so, TF recognizes they have already experienced many of the described responsibilities as the assistant nurse manager of the unit. TF also realizes their graduate studies have prepared them well, as they are familiar with most of the defined leadership concepts and proficient in many of the listed competencies. While speaking to the seasoned nurse managers from the other units, TF feels comforted by their words as they too had felt apprehensive about taking on their roles in the beginning. Moreover, they shared with TF the organizational leadership courses, certifications, and conferences they felt helped them develop as managers the most. These discussions have bolstered TF's confidence, and TF eagerly accepts the promotion.

DISCUSSION QUESTIONS

1. Describe how TF can learn more about the scope and responsibilities of a nurse manager.
2. What are the benefits of TF obtaining a board certification in a nursing specialty?
3. List three additional methods in which TF could hone their leadership skills.

STRATEGIC MANAGEMENT: FACILITATING CHANGE

With the onslaught of the global COVID-19 crisis, hospitals and healthcare facilities have had to enact contingency plans and source new economic, practical, and life-saving ways to accommodate the ever-changing factors involved with the pandemic. Such factors include the following: the inordinate number of sick patients admitted, staffing shortages due to absenteeism and sick leave, and the limited provision of supplies, specifically personal protective equipment (PPE). Being able to balance resources and staffing needs while still following the best practices to maintain optimal patient care is the hallmark of a proficient manager. An essential tool nurse managers often utilize to meet organizational goals with the resources available, even during a crisis, is a concept called strategic management.

Strategic management can be described as the overall process of an organization's decisions, actions, and utilization of resources, to achieve desired levels of performance, facilitate competitive advantage, and outperform other organizations (Jasper & Crossan, 2012; Kong, 2008). Organizational success relies on the nurse manager's understanding of strategic management and the ability to formulate an effective strategic plan to guide the process.

A well-crafted and clearly communicated strategy not only increases the likelihood of successful implementation but improves profitability and enhances team satisfaction (Fry & Baum, 2016).

A strategic nursing plan establishes a roadmap for the achievement of future goals and provides the specific direction teams need to follow; it is a critical component of strategic management and ensures quality patient care and the best possible patient outcomes (Lal, 2020). Moreover, strategic planning helps focus resource allocation on key initiatives and enables priorities to be clearly defined (Schaffner, 2009).

Various actions are involved when devising a nursing strategic plan. These actions include forming a strategic planning team, creating a shared vision with goals, understanding the current state of nursing services, conducting a gap analysis based on the current state, developing tactics and plans for implementation, and evaluation (Drenkard, 2012). An integral first step in strategic planning is the appointment of a strategic planning committee. Makeup of the planning committee should consider the key stakeholders potentially impacted by the project and be inclusive of as many disciplines and nursing levels as needed to ensure diverse perspectives and insights (Lal, 2020). This committee will help create a shared vision with defined goals and guide the entire strategic process.

Subsequently, an assessment of the current state of nursing services, and a gap analysis, should be performed as parts of the strategic nursing plan. Pertinent nursing indicators such as quality data, staffing ratios, and patient experience scores should be reviewed to determine the current state, as well as what would be needed to achieve the desired vision and goals. Additionally, the strategic planning committee can employ a strategic planning technique and complete a SWOT (strengths, weaknesses, opportunities, threats) analysis of the planned project. Conducting a SWOT analysis of the planned project can help build on strengths, address weaknesses, leverage opportunities, and identify internal and external threats to the plan (Mallon, 2019; Schaffner, 2009).

The final steps involved in a strategic nursing plan are communication, implementation, and evaluation. Proper communication of the strategic plan to identified key audiences is paramount to the plan's success. To ensure adequate communication dissemination, consider creating a succinct one page summary of the plan, as well as utilizing multiple modes of communication including email, staff meetings, nursing leadership forums, and townhall meetings (Schaffner, 2009). Successful plan implementation largely depends on the accountability of team members. It is important to assign accountability for the completion of specific initiatives to specific members of the team (Fry & Baum, 2016). Lastly, an evaluation process should include outcome-related metrics for each plan goal to accurately evaluate whether the vision of the strategic plan is being reached (Drenkard, 2012).

Even in the wake of a pandemic, the development of a strategic nursing plan can help assist nurse managers navigate the ever-changing landscape of healthcare (Campbell, 2020) and provide their teams with the necessary guidance to adapt to the change. Nurse managers are often frustrated with their perceived limited ability to effect change in the organizations. However, as the largest managerial group in healthcare settings, nurse leaders can leverage this power in numbers and ensure the values and beliefs of managerial strategy are aligned with the patient-focused culture of nursing (Jasper & Crossan, 2012).

⬡ CASE SCENARIO

A NURSE MANAGER LEADING THE TEAM THROUGH TRANSFORMATION OF THE MEDICAL–SURGICAL UNIT

SITUATION

The COVID-19 pandemic has reached the doors of a local community hospital with the admission of its first COVID-19 positive patient. During an emergent nursing enterprise meeting, JM, the nurse manager of a 35-bed medical–surgical unit, is tasked with transforming the unit into the hospital's designated COVID-19 unit. The unit design will need to be equipped with "clean" and "dirty" zoned areas for infection control purposes. Effective immediately, all COVID-19 positive patients will be admitted to JM's unit until full census capacity is reached. JM's unit team members have been feeling apprehensive due to the circulating rumors that a specific unit will be appointed as the hospital's designated COVID-19 unit. What steps should JM take to ensure the team is physically and mentally prepared to embrace the challenge of being the hospital's COVID-19 designated unit?

APPROACH

As there are already rumors circulating the organization regarding the designation of a COVID-19 unit, JM's first step in managing the directive should focus on communicating the information to the team. JM should immediately consider conducting an ad hoc team meeting to inform them of their unit's COVID-19 designation and listen to any of the team's concerns and suggestions. The information should also be shared via email, especially for staff unable to join the ad hoc meeting. JM's next steps should then include the formation of and recruitment for a strategic planning committee. Committee members will then formulate a strategic nursing plan to guide the implementation of the unit's COVID-19 designation.

OUTCOME

Upon receiving the directive to transform the nursing unit to the hospital's main COVID-19 designated unit, JM calls for an impromptu meeting to communicate this to the team. Team email communication regarding the directive is delegated to the assistant nurse manager to complete. During the meeting, JM recruits staff volunteers to participate in an interdisciplinary, strategic planning committee; representatives from other departments such as the hospitalist physician team, infection control, supply team, environmental services, facilities, and patient services also join. The committee creates a strategic nursing plan outlining the process steps needed to prepare the unit. Upon completion, the plan is shared with all involved stakeholders.

Guided by the strategic nursing plan, the team moves forth to complete the listed action items. Unit corridors are assigned either "clean" or "dirty" zones. The facilities team applies colored tape to the unit floor to provide clear visual cues to differentiate the two zones, red tape for dirty and green tape for clean. The supply team then stocks additional PPE for use in the dirty zone. Staff caring for patients in the dirty zone can better preserve PPE as they do not have to don and doff PPE, except for gloves, after leaving each patient room. Although initially apprehensive about their unit's COVID-19 designation, JM's team adhered to the process steps outlined by the strategic plan, and the unit transformation proceeded seamlessly.

DISCUSSION QUESTIONS

1. Briefly describe the concept of strategic management.
2. List at least three key disciplines/stakeholders impacted by this directive.
3. How can JM evaluate the effectiveness of the unit as the hospital's COVID-19 designated unit?

RELATIONSHIP MANAGEMENT AND INFLUENCING BEHAVIORS: MANAGING CONFLICT

High-performing nurse managers in acute care settings have been linked to improved nursing care, fewer adverse events (AEs), and improved patient outcomes (Grubaugh & Flynn, 2018). These nurse managers positively influence individual behaviors, develop authentic connections, and competently manage team relationships. Managing such relationships includes learning how to effectively manage conflict within the healthcare environment.

Due to the dynamic and complex nature of healthcare, instances of conflict in healthcare organizations are inevitable (McKibben, 2017). As such, conflict management is an essential leadership competency for nurse managers. Gaining a basic understanding of what conflict is and why it occurs can help prepare nurse leaders on how to circumvent and manage conflict situations (Ellis & Abbott, 2012). Consequences of poorly managed or unresolved conflict include higher stress levels, increased nurse turnover rate, decreased productivity, patient dissatisfaction, breakdowns in trust, and diminished quality of care (Gokoglan & Ozen Bekar, 2021; Grubaugh & Flynn, 2018; Kayser & Kaplan, 2020). Conversely, effective conflict resolution promotes critical thinking, team building, innovative ideas, and a healthy work environment (Ronquillo et al., 2020).

Conflict can be defined as a disagreement with oneself, or real or perceived differences between individuals with differing values, ideas, and goals (Abd-Elrhaman & Ghoneimy, 2018; Piryani & Piryani, 2019). Several types of conflict situations can occur in hospital settings, including interpersonal, intra-group, inter-group, and organizational conflict. Interpersonal conflicts occur between two or more persons whose beliefs and values are incompatible. Intra-group conflicts occur within an established group and may emerge due to changes within group member roles and/or lack of support. Inter-group conflicts occur between groups with differing goals, and organizational conflicts occur when there is discord regarding policies and procedures, and/or informally accepted norms of behaviors and communication patterns (Abd-Elrhaman & Ghoneimy, 2018).

According to a 2009 survey conducted by the Center for American Nurses to identify conflict challenges encountered by nurses, the most common type of conflict experienced in the workplace involved interpersonal conflicts (Johansen, 2012). Interpersonal conflicts can occur among nurse colleagues, nurses and patients/visitors, nurses and physicians, and nurses and managers. Precipitating factors of conflict include poor communication, power differentials between various positions, and incivility (Kim et al., 2017).

Depending on the nature of the conflict, nurse managers can utilize various approaches to conflict resolution. Thomas-Kilmann identified five varying styles of conflict management based on an individual's level of assertiveness and cooperativeness. The five management styles are titled avoiding, accommodating, compromising, competing, and collaborating (Kilmann, n.d.; McKibben, 2017; Piryani & Piryani, 2019). The avoiding style delays dealing with the immediate conflict, and is essentially a lose-lose approach, as no party's concerns are met. Accommodators generally neglect one's own concerns to accommodate those of others. Compromising individuals negotiate to find a suitable middle ground, while a competing style is adopted when an unquestionably correct side exists. Lastly, the collaborating style attempts to merge perspectives to generate an integrated solution to which all parties feel satisfied (McKibben, 2017; Piryani & Piryani, 2019).

Additional strategies to support conflict resolution include abiding by predetermined ground rules for the discussion, as well as establishing the content and context in which the dispute occurred. Openly contrasting the different views and opinions held can also help distinguish whether the conflict is a healthy debate or a harmful situation (Ellis & Abbott, 2012). Moreover, engaging in practice simulations and role-playing of potential conflict situations can help prepare nurse leaders to deal with conflict (Choudhary, 2018). By effectively managing conflict, nurse managers influence teamwork, foster collaborative partnerships, and promote healthier work environments.

● | CASE SCENARIO
A NURSE MANAGER'S ROLE IN RESOLVING CONFLICT
SITUATION

As the nurse manager of a 30-bed surgical unit, AM facilitates the unit's daily interdisciplinary rounds (IDR) during which multiple disciplines convene to collaborate and discuss effective treatment interventions and discharge plans for each patient. The IDR participants include the unit nurses, physicians, physical therapist, dietician, and care coordinator. During the discussion of a specific patient who for the last couple of days has been having breakthrough postoperative pain, the primary nurse suggests increasing the dose of the patient's pain medication or treating the patient with an additional pain medication because the patient's current pain medication, Percocet, has not been controlling the patient's pain throughout the day. This is the second shift the primary nurse has cared for the patient; thus, the nurse has witnessed the patient's breakthrough pain on more than one occasion. The physician disagrees with the primary nurse's suggestion and indicates the current pain management regimen should be more than enough to control the patient's pain. The physician refuses to add another pain medication to the patient's treatment plan and requests moving on to discuss the next patient. What should AM do as the facilitator of the IDR meeting?

APPROACH

Having been a nurse manager for over 10 years, AM has facilitated many IDR meetings and experienced all types of conflict situations in the work environment. Fortunately, AM is well-versed in various styles of conflict management and has implemented different styles to resolve conflict, depending on the situation. In this particular example, the unit IDR meeting is running over on time, with more than half of the patients still requiring discussion. As such, AM has decided to utilize the compromising style of conflict management that seeks to find a middle ground between involved parties.

OUTCOME

To resolve most conflicts, AM typically prefers utilizing the collaborating style of conflict management that focuses on having all participants provide their perspectives on the situation to come up with a mutual resolution. Nonetheless, as time is not permitting, AM decides to employ the compromising style to facilitate IDR flow. AM interjects the conversation, reiterates the patient's more than one instance of breakthrough pain, and suggests the physician reassess the patient's pain status after IDR. The decision to either increase the patient's pain medication dosage or add another pain reliever to treat the patient's breakthrough pain can be determined after patient reassessment.

DISCUSSION QUESTIONS

1. What type of conflict best describes the listed situation?
2. Name another conflict management style AM could have utilized to manage the situation.
3. List three healthcare-related consequences that could occur from poorly managed conflicts.

COMMUNICATION AND RELATIONSHIP BUILDING

Competencies that are described in the following case scenario include creating academic partnerships to ensure a qualified workforce for the future, collaborating with nursing programs to provide required resources, collaborating to investigate care delivery models across the continuum, and determining current and future supply and demand for nurses to meet their care delivery needs (AONE & AONL, 2015a).

A Task Force on Academic-Practice Partnership was created by the AONE in collaboration with the AACN. The Partnership's goal is to enhance the academic and practice partnerships, advance nursing practice, and improve public health. The Task Force recommended that nursing schools and their hospital partners should collaborate to develop programs that enhance student competencies in the delivery of healthcare. Alignment of students' academic preparation to the current needs in actual healthcare settings is critical for students to transition effectively from academia to practice (AACN, n.d.).

College students surveyed by Northeastern University reported that practical experiences such as internships and hands-on learning opportunities allow them to gain the required skills to transition successfully into their careers (News@Northeastern, 2014).

● CASE SCENARIO
CREATING ACADEMIC PARTNERSHIPS

SITUATION

A large hospital system in a major metropolitan area has several nursing school affiliations. Students who are pursuing bachelor's, master's, or doctoral degrees in nursing participate in clinical rotations at the system hospitals. These students create a pipeline for the system's future hires.

At the onset of the COVID-19 pandemic in March 2020, clinical rotations were suspended for several reasons including rapidly evolving knowledge of the COVID-19 virus, rapid rate of infections and death, lack of PPE, concern for student safety, and lack of staff to precept students due to patient surge. As the COVID-19 surge continued at an overwhelming pace, the need to support clinical nurses at the bedside became critical. Nurses were very stretched with their patient load assignments and were caring for extremely high acuity patients. Staffing was very hectic to say the least.

APPROACH

As days progressed, it was evident that the hospital system needed to work with its nursing school partners to determine the feasibility of senior nursing students working at the hospital as nurse technicians supporting clinical nurses at the bedside. Several discussions were held between senior nursing leaders of the hospital and its major nursing school partner; the goal was to explore innovative ways to allow nursing students to continue clinical exposure while working as nurse technicians at the hospital. The hospital system's major nursing school partner surveyed senior nursing students to determine their interest in working as nurse technicians at the hospital; almost 100 senior nursing students volunteered to work as nurse technicians. These senior nursing students were provided orientation and clinical competencies needed to take care of COVID-19 infected patients. They functioned as clinical support to the frontline staff performing functions such as taking vital signs, performing basic health screenings, performing patient rounding, and assisting nurses with patient care activities. The nursing students' support proved to be invaluable.

OUTCOME

A strong partnership between academia and practice was critical in implementing innovations in nursing practice, particularly during the pandemic. Not only did it provide an opportunity for nursing students to experience real life scenarios caring for patients with COVID-19, but their exposure to extremely high acuity patients enabled them to use their critical thinking skills in a fast-paced setting environment. Students also gained an appreciation of the importance of interprofessional collaboration and team effort. In addition, these students became the hospital's pipeline for recruitment into critical nursing positions with the benefit of requiring fewer clinical orientation hours once hired into clinical nurse positions.

DISCUSSION QUESTIONS

1. Why is it critical to have a strong partnership between academia and practice?
2. Identify an innovative partnership that nursing schools and hospitals implemented at the height of the pandemic.

PROFESSIONALISM

Competencies that are described in the following case scenario include promoting leader and staff participation in lifelong learning and educational achievement, coaching others in developing their own career plans, and contributing to the advancement of the profession (AONE & AONL, 2015a).

In today's complex and competitive environment, organizations need to focus on human capital and leverage their people or workforce to achieve their goals. Investing in higher education to increase the organization's workforce intellectual capital is the most important driver of value creation and organizational success (Chang et al., 2008). The effects of higher education were found to be associated with increased evidence-based practice (Johansson et al., 2010). Critical thinking is a highly valued educational outcome resulting from higher and professional education.

Human capital is the most valuable resource in an organization. Therefore, it is important to attract and retain qualified workers. To achieve this goal, one of the HRM strategies is to provide tuition reimbursement and incentives to its workforce.

 CASE SCENARIO

PROFESSIONALISM

SITUATION

One of the recommendations released by the Institute of Medicine (IOM) report in 2010 on the future of the nursing profession is to encourage nurses to achieve higher levels of education to advance the nursing profession. Higher education and training allow nurses to feel confident in being full partners with physicians and other healthcare professionals in redesigning healthcare (Redman et al., 2015).

In alignment with the IOM's recommendation to increase the number of doctorate-prepared nurses by 2020, a nurse executive at a large healthcare system envisioned that nurse leaders in their organization will attain the highest level of nursing education. At the time of the IOM report, there were fewer than five nurse leaders with a doctorate degree in the organization.

APPROACH

The nurse executive researched several nursing schools that offered a doctorate nursing program with flexibility for nurse leaders to pursue their doctorate education while working full time. A partnership with a prestigious nursing school that met the hospital employee's and the school faculty's requirements was successfully established. A year later, the first cohort of 12 nurse leaders enrolled in the DNP program with a major focus on nursing leadership development. The organization provided some financial support and scheduling flexibility for the nurse leaders to pursue their studies. Ongoing recruitment of nurse leaders to participate in the doctorate program was enabled through in-person meetings between the school faculty and the organization's nurse executive, information emailed to nursing leadership about the program, and modeling nurse leaders who successfully completed the program. These nurse leaders discussed their positive experiences related to learning innovative nursing leadership concepts, their ability to network with colleagues globally, and their professional confidence and joy in achieving the highest level of nursing education.

OUTCOME

Six years following the program initiation, the number of doctoral prepared nurses in the organization increased from five to more than 40. Several nurses conducted, completed, and published nursing research in peer-reviewed journals. In addition, there has been an increase in podium presentations and poster presentations by the organization's nurses both nationally and internationally. Highlighting the organization's workforce achievements leads to positive perception by internal and external stakeholders. This promotes hospital branding, thereby attracting more qualified talents to the organization.

DISCUSSION QUESTION

1. Identify two transformational leadership characteristics displayed by the nurse executive that support the NEC of professionalism.

KNOWLEDGE OF THE HEALTHCARE ENVIRONMENT

Competencies that are described in the following case scenario include developing new delivery models, assessing the effectiveness of delivery models, and taking action when opportunities exist to adjust operations to respond effectively to environmental changes in economic elements (AONE & AONL, 2015a).

Organizations use different staffing models to assess their staffing requirements and staffing skill mix based on ADC, patient acuity, and financial capacity. With limited financial resources and increased regulatory requirements, organizations need to use resources more effectively and efficiently (Arena et al., 2009). Leveraging and managing human capital effectively is critical to improve organizational performance (Schiuma & Lerro, 2008).

 CASE SCENARIO

KNOWLEDGE OF THE HEALTHCARE ENVIRONMENT

SITUATION

The strain on staffing during the pandemic surge was enormous. Patients infected with COVID-19 presented themselves in the ED in high volume and at a rapid pace. Patient acuity and mortality were high. Patients were in dire need of oxygenation and most required mechanical ventilation. COVID-19 infected patients were considered critically ill patients and required the expertise of trained personnel in critical care nursing.

Information about the disease was constantly evolving, causing anxiety and fear among staff. Exposure to COVID-19 infected patients was high, which led to many personnel being placed on quarantine. With the mandate to increase ICU-bed capacity to handle COVID-19 patients, a new staffing model was developed by a large health system to manage the surge.

APPROACH

It should be noted that several executive orders issued by the state's governor at the onset and during the stages of the pandemic facilitated nursing practice exemptions, scope of practice was expanded for several healthcare disciplines, and out-of-state licenses were honored for a limited period of time. With these executive orders, a new staffing model was developed in the ICU and medical–surgical areas where different levels of staff were stacked in pyramid style to deliver safe patient care. Each personnel member in the pyramid has a clearly defined role and responsibilities driven by their set of competencies. In the ICU pyramidal model, the anesthesiologist or the certified nurse anesthetist is at the top of the pyramid directing the care of their assigned patients. Next on the pyramid is the ICU RN, followed by a step-down nurse, a medical–surgical nurse, and a technician or nursing assistant at the base of the pyramid. Each staff member has a unique important role, but the pyramid functions as one team. Nursing professional development provided training on the different competencies needed by nursing staff to deliver safe patient care in this new environment. This pyramidal model enabled the team to safely stretch their assignments. A team in the pyramidal model could manage four acutely ill ICU patients as compared to one or two ICU patients per RN in a nonpandemic setting.

Additionally, the pyramid team could care for eight to 10 medical–surgical patients as compared to four to five patients per RN outside of this model.

OUTCOME

Interdisciplinary collaboration and teamwork were critical to the care of the patients during the pandemic. The ability to form new models of care during emergencies was necessary to meet the need of the organization. Ongoing education and training of nurses were part of the department of nursing and organization's strategy to ensure that nurses were competent to take care of highly acute critical care patients. Clinical nurses and advanced practice nurses functioned at the highest level of their education and training without barriers, facilitated by the governor's executive orders.

DISCUSSION QUESTION

1.   What considerations should be taken when creating new staffing models?

SYSTEMS THINKING IN LEADERSHIP

Competencies that are described in the following case scenario include addressing ideas, beliefs, or viewpoints that should be given serious consideration; providing visionary thinking on issues that impact the healthcare organization; promoting systems thinking as an expectation of leaders and staff; and considering the impact of nursing decisions on the healthcare organization as a whole (AONE & AONL, 2015a).

In today's dynamic and competitive healthcare environment, it is important to nurture and develop systems thinking as a leadership competency. Systems methodology looks at organizations as an open sociocultural system, capable of organizing itself through their culture, diversity, and people performance (Gharajedaghi, 2006). It is a predictor of leadership performance for effective decision-making, organizational performance, and ongoing learning (Palaima & Skar-auskiene, 2010). Systems thinking includes looking at a larger picture to understand the complexities of the situation, prioritize what is important, manage effectively, and make informed decisions that positively impact the organization's people performance, quality performance, and financial performance.

◆ CASE SCENARIO

SYSTEMS THINKING IN LEADERSHIP

SITUATION

As described thus far, the COVID-19 pandemic created an urgent clinical situation for patients, clinicians, healthcare organizations, and city, state, and federal governments. Immediate, definitive, and often unproven action was required to mitigate the pandemic's devastating effects on the population. The challenge was to plan for an onslaught of urgent care needs, both in the EDs and the ICUs, while facing a variety of unknown variables including, but not limited to, patient volume, pace of patient influx, bed capacity, how to quickly expand bed capacity, equipment volume and how to quickly obtain more (e.g., respirators), staffing, staff competency, regulatory changes, therapeutics (or lack thereof), communication throughout the organization, and PPE requirements and availability.

APPROACH

As described by Trbovich, systems thinking "centers on the dynamic interaction, synchronization, and integration of people, processes and technology.... [It] helps identify the critical relationships and connections often missed or undervalued that are pivotal to a successful implementation effort" (Trbovich, 2014, p. 31). The author outlines a five-step approach to actualizing systems thinking: apply a holistic approach to solving problems, define approaches to evaluating and understanding system-wide effects, identify and nurture great systems thinkers, apply a positive approach to identify leverage points, and create a culture of systems thinking.

While the original intent of the 2005 joint report from the National Academy of Engineering and the IOM was to recommend systems thinking application in order to improve healthcare (Reid et al., 2005), the CNE and the organization clearly actualized a systems thinking approach in response to the COVID-19 pandemic. As discussed previously, the nurse executive developed innovative programs with a school of nursing and recruited nursing students to work as nurse technicians. Furthermore, the nurse executive quickly created a 24/7 corporate nursing command center to serve as a focal point of communication around issues concerning, but not limited to, nurse staffing, staff redeployment with corresponding competency assessment and evaluation, coordinating the nursing department's response to regulatory changes and survey requirements, and collaborating with the hospital's departments in managing bed-surge capacity. The command center exemplified a definitive approach to evaluating and understanding system-wide needs and the effects decisions made in a rapidly changing environment.

In the context of the pandemic, the organization did not need to identify and nurture great systems thinkers. Instead, great systems thinkers rose to the occasion, offering their services 24/7, filling any identified need before being asked, and having leaders serve as role models to their staff. No one raised an objection by stating "that's not my job." Once a need was identified, everyone worked together to place the best level resource at the appropriate level of care.

OUTCOME

The net effect of the organization's COVID-19 pandemic management was the advancement of a culture of systems thinking. Multidisciplinary cooperation was the norm and new work styles were normalized (i.e., remote work with Zoom and Webex meetings). As the pandemic progressed, both in terms of the first wave peaking and the second wave appearing, multidisciplinary communication was the norm, born out of necessity and the desire to collectively manage the pandemic and reduce mortality. New therapies and treatment modalities were identified and implemented, requiring extensive communication and cooperation at all levels of care.

DISCUSSION QUESTIONS

1. Why is systems thinking an important competency for nurse executives?
2. Is systems thinking limited to AE reduction?
3. Are systems thinkers born, nurtured, or both?

WHAT EVERY NURSE EXECUTIVE NEEDS TO KNOW ABOUT HUMAN RESOURCES

Human capital is the most important asset for organizational success. To achieve organizational priorities and strategic goals, nurse executives should develop innovative HRM strategies and programs that support the ongoing development of their workforce. In addition, nurse executives should engage in life-long learning to enhance their competencies.

Today's environment is very complex and organizational changes are evolving more rapidly than ever due to internal and external factors. Leaders are faced with situations that require them to be agile and be able to forecast and scan the environment quickly. They must take into consideration the impact on people and the organization overall for any decisions made. Systems thinking involves understanding the complexity of social systems that is dynamic (Senge et al., 2007). It enables the leader to view the organization as a whole, understand the complexity of the problem, and handle the problem effectively (Senge, 1990). It is vital for nurse executives to develop systems thinking competency, especially as they lead the creation of a nursing strategic plan. Such plans serve as a blueprint for nursing to lead the way in maximizing people development, promoting patient safety, and contributing to the organization's financial performance.

Healthcare organizations strive to be an employer and provider of choice. Nurse executives, in partnership with human resources and other interdisciplinary departments, need to focus on innovative personnel management practices that increase employee satisfaction, employee retention, and diversity in hiring practices free from racism and bias. The *Future of Nursing Report 2020–2030* calls for achievement of health equity built on strengthened nursing capacity, diversity, and expertise (Wakefield et al., 2021). Nurse executives need to partner with other health disciplines in their respective organizations to ensure that patients and their workforce have access to screenings and treatments regardless of race, gender, and financial status.

Educational programs and processes should be put in place to address racism not only in the workforce environment but also in the community. Examples of innovative practices include high involvement work practices, cross functional trainings, robust tuition reimbursement for staff who want to pursue higher education, partnerships with schools in developing programs that are easily accessible for full-time employees, creating programs on diversity and inclusion, and staff incentives for performance.

Leaders influence the behaviors and mindset of the workforce; therefore, they need to focus on development of their people who ultimately carry out the strategy. A sound HRM strategy increases the organization's capacity to manage its culture and strategy in order to achieve its goals (Monavvarian & Khamda, 2010).

WHAT EVERY NURSE MANAGER NEEDS TO KNOW ABOUT HUMAN RESOURCES

To facilitate the achievement of organizational goals, nurse managers should be proficiently skilled in HRM. Key components of HRM are employee recruitment and retention, training and development, and performance appraisal. It also includes understanding the required qualifications for specific roles and the various factors involved to ensure adequate staffing. Nurse managers who can effectively manage human resources optimize nursing care and influence positive patient outcomes.

As the cornerstone of healthcare organizations, nurse managers need to be educationally prepared and competent in their roles. This includes proficiency in leadership competencies such as financial management and HRM, strategic planning, performance improvement, influencing behaviors and relationships, and cultural diversity. To uphold nursing as the most trusted profession in the nation, nurses, and especially nurse leaders, must be professionally accountable to continually seek professional growth and development opportunities to keep current in the dynamics of healthcare.

KEY POINTS

- Comprehension of the importance of adequate staffing, combined with the selection of appropriately skilled personnel, is paramount in providing optimal patient care.
- Effective management of team relationships and conflict situations in the healthcare environment has been linked to improved patient care and outcomes.

■ Nurse leaders are professionally held accountable to continually seek out educational and developmental opportunities in order stay current in healthcare's ever-evolving landscape.

■ Leveraging and managing human capital is critical to improve organizational performance. Innovative HRM practices should be incorporated in defining priorities and strategic goals for organizations.

■ Organizational changes are rapidly evolving due to internal and external factors. Leaders need to be systems thinkers, forecast changes, and be able to make decisions quickly and effectively, taking into consideration the impact on people and the organization overall for any decisions made.

■ Alignment of students' academic preparation to the current needs in actual healthcare settings is critical for students to transition effectively from academia to practice. Well-planned HRM practices to support students' transitions to professional practice is vital to increase productivity and staff retention.

SUMMARY

Concerning nurse managers, HRM typically pertains to the recruitment, orientation, and retention of staff. HRM also consists of establishing staffing plans, comprehending employee roles/responsibilities/scope of practice, and understanding organizational policies and procedures. Nurse leaders should have a clear understanding of these areas, as well as develop financial acumen, and gain proficiency in conflict and strategic management. Nurse managers adept at HRM are better equipped at successful operation of their nursing units.

Effective HRM is a critical component to the nurse manager's and nurse executive's roles. More than ever, nurse leaders need to be strategic and agile in developing human resources strategies that meet the organizational goals. In developing the nursing strategic plan, nurse leaders should consider strategies that have a positive impact on the quality of work by the staff, organization, and patients. Current critical nursing challenges should be addressed such as short staffing, developing innovative staffing models, recruitment and retention strategies, diversity, racism and inclusion, staff engagement, patient and family engagement, quality and patient safety, operational excellence, technology and innovations, research, and nursing education.

As nurse executives and nurse managers, it is important to understand and practice effective HRM strategies that support organizational goals. HRM practices that focus on development of people lead to greater employee satisfaction, low turnover, and high-quality patient care. Thus, it is critical nurse executives and nurse managers have the necessary skills and competencies to lead their staff effectively.

END-OF-CHAPTER RESOURCES

⬡ DISCUSSION QUESTIONS

1. Why is systems thinking an important competency for nurse executives?
2. How can nurse executives operationalize key components of the *Future of Nursing 2020–2030* report, such as diversity and racism, in their organization?
3. How can formulating a strategic nursing plan assist in the implementation of an organizational directive?
4. As nurse leaders have limited spare time, what are the most time-efficient learning modalities in which nurse managers can still develop professionally?
5. What methods can nurse managers utilize to practice varying styles of conflict management?

REFERENCES

Abd-Elrhaman, E. S. A., & Ghoneimy, A. G. H. (2018). The effect of conflict management program on quality of patient care. *American Journal of Nursing Science*, 7(5), 192–201. https://doi.org/10.11648/j.ajns.20180705.16

American Association of Colleges of Nursing. (n.d.). Guiding principles for academic-practice partnerships. Retrieved June 12, 2022, from https://www.aacnnursing.org/Academic-Practice-Partnerships/The-Guiding-Principles

American Association of Colleges of Nursing. (2019, March). *Academic progression in nursing: Moving together toward a highly educated nursing workforce*. https://www.aacnnursing.org/News-Information/Position-Statements-White-Papers/Academic-Progression-in-Nursing

American Nurses Association. (n.d.). *Scope of practice*. https://www.nursingworld.org/practice-policy/scope-of-practice

American Nurses Association. (2018, July). *ANA leadership: Competency model*.https://www.nursingworld.org/~4a0a2e/globalassets/docs/ce/177626-ana-leadership-booklet-new-final.pdf

American Organization of Nurse Executives & American Organization for Nursing Leadership. (2015a). AONL nurse executive competencies. https://www.aonl.org/system/files/media/file/2019/06/nec.pdf

American Organization of Nurse Executives & American Organization for Nursing Leadership. (2015b). AONL nurse manager competencies. https://www.aonl.org/system/files/media/file/2019/06/nurse-manager-competencies.pdf

Arena, M., Arnaboldi, M., Azzone, G., & Carlucci, P. (2009). Developing a performance measurement system for university central administrative services. *Higher Education Quarterly*, 63(3), 237–263. https://doi.org/10.1111/j.1468-2273.2008.00415.x

Arnold, K. (2017). Transformational leadership and employee psychological well-being: A review and directions for future research. *Journal of Occupational Health Psychology*, 22(3), 381–393. https://doi.org/10.1037/ocp0000062

Boston-Fleischhauer, C. (2020). Chief nurse executive readiness for the here and now. *The Journal of Nursing Administration*, 50(6), 307–309. https://doi.org/10.1097/NNA.0000000000000889

Campbell, R. J. (2020). Change management in health care. *The Health Care Manager*, 39(2), 50–65. https://doi.org/10.1097/HCM.0000000000000290

Chang, S.-C., Chen, S.-S., & Lai, J.-H. (2008). The effect of alliance experience and intellectual capital on the value creation of international strategic alliances. *Omega*, 36(2), 298–316. https://doi.org/10.1016/j.omega.2006.06.010

Choudhary, L. (2018). Educational strategies for conflict management. *Nursing2021*, 48(12), 14–15. https://doi.org/10.1097/01.NURSE.0000547734.74555.3c

Davis, C. (2017). The importance of professional accountability. *Nursing Made Incredibly Easy*, 15(6), 4.

Dewald, G., & Reddy, N. (2020). Becoming a successful nurse manager. *Nephrology Nursing Journal*, 47(3), 259–265. https://doi.org/10.37526/1526-744X.2020.47.3.259

Drenkard, K. (2012). Strategy as solution: Developing a nursing strategic plan. *JONA: The Journal of Nursing Administration*, 42(5), 242–245. https://doi.org/10.1097/NNA.0b013e318252efef

Ellis, P., & Abbott, J. S. (2012). Strategies for managing conflict within the team. *British Journal of Cardiac Nursing*, 7(3), 138–140. https://doi.org/10.12968/bjca.2012.7.3.138

Fennimore, L., & Warshawsky, N. (2019). Graduate leadership education for nurse leaders—needed now more than ever. *Journal of Nursing Administration*, 49(7–8), 347–349. https://doi.org/10.1097/NNA.0000000000000765

Feringa, M. M., De Swardt, H. C., & Havenga, Y. (2018). Registered nurses' knowledge, attitude, practice and regulation regarding their scope of practice: A literature review. *International Journal of Africa Nursing Sciences*, 8, 87–97. https://doi.org/10.1016/j.ijans.2018.04.001

Fry, A., & Baum, N. (2016). A roadmap for strategic planning in the healthcare practice. *Journal of Medical Practice Management*, 32(2), 146–149.

Ganz, F. D., Toren, O., & Fadlon, Y. (2016). Factors associated with full implementation of scope of practice. *Journal of Nursing Scholarship*, *48*(3), 285–293. https://doi.org/10.1111/jnu.12203

Gharajedagh, J. (2006). *Systems thinking: Managing chaos and complexity*. Elsevier.

Gokoglan, E., & Ozen Bekar, E. (2021). The relationship between nurse managers' personality traits and their conflict management strategy preferences. *Journal of Nursing Management*, *29*, 1239–1245. https://doi.org/10.1111/jonm.13262

Goodyear, C., & Goodyear, M. (2018). Career development for nurse managers. *Nursing Management*, *49*(3), 49–53. https://doi.org/10.1097/01.NUMA.0000530429.91645.e2

Grubaugh, M. L., & Flynn, L. (2018). Relationships among nurse manager leadership skills, conflict management, and unit teamwork. *The Journal of Nursing Administration*, *48*(7/8), 383–388. https://doi.org/10.1097/NNA.0000000000000633

Gunawan, J., Aungsuroch, Y., & Fisher, M. L. (2019). Competence-based human resource management in nursing: A literature review. *Nursing Forum*, *54*(1), 91–101. https://doi.org/10.1111/nuf.12302

Halm, M. (2019). The influence of appropriate staffing and healthy work environments on patient and nurse outcomes. *American Journal of Critical Care*, *28*(2), 152–156. https://doi.org/10.4037/ajcc2019938

Heydari, A., Kareshki, H., & Armat, M. R. (2016). Is nurses' professional competency related to their personality and emotional intelligence? A cross sectional study. *Journal of Caring Sciences*, *5*, 121. https://doi.org/10.15171/jcs.2016.013

Hunt, P. S. (2018a). Developing a staffing plan to meet inpatient unit needs. *Nursing Management*, *49*(5), 24–31. https://doi.org/10.1097/01.NUMA.0000532326.62369.9b

Hunt, P. S. (2018b). Professional growth is a personal responsibility. *Nursing Management*, *49*(9), 5–6. https://doi.org/10.1097/01.NUMA.0000544465.45119.12

International Council of Nurses. (2009). *Guidelines on planning human resources for nursing*. http://www.who.int/

Jasper, M., & Crossan, F. (2012). What is strategic management? *Journal of Nursing Management*, *20*(7), 838–846. https://doi.org/10.1111/jonm.12001

Johansen, M. L. (2012). Keeping the peace: Conflict management strategies for nurse managers. *Nursing Management*, *43*(2), 50–54. https://doi.org/10.1097/01.NUMA.0000410920.90831.96

Johansson, B., Fogelberg-Dahm, M., & Wadenstein, B. (2010). Evidence-based practice: The importance of education and leadership. *Journal of Nursing Management*, *18*, 70–77. https://doi.org/10.1111/j.1365-2834.2009.01060.x

Johns Hopkins Nursing. (2021, January 22). *Nurses are the "most trusted profession" for 19 years in a row*. On the Pulse. https://magazine.nursing.jhu.edu/2021/01/nurses-are-the-most-trusted-profession-for-18-years-in-a-row

Kabene, S. M., Orchard, C., Howard, J. M., Soriano, M. A., & Leduc, R. (2006). The importance of human resources management in health care: A global context. *Human Resources for Health*, *4*(1), 1–17. http://doi.org/10.1186/1478-4491-4-20

Kayser, J. B., & Kaplan, L. J. (2020). Conflict management in the ICU. *Critical Care Medicine*, *48*(9), 1349–1357. https://doi.org/10.1097/CCM.0000000000004440

Kilmann, R. H. (n.d.). A brief history of the Thomas-Kilmann conflict mode instrument. Retrieved July 6, 2021, from https://kilmanndiagnostics.com/a-brief-history-of-the-thomas-kilmann-conflict-mode-instrument/

Kim, S., Bochatay, N., Relyea-Chew, A., Buttrick, E., Amdahl, C., Kim, L., & Lee, Y. M. (2017). Individual, interpersonal, and organisational factors of healthcare conflict: A scoping review. *Journal of Interprofessional Care*, *31*(3), 282–290. https://doi.org/10.1080/13561820.2016.1272558

Kong, E. (2008). The development of strategic management in the non-profit context: Intellectual capital in social service non-profit organizations. *International Journal of Management Reviews*, *10*(3), 281–299. https://doi.org/10.1111/j.1468-2370.2007.00224.x

Kouzes, J., & Posner, B. (2012). *The leadership challenge*. Jossey-Bass.

Kutney-Lee, A., Germack, H., Hatfield, L., Kelly, M. S., Maguire, M. P., Dierkes, A., & Aiken, L. H. (2016). Nurse engagement in shared governance and patient and nurse outcomes. *The Journal of Nursing Administration*, *46*(11), 605. https://doi.org/10.1097/NNA.0000000000000412

Lal, M. M. (2020). Why you need a nursing strategic plan. *Journal of Nursing Administration*, *50*(4), 183–184. https://doi.org/10.1097/NNA.0000000000000863

Mallon, W. T. (2019). Does strategic planning matter? *Academic Medicine*, *94*(10), 1408–1411. https://doi.org/10.1097/ACM.0000000000002848

Monavvarian, A., & Khamda, Z. (2010). Toward successful knowledge management: People development approach. *Business Strategy Series, 11*, 20–42. https://doi.org/10.1108/17515631011013096

McKibben, L. (2017). Conflict management: Importance and implications. *British Journal of Nursing, 26*(2), 100–103. https://doi.org/10.12968/bjon.2017.26.2.100

News@Northeastern. (2014, November 18). *'Generation Z' is entrepreneurial, wants to chart its own future.* Northeastern University. http://news.northeastern.edu/2014/11/18/generation-z-survey

Northeastern University. (2014). *Innovation imperative: Portrait of generation Z.* https://news.northeastern.edu/2014/11/18/generation-z-survey/

O'Grady, T. P., & Clavelle, J. T. (2021). Transforming shared governance: Toward professional governance for nursing. *JONA: The Journal of Nursing Administration, 51*(4), 206–211. https://doi.org/10.1097/NNA.0000000000000999

Palaima, T., & Skaržauskienė, A. (2010). Systems thinking as a platform for leadership performance in a complex world. *Baltic Journal of Management, 5*(3), 330–355. https://doi.org/10.1108/17465261011079749

Piryani, R. M., & Piryani, S. (2019). Conflict management in healthcare. *Journal of Nepal Health Research Council, 16*(41), 481–482. https://doi.org/10.33314/jnhrc.v16i41.1703

Prado-Inzerillo, M., Fitzpatrick, J., & Clavelle, J. (October 2018). Leadership practices and engagement among Magnet® hospital chief nurse officers. *The Journal of Nursing Administration, 48*(10), 502–507. https://doi.org/10.1097/NNA.0000000000000658

Redman, R., Pressler, S., Furspan, P., & Potempa, K. (2015). Nurses in the United States with a practice doctorate: Implications for leading in the current context of healthcare. *Nursing Outlook, 63*(2), 124–129. https://doi.org/10.1016/j.outlook.2014.08.003

Reid, P. P., Compton, W. D., Grossman, J. H., & Fangiang, G. (Eds.). (2005). *Building a better delivery system: A new engineering/health care partnership.* National Academies Press. https://www.ncbi.nlm.nih.gov/books/NBK22832/pdf/Bookshelf_NBK22832.pdf

Ronquillo, Y., Ellis, V. L., & Toney-Butler, T. J. (2020). *Conflict management.* StatPearls. https://pubmed.ncbi.nlm.nih.gov/29262184/

Schaffner, J. (2009). Roadmap for success: The 10-step nursing strategic plan. *Journal of Nursing Administration, 39*(4), 152–155. https://doi.org/10.1097/NNA.0b013e31819c9d28

Schiuma, G., & Lerro, A. (2008). Knowledge-based capital in building regional innovation capacity. *Journal of Knowledge Management, 12*(5), 121–136. https://doi.org/10.1108/13673270810902984

Schlaak, M. E. (2019). From nurse to nurse manager. *AAACN Viewpoint, 41*(2), 1–14. https://www.aaacn.org/viewpoint

Senge, P. (1990). *The fifth discipline.* Currency Doubleday.

Senge, P. M., Lichtenstein, B. B., Kaeufer, K., Bradbury, H., & Carroll, J. S. (2007). Collaborating for systemic change. *MIT Sloan Management Review, 2*, 44–54. https://sloanreview.mit.edu/article/collaborating-for-systemic-change

Sherman, R. O. (2017). *Transcending your comfort zone.* American Nurse Today. https://www.myamericannurse.com/wp-content/uploads/2017/09/ant9-Comfort-Zone-824.pdf

Trbovich, P. (2014). Five ways to incorporate systems thinking into healthcare organizations. *Biomedical Instrumentation & Technology, 48*(s2), 31–36. https://doi.org/10.2345/0899-8205-48.s2.31

Van Wicklin, S. A. (2021). Determining scope of practice. *Plastic Surgical Nursing, 41*(1), 40–42. https://doi.org/10.1097/PSN.0000000000000354

Wakefield, M. K., Williams, D. R., Le Menestrel, S., & Flaubert, J. L. (Eds.). (2021). *The future of nursing 2020–2030: Charting a path to achieve health equity.* National Academies Press. https://nam.edu/publications/the-future-of-nursing-2020-2030

SECTION VI

HEALTHCARE FINANCE AND BUDGETING

CHAPTER 18

MACRO COMPONENTS OF HEALTHCARE FINANCING

Nathanial Schreiner and Todd Nelson

"No society can surely be flourishing and happy, of which the far greater part of the members are poor and miserable."

Adam Smith

LEARNING OBJECTIVES

- Identify regulation and payment issues that affect an organization's finances.
- Describe an individual organization's payor mix, Case Mix Index (CMI), and benchmark database.
- Align care delivery models and staff performance with key safety and economic drivers (e.g., value-based purchasing, bundled payment).
- Formulate strategies to adjust operations to respond effectively to environmental changes in economic elements.

INTRODUCTION

Healthcare financing in the United States, specifically related to regulation and reimbursement, is a complex, dynamic phenomenon affecting clinical nursing care. For instance, despite spending the highest amount of total gross domestic product (GDP) on healthcare in the world, the United States has inferior health outcomes compared to other developed countries (Organisation for Economic Co-Operation and Development [OECD] Health Statistics, 2021). In fact, other developed countries only spend 8.6% of their GDP on average on healthcare as compared to the United States spending of 17% (OECD Health Statistics, 2021). This discrepancy between the cost and value of healthcare in the United States has prompted the government, which is the largest single payor of healthcare goods and services within the United States, to reevaluate how they reimburse healthcare in this country. This shift toward quality, often referred to as value-based, care has changed how healthcare facilities and providers deliver, document, track, and are ultimately reimbursed for the service of healthcare provided to patients. In this chapter, we aim to discuss the macroeconomics of healthcare financing, examining how monetary healthcare policy affects how hospitals and providers are reimbursed for services rendered. Moreover, we will examine how nurse executives and managers are affected and effect healthcare financing.

ECONOMIC PRINCIPLES

Economics, at its most basic level, revolves around principles of supply and demand, and this is true even when applied to the consumption of health and healthcare. Other economic principles, such as opportunity cost (what one is willing to give up in order to get something else), the assumption of rational decision-making, or the transparency of information, make up a myriad of factors that are used to predict why one chooses to seek healthcare. Entire books are devoted to fully describing the economics of health and healthcare, but, within this chapter, we are interested in how macroeconomic principles affect healthcare financing in the United States. Specifically, we examine: (a) What are the economic principles affecting healthcare financing? (b) How do these principles determine healthcare financing? and (c) What do nurse executives and managers need to understand about these principles in the context of healthcare financing?

To introduce and define economic principles integral to healthcare financing, we will first discuss these principles in terms of a simple consumer purchase, in this case, a television. When deciding to purchase a new television, a consumer would first need to have a reason for seeking out a new television (e.g., old one is broken, does not have the new bells and whistles, too small for a given room).

One fundamental economic principle assumes that consumers are rational decision makers. The *assumption of rational decision-making* posits that a consumer will make the best choice to meet their own demands given one's financial constraints. Thus, after realizing the demand for a new television exists, the consumer, based on assumption of rational decision-making, would potentially examine all available information (e.g., specifications, pricing, performance, warranty) on televisions to make an informed decision that best meets their needs.

In order to make this decision, the amount of information available to the consumer will directly affect their ability to make the most rational choice. The amount of information available to the consumer is known as *transparency*. The information on television specifications, performance, warranties, and pricing is ubiquitous thanks to the internet; thus, there is a high level of transparency of information guiding the consumer's decision of which television to purchase.

After thoroughly researching televisions, the consumer will potentially purchase one based on their needs. The *scarcity of resources* is the first factor a consumer will account for. Economists view time as the most scare resource. Thus, an individual must give up their time to get another resource. From the prospective of the consumer, they give up their time to work, thereby earning a wage; thus, money is the most scare resource in this scenario. This wage, represented in units of dollars, will determine the opportunity cost of the television. *Opportunity cost* is defined as what a person is willing to give up in order to get something else; in other words, how much money am I willing to give up in order to get the product (in this case, a television) I am most interested in purchasing? Finally, a consumer will use all these factors to establish the marginal analysis associated with purchasing the television. *Marginal analysis* is the process in which the consumer balances the cost of a product in relation to the benefit of the next, or marginal, unit. Thus, in our example, the consumer asks, "Does a television with a larger screen or more high-end features warrant a higher price?"

Now, you might be wondering, do these principles affect healthcare financing? As stated in the introduction, the dynamics of the U.S. healthcare system are far more complex than the decision-making process involved with purchasing a television. However, these principles still apply, albeit from a macroeconomic level, especially when factoring in governmental regulation, which is less straightforward. The first macroeconomic principle affecting healthcare financing in the United States we explore is gross GDP.

GROSS DOMESTIC PRODUCT AND HEALTHCARE SPENDING IN THE UNITED STATES

GDP is the totality of all goods and services produced within a country for a given year. The calculation of GDP takes into account consumer consumption (the largest component of GDP); investments, which are defined as the purchasing of new capital goods (e.g., a new medical office building or a telemetry system); government expenditures (e.g., Medicare and Medicaid programs); and exports (e.g., agricultural goods, such as soy sent to China), while subtracting the total amount of goods and services imported from other countries. In short, the GDP is an economic benchmark of how economically successful a country is. As depicted in Table 18.1, the United States leads the world in GDP.

TABLE 18.1: Top 10 Countries by Nominal GDP at Current U.S. Dollar Exchange Rates

Country	Nominal GDP (in trillions)	PPP Adjusted GDP (in trillions)	Annual Growth (%)	GDP Per Capita (in thousands)
United States	$21.43	$21.43	2.2	$65,298
China	$14.34	$23.52	6.1	$10,262
Japan	$5.08	$5.46	0.7	$40,247
Germany	$3.86	$4.68	0.6	$46,445
India	$2.87	$9.56	4.2	$2,100
United Kingdom	$2.83	$3.25	1.5	$42,330
France	$2.72	$3.32	1.5	$40,493.9
Italy	$2.00	$2.67	0.3	$33,228.2
Brazil	$1.84	$3.23	1.1	$8,717
Canada	$1.74	$1.93	1.7	$46,195

GDP, gross domestic product; PPP, purchasing power parity.

Source: Data from World Bank Group. (2021). GDP, PPP (current international $) – United States. The World Bank: Data. Retrieved July 19, 2022, from https://data.worldbank.org/indicator/NY.GDP.MKTP.PP.CD?locations=US.

TABLE 18.2: Healthcare Coverage in 2019

Source	Enrollment (millions/percentage of U.S. population)
Insured	293 (90.8%)
Private health insurance—Group	179 (55.4%)
Private health insurance–Non-group	42 (13.1%)
Medicare	58 (18.1%)
Medicaid/CHIP	64 (19.8%)
Military—TRICARE	9 (2.7%)
Military—VA Care	7 (2.2%)
Uninsured	30 (9.2%)

Notes: Individuals may have more than one type of coverage at a time (e.g., Medicare and Medicaid). Therefore, estimates by type of coverage are not mutually exclusive. CHIP, The State Children's Health Insurance Program. Medicaid/CHIP coverage estimate also includes all means-tested public coverage, such as state and locally financed public coverage.

Source: U.S. Census Bureau. (2020, September). *Health insurance coverage status and type of coverage by state—all persons: 2008 to 2019.* Table HIC-4_ACS. https://www.census.gov/data/tables/time-series/demo/health-insurance/historical-series/hic.html.

Thus, U.S. GDP indicates that U.S. citizens and companies, as well as the government, have strong purchasing power toward goods and services, including healthcare. The first caveat in healthcare we must address is the fact that few individuals pay for healthcare directly. In 2019, 90.8% of all people in the United States had some form of healthcare coverage; thus, healthcare is rarely financed directly by individual consumption. Instead, private or governmental insurance mechanisms are responsible for the majority of healthcare financing. In Table 18.2, we see that insurance provided by employers (both group and non-group) make up 68.5% of all individuals insured in the United States. Additionally, the U.S. government provides coverage for the remaining 22.3% of those individuals who are insured.

Nonetheless, in the U.S. healthcare system, there are three consumers of healthcare: private health insurance companies, the U.S. government, and individuals. The next section discusses how healthcare in the United States is financed.

HEALTHCARE REIMBURSEMENT IN THE UNITED STATES

As depicted in our television example, the payment for a good or service is relatively simple. A person has a need, determines what they are willing to give up to get that need satisfied, and then pays for the product. Conversely, traditionally within healthcare, a patient obtains services before payment is rendered to the provider. This reimbursement type is known as *fee-for-service*. To make the financing of healthcare even more complicated, as introduced in the previous section, most individuals do not pay for healthcare directly, with over 90% of Americans having some sort of private or governmental insurance. In short, most individuals in the United States pay insurance premiums and deductibles while incurring the cost of noncovered expenditures (e.g., cosmetic procedures). Thus, to describe the financing of healthcare in the United States, this chapter focuses on reimbursement from two payor sources: the U.S. government and private insurance.

U.S. GOVERNMENT REIMBURSEMENT

When it comes to the impact on the delivery of healthcare in the United States, the government is the 500-pound gorilla in the room. As stated previously, the U.S. government is the largest single consumer and payor of healthcare services in the United States. From an economic standpoint, being the largest consumer and payor of healthcare services would allow the government to negotiate the price of consumed healthcare services more effectively than smaller entities, such as a private insurance company. But the U.S. government does not need to rely on negotiation; instead, it has the power of administrative regulation. Thus, it has—and uses—this ability to set payments for services rendered by healthcare systems.

How the U.S. government determines the reimbursement rates for services rendered by healthcare systems is another complicated process. In a simplified form, the rate of reimbursement has relied upon provider/system documentation of the *International Classification of Diseases*, or *ICD-10*, codes, which are used to explain a diagnosis, and Current Procedural Terms, or *CPT*, codes, which are used to describe procedures that healthcare systems provide during the care of a patient. *ICD-10* codes are World Health Organization (WHO)-developed classifications of morbidity and mortality data allowing for interpretation and use in statistical health reporting as well as a decision support tool for resource allocation, reimbursement, clinical guidelines, and so on. CPT codes reflect medical, surgical, and diagnostic procedures associated with the care rendered to a patient based on their diagnosis-driven *ICD-10* codes.

These codes are used to determine a diagnostic-related group, or *DRG*, which determines the payment a healthcare system receives for treating the patient. Furthermore, the more DRGs a patient falls under, the higher amount of reimbursement the healthcare system will receive. The U.S. government also takes into account variations between patients and the healthcare system. For instance, Medicare makes additional payments to healthcare systems for capital costs, outlying cases, medical education, and indigent and/or Medicaid patients.

U.S. GOVERNMENT PAYOR SOURCES

The U.S. federal government provides healthcare funding through Medicare, Medicaid, and the Veterans Administration (VA) program. Table 18.2 breaks down the number of Americans receiving benefits from these three programs.

The Medicare program funds healthcare coverage for eligible adults aged 65 and over, as well as individuals with certain disabilities (Centers for Medicare & Medicaid Services [CMS], 2021a). This coverage is provided through four parts: A, B, C, and D. Part A provides inpatient/hospital coverage; Part B provides outpatient/medical coverage; Part C allows recipients to participate in the Medicare Advantage plans, in which private insurers (e.g., health maintenance organization [HMO], preferred provider organization [PPO]) contract with the federal government to provide healthcare services for a fixed rate; and Part D provides prescription drug coverage. Furthermore, all Medicare recipients are required to pay a monthly premium for Part B and some recipients pay a premium for Part A.

The Medicaid program funds healthcare coverage for eligible low-income adults, children, pregnant women, older adults, and people with disabilities (Medicaid.gov, 2021). Whereas Medicare is a federally funded program, Medicaid is funded both by federal and state entities, with funding administered by each state following federal guidelines. At the state level, eligibility for Medicaid is set based on each state's poverty level. Additionally, through the Children's Health Insurance Program (CHIP), children can receive healthcare through Medicaid even though their family is ineligible for Medicaid based on earned income.

The VA is a federally funded and administrated program that provides healthcare to military veterans. The system is comprised of 171 medical centers and 1,113 outpatient centers across the nation (Veterans Health Administration, 2022).

THE IMPORTANCE OF CASE MIX INDEX TO HEALTHCARE FINANCING

The Case Mix Index (CMI) is a valuable financial and clinical metric that healthcare systems use to estimate reimbursement from patients who are insured by Medicare and Medicaid. The CMI analyzes the relative severity of a patient population, which is directly proportional to DRG payments from Medicare and Medicaid. CMI is calculated by summing all the relative DRG weights for that specific fiscal period (e.g., month, quarter, year) and dividing that summed total by the total number of Medicare and Medicaid discharges for that specific period (CMS, n.d.). A higher CMI indicates a greater severity of illness of patients treated at that facility, resulting in a higher use of resources, thereby resulting in a higher rate of reimbursement.

PRIVATE INSURANCE REIMBURSEMENT

As alluded to in the previous section, private insurance lacks the administrative regulatory power of the U.S. government; thus, it must rely on negotiation with healthcare providers to determine reimbursement. The price a private insurer will negotiate to pay a healthcare system is a function of healthcare market dynamics. This health market dynamic is relative to market power held by the healthcare system relative to that of the private insurance entity; thus, healthcare systems with greater market power in a given area can leverage that power, thereby negotiating higher payments from private insurance. According to an analysis (Lopez & Neuman, 2020) of published, peer-reviewed articles comparing Medicare to private insurer payments, private insurers paid nearly double the Medicare rates for all hospital services (199% of Medicare rates, on average), with private insurance rates varying from 141% to 259% of Medicare rates across the reviewed studies.

THE IMPACT OF PAYOR MIX ON HEALTHCARE REIMBURSEMENT

Based on the difference in reimbursement between private insurers and U.S. government plans, such as Medicare and Medicaid, one can surmise having more privately insured patients will result in stronger healthcare system profits. Thus, this mix of payor sources, which is known as *payor mix*, is an important healthcare metric directly related to the financial health of a healthcare system. Payer mix is calculated as a percentage of those patients who have government health insurance versus private health insurance. Thus, the lower one's payor mix is (which is expressed as a percentage), the more profitable the health system will be. For example, Frenz (2020) demonstrated that hospitals need an *operating margin*, which is calculated by subtracting operating expenses from total revenue, of 2.5% to remain solvent. Those hospitals with a payor mix of 70% or less reached this 2.5% operating margin 80% of the time, while those with a payor mix of greater than 70% only reached this 2.5% operating margin 63% of the time, indicating that these hospitals struggled to maintain financial solvency.

◼ WHAT EVERY NURSE MANAGER NEEDS TO KNOW ABOUT HEALTHCARE REIMBURSEMENT

Understanding one's payor mix is important for nurse managers because it is one major index of a hospital system's financial health that has major implications to reimbursement but is something that is not readily clinically transparent or relatable. From a nursing perspective, a hospital could be at inpatient capacity, causing patients to be admitted to the ED; thus, from a care delivery/clinical standpoint, the hospital should be profitable. However, due to a reimbursement derived from that hospital's payor mix, clinical care provided does not equate to equal profits. The ability of a nurse manager to explain how payor mix affects reimbursement to clinical staff can alleviate misconceptions arising from high clinical census/acuity that do not align with hospital profitability. The nurse manager who also understands payor mix can also better justify clinical needs (e.g., equipment, staffing) in relation to operating margin.

◼ WHAT EVERY NURSE EXECUTIVE NEEDS TO KNOW ABOUT HEALTHCARE REIMBURSEMENT

A nurse executive needs to understand payor mix from an organizational perspective, whereas the nurse manager's understanding of payor mix is applicable at a unit level. While current payor mix will affect clinical services currently rendered within a healthcare organization, forecasted fluctuations in these levels should help determine clinical decisions at an organizational level. For instance, if there is an identified need for an expanded service line (e.g., trauma designation for the ED), a major determining factor of moving forward with this capital commitment is the forecasted payor mix associated with this change in clinical dynamics. Thus, will the return on investment (ROI), which is determined by the volume of additional patients multiplied by the average reimbursement for services rendered (i.e., payor mix), offset the cost of adding the service (e.g., construction, staffing, resources, training)? Current and forecasted payor mix is a financial index that can help a nurse executive make a fully informed clinical decision based on a quantified metric associated with current and future viability of a healthcare organization.

⬢ CASE SCENARIO

PAYOR MIX SCENARIO A

SITUATION

The government has just announced that they are expanding the Affordable Care Act (ACA) in order to provide increased comprehensive coverage to a larger pool of individuals at a lower cost through an increase in government subsidies. How might this change in privately insured patients affect the associated payer mix at a hospital?

APPROACH

The nurse manager or nursing executive would need to examine the current payor mix focusing on previously uninsured or Medicaid patients to estimate the potential increase in revenue based on how many of these individuals would be expected to be covered by the changes in ACA coverage. The nurse manager would focus on payor mix associated with their individual unit, while the executive would look across their service line or all clinical units in respect to forecasting a change in revenue.

OUTCOME

The increase in privately insured patients should improve the payor mix of patients served at the hospital, thus positively affecting the operating margin of the hospital.

DISCUSSION QUESTION

1. From a revenue perspective, what may be the clinical impact of changes in payor mix?

⬢ CASE SCENARIO

PAYOR MIX SCENARIO B

SITUATION

You are the manager of ambulatory care services at a rural teaching hospital. Resident physicians at one of the ambulatory clinics you oversee state there is a population need for expanded surgical consultations. Patients wait for up to 6 weeks before they can be seen at this particular clinic. This specific surgical clinic sees uninsured or Medicaid patients requiring general surgical consultation or follow-up. Patients are required to pay a minimum fee-for-services, although services are rendered on an income-based sliding scale, with most patients paying pennies on the dollar compared to privately insured patients. Based on the patient population provided earlier, how do you reply to the resident's inquiry into expanding consultation services at the clinic based on your knowledge of payor mix?

APPROACH

The manager would be best served approaching the resident's inquiry by first recognizing the needs of the patient population served by the clinic and then introducing that the capacity of the clinic in meeting those needs is limited due to the financial constraints associated with the low reimbursement associated with the patients treated.

OUTCOME

Due to the payor mix of the population of the patients seen at the surgical clinic, the hospital system writes off and accounts the majority of services provided at the clinic as charity care. The hospital system is committed to serving the healthcare needs of the community, but also balancing these patient needs with the fiscal responsibility in order to serve the needs of other patient populations.

DISCUSSION QUESTION

1. A common point of contention between clinical staff and hospital administration is the disconnect between maximizing profit and maximizing patient care. How might the nurse leader address this issue with staff?

⬢ CASE SCENARIO

PAYOR MIX SCENARIO C

SITUATION

You are the director of nursing (DON) at a long-term care facility. Your administrator let you know that corporate has decided to apply for a Medicaid waiver in order to start accepting Medicaid residents. Based on your knowledge of payor mix, how could this decision affect facility reimbursement? Additionally, could this change in payor mix affect clinical operations?

APPROACH

The DON discusses with the administrator the forecasted change in the facility's CMI. Within this discussion, the DON should take into account current facility occupancy rates as well. Thus, the DON needs to ask the question: "Is the facility currently at full capacity or was the application for the Medicaid waiver in response to unfilled beds within the facility?"

DISCUSSION QUESTION

1. Based on this scenario, is CMI or volume the more important factor in moving forward with the Medicaid waiver? Can there be a financially beneficial outcome within this situation?

CASE SCENARIO

PAYOR MIX SCENARIO D

SITUATION

You are the program director of emergency services. In a meeting with your chief nursing officer (CNO), they tell you to collaborate with the marketing and finance departments on developing a budget for becoming a certified chest pain center with percutaneous coronary intervention. What metrics should you ask the marketing and finance departments for to help inform your operational budget?

APPROACH

As the director, you should work the marketing and finance departments to obtain financial metrics, such as forecasted payor mix and CMI, as well as the project increase in patient volume associated with the estimated demand for the new service.

DISCUSSION QUESTION

1. If the volume of patients, CMI, and overall payor mix does not appear to offset the cost of adding and continuing to operate this new service, how should the director approach the CNO? How should the director use their knowledge of metrics that determine hospital reimbursement in their response to the CNO?

A SHIFT TOWARD VALUE-BASED HEALTHCARE

We now examine how value, or the quality of care, intersects these two entities when determining healthcare financing. When revisiting Table 18.1, one would assume, based on the economical principle of marginal analysis, that the United States would be leading the world in health outcomes related to the vast amount of GDP expenditures. But here lies the disconnect: Despite spending the highest amount of GDP in the world on healthcare services, the United States has poor healthcare outcomes in comparison to other developed countries which spend far less money on healthcare, as depicted in Figure 18.1.

An analysis conducted by the Commonwealth Fund (2021) found that U.S. healthcare ranks last overall in comparison with other high-income countries. This analysis compared the United States to other developed countries using healthcare indicators of access, care process, administrative efficiency, equity, and outcomes and found the United States ranked last among all countries except in the category of care process (Commonwealth Fund, 2021). Table 18.3 presents a synopsis of these findings.

These reports indicate that the consumer of healthcare, whether the payor is the government, private insurer, or individual, is not getting "value" for what they paid for. Thus, the opportunity cost of U.S. healthcare is poor; the payor gives up the most (in dollars) to get poor outcomes as compared to other developed countries. There are many reasons for this disconnect between value and cost within U.S. healthcare: high cost of care (e.g., innovation in medical technology and pharmaceuticals), lack of insurance coverage, a lack of transparency (i.e., information related to the cost and quality of services rendered), a lack of access to care (e.g., primary care and specialists), and preventable medical errors (Kumar et al., 2011; LiPuma & Robichaud, 2020; Shmerling, 2021). Thus, to address many of these identified

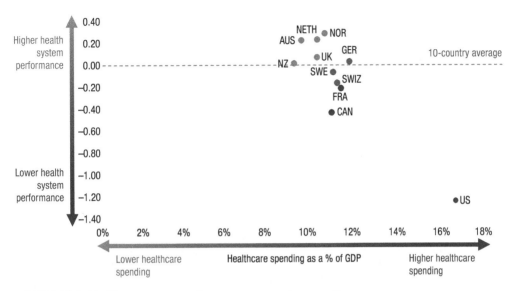

FIGURE 18.1: Healthcare system performance compared to spending.

AUS, Australia; CAN, Canada; FRA, France; GDP, gross domestic product; GER, Germany; NETH, Netherlands; NOR, Norway; NZ, New Zealand; SWE, Sweden; SWIZ, Switzerland; UK, United Kingdom, US, United States.

Source: Reproduced with permission from Schneider, E. C., Shah, A., Doty, M. M., Tikkanen, R., Fields, K., & Williams, R. D., II. (2021, August). *Mirror, mirror 2021: Reflecting poorly: Health care in the U.S. compared to other high-income countries.* Commonwealth Fund. https://doi.org/10.26099/01DV-H208.

TABLE 18.3: Healthcare System Performance Rankings

	AUS	CAN	FRA	GER	NETH	NZ	NOR	SWE	SWIZ	UK	US
Overall ranking	3	10	8	5	2	6	1	7	9	4	11
Access to care	8	9	7	3	1	5	2	6	10	4	11
Care process	6	4	10	9	3	1	8	11	7	5	2
Administrative efficiency	2	7	6	9	8	3	1	5	10	4	11
Equity	1	10	7	2	5	9	8	6	3	4	11
Healthcare outcomes	1	10	6	7	4	8	2	5	3	9	11

AUS, Australia; CAN, Canada; FRA, France; GER, Germany; NETH, Netherlands; NOR, Norway; NZ, New Zealand; SWE, Sweden; SWIZ, Switzerland; UK, United Kingdom; US, United States.

Source: Reproduced with permission from Schneider, E. C., Shah, A., Doty, M. M., Tikkanen, R., Fields, K., & Williams, R. D., II. (2021, August). *Mirror, mirror 2021: Reflecting poorly: Health care in the U.S. compared to other high-income countries.* Commonwealth Fund. https://doi.org/10.26099/01DV-H208.

issues within the U.S. healthcare system, a shift toward a "value-based" healthcare delivery and reimbursement model was implemented.

Porter (2010) defined value in healthcare as outcome dependent; thus, value should be determined by outcomes achieved and not the volume of services rendered, nor by the process of care utilized to achieve these outcomes. Thus, in value-based healthcare, the ability of healthcare agencies to meet the demands of consumers of care is the central tenet (Porter, 2010). In the most basic form, value in healthcare is calculated by determining quality, measured via health outcomes, divided by the cost of achieving those outcomes (Porter, 2010).

Thus, the better the outcome achieved in the most efficient way (e.g., costing less), the higher the value. This value-based philosophy has been adopted by the U.S. government and private insurers to improve health-related outcomes of those they insure; thus, hospital systems are now paid for performance and not by volume as they were in the past. Furthermore, the use of health-related metrics, such as hospital-acquired infections and inpatient falls, allows the payors to withhold financial reimbursement for preventable medical errors or poor performance related to health outcomes, such as high readmission rates.

THE TRIPLE/QUADRUPLE AIM

The *Triple Aim* is a healthcare reform initiative focused on tackling three identified concerns facing the U.S. healthcare system: improving the experience of care, improving the health of populations, and reducing per capita costs of healthcare (Berwick et al., 2008). The Triple Aim is often referred to as the *Quadruple Aim* after an additional focus on reducing clinician and staff burnout was added to this initiative (Bodenheimer & Sinsky, 2014; Sikka et al., 2015).

The Institute of Healthcare Improvement (IHI) is the organization responsible for implementing the Quadruple Aim, although hospital outcomes associated with the Quadruple Aim are reported to nonprofits, such as the Leapfrog Group; governmental agencies, including the CMS; and accrediting bodies, like The Joint Commission (TJC). Thus, the Quadruple Aim's focus on quality has permeated the healthcare industry with metrics tied to healthcare system accreditation and reimbursement. For instance, due to this shift toward value driven by the Quadruple Aim, TJC expectations of hospital quality metrics include their relevance to patient safety or quality of care, contribution to positive health outcomes to patients, meeting or surpassing regulatory standards, and accuracy and ease of quantification. The establishment of the mandated reporting of quantified, quality-related healthcare metrics increased the transparency of how healthcare systems delivered care to patients, thus justifying the cost of care to the payor (Park et al., 2018). This value-based methodology rooted in clinical quality allowed the U.S. government to establish quality benchmarks that would affect hospital reimbursement.

THE IMPORTANCE OF CLINICAL QUALITY TO HEALTHCARE FINANCING

Clinical quality has always been a priority of healthcare providers, but now, clinical quality is a primary indicator of a healthcare system's financial viability. The CMS uses these quality metrics to rate hospitals using a Star Rating system and makes this Star Rating public knowledge via the *Hospital Compare* website (CMS, 2021b). The calculation of the Star Rating is a complicated process. Simplified, healthcare systems first submit clinical quality metrics to a myriad of CMS programs: Inpatient Quality Reporting (IQR), Outpatient Quality Reporting (OQR), Hospital Readmission Reduction Program (HRRP), Hospital Acquired Conditions (HAC) Reduction, and Hospital Value-Based Purchasing (HVBP). Then the CMS standardizes quality measures from each hospital, allowing comparison between hospitals. Scores are then grouped into five broad categories: mortality, safety of care, readmission, patient experience, and timely and effective care. These grouped scores are averaged and then a specific weight is applied to each group. Then hospitals are placed in like-groupings and split into five groups, which determine a hospital's Star Rating.

This public, searchable Star Rating affects healthcare reimbursement from two perspectives. First, the Star Rating is a consumer tool. It improves consumer transparency of quality in terms of care rendered to patients; thus, it allows them to choose a facility that demonstrates high value (i.e., quality/cost). Prospective patients are thereby better informed on the quality versus cost of the service and can make an informed decision based on this information. For instance, by applying the assumption of rational decision-making, a patient will seek out information on healthcare facilities that provide the best care in relation to that cost of care. A rational consumer of healthcare would choose the highest rated facility in order to secure the best care for their healthcare needs.

Second, the CMS uses these metrics to reimburse healthcare systems. Some reimbursement programs are voluntary, such as Accountable Care Organizations, in which healthcare organizations are fiscally rewarded for efficient high-quality care while keeping the cost of care manageable. Other reimbursement programs are involuntary, such as the Hospital Based Value Purchasing Program, in which 2% of Medicare dollars are withheld and hospitals are allotted a certain amount of this withheld reimbursement based on quality achievement and improvement, with poorer performing facilities having a greater portion of this 2% withheld. When recalling the 2.5% operating margin as a rule-of-thumb determining the fiscal solvency of a healthcare system, having a portion or all of 2% of Medicare dollars withheld could have significant fiscal, and ultimately clinical, ramifications, especially to those facilities who serve a high proportion of Medicare patients.

As introduced in an earlier section of this chapter, healthcare reimbursement was based on a fee-for-services model, which has also been referred to as a disease treatment model, in which quantity of services was the driving mode of fiscal opportunity for the healthcare system. With the emergence of an emphasis on quality and cost containment, alternative methods of reimbursement, namely *bundled payments*, are becoming a standard of healthcare reimbursement. Instead of separate payments made across the continuum of care, a single payment is made to the hospital system. This single payment encourages all actors participating in the care of the patient (e.g., inpatient, post-acute, outpatient, physicians) to coordinate care delivery, thus aligning treatment and health goals of the patient in order to maximize efficiency. According to the American Hospital Association (AHA), 31% of U.S. community hospitals participated in bundled payment models during 2019 (AHA, 2021). Bundled payments are another example of how the expectation of quality care has been relegated to healthcare systems and providers; thus, healthcare systems and providers are now exposed to financial risk associated with poor patient outcomes. As a result, healthcare systems, especially those that participate in ACOs or receive bundled payments, are best served by adopting a healthcare model of promoting preventive healthcare, as the risk associated with poorly managed care has financial ramifications to these institutions.

◼ WHAT EVERY NURSE MANAGER NEEDS TO KNOW ABOUT CLINICAL QUALITY'S IMPACT ON HEALTHCARE REIMBURSEMENT

This is where the rubber meets the road, especially in acute, sub-acute, and long-term care settings. Nursing is the fulcrum by which patient care revolves; thus, if nursing is informed, empowered, engaged, and competent in providing quality, cost-effective care, patient outcomes will reflect this dedication to clinical quality. A nurse manager should be able to understand and articulate clinical benchmarks through analysis of benchmark utilization reports affecting healthcare reimbursement.

Broadly speaking, *benchmarking* is the practice of making structured comparisons of processes linked to outcomes to determine best clinical practice. For instance, determining factors of the CMS HVBP Program are heavily clinically oriented: 25% clinical outcomes, 25% person and community engagement, 25% safety, and 25% efficiency and cost reduction (CMS, 2021c). Benchmark utilization reports should focus on clinical outcomes (e.g., core measures), patient satisfaction (e.g., Hospital Consumer Assessment of Healthcare Providers and Systems [HCAHPS] scores), patient safety (e.g., fall rate, hospital-acquired infection rate), and cost reduction (e.g., readmission rates; Ettorchi-Tardy et al., 2012). These benchmarks serve as a quantitative guide that allows the nurse manager to drill down into the qualitative, or operational, minutia. Benchmark utilization is an essential tool for quality assurance (QA), a catalyst for staff-driven quality improvement (QI) initiatives, and the foundation for policy creation and remediation at the unit level. Clinical benchmarks also serve as an early warning sign of operational issues, such as the impact of inadequate staffing on the quality of care, or a change in operational needs, such as an influx of patients with higher acuity or specialized, care-intensive diagnoses. A successful nurse manager should be able to interpret these clinical benchmarks, educate the clinical and fiscal importance of these benchmarks to their staff, and incorporate these benchmarks into continuous, staff-driven, unit-based, quality assessment/improvement. This attention to clinical quality driven by benchmarking at the unit level will support the overall fiscal viability of any healthcare system.

 ## WHAT EVERY NURSE EXECUTIVE NEEDS TO KNOW ABOUT CLINICAL QUALITY'S IMPACT ON HEALTHCARE REIMBURSEMENT

Every nurse executive should understand the dynamics among clinical quality, reimbursement, and the fiscal viability of a healthcare system. Whereas the nurse manager focuses on clinical quality at a unit level, the nurse executive needs to examine, interpret, and influence clinical quality indicators and benchmarks from an organizational level. The nurse executive should rely on these benchmarks to justify current operational budgets and future clinical investments or programs. Furthermore, quarterly or yearly changes in these benchmarks indicate the success of QA/QI projects and initiatives when trending toward mandated or organizational goals, or the need for a root-cause analysis in order to address substandard performance associated with specific clinical benchmarks. The nurse executive's ability to fluently interpret how clinical benchmarks impact a healthcare system's financing allows the individual to align clinical needs and concerns to the fiscal well-being of the healthcare system using value-driven metrics, thereby promoting and supporting both the fiscal and clinical goals of the institution.

⬡ CASE SCENARIO

VALUE-BASED CARE SCENARIO A

SITUATION

You are the new manager of a medical–surgical floor. You would like your staff to develop clinical QA/QI projects as part of your hospital's clinical ladder initiative. Your staff would like your input on what the QA/QI projects should focus on. What clinical areas should you suggest your staff to focus on when developing QA/QI projects?

APPROACH

This situation presents you the unique opportunity to align clinical processes and patient outcomes with supporting the fiscal success of the hospital. You should not only use clinical benchmarks to determine what QA/QI project is of high priority, you should also engage the staff by soliciting their observations and ideas while also being mindful of your available resources to allocate to potential projects.

DISCUSSION QUESTION

I.   What if staff suggestions differ from what the clinical benchmark utilization indicates should be taken on as the QA/QI project? What criteria should you as the manager prioritize to guide your decision of which project to choose?

⬡ CASE SCENARIO

VALUE-BASED CARE SCENARIO B

SITUATION

You are the bed-coordinator/nursing supervisor for a 100-bed hospital. A nursing-driven, research-based QI initiative is to expedite the admission of patients from the ED to inpatient floors. This initiative was created due to the identification of above-average complications, including death, associated with prolonged stays in the ED. One evening, the ED is very busy, and you assign an ICU multiple patients at once due to their bed availability. The ED charge nurse calls you and informs you that the ICU is refusing to take multiple patients. When you arrive in the ICU, the staff tells you that it is unfair that they are getting all of these admissions and "The bottom line is more important than good patient care!" How do you respond to the pushback from the ICU staff?

APPROACH

You should incorporate your knowledge of clinical benchmarking (i.e., avoidable patient complications) and recent scientific evidence suggesting that prolonged stays in the ED after disposition to the floor increases the risk for poor health outcomes (i.e., increasing patient morbidity and mortality) in order to breach this impasse between nurses.

DISCUSSION QUESTION

1.   What happens if the ICU continues to push back on future admissions during the evening? How should you approach the situation or what additional actions should be taken?

KEY POINTS

- Unlike other goods and services, or even similar services in other countries, spending more on healthcare in the United States has not led to improved outcomes or higher quality.
- Understanding consumer behavior as it relates to the purchase of healthcare services is challenging due to a number of factors such as lack of transparency in cost data, lack of understanding and accepted definition of quality, and third-party payor involvement in the middle of the process.
- The intersection between cost, quality, and satisfaction are all factors considered in the shift to value-based care.
- Reimbursement rates and methodologies differ based on who is the ultimate payor for services—and understanding how those rates are established, affected, and adjusted by various clinical factors is key to understanding overall payment.
- The impact of clinical practice on quality measures, and therefore payment, has the ability to increase the collaboration and influence with financial colleagues.

SUMMARY

Although healthcare financing is exponentially more complex than a simple consumer transaction, as demonstrated throughout the chapter, economic principles that explain and guide consumer decisions are relevant and have significant influence on the financing of healthcare organizations. Due to a misalignment between cost and quality, payors have shifted how they reimburse healthcare organizations, moving from a quantity, fee-for-service, illness-driven model to a preventive care-driven model, in which value for both the patient and payor, in terms of outcomes and efficiency, are expected and in which exceeding expectations receive additional monetary reimbursement. Nurse managers and executives need to be familiar with current healthcare reimbursement policy, demonstrate understanding of payor mix and associated metrics (i.e., CMI), and develop unit and/or organization clinical policies, staff education and training, and QA/QI projects that focus on clinical-based, quality-driven benchmarked outcomes that affect the financial viability of a healthcare organization. As reimbursement for healthcare becomes even more dependent of the quality of patient outcomes, nursing now is placed in a unique and equally important position to assume a major role in the financial success of any healthcare organization.

END-OF-CHAPTER RESOURCES

◯ DISCUSSION QUESTIONS

1. Based on the economic principles presented in the chapter, how does the consumer decision to seek healthcare differ from an emergent situation (ST-elevated myocardial infarction) as compared to a non-emergent situation (cataract surgery)?

2. How does a shift in payor mix affect financial reimbursement for a healthcare entity?

3. How did the fee-for-service reimbursement model contribute to the disconnect between cost and quality in U.S. healthcare?

4. What are the three components of the Triple Aim?

5. How does value-based care align clinical and financial outcomes within the healthcare setting?

6. How does clinical quality measured by benchmarked patient outcomes contribute to healthcare financing?

 A robust set of instructor resources designed to supplement this text is located at http://connect.springerpub.com/content/book/978-0-8261-7795-7. Qualifying instructors may request access by emailing textbook@springerpub.com.

REFERENCES

American Hospital Association. (2021). *Bundled payment: AHA*. American Hospital Association. https://www.aha.org/bundled-payment

Berwick, D. M., Nolan, T. W., & Whittington, J. (2008). The Triple Aim: Care, health, and cost. *Health Affairs, 27*(3), 759–769. https://doi.org/10.1377/hlthaff.27.3.759

Bodenheimer, T., & Sinsky, C. (2014). From Triple to Quadruple Aim: Care of the patient requires care of the provider. *The Annals of Family Medicine, 12*(6), 573–576. https://doi.org/10.1370/afm.1713

Centers for Medicare & Medicaid Services. (n.d.). *Case Mix Index*. CMS.gov. https://www.cms.gov/Medicare/Medicare-Fee-for-Service-Payment/AcuteInpatientPPS/Acute-Inpatient-Files-for-Download-Items/CMS022630

Centers for Medicare & Medicaid Services. (2021a, December 1). *Hospital compare*. CMS.gov. https://www.cms.gov/Medicare/Quality-Initiatives-Patient-Assessment-Instruments/HospitalQualityInits/HospitalCompare

Centers for Medicare & Medicaid Services. (2021b, December 1). *Hospital value-based purchasing program*. CMS.gov. https://www.cms.gov/Medicare/Quality-Initiatives-Patient-Assessment-Instruments/HospitalQualityInits/Hospital-Value-Based-Purchasing

Centers for Medicare & Medicaid Services. (2021c, January 19). *2019 Medicare enrollment section*. CMS.gov. https://www.cms.gov/research-statistics-data-systems/cms-program-statistics/2019-medicare-enrollment-section#Total

Commonwealth Fund. (2021). *Mirror, mirror 2021: Reflecting poorly*. from https://www.commonwealthfund.org/publications/fund-reports/2021/aug/mirror-mirror-2021-reflecting-poorly.

Ettorchi-Tardy, A., Levif, M., & Michel, P. (2012). Benchmarking: A method for continuous quality improvement in health. *Healthcare Policy, 7*(4), 101–119. https://doi.org/10.12927/hcpol.2012.22872

Frenz, D. A. (2020, March 20). What's your payer mix? *Today's Hospitalist*. https://www.todayshospitalist.com/insurer-payer-mix/

Kumar, S., Ghildayal, N. S., & Shah, R. N. (2011). Examining quality and efficiency of the US healthcare system. *International Journal of Health Care Quality Assurance, 24*(5), 366–388. https://doi.org/10.1108/09526861111139197

LiPuma, S. H., & Robichaud, A. L. (2020). Deliver us from injustice: Reforming the U.S. healthcare system. *Journal of Bioethical Inquiry*, 17(2), 257–270. https://doi.org/10.1007/s11673-020-09961-2

Lopez, E. F., & Neuman, T. (2020, May 1). *How much more than Medicare do private insurers pay? A review of the literature*. Kaiser Family Foundation. https://www.kff.org/medicare/issue-brief/how-much-more-than-medicare-do-private-insurers-pay-a-review-of-the-literature/

Medicaid.gov. (2021). *Medicaid*. https://www.medicaid.gov/medicaid/index.html

Organisation for Economic Co-operation and Development Health Statistics. (2021). *Health at a glance 2021: OECD indicators*. https://www.oecd.org/health/health-data.htm

Park, B., Gold, S. B., Bazemore, A., & Liaw, W. (2018). How evolving United States payment models influence primary care and its impact on the Quadruple Aim. *The Journal of the American Board of Family Medicine*, 31(4), 588–604. https://doi.org/10.3122/jabfm.2018.04.170388

Porter, M. E. (2010). What is value in health care? *New England Journal of Medicine*, 363(26), 2477–2481. https://doi.org/10.1056/nejmp1011024

Shmerling, R. (2021, July 13). *Is our healthcare system broken?* Harvard Health. https://www.health.harvard.edu/blog/is-our-healthcare-system-broken-202107132542

Sikka, R., Morath, J. M., & Leape, L. (2015). The Quadruple Aim: Care, health, cost and meaning in work. *BMJ Quality & Safety*, 24(10), 608–610. http://dx.doi.org/10.1136/bmjqs-2015-004160

Veterans Health Administration. (2022, May 24). *Veterans Health Administration*. Retrieved June 12, 2022, from https://www.va.gov/health

CHAPTER 19

DEVELOPING FINANCIAL ACUMEN FOR NURSE LEADERS

Deborah J. Stilgenbauer

"Leadership and learning are indispensable to each other."

John F. Kennedy

LEARNING OBJECTIVES

- Describe current trends and challenges in healthcare as related to financial resources.
- Identify key dimensions of financial stewardship for nurse leaders.
- Analyze outcomes of key assumptions in budget development.
- Evaluate various budget calculations for management of resources.

INTRODUCTION

Healthcare today is extremely complex. Globally, healthcare organizations are facing the challenges of higher cost for providing care and increased cuts in reimbursement (Asamani et al., 2016). Optimal financial performance of an organization requires a combination of strategy, operational efficiency, and environmental conditions (Moseley, 2017). Current healthcare settings provide the nurse leader with many competing priorities and endless decision-making opportunities. Acutely ill patients, shorter lengths of stay, advancing technology, focus on patient and employee engagement, quality indicators, and patient outcomes are daily concerns. Staffing is a daily challenge in every healthcare setting and the most time-consuming responsibility nurse leaders contend with.

Almost every decision made by nurse leaders has a financial implication. The nurse leader's role has changed significantly and now includes human and financial management (Naranjee et al., 2019). Schedule management, over- or understaffing, poor patient outcomes, lack of focus on engagement, and turnover all affect financial performance. The scope of nurse executives and leaders includes management of as much as 50% of a hospital budget (Brydges et al., 2019). Management of the nursing resources has a significant effect on the overall financial health of an organization.

Outside influences, regulatory agencies, the Affordable Care Act (ACA), the Centers for Medicare & Medicaid Services (CMS), Hospital Consumer Assessment of Healthcare Providers and Systems (HCAHPS), and Value-Based Purchasing (VBP) focus on patient outcomes, patient experience and affect reimbursement. VBP applies to services paid by Medicare and shifts the healthcare delivery system from disease management to disease prevention (Aroh et al., 2015). Since the advent of VBP and HCAHPS, the direct relationship between nursing practice and reimbursement is transparent. Under VBP, metrics are collected, and higher performing hospitals receive higher payments compared to lower performing hospitals (Aroh et al., 2015).

The connection between reimbursement and practice results in organizations being laser focused on quality, as well as cost reduction, and the nurse leader is at the forefront.

Understanding and knowledge of healthcare costs provide insight into challenges confronting nurse leaders (Naranjee et al., 2019).

Reimbursement from payors, government, commercial insurers, or self-pay cover the expenses of providing care and paying the bills. If revenue exceeds expenses, the dollars can be reinvested in additional staffing, new equipment, technology, and so on. Conversely, if revenue does not cover the cost of expenses, an organization must carefully review expenses and make adjustments.

Chief nurse executives (CNEs), chief nursing officers (CNOs), and nurse leaders at all levels must understand the elements of finance as it pertains to the practice setting and understand how to advocate for and manage the resources. Clinical nurses are often unaware of the role their practice has on an organization's finances. Nurse leaders play a critical role in the education of frontline staff regarding how their practice affects the financial health of the organization.

Hospital-acquired conditions (HACs) can have serious implications for patients and may result in reduction or nonpayment for services. The unit level leader's role is to engage staff, seek their input, and develop strategies for addressing issues of financial concern.

Hospital-acquired pressure injuries (HAPIs), catheter-associated urinary tract infections (CAUTIs), central line-associated bloodstream infections (CLABSIs), and falls resulting in injuries are conditions that can be avoided. Nursing has an opportunity to influence value-based payment by implementing quality improvements and providing care that is evidence based in clinical and patient experience domains (Aroh et al., 2015).

Nurse executives must align with nurse leaders at all levels including frontline staff to be successful at financial management. Nursing staff are delivering care; their practice determines patient outcomes, the use of supplies, and productivity. Managing the finances, and making prudent decisions that positively impact expenses, leads to collaboration and mutual respect with finance colleagues. Finance executives respect nurse leaders who understand and make finances a key responsibility of their role and listen closely to what they have to say. Nurse leaders need to be at finance meetings as it relates to their span of control to understand and speak the language of finance colleagues. Nurse leaders become empowered to work with finance executives and provide evidence to support the needed resources to improve patient care.

Nurse leaders are chief executive officers (CEOs) of small companies (patient care units, clinics, divisions) that make up a larger organization. Many unit leaders are managing multimillion dollar budgets for units made up of personnel that perform different functions with one goal, the provision of care and the best patient outcomes. Nurse executives are stewards of hundreds of millions of dollars in their roles as vice presidents, CNEs, CNOs, directors of nursing, or any of the many titles that make up the table of organization (T of O).

The focus of the chapter is to examine different types of budgets, stages of the budget development, and management. There are various models and timelines for developing a budget; however, all have similar critical elements. Regardless of the model, it is critical for nurse leaders to have input and understand what is included, how it is determined, and provide quantitative data to support requests. Once the budget is developed, it must be implemented and managed. Financial and operational reports provide useful information related to budgeted versus actual expense. Variances will need to be analyzed and explained to senior leadership and the finance department. There are controllable and uncontrollable factors that affect expense, so ongoing review is necessary. Educating frontline staff about practice and decisions that affect expense will support the nurse leader and the financial goal of the organization.

CONCEPTS OF THE BUDGET PROCESS

WHAT IS A BUDGET?

A budget is a plan for procuring resources to allocate in a finite period, usually 1 year. The assumptions are based on historical data and forecasting trends.

The budget is one of the most important administrative tools for a nurse leader and an organization; it is a road map to support the organization as it seeks to achieve financial health. As nurses, we do not like to think of healthcare as a business; however, there is tremendous overhead. For example, labor is 65% of overall expense. There are also supplies, equipment, utilities, insurance, and dollars available for contingencies. In 2020, a global pandemic affected healthcare systems around the world. The economic effect on organizations was beyond most contingency plans. Across the county and world, we watched acute care hospitals increase capacity in some cases by 50% to 100%. The increase in volume required additional staffing, medications, oxygen, and supplies. Many organizations received relief dollars from the Federal Emergency Management Agency (FEMA); however, to be better prepared, organizations will have to incorporate lessons learned from COVID-19 into future budgets.

The types of budgets nurse leaders develop focus on labor and supply expense associated with a patient care unit, service, or division. Budgeting consists of three phases: planning, implementation, and management. The planning phase occurs 6 to 9 months prior to implementation. Countless variables are considered in this phase, many out of the control of the nurse leader, such as patient volume, changes in patient population, new technologies, turnover, and leaves of absence (LOAs). Nurse leaders hold the key to monitoring and tracking variables and can use historical data and trends to plan for the coming year budgets. One example is an ICU that has a cyclical resignation trend. There is a cadre of RNs hired into positions in the ICU each year who ultimately want to apply to a nurse anesthetist (NA) program. One of the requirements for the program is 2 years of experience working in an ICU. The nurse leader can track the 2-year anniversaries of the nurses who plan to attend an NA program in a specific year and anticipate the resignations. The vacancy information is used when budgeting overtime (OT) or orientation expenses for the coming year.

Everything cannot be anticipated for budget preparation in the healthcare environment; however, the more data nurse leaders have to support the unit needs, the better equipped they are for developing a budget that is appropriate for the coming year.

The finance department is data driven, and for that reason nurse leaders need to be able to support budget proposals with data. Anecdotal notes with quantitative data plus information from available reports are excellent sources of information that empower the nurse leader to project and advocate for resources. Evidence-based findings and best practices should also be considered when planning the budget. The finance team in most cases does not understand the complex side of patient care or medical terminology. Nurse leaders must learn how to articulate clinical situations and findings in a manner that the finance team understands (Rosenthal & Stilgenbauer, 2015). In turn, nurse leaders need to understand and be comfortable using the finance terms and to cultivate relationships with finance colleagues. In addition, they need to be able to translate clinical conditions into language the finance team understands (Rosenthal & Stilgenbauer, 2015). At the end of the chapter, there is a glossary of financial terms; understanding the meaning and being able to use the terms during discussions with finance colleagues are vital.

The overall budget process takes 6 months: preparation starts in July and ends in December. There are multiple levels of approval: unit leaders to the director, to the CNO, the finance team, senior leadership, and finally the board of trustees. At any point in the process, the proposed budget may be returned for modifications or additional information if requested. Regardless of the budget process utilized at an organization, the goal is to identify the appropriate resources required to provide patient care and the supplies to support their work.

TYPES OF BUDGETS

There are four types of budgets: revenue, expense, operating, and capital. The overall organization's annual budget will include all four types of budgets. There are revenue budgets based on centers that charge for services, such as infusion centers, perioperative services, ambulatory surgery, radiology, and laboratory. The revenue budget is based on revenue center volume projections (i.e., number of cases, procedures, visits) for the coming year and payor mix (Medicare, Medicaid, commercial). Expense centers, patient care units, environmental services, social work, care coordination, and facilities expenses are included in room and board charges. Expense budgets identify other costs related to providing services that do not include labor or supply expenses. Operating budgets include the cost of salary expense as well as non-salary items; for example, medical–surgical supplies. The capital budget includes large purchases and equipment that cost over a designated price (i.e., beds, CT scanners, robotic surgical devices); information technology (IT) upgrades and building renovations are also funded through the capital budget.

Revenue must cover the costs of services provided. The operating budget needs to be adequate to fund expenses and contingencies (Zaichkin, 2018). For any organization to be financially solvent, revenue must be higher than expenses, so the organization has profits to reinvest in infrastructure, technology, staffing, benefits, and capital expenditures.

The remaining parts of the chapter focus in depth on the capital and operating budgets, the primary budgets nurse leaders are involved with. The financial responsibility of nurse leaders has three components: developing a budget, implementation, and managing resources.

CAPITAL BUDGETS

The capital budget is a multiyear plan, with specific dollar amounts allocated for each year. Capital budgets are usually controlled centrally, and requests are prioritized. At times, organizations may use capital funds for a large project; for example, to replace the entire fleet of beds. Most organizations have a policy that dictates the specific criteria related to capital purchases. The specifics include the dollar amount that exceeds a figure determined by the organization and the expenditure must have an extended utilization period. Lastly, the items purchased must have an economic value for a specified number of years and depreciate in value. The dollars are usually apportioned to senior vice presidents and then distributed to department heads. Capital budgets provide nurse leaders with the opportunity to purchase specific items needed on a patient care unit. A bariatric unit may need specific scales and beds to care for the patients on the unit, while a neonatal ICU (NICU) may need Arctic Suns. The CNO may choose to purchase intravenous (IV) pumps for all of the ICUs. A portion of the dollars are usually kept in reserve for contingencies. Nurse leaders should always have a list of items that fit the guidelines for capital requests ready to submit. If the money is not used by the end of the year, nurse leaders may be asked what remains on their list.

OPERATING BUDGETS

The operating budget is an annual plan for salary and supply expenses associated with the provision of patient care. Healthcare is labor intensive; therefore, the personnel or salary portion of the budget is the largest expense (Marquis & Huston, 2021). Fixed costs are expenses that do not change regardless of volume of a unit or cost center; for example, utilities, maintenance, and insurances. Certain departments fall into fixed expenses (e.g., human resources, finance, legal departments). Variable costs will increase or decrease in relationship to volume; these costs include things such as drugs, medical–surgical supplies, food and nutrition, linen, and labor.

BUDGET PROCESS

PLANNING AND DEVELOPMENT OF OPERATING BUDGET

The budget process begins when Finance sends a memo outlining budget assumptions and a timeline. In preparation, RN leaders should be reviewing monthly financial reports, staffing reports, volume metrics, vacancy, turnover statistics, and workload (if available). Conversations with physician partners can provide insight into the expansion of services. Budget development, regardless of the clinical setting, involves fundamental elements, such as volume projections, measurement of productivity, and staffing requirements. Projecting staffing requirements is the most complex element and varies by clinical setting. Staffing for the acute care, ambulatory care, and medical group practices are vastly different because of the specific work being done in each setting.

There are two components to the operating budget: supply and salary.

SUPPLY BUDGET, ALSO KNOWN AS THE OTHER THAN PERSONNEL SALARY BUDGET

The supply budget is less complex than the salary budget and requires less analysis because it is developed using a formula. The supply budget is often referred to as OTPS (other than personnel salary). The budget encompasses medical–surgical supplies, blood products, medical gases, pharmacy charges, conferences, consulting fees, leases, and other non-salary items. The projected OTPS budget can be determined in several ways. One process is based on 6 months of utilization, which is annualized, with an anticipated inflation factor. Additional dollars are added to cover increases in volume related to anticipated new programs.

In both the salary and OTPS budgets, input from the nurse leaders is imperative. They are the unit or service expert and should play an intricate role in the budget process. Nurse leaders are aware of changes in patient populations, new modalities, new programs, growth of current service lines, construction projects, and changes in technology. One example is the introduction of midline catheters, a product introduced to reduce the number of central lines. The finance team may not be aware of or understand the connection between clinical advances and the potential increase in expense. In this example, the year midline catheters are introduced a complete line of catheters is stocked, increasing the OTPS expense. The decrease in use of central line catheters will not be immediately apparent and will take time to be recognized. The nurse leaders can alert the finance team and ensure the budget includes the additional expense related to product enhancements or replacements that may affect the projected OTPS budget.

It takes a village; nurse leaders need to engage the nursing staff to identify waste reduction efforts. Frontline staff utilize supplies in most cases without knowing the cost of the item. For example, items taken into an isolation room must be discarded when the patient is discharged, which may total as much as $500 worth of supplies. Nurses fill their pockets with items to save redundant trips to the utility room with no thought given to the associated expense. Education and awareness of the prices of items can support the team to make cost effective decisions.

The supply budget is straightforward if there are no major adjustments from the prior year. There is usually a calculation based on utilization and an inflation percentage added. All clinical settings utilize a similar format.

SALARY BUDGET

The salary budget includes the number of full-time equivalents (FTEs) needed to provide care and the associated salary dollars. One FTE (1.0) is typically paid for 1,950 or 2,080 hours annually. Employees can be classified as full time or part time (working a fraction of the full-time hours). The budget is the sum of FTEs and the associated salary. The actual number of positions may differ from the number of FTEs budgeted because of part-time positions. The budget should also include merit and cost of living increases projected by the organization for the coming year. There are different processes for determining the salary budget. Check with the organization's finance colleagues to understand how the salary budget is determined.

There are two methodologies for the determination of salary dollars:

- The actual salary of staff budgeted in the cost center is added together to determine the salary budget.
- The average salary for each job code in a cost center is used and multiplied by the number of FTEs in the job code.

In both examples, the salary budgets are based on the individuals in the cost center (CC), department, or service line. Monitoring the position control, which is a roster of individuals in the CC, must be accurate so the appropriate salary dollars are included in the CC budget. The topic of position control will be explained more fully in the Budget Management: Financial Stewardship section of the chapter. The salary budget should include dollars allocated to OT and/or agency expenses to cover LOAs, vacancies, and volume fluctuations. The process for budgeting OT and agency expenses differs by organization and needs to be included in the budget. Historical data related to LOAs, vacancies, orientation, and current run rate (utilization) of OT should be analyzed to project the amount of OT dollars needed for the coming year. Areas that remain open on holidays need to calculate the number of staff working each holiday and determine the amount of OT that will be needed to pay staff at a premium rate, sometimes referred to as structural OT.

To recap, the salary budget is a combination of all earning types for the FTEs budgeted in a specific CC. Earning types include base salary rates, differentials, certifications, bonuses, OT, agency dollars, and projected cost of living and merit increases.

Ambulatory care associated with medical centers follow the same budget timeline and have the benefit of the same financial reports to review. Budget development for ambulatory care is complicated as each individual clinic type needs to be assessed and incorporated into one cohesive budget. Budget preparation for ambulatory care will be outlined in more detail at the end of the "Budget Process" section.

DETERMINATION OF FULL-TIME EQUIVALENTS

Projecting the accurate number of staff to provide patient care is a fundamental and critical element of the budgeting process. There are different methodologies for determining the number of FTEs, using volume metrics, hours per patient day (HPPD), a coverage factor (CF), nurse-to-patient ratios, staffing by teams (ED), or rooms in perioperative and procedural areas. Ambulatory care will use number of visits, hours of operation, and provider case load, as well as acuity of care. There are common metrics used in all methodologies; benchmarking and skill mix are also factored into the budget process.

Volume Projection

One of the key metrics at the foundation of the budgeting process is volume. Regardless of the type of service, a volume baseline must be identified. It can be based on the current year's run rate of patient days, procedures, or clinic visits for a specified period of time. This becomes the starting point and is adjusted by forecasted growth and erosion. The finance department usually supplies the growth and erosion projections. The addition of new physicians, growing practices, and new programs must be added to the baseline to ensure the FTEs are added. Erosion occurs when physicians leave the organization, procedures are transitioned to the outpatient setting, or a program ceases, causing a decrease in the project volume. Volume metrics for inpatient settings are measured in patient days, perioperative measure cases, catheterization lab measures, number of procedures, and ambulatory care visits. All service departments must then understand if there is growth or erosion that will be applied to the baseline volume metric.

Unit reorganization, relocation, and/or plans to convert a unit to a different service type need to be considered into the volume assumptions as well. Knowledge of changes in unit type and reorganization are pieces of information the nurse leaders are usually aware of and should be shared during the volume discussion.

Inpatient units focus on average daily census (ADC) calculated by dividing the number of patient days by the period you are reviewing.

Example: Converting Patient Days to Average Daily Census

- 9,125 patient days in 1 year (365 days)
- ADC = 9,125(patient days) / 365 (1 year) = 25

The ADC for the inpatient unit is 25 and will be utilized in the calculation to determine number of FTEs. ADC is an average; there will be some days the actual census will be higher or lower. Non-census departments and areas start with a similar calculation using the metric that is appropriate for the area.

 ## CASE SCENARIO

IMPACT OF NOT REPLACING DEPARTING SURGEON

A cardiac surgeon has decided to depart the medical center for other opportunities. The annual number of cases they performed was 170. Using 7 days as the average length of stay (number of days patients are in the hospital) for each patient calculates to 1,190 days, divided by 365 is 3.3 ADC. ADC equates to number of patients in beds per day. The decision is to not replace the surgeon with another doctor.

DISCUSSION QUESTIONS

1. As a result of the surgeon leaving, what are the immediate and downstream effects?
2. Why do you think the medical center has chosen not to replace the cardiac surgeon?

There may need to be an adjustment in the ADC because of seasonality. On a burn unit, the census is lower during spring and summer months and higher in the fall and winter. The census fluctuation creates a staffing challenge for the nurse leader; however, it is critical the ADC calculation includes the period when the census is highest. If you are reviewing a partial year, the denominator is equal to the sum of the days in the months you are including.

Patient care units are staffed 24/7; all other non-census CC must determine the number of FTEs needed to cover the hours and days of operation as well as nonproductive time. Inpatient units need to determine the number of FTEs required to cover a unit for the projected ADC for 356 days. All other departments or facilities will use calculations associated with hours and days of operation. Peri-op and procedural areas will calculate the number of rooms, as well as the hours and minutes each room is in service, plus the time it takes to turn the room around and break relief. The ED may staff by teams (gold team, blue team, etc.) or areas to cover such as triage, pediatrics, and/or admitted patients waiting for bed assignments. Boarders are admitted patients waiting for an inpatient room assignment due to high occupancy rates. EDs also flex the number of RNs and techs scheduled by hour of the day, the busiest time being 11:00 a.m. through midnight. Shifts are staggered to provide coverage during the busiest time.

Ambulatory and outpatient departments have to project volume; an essential factor in cludes hours of operation for each of the different clinics.

Productivity and Benchmarks

Once the volume metric has been established, determining a metric for intensity of care is the next element essential to the budget. Workload variables include number and acuity of patients, staffing patterns, staff competency, and skill mix. Productivity and classification systems can be useful but may not capture the full complexity of care. Healthcare efficiency is a significant policy concern, whereas nursing quality and safety indicators are viewed as a gauge for efficiency (Yankovsky et al., 2016). National benchmark data compares average nursing worked hours for comparable units. The National Database of Nursing Quality Indicators (NDNQI) and Action OI are two examples. System organizations can use internal benchmarks to standardize hours of care across sites. There are different acronyms that identify the number of hours of care a patient receives in 24 hours: WHPPD (worked hours per patient day), NCH (nursing care hours), and HPPD. For the purposes of this chapter, the term HPPD will be utilized for inpatient- or census-driven units as a measurement of the care patients receive in 24 hours. Non-census areas do not use HPPD, but instead may use hours per unit of service.

HPPD is defined as the number of hours of nursing care a patient receives in a 24-hour period. The calculation can vary by organizations related to who is included in the calculation. The calculation may include the worked hours (productive hours) of all job titles in the CC (direct and indirect) or just the job titles of individuals who provide direct care called caregivers. It is very important to understand if the budgeted HPPD includes only caregiver productive hours or productive hours for all staff on the CC. If direct and indirect hours are included in the HPPD calculation, the actual hours of direct care will be less than the calculation.

There are several national databases that can provide data for clinical areas comparing peer groups, and large multisite organizations can utilize internal benchmarks for like units across campuses. System CNOs are tasked to standardize internal benchmarks and staffing across the system (Gavigan et al., 2016). HPPD will vary by service type; the HPPD for a medical–surgical unit will be different than that for an ICU, mother–baby, or pediatrics unit. The HPPD and the ADC are two of the essential metrics used in the budget process for inpatient units.

If RN-to-patient ratios are utilized to determine FTEs, there must be an organizational agreement on ratios by service. Generally, the medical–surgical ratio is one nurse to five patients, whereas in the ICU it is one nurse to two patients. Benchmarks are useful to standardize the ratios. Once the ratio is determined and the nurse leader knows the number of RNs per shift, the coverage factor before CF can be applied to determine the total number of FTEs needed.

The following calculation can be used to determine the HPPD being provided once you know the ADC and the number of RNs per shift from the ratios.

Example: Calculating Hours per Patient Day RN-to-Patient Ratios

In a medical–surgical unit, budgeted ADC 30 with 1:5 nurse-to-patient ratio, nurses work 12-hour shifts, assistive personnel (APs) work 7.5-hour shifts.

- Six RNs work day shift; productive hours are 12
- Six RNs work night shift; productive hours are 12
- Two APs work day, evening, and night shift; productive hours 7.5
- Shift length excludes paid mealtime
- Staffing

$$\text{Day} \quad \text{Night} \quad \text{AP day} \quad \text{AP eve} \quad \text{AP night}$$
$$(6 \times 12) + (6 \times 12) + (7.5 \times 2) + (7.5 \times 2) + (7.5 \times 2) / 24 = 7.8 \text{ (HPPD)}$$

The calculations and examples throughout the chapter cite RNs as the primary caregivers; however, it is noted LPNs may also apply to caregiver calculations.

Coverage Factor/Benefit Relief Factor

The third important element for determining the FTEs budget is a CF or benefit relief factor (BRF). The CF calculates the number of FTEs required to maintain staffing levels during hours of operation and will differ depending upon the setting. Inpatient units will have a CF to provide the same level of staffing 24/7. Perioperative services, procedural suites, and dialysis centers are more complex because of varied hours of operation (full staffing Monday through Friday, reduced staffing Saturday, and closed on Sundays and holidays). The areas may use an on-call team to cover for emergencies.

Depending upon the organization, the amount of CF calculated in the budget for nonproductive time can vary. Most CF includes vacation, personnel days, holidays, sick days (full sick or partial), continuing education (CE), and days off. Nurse leaders should understand the number and type of days budgeted by the organization. Some organizations use a percentage of total paid hours as the CF. On average, a full-time employee is paid 1,950 or 2,080 hours per year, depending upon the organization's definition of "standard hours." If the employee works 37.5 hours per week, the annual paid hours are 1,950; if paid 40 hours per week, the annual paid hours are 2,080. These paid hours include both productive hours (hours directly related to patient care) and nonproductive hours (hours not associated with patient care and benefit time). As mentioned, the CF will vary by organization and can account for 16% to 19% of the total annual paid hours. In addition, when figuring out staffing, for units that require coverage for hours of operation beyond Monday–Friday 9 to 5, coverage for days off must also be included.

Example: Conversion of Nonproductive Hours to Days

An FTE is paid 1,950 hours annually. Of the 1,950 hours, a percentage is considered nonproductive, and the remaining hours are productive. Productive hours are those related to the time you are working. Nonproductive time is usually referred to as benefit or paid time off (PTO) and is part of the paid 1,950 hours.

In Table 19.1, all FTEs (1.0) are budgeted for the same number of hours of nonproductive time. Shift length will determine the number of days because when flex time staff (12-hour shift) uses vacation, 12 hours are utilized for each day. The nonproductive time in this example totals 330 hours or 17% (330 / 1,950) of paid time. Organizations can use a percentage for each CC or use the actual utilization of nonproductive time by CC. For example, a CC with low use of sick time will budget a lower percentage of nonproductive time to calculate needed FTEs. A unit may have many staff with high years of seniority, in which case the staff may be accruing more than the usual 4 weeks of vacation. The additional vacation weeks need coverage, and the following calculation will provide the FTEs needed to cover the additional vacation weeks.

Example: Adjusting Coverage Factor for Additional Vacation Accrual

In the NICU, 10 RNs are accruing 5 weeks of vacation, resulting in an additional 50 weeks of vacation for the NICU.

- 10 nurses × 1 additional week
- 1 week = 37.5 hours × 10 RNs = 375 hours
- 375 hours / 1,950 (1.0 FTE) = 0.2 FTE

The calculation provides justification to add dollars or 0.2 FTEs to cover the additional coverage for vacation for the 10 RNs. One option is to hire a per diem nurse to cover the additional vacation time.

Per diem nurses work approximately 390 hours per year or a 0.2 FTE status. The per diem does not accrue benefits and is able to work at their convenience and when needed by the facility.

Units that are open 24/7 including holidays will have to factor in coverage for staff's regular days off. Full-time staff working 7.5 hours work 5 days per week and have 2 regular days off per week, or an additional 104 days per year that require coverage. Staff working 12-hour shifts are off 4 regular days per week and need to be backfilled 208 days per year. The CF for a 7.5-hour shift in this example is 1.69, which may vary depending upon the nonproductive time the organization budgets (Table 19.2).

Example: 7.5-Hour Shift, How Many Full-Time Equivalents Are Required?

- Desired staffing is 5 RNs working 7.5 hours (day, evening, and night shift)
- 5 RNs per shift × 1.69 (CF) = 8.45 FTEs per shift
- 8.45 FTEs × 3 (day, evening, night shifts) = 25.35 total FTEs

TABLE 19.1: Calculating Nonproductive Hours

Nonproductive Hours	7.5-Hour Shift	12-Hour Shift
Vacation	150 hours (20 days at 7.5 hours)	(12.5 days at 12 hours)
Holiday	60 hours (8 days at 7.5 hours)	(5.1 days at 12 hours)
Personal time	30 hours (4 days at 7.5 hours)	(2.7 days at 12 hours)
Sick time	90 hours (12 days at 7.5 hours)	(7.5 days at 12 hours)

TABLE 19.2: Nonproductive Time Converted to Coverage Factor

Type	Annual Nonpro-ductive Accrual in Hours	Hours Converted to Days		
		7.5-Hour Shift	10-Hour Shift	12-Hour Shift
Vacation (days)	150	20	12	12.5
Holiday (days)	60	8	6	5
Personal (days)	30	4	3	2.5
Sick (days)	90	12	9	7.5
CE (days)	15	2	1.5	1.25
Days off coverage		104	156	208
Total nonwork days		150	187.5	236.8
Work days		215	177.5	128.4
Coverage factor		0.69	1.1	1.8
Plus person being covered		1.69	2.06	2.8

CE, continuing education.

Example: 12-Hour Shift, How Many Full-Time Equivalents Are Required?

- Desired staffing is 5 RNs working 12 hours (day and night shift)
- 5 RNs per shift × 2.8 (CF) = 14.0 FTEs per shift
- 14.0 FTEs × 2 (day, night shifts) = 28.0 total FTEs

● CASE SCENARIO

STAFFING A NEW ONCOLOGY UNIT

You have been asked to open an oncology unit. The desired staffing is 5 RNs per shift. You are considering if the RNs should work 7.5-hour or 12-hour shifts.

DISCUSSION QUESTIONS

1. Is either shift length beneficial to patient care based on patient needs or unit flow?
2. Based on the previous calculations, is there a financial benefit for the RNs to work either 7.5 hours or 12 hours shifts? If so, why?
3. Are there other considerations for choosing one shift length over the other?

The budget for an area closed on weekends and holidays (for example, the endoscopy suite) will have a different CF for nonproductive time. Holidays and regular days when the unit is closed will have to be eliminated from the CF for staff working a standard 7.5-hour shift. If staff are working 12-hour shifts, days off will have to be incorporated into the calculation.

Hours per Patient Day

Example: Full-Time Equivalent Calculation Using Hours per Patient Day and Coverage Factor for 24/7 Unit

To determine the number of FTEs required for an inpatient medical–surgical unit with a census of 30 and an HPPD of 7.59, use the following:

- 30 × 7.59 (HPPD) × CF 1.69 / shift length 7.5 hours = 51.3 FTEs
- 30 × 7.59 (HPPD) × CF 2.8 / shift length 12 hours = 53.1 FTES

Flex time paid for 12-hour shifts requires more FTEs than 7.5-hour shifts in the calculations for the same level of care because of the 4 days off per week. A modification for changing the flex schedules from 12 hours to 11.5 hours per shift requires RNs to work an additional shift every 4 weeks. This reduces the days off by 13 per year for each RN, reducing the coverage needed for days off to 195 per year. Depending on how the organization pays, the additional shift may incur OT in the week the fourth shift is scheduled. To avoid OT, organizations have adopted a smoothing process by paying the hours for the additional shift over two pay periods, usually 4-week periods. In the example, the number of FTEs from the calculation is the budgeted caregiver FTEs required to provide 7.59 hours of care to 30 patients 365 days per year. Higher census and increased patient acuity may require day-to-day staffing to be flexible, using float pool nurses or per diems. Conversely, when census is lower than ADC, floating to another unit, approving benefits, or CE time are all methods for managing the budget.

Caregivers provide direct patient care and include licensed nurses, RNs, LPNs, and APs (nurse aides and techs). Once the total number of FTEs needed is determined, the next step is to determine the skill mix among the caregiver job codes.

Skill Mix

Skill mix refers to the percentage of caregivers that are RNs compared to non-licensed caregivers (APs). Medical–surgical units may have a skill mix of 65% RN caregivers compared to 35% non-licensed caregivers; an ICU, however, will have a skill mix of 90% RNs and that number could be higher. Rehab units will have a lower RN skill mix at 60% to 40% non-licensed. Behavioral health units have mental health workers helping with groups and rehab units have nursing attendant techs who assist with getting patients to meals and physical therapy.

Example: Calculating Skill Mix for Assistive Personnel

In the previous example of the medical–surgical unit, the caregiver FTE budget total was 51.3 FTEs.
Percentage of licensed caregivers is 65% for this example:

- $51.3 \times 65\% = 33.35$ RN FTE caregivers
- $51.3 \times 35\% = 17.96$ AP caregivers

The daily shift-to-shift staffing must be aligned with the budgeted caregivers and actual census. The CF can be utilized to figure out the shift-to-shift staffing. In the previous example, the budgeted caregivers are 51.3 multiplied by the skill mix to determine the breakdown between the number of licensed and non-licensed caregivers.

⬡ CASE SCENARIO

DETERMINING SKILL MIX

Skill mix is the percentage of RNs or AP FTEs compared to the total calculated FTEs required to care for a specific type and number of patients.

You are developing a budget for a subacute rehab unit. The calculated FTEs are 27.5 FTEs. The next step is determining the skill mix. You talk with your colleagues from a medical–surgical unit where the skill mix is 70/30, from an ICU where the skill mix is 90/10, and finally from behavioral health, where the skill mix is 60/40.

DISCUSSION QUESTIONS

1. Why is there such a difference in the skill mix among the types of units?
2. What should the skill mix be for the rehab unit and why?

Example: Daily RN Staffing

Licensed caregivers working a 7.5-hour shift:

- $33.35 / 1.69 = 19.7$ RNs to cover 3 shifts in 24 hours
- $19.7 / 3$ (shifts) $= 6.5$ RNs per shift

The daily staffing pattern could be 6 RNs per shift; the fraction in the calculation allows for flexibility. A seventh RN could be staffed if there is a day with increased activity; for example, on a surgical unit, if Wednesday typically has a high number of orthopedic surgeries, flexing staffing to seven nurses to support increased activity is beneficial. Also, if the schedule works out to have seven RNs, an additional holiday or CE day can be approved.

Example: Daily Staffing for Assistive Personnel Caregivers

Non-licensed caregivers working 7.5-hour shifts:

- 17.96 / 1.69 = 10.6 non-licensed caregivers to cover 3 shifts in 24 hours.
- 10.6 / 3 (shifts) = 3.5 APs per shift

The staffing pattern is 3 APs per shift, and the fraction allows for flexibility, perhaps to cover a patient on 1:1 watch. A staffing matrix or guideline should be developed with fluctuating census points that maintain the level of care and serve as a guide for shift-to-shift staffing. This staffing grid serves as a reference for the charge nurse and off-shift administrators. In the example in Table 19.3, HPPD and skill mix remain the same; the staffing pattern adjusts to the changes in the census. At a census of 32 (above the budgeted census of 30), additional resources are needed; for example, 7 RNs and perhaps 4 APs. In the example, the seventh RN may be already scheduled (based on the calculation), or OT, a float nurse, or per diem may be required. Conversely, at a census of 24, the staffing pattern can be adjusted down to 5 RNs.

The staffing grids or matrix are used as a guide; however, professional judgment must also be involved in staffing decisions and include consideration of all pertinent factors.

The budgeted FTEs can be manipulated to change the staffing pattern (i.e., by changing the skill mix %). If the RN skill mix is increased, the number of RNs per shift will increase. Permanent changes in skill mix should always be done during the budget process as increasing the professional skill mix will increase the salary expense.

A temporary change in skill mix in response to an unusual clinical situation is always an option for staffing; however, if the number of nurses increases, the number of APs should be adjusted to offset the increased salary expense when possible. Budgeted salary dollars are based on the budgeted FTEs in each job code in the CC.

Ambulatory care settings provide a critical service along the continuum of care. Treatment, education, and follow-up have a key impact on hospital readmission. The ambulatory budget preparation will include the same elements as previously reviewed; however, there are nuances to each of the components. Ambulatory care is made up of individual clinics that cover all clinical specialties; for example, medicine, endocrine, pediatrics, obstetrics, and so on. The skill mix among the clinics differs depending upon the acuity of the patient and the care requirements. Determination of staffing also includes evaluation of the providers' (MDs and APRNs) case load.

Volume determination is related to the number of annual visits each clinic tracks. *FTE* determination includes volume, hours of operation for each clinic, and type of care provided (assessments, education, vaccination, dressings, and venipuncture). *Benchmarking* provides data related to room turnaround and number of patients seen per hour. The Medical Group Management Association (MGMA) is a national organization specializing in research, education, staffing, and benchmarking for ambulatory care. *Skill mix* includes APRNs, RNs, LPNs, and medical assistants. *Productivity* involves the number of rooms to cover and patient type (geriatrics vs. infusions). *CF* is calculated to be sure there is coverage for nonproductive time. If the staff is responsible for nonpatient-facing tasks (i.e., instrument sterilization), the time needs to be quantified and included in staffing calculations.

Although the ambulatory care budget is submitted as a whole, it includes an FTE calculation for each clinic (Table 19.4).

The annual visits are multiplied by time for each visit (15 minutes). Minutes are then converted to hours, and hours divided by 1,950 (the hours paid to a full-time FTE).

TABLE 19.3: Staffing Grid (Matrix)

				Census Adjusted Flexible Staffing Pattern for 7.5-Hour Shift						
Census	HPPD	Relief Factor	Total FTEs	Total Number RN FTEs @ 65% Skill Mix	RN Skill Mix (% HPPD)	RN Coverage for 24 Hours	Nurses per Shift	Total Number AP FTEs at 35% Skill Mix	AP for 24 Hours	AP per Shift
32	7.59	1.69	54.7	35.6	65	21.0	7.0	19.16	11.33	3.8
30	7.59	1.69	51.3	33.4	65	19.7	6.5	17.96	10.63	3.5
28	7.59	1.69	47.9	31.1	65	18.4	6.1	16.76	9.92	3.3
26	7.59	1.69	44.5	28.9	65	17.1	5.7	15.56	9.2	3.1
24	7.59	1.69	41.0	26.7	65	15.8	5.3	14.37	8.5	2.8

AP, assistive personnel; FTE, full-time equivalent; HPPD, hours per patient day.

TABLE 19.4: FTE Calculation for Ambulatory Care

Clinic Name	Annual Visits	Average Length of Visit in Minutes[a]	Annual Visit Minutes Utilized	Annual Visits in Hours	FTEs
Medicine	27,300	15	409,500	6,825	3.50
Allergy	2,184	15	32,760	546	0.28
Obstet-rics	16,380	30	491,400	8,190	4.20
Totals	45,864				7.98
				FTEs include CF	11.17

[a]New patient visit time increased to 30 minutes.
Note: Calculations are based on average room turnover, hours, and actual visit time.
FTE calculation: Annual visits × Average length of visits in minutes = Annual visit minutes utilized
Annual visit hours = Annual visit minutes utilized / 60
FTEs = Annual visit hours / 1,950
CF, coverage factor; FTE, full-time equivalent.

CF is 1.4 because only benefit time needs to be covered, no weekends. The example is based on 7.5-hour shifts and a Monday to Friday schedule. The skill mix will be determined by the acuity of the clinic and the skill level required; an obstetrics (OB) clinic must be staffed with RNs because of the assessment component of the visit.

APRNs need to understand how to calculate the correct number of APRNs needed to cover a service or manage/work in a clinic or medical practice.

The first element in every setting for calculating FTEs is volume. In an acute care setting, the APRNs often cover a service. They have 24-hour responsibility as providers to cover medical needs of the patient in the specific service. APRNs can also partner with MDs to cover office hours, post-op visits, and education. In ambulatory care, APRNs as providers carry a case load and can manage the clinical staff.

Staffing calculation for APRNs in acute care include volume (case load), hours requiring coverage, and CF plus other responsibilities (coaching residents in specialty areas, and documentation). APRNs can work 7.5-hour or 12-hour shifts (Table 19.5).

Assume APRNs cover a 20-bed orthopedic unit 24/7, working 12-hour shifts. The case load is 10 patients, and there is one APRN who works with surgeons to facilitate discharges and cover emergencies on day shift only.

Twenty patients require two APRNs on the day and night shifts, making a total of four, plus one to cover surgical time plus facilitate discharges and admissions on the day shift. We know from the previous section that the CF to use for 12-hour shifts is 2.8. Therefore, FTE requirements for day shift 2.8 times 3 = 8.4 plus night shift 2.8 times 2 = 5.6 (Table 19.6). Total FTEs required to staff 3/2 including CF is 14.0.

TABLE 19.5: Calculation to Determine Number of APRN FTEs

APRN FTE Calculation		
Coverage Required	Per Shift	w CF
Days Monday–Sunday	3	8.4
Nights Monday–Sunday	2	5.6
Total FTEs with coverage		14

FTE, full-time equivalent.

TABLE 19.6: Ambulatory Care APRN FTE Calculation

APRNs	Average Number of Patients Seen per Day = 12 (Combination New Patients + Revisits)					Total
Volume	36 visits	48	36	36	48	
	Monday	Tuesday	Wednesday	Thursday	Friday	
APRNs per day	3	4	3	3	4	17
Total number of NPs for week coverage						17
Coverage factor 1.4 (no weekend coverage needed)						23.8

Note: Assumption: The APRNs work 8-hour shifts Monday to Friday.
CF, coverage factor; FTE, full-time equivalent.

BUDGET MANAGEMENT: FINANCIAL STEWARDSHIP

The operating salary budget should include the number of FTEs required to provide a level of patient care for a specific number of patients, with coverage for nonproductive time. Healthcare is not a typical industry, and mitigating events requires the utilization of resources to be nimble. It is important for nurse leaders to understand contributing factors that may or may not justify overspending or underspending. Census above the budgeted ADC may require additional nursing resources, which is a justified reason to add expense. New CE requirements and higher patient acuity are also reasons to staff above the budgeted guidelines. Understanding why there is an unfavorable variance is very important and requires routine tracking of justifications.

Posting an unbalanced schedule with too many staff scheduled Wednesday and not enough Saturday, thereby requiring OT, is not acceptable. Factors that influence expense include fluctuating census, increased or decreased patient needs, vacancy management, turnover, balanced schedule development, vacation smoothing, habitual missed meal breaks, and management of patients on one-to-one watch.

Nurse leaders need to make difficult decisions at times to be effective financial stewards. Educating staff about how their practice contributes to the overall financial health of the organization is important. Connecting the dots related to reimbursement, clinical outcomes, HCAHPS scores, and nursing practice are key points that must be communicated at staff meetings.

REPORTS

Financial reports are an essential part of financial accountability. Having access and understanding the information each report contains is the roadmap to explaining variances. Most organizations have financial systems that produce payroll reports by pay period or monthly. The reports track expenses compared to budget, for both salary and OTPS. The financial reports are a retrospective view of spending for a specified period. Nurse leaders are juggling a multitude of challenges and may find it difficult to remember what happened 2 to perhaps 6 weeks earlier, contributing to an unfavorable variance. Being ahead of the monthly reports, developing a day-to-day method of collecting data that supports variance explanation, can be very helpful when preparing justification (Rosenthal & Stilgenbauer, 2015).

An unfavorable variance, spending in excess of the budget, usually requires an explanation or justification to the finance department. There are variance explanations resulting from uncontrollable circumstances, such as a census higher than the budget or high numbers of employees on paid LOA. There are variances that result from situations that are controllable, such as creation of an unbalanced schedule: too many approved vacations, insufficient coverage on weekends, and staffing above the recommended number of staff per shift. Because there are numerous unplanned reasons that affect your ability to provide staffing aligned with the budget, it is important to control as many factors as possible that trigger the need to use premium labor. Managing day-to-day operations, shift-to-shift staffing, bed utilization, and supply waste are areas that need to be closely and frequently monitored.

STAFFING

The budget for an inpatient unit, as discussed earlier in the chapter, is based on a budgeted ADC/HPPD or RN-to-patient ratios. Non-census areas, such as EDs, perioperative and procedural departments, and ambulatory clinics, also develop budgets based on volume metrics and CFs. The nurse leader has a responsibility to both patients and staff to create a schedule that has the appropriate number of staff working each shift to provide patient care and support staff satisfaction.

The first step is to create and implement a staffing guideline or matrix, reviewed earlier in Table 19.3. The starting point is the budgeted ADC/volume metric, which should identify the number of RNs and unlicensed staff for that census point. If the RN-to-patient ratios are used, the matrix should address census points when the staffing changes. If ratios are not used, the matrix should be aligned with the budgeted ADC and HPPD. An example of how to determine the shift staffing was reviewed previously in the chapter. The matrix supports decisions made related to staffing when the unit leadership is not present and assists staff in understanding shift assignments. Noncensus areas should create staffing guidelines or matrix grids that are flexible and align with actual volume or hours of operation.

DEVELOPMENT OF A BALANCED SCHEDULE

The schedule is developed for a specified period—4 to 6 weeks. Using the staffing matrix as a guide for scheduling, the appropriate number of RNs and AP staff per shift are assigned each day. Schedule planning includes employee requests for days off, planned vacations, and planned LOAs and CE time. Organizations usually have staffing policies or standardized processes with timelines for submission of requests. Collective bargaining agreements (CBAs) may also contain language regarding request submission. CBAs are found in unionized organizations and the language only applies to the members of the bargaining unit based on agreed upon job codes.

Most organizations have an HR policy with language governing vacation accrual and approval processes. In organizations with CBAs, there will be specific language related to vacation approval. In many cases, the vacation process requires staff to request vacation for a designated period, most often within a calendar year. The approval process is usually based on seniority. Vacation planning is essential to the development of a balanced schedule; not only is it an important element of managing a budget, but it is also important for staff satisfaction. Fair and smooth vacation planning is a major staff satisfier. Nurse leaders are the gatekeepers to this important process and must determine the number of staff that can have approved vacations per week.

The following calculation can be utilized to determine the number of weeks a nurse leader should approve per week by job code.

Example: How to Determine the Number of Vacations to Approve per Week

- A unit with 20 RNs: 10 accrue 4 weeks of vacation, and 10 accrue 5 weeks, for a total of 90 weeks.
- $(10 \times 4) + (10 \times 5) = 90$ weeks of vacation to be scheduled per year.
- 90 weeks / 52 (the number of weeks in a year) = 1.76 or 2 approved vacations per week.

Keep in mind, two vacations approved per week is spread across all shifts. There are also holidays, personal days, and potentially CE days that also need to evenly be approved as well. Vacation planning is one of the controllable elements in staffing and budget management.

PTO, which combines all nonproductive time into one bucket, is used by some organizations in lieu of specific titles for nonproductive time. The calculation to determine number of PTO weeks to approve varies from the previous calculation.

Example: How to Determine the Amount of Time Off to Approve Using PTO

- Total hours accrued per year for one RN is 330 minus 90 hours of sick time (sick time should not be a scheduled day off with few exceptions)
- 330 − 90 = 240 hours to approve
- 240 / 37.5 (hours paid per week) = 6.4 weeks per RN
- 20 (nurse FTEs budgeted on unit) × 6.4 = 128 total weeks
- 128 / 52 (weeks per year) = 2.4 (2 to 3 PTO requests approved per week)

This calculation encompasses all nonproductive time: vacation, holiday, personal, and CE. There are scheduling and staffing systems available that support nurse leaders in the schedule creation process.

Once the schedule is approved and posted, there are always changes that need to be made related to LOAs, vacancies, mutual switches, and sick time. Keeping up with the changes is an ongoing task that must be done correctly so you can anticipate who will be coming to work each day. This information is also tied to payroll.

Most inpatient units require the same number of nurses 24/7; however, there are units that may benefit by flexing the number of staff, depending upon the day of the week, season, and/or occupancy rate. For example, a cardiothoracic (CT) ICU may adjust staffing based on the operating room (OR) schedule. The CT surgeons may perform a higher number of cases on Monday, Wednesday, and Friday. Balanced staffing would call for 15 RNs per shift; however, based on the surgical schedule, 14 RNs can be scheduled on Tuesday, Thursday, and Sunday, and 16 on Monday, Wednesday, and Friday. Flexible hours may also help with scheduling the correct number of nurses to meet the patients' needs. If there are high numbers of admissions in the afternoon or late surgical cases, the facility can establish a swing shift. Instead of all nurses having the same start time, an RN can be assigned to work a shift that has hours that overlap two shifts.

Inevitably, there will be days on the schedule when there is a gap. When considering how to fill the gap, think of the expense associated with the options. Floating from another unit, float pool staff, and choosing a part-time employee are the least expensive choices. Per diem staff are next and are usually paid at a higher hourly rate, and finally OT, or agency staff, is the highest-cost option.

POSITION CONTROL

Position control is management of budgeted FTEs in a CC that are associated with a position number in the human resource system. Each position identifies an employee by name, job title, and FTE status. There is a roster or report of budgeted positions for each CC. Vacancy management is the third element essential to financial oversight. Turnover is inevitable and constant; although the literature identifies contributing causes and recommendations related to reducing turnover, this chapter focuses on the financial impact of vacancy management.

To reiterate, the salary budget provides the number of FTEs and associated dollars required to care for a specified number of patients during hours of operation. Position control is the management of the FTEs, which are converted to positions and job codes. There can be more positions than FTEs with a combination of full-time (1.0) and part-time (less than 1.0) positions. However, the FTE total of all positions added together must not exceed the number of budgeted FTEs.

Nurse leaders should be reviewing the positional control roster monthly. Anticipating upcoming vacancies is an excellent practice. Earlier in the chapter, the example of the ICU RN expecting to stay for 2 years before attending NA school is a perfect example of using foresight. The process of sourcing new candidates can be lengthy. The steps to hiring an RN include review of initial documents, multiple interviews, background checks, references, making an offer, and identifying an orientation date, which can take 2 months. The nurse may be in orientation 6, 8, or maybe 12 weeks before being a productive caregiver.

Developing a collegial relationship with the talent acquisition staff is very beneficial. Regular meetings reviewing filled and current vacancies enable them to source the best candidates to meet the needs of the unit. Being proactive when working with talent acquisition and anticipating resignations and other departures on an ongoing basis allows them to cultivate a pipeline of potential candidates who are readily available.

Vacancies leave gaps on the schedule that need to be covered. The longer the position is vacant, the more difficult it becomes to use the less expensive option. It is important for nurse leaders to remain knowledgeable about the number of vacancies and be proactive in filling the positions. The financial impact of backfilling the vacancies will be determined by the type of staff utilized. The longer the vacancies are replaced at the higher hourly rate, the greater the variances between budget and actual spend.

Position control can also be a method used to effectively manage decreases in the census compared to the budget. An example is a pediatric heart surgeon who leaves the organization, causing a decrease in the actual census in the pediatric ICU. Good financial management would be to monitor the actual census and perhaps hold off on filling all vacancies until the census starts to rebound. Another example of why you may not fill vacancies at 100% is when the unit has seasonal fluctuations. For example, a burn unit in the northeast will have a higher census during winter months. To be proactive, as spring approaches, the nurse manager may begin to leave positions vacant until August when they will begin working with talent acquisition to fill vacancies when anticipating a rebound in the census. If vacancies are utilized in budget management, it would be important for the unit leader to inform finance there was a deliberate choice to leave positions vacant during seasonal decreases in census.

OFF BUDGET CYCLE RESOURCE REQUESTS

The annual budget is developed months prior to implementation. Much thought and consideration was used in anticipating what may happen in the coming year. By nature of healthcare, there are always the unexpected scenarios that require resources. Most organizations have a process for addressing the unexpected, depending upon the issue. For example, a temporary increase in volume may be addressed by using OT and creating a justified variance. However, a permanent increase in volume related to a new physician joining the team requires a different remedy. Large organizations have financial planning teams that identify the increases in volume from new business. There may be the need for additional resources that require nurse leaders to present the request to the finance department. Business planning is the process a nurse leader can utilize to request additional resources. For example, suppose a clinical decision is made to have a NICU nurse attend complex deliveries. The current NICU budget does not support floating a nurse to labor and delivery (L & D) every shift. The nurse leader of the NICU must develop a business plan and present the case as to why the budget should be increased by an additional RN per shift. If OT is being used to cover the NICU nurse floating to L & D, the nurse leader can calculate the cost of the OT compared to the cost of hiring FTEs and include that in the presentation.

Additional resources can also include clinical specialty roles that are not calculated in the usual caregiver formulas, such as an additional wound care nurse. The plan has to be specific and include the value the position will bring to the organization. Always include data to support the request. For example, suppose a new gastrointestinal (GI) surgeon joined the team and the number of ostomies increased. There is also an increase in pressure injuries, identifying the need for an additional wound care RN. Data related to increasing rates of HAPI should be included in the plan as well as the potential loss of reimbursement to the organization related to HAPI. Calculations are needed to determine the number of FTEs being requested and the value added, as well as adjustments that may be needed, in this case a potential reduction in reimbursement due to HACs. The plan should include the desired outcome, be informative, and be data-driven. Do not be discouraged if your request is not approved on the first try. Utilize the feedback to strengthen your plan for another attempt, always putting the patient at the center of the plan.

◼ WHAT EVERY NURSE EXECUTIVE NEEDS TO KNOW ABOUT FINANCIAL ACUMEN

Nurse executives have a scope that can span a single facility or a system-wide enterprise. Regardless of the size of the scope, the competencies for nurse executives are the same.

Knowledge of the healthcare environment, professionalism, communication, relationship management, and business skills (American Organization of Nurse Executives [AONE] & American Organization for Nursing Leadership [AONL], 2015a) are required competencies. There are individual competencies within four domains that encompass skills that have financial impact. Certainly, the ability to develop and manage budgets, use business models, advocate for additional resources, and educate the care team of the financial impact of practice decisions are competencies under business skills. Human resource management (HRM) and strategy include endorsing nursing business cases. Nurse executives must set the tone, be role models for professionalism and clinical excellence, and be confident when making difficult decisions. CNEs and CNOs are members of the senior administrative team of the organization and can be very influential in representing nursing. By understanding the healthcare climate, as well as the financial processes for budgeting and resource management, the CNE and CNO can be mentors and impart their knowledge to the nursing management team.

◼ WHAT EVERY NURSE MANAGER NEEDS TO KNOW ABOUT FINANCIAL ACUMEN

Nurse leaders with financial management knowledge can engage staff to identify cost efficiencies at the point of care (Waxman & Massarweh, 2018). Nurse manager competencies identified by AONL have three domains: the science, the leader within, and the art (AONE & AONL, 2015b). The science domain encompasses financial management, HRM, performance improvement, and foundational thinking skills. The four competencies can impact financial performance and be used as a road map for finance management education. Nurse managers are the closest manager to the point of care, where most of the healthcare costs are spent. Nurse managers are the intermediary between caregivers and nurse executives, putting them in a formidable position. Nurse managers can impart the organizational strategic plans, goals, and values to frontline staff, and develop strategic plans, goals, and values for the specific unit they are accountable for. Financial health of an organization starts with fiscal management at the unit level by the nurse manager. "Nurses make up the single largest component of human capital within healthcare organization . . ." (Welton & Harper, 2016, p. 7). Nurse managers, directors, vice presidents, and senior vice presidents are accountable to patients, staff, and the organization for the immense budgets they develop, implement, and manage.

KEY POINTS

- Healthcare is complex. There are many influences, both external and internal, that nurse leaders must manage and understand. One of the competing priorities is developing and managing a budget.
- There are four types of budgets. The operating and OTPS budgets are the primary budgets most nurse leaders develop, implement, and manage.
- There are sequential steps to developing a budget. Collecting historical and new data is extremely important to substantiate the request for resources. Construct the budget one step at a time.

- Educate staff about the budget process. Their understanding of the process and limitations can facilitate implementation and management of the approved budget.

- Nurse leaders need to be at the table during budget discussions. Using financial terminology, data, and understanding, the financial climate of the organization will give nurse leaders the confidence to advocate for resources to care for patients and staff.

SUMMARY

Globally, healthcare is faced with challenges related to rising costs and reductions in reimbursement (Asamani et al., 2016) Nurse leaders must manage resources judiciously with innovative approaches to financial challenges (Naranjee et al., 2019).

Finance is a complex process, especially in healthcare, which must consider current reimbursement trends, the focus on quality, efficiencies, and external influences. Research suggests nurse managers are lacking financial management skills and learn by trial and error (Naranjee et al., 2019). A study assessing the financial literacy of executive nurse leaders suggests there is a gap in education and a difference in focus between novice and expert executive nurse leaders (Brydges et al., 2019).

Organizations approach the budget process using different methodologies, terminologies, and timelines. However, there are common elements and stages in the process. It is important that nurse leaders are involved and understand the process and what is included in each stage of the plan. Financial planning is a learned skill and improves with practice (Marquis & Huston, 2021).

Cultivating financial acumen may not come without a lot of effort, but remember your journey as a novice nurse. As a nurse leader, you can develop skills that support the organization's financial health. According to the American Hospital Association (AHA; 2016) almost 30% of hospitals in the United States have had a negative operating margin in each of the last 15 years. A financially secure organization can reinvest in resources—staff, supplies, and equipment—ultimately supporting clinical staff in their work. Take it step by step and develop relationships that can support your learning process. If a finance colleague is interested in your patient experiences, invite them on rounds. Help the talent acquisition coworker who wants to find great candidates to fill vacancies. Befriend a nurse leader colleague who is a financial expert and have regular meetings to review and discuss reports. Nurse leaders have an opportunity to make a difference by securing and managing resources to improve patient care and foster employee engagement.

END-OF-CHAPTER RESOURCES

◆ DISCUSSION QUESTIONS

The nurse manager of a medical–surgical unit has a budgeted ADC of 20. A new vascular surgeon has been admitting patients to the unit, which is requiring an increase in nursing care to treat these additional patients. The current budgeted HPPD is 7.59. You have been monitoring the number of patients with the higher acuity in anticipation of budget planning.

You have been reviewing reports, and over the past 6 months since the surgeon came on board you notice an unfavorable salary variance. You also have been tracking the actual census, and the ADC on average remains at 20; however, six of the patients have higher acuity.

You are proposing the configuration of the unit is changing to a blended model with an overall ADC of 20. The blend is 70% medical–surgical (14) ADC and 30% stepdown (6 ADC). You need to discuss the issues with the nurse leader you report to.

1. What discussion points should you plan to cover?

2. Will there be a need for additional FTE caregivers to care for the change in acuity? If so, how many FTEs?

3. Have you been staffing above the staffing guideline using OT?

4. The assumption is you are using OT to cover the additional clinical requirements. Financial reports indicate for the 6-month period OT expense is $125,000, which is unfavorable to the budget. What are your recommendations? Compare the cost of OT used over the past 6 months with the cost of hiring the additional RNs.

5. Develop a revised staffing grid.

◉ LEARNING EXERCISES FOR STUDENTS

LEARNING EXERCISE 1

A new patient care unit is being proposed to consolidate adult rehab patients currently scattered in the medical–surgical units. Based on reports, the average number of rehab patients in the hospital at all times is 15. The proposed HPPD will be 6.5, whereas the skill mix is 75% RN and 25% AP. RNs work 12-hour shifts and APs work 7.5-hour shifts.

1. Calculate the total number of FTEs required to provide 5.68 HPPD to 15 patients.

2. Calculate the skill mix. How many RNs will be budgeted among the total FTEs? How many APs will be budgeted as part of the total?

3. Based on the number of RN FTEs, what will be the optimum RN staffing number for 15 rehab patients per shift? How many APs will be budgeted per shift?

LEARNING EXERCISE 2

After calculating the ADC, the finance department provided the volume projections related to service. Complete the ADC projections for oncology, behavioral health, and medicine.

Service Volume Projections for 2022				
Service	Cases	Length of Stay (Days)	Total Days	ADC
Cardiac surgery	100	8	800	2.2
Orthopedics	700	5	3,500	9.6
Peds	500	4	2,000	5.5
OB/GYN	300	3	900	2.5
Oncology	150	7		
Behavioral health	50	14		
Medicine	500	7.5		

ADC, average daily census.

LEARNING EXERCISE 3

Complete the following staffing grid for all census points (empty cells shaded in purple).

Census-Adjusted Flexible Staffing Pattern for 7.5 Hours Shift									
A	B	C	D	E	F	G	H	I	J
Census	HPPD	Relief Factor	Total FTEs	Total # RN FTEs at 70% Skill Mix	RN Coverage for 24 hours	RNs per Shift	Total # AP FTEs at 30% Skill Mix	AP for 24 Hours	AP per Shift
36	7.59	1.69							
34	7.59	1.69							
32	7.59	1.69	54.7	38.3	22.7	7.6	16.42	9.72	3.2
30	7.59	1.69	51.3	35.9	21.3	7.1	15.39	9.11	3.0
28	7.59	1.69	47.9	33.5	19.8	6.6	14.37	8.50	2.8
26	7.59	1.69	44.5	31.1	18.4	6.1	13.34	7.9	2.6
24	7.59	1.69							
22	7.59	1.69							
20	7.59	1.69							

◑ GLOSSARY OF KEY TERMS

- **Available beds:** The number of beds that can be used for patients.
- **Average daily census (ADC):** The average number of patients per day in a hospital or patient care unit over a given period; admitted patients and outpatients are counted separately. The ADC is calculated using the number of patients in beds at midnight or another specified time of day totaled and divided by the specified period. For example, the ADC of a unit for 1 month would be calculated by adding up the number of patients in the bed at midnight for each day of the month and dividing by the number of days in the month.
- **Benchmark:** Comparing business processes, levels of care, and performance metrics to industry best practices; examples: NDNQI, Action OI, Prospect.
- **Benefit relief factor/coverage factor:** A calculation to determine the additional number of FTEs needed to cover the total benefit time and days off to maintain the direct patient care hours or staffing levels.
- **Caregiver:** Term associated with employees with a job title indicating they provide direct patient care in a department (e.g., RN, LPN, nursing attendant, ICU tech).
- **Cost center (CC):** A department within an organization. The manager of a CC is responsible for costs associated with salary and supplies, which are charged to a CC through the organization's financial systems. Each patient care unit is considered a CC.
- **Erosion:** Reduction in volume, which can be related to closure of a program, physician loss, or changes in procedures from inpatient to outpatient, reducing census.
- **Full-time equivalent (FTE):** A term utilized in budgeting and position control. An employee working 1,950 or 2,080 hours per year is considered full-time (1.0 FTE). Employees who are classified as part time will work less than the definition for full time and be considered a fraction of 1.0 FTE.

- **Fixed FTE:** A job code that has fixed value and will not change as volume fluctuates.
- **Hours per patient day (HPPD):** The average number of hours of care a patient received in a 24-hour period. The HPPD will vary by service line. For example, the HPPD for a medical–surgical unit will be different than for an ICU. HPPD is synonymous with nursing care hours (NCH).
- **Job code:** Every job in an organization has a title and code (number) used in human resources and financial systems.
- **Licensed beds:** Number of beds licensed by the Department of Health (DOH) by specialty.
- **Nurse-to-patient ratio:** Number of patients being care for by one nurse.
- **Payor mix:** Organizations are reimbursed by different payors (i.e., Medicare Medicaid, and commercial insurers). Payor mix identifies percentages each payor represents compared to the total revenue.
- **Productive hours:** Paid hours worked while providing patient care.
- **Nonproductive hours:** Paid hours associated with time off, or may be time associated with worked hours that are nonpatient facing (e.g., meetings or CE classes).
- **On call:** Staff who are paid a percentage of their wages for being available to come to work when called. Utilized for areas that are not staffed 24/7 but have emergencies (e.g., perioperative, catheterization lab, dialysis units).
- **OTPS budget:** OTPS (other than personal salaries); a portion of the operating budget associated with a CC that includes nonsalary expenses (e.g., supplies, equipment, pharmaceuticals, and temporary help).
- **Paid time off (PTO):** A method for accruing annual nonproductive time. All types of benefit time hours are combined and utilized throughout the year.
- **Pay period:** A specified period of time that staff are paid for, which can vary by organization; 7 and 14 days are the most common.
- **Position control:** A process of monitoring the number of filled and vacant positions in an organizational unit (CC). Also referred to as the table of organization (T of O).
- **Skill mix:** A term used to describe the percentage of licensed personnel compared to unlicensed direct caregivers; usually compares the number of registered nurses to the number of nursing aides/techs.
- **Staffed beds:** Number of beds that can be covered by the budgeted number of staff.
- **Unit of service:** A metric utilized to capture productivity and cost in non-inpatient CCs.

A robust set of instructor resources designed to supplement this text is located at http://connect.springerpub.com/content/book/978-0-8261-7795-7. Qualifying instructors may request access by emailing textbook@springerpub.com.

REFERENCES

American Hospital Association. (2016). *Trendwatch chartbook: Trends affecting hospital and health systems.* American Hospital Association.

American Organization of Nurse Executives & American Organization for Nursing Leadership. (2015a). Nurse executive competencies. https://www.aonl.org/system/files/media/file/2019/06/nec.pdf

American Organization of Nurse Executives & American Organization for Nursing Leadership. (2015b). Nurse manager competencies. https://www.aonl.org/system/files/media/file/2019/06/nurse-manager-competencies.pdf

Aroh, D., Colella, J., Douglas, C., & Eddings, A. (2015). An example of translating value-based purchasing into value-based care. *Urologic Nursing, 35*(2), 61–74. https://doi.org/10.7257/1053-816X.2015.35.2.61

Asamani, J. A., Naab, F., Ofei, A. M. A., & Addo, R. (2016). Do leadership styles influence productivity? *British Journal of Healthcare Management, 22*(2), 83–91. https://doi.org/10.12968/bjhc.2016.22.2.83

Brydges, G., Krepper, R., Nibert, A., Young, A., & Luquire, R. (2019). Assessing executive nurse leaders' financial literacy level: A mixed-methods study. *The Journal of Nursing Administration, 49*(12), 596–603. https://doi.org/10.1097/NNA.0000000000000822

Gavigan, M., Fitzpatrick, T. A., & Miserendino, C. (2016). Effective staffing takes a village: Creating the staffing ecosystem. *Nursing Economic$, 34*(2), 58–65. PMID: 27265946.

Marquis, B. L., & Huston, C. J. (2021). *Leadership roles and management functions in nursing (10th ed.).* Wolters Kluwer.

Moseley III, G. B. (2017). Managing health care business strategy. Jones & Bartlett Learning.

Naranjee, N., Sibiya, M. N., & Ngxongo, T. S. P. (2019). Development of a financial management competency framework for nurse managers in public health care organizations in the province of KwaZulu-Natal, South Africa. *International Journal of Africa Nursing Sciences, 11*, 100154. https://doi.org/10.1016/j.ijans.2019.100154

Rosenthal, N., & Stilgenbauer, D. (2015). Demystifying finance in perioperative nursing. *OR Nurse, 9*(2), 10–14. https://doi.org/10.1097/01.ORN.0000460907.96093.39

Waxman, K. T., & Massarweh, L. J. (2018). Talking the talk: Financial skills for nurse leaders. *Nurse Leader, 16*(2), 101–106. https://doi.org/10.1016/j.mnl.2017.12.008

Welton, J. M., & Harper, E. M. (2016). Measuring nursing care value. *Nursing Economic$, 34*(1), 7–14. PMID: 27055306.

Yankovsky, A., Gajewski, B. J., & Dunton, N. (2016). Trends in nursing care efficiency from 2007 to 2011 on acute nursing units. *Nursing Economic$, 34*(6), 266–276. PMID: 29975489.

Zaichkin, D. (2018). Budget principles for nurse leaders. In C. R. King, S. O. Gerard, & C. G. Rapp (Eds.), *Essential knowledge for CNL and APRN nurse leaders* (pp. 217–244). Springer Publishing Company.

SECTION VII

GOVERNANCE

CHAPTER 20

BOARD LEADERSHIP AND RESPONSIBILITIES

Kimberly J. Harper and Laurie S. Benson

"Leadership is showing up and using your voice."
Claire Fagin, PhD, RN, FAAN (Moore Foundation, 2015)

LEARNING OBJECTIVES

- Identify competencies that nurses contribute to effective board service.
- Describe how specific nurse competencies prepare one for service within a variety of governance levels and types of boards.
- Analyze specific types of boards where nurses could serve.
- Evaluate intrinsic and extrinsic rewards board service brings to the individual nurse.

INTRODUCTION

THE CASE FOR BOARD LEADERSHIP FOR NURSES

Governance is an extension of leadership. To ensure health equity for all, nurses must chart a personal and professional path that provides a platform to raise their leadership voices in new ways. Nurse leaders must embrace the abundance of opportunities to serve in board roles to influence and shape strategies and policies. As boards of all types are seeking to diversify their board composition, nursing leaders at all levels are uniquely and ideally suited to answer the call to contribute to the collective effectiveness and impact of a wide variety of boards, appointments, and commissions. By applying the knowledge and skills gained through education and practice, nurses bring a much-needed perspective to boards.

Pam Rudisill stated that

In today's current environment amidst the pandemic, there has never been more awareness, recognition, and visibility of the importance of including the nursing perspective in all settings, including the boardroom. While the most recent data continues to reflect a small percentage of nurses who serve as voting members on health systems and hospital boards, the dynamics are certainly shifting for pragmatic and altruistic reasons. This presents a time of great opportunity for hospitals and health systems to consider and invite the voice of nursing to serve in diverse governance roles within their organizations. (Sanford, 2021, para. 11)

WHY NURSES?

All boards benefit from the unique perspective of nurses to achieve the goals of improved health and efficient, effective healthcare systems at the local, state, and national level. Nurses bring a special set of skills including leadership, quality and process improvement, communications, human resource utilization, strategic planning, finance, teamwork, research, systems thinking, and change theory. While these skills are essential in practice, they are also extremely relevant in the boardroom. Boards function as a collective body, with no one board member having all these skills. Yet nurses are well versed in most of these critical skills and thus are able to provide a level of experience, expertise, and evidence-based perspective, which allows them to optimally contribute to boardroom discussions and decision-making.

In March of 2018, nursing students at Illinois State University Mennonite College of Nursing Leadership Academy were asked, "Why do you think nurses should serve on boards?" (Benson, 2018). The following is a sample of their responses to the question:

- "To create cultures of safety, in a variety of settings, in which individuals would have nurses advocating for them throughout the decision-making process."
- "Nurses should be able to serve on boards because they make a huge impact in their community and overall patient care. They are highly skilled professionals, and their input is crucial in decision-making for an overall improvement in healthcare."
- "Nurses have frequent exposure to a variety of issues in healthcare and have the knowledge and experience to help lead these boards in creating better patient and community outcomes."
- "It's important to stay involved and be included in decision-making processes."
- "We represent the majority of the medical community and are influenced by changes in not only hospital policies, but also community and governmental policies."
- "I believe nurses should serve on boards because they are the front line in hospitals. Nurses are always acting as patient advocates and can do the same while serving on a board. They can make changes that could impact patient care in positive ways."

These students clearly understood the "why" that compels nurses at all levels to claim their purpose and passion to serve on a board where they live, work, or pursue their education. For these reasons, and many more, nurses should consider where they might serve early in their careers and incorporate board membership as an integral part of their nursing leadership development.

All boards would benefit from adding the voice of a nurse to the discussions and decision-making. The impact of bringing that voice forward will be evident through better decisions relating to all aspects of healthcare in our communities and nation. To reach this point, nurses must identify and accept that board service is an extension of leadership, search out an appropriate board that aligns with their values and passion, and surround themselves with all the resources and support needed to be successful.

Lawrence W. Vernaglia, Partner, Foley & Lardner LLP, said it well when he stated, "The involvement of their nurse executives in high-profile community boards builds credibility and enhances the reputation for the organizations that employ them. Serving on community boards, nurses are extending the reach and reputation of the hospital beyond the clinical environment in helping shape policy and strategy decisions that impact these critical areas of patient care across the continuum of care" (Benson & Harper, 2017, p. 2).

WHY NOW?

The landmark 2011 Institute of Medicine (IOM; now the National Academy of Medicine [NAM]) report titled *The Future of Nursing: Leading Change, Advancing Health* recommended increasing the number of nurse leaders in pivotal decision-making roles on boards and commissions that work to improve the health of everyone in America. The report's recommendation number seven focused on both educating nurses to lead and ensuring that leadership positions are available for nurses. That necessary preparation was further defined as, "Nurses, nursing education programs, and nursing associations should prepare the nursing workforce to assume leadership positions across all levels, while public, private, and governmental health care decision makers should ensure that leadership positions are available to and filled by nurses" (IOM, 2014, p. 14). Based on this important recommendation, many changes were introduced to the profession of nursing. One of those was a national, organized effort to support the concept of nurses serving on boards to improve the health of their communities and the nation.

In May of 2021, the National Academy of Science, Engineering, and Medicine (NASEM) released *The Future of Nursing 2020–2030: Charting a Path to Achieve Health Equity* (Wakefield et al., 2021). The new report serves as a roadmap for nurses to engage individually and collectively to improve health for all. Nursing leaders at all levels are needed to lead change and shape policies that address the social determinants of health (SDOH) and the many inequities in the system and in our communities. These policies are needed to achieve health equity in all settings, including the boardroom. Recommendations in the 2020–2030 report target increasing diversity, adding SDOH to the curricula of schools of nursing, supporting the well-being of nurses, removing barriers to practice, and valuing the nursing contributions to achieve health equity across all systems. The critical role of nursing leadership is an integral part of the entire report, but is addressed most specifically in the following recommendations:

- *1.6 External to nursing organizations: Increase the number and diversity of nurses.*
  - "Increase the number and diversity of nurses, especially those with expertise in health equity, population health, and social determinants of health on boards and in other leadership positions within and outside of health care (e.g., community boards, housing authorities, school boards, technology-related positions)." (Wakefield et al., 2021, p. 359)

- *2.9 Include nursing expertise when health-related multisector policy reform is being advanced.*
  - "Representatives of social sectors, consumer organizations, and government entities should include nursing expertise when health-related multisector policy reform is being advanced." (Wakefield et al., 2021, p. 361)

- *7.1 Nursing education programs, including continuing education, and accreditors and the National Council of State Boards of Nursing should ensure that nurses are prepared to address social determinants of health and achieve health equity.*
  - "Prepare all nursing students to advocate for health equity through civic engagement, including engagement in health and health-related public policy and communication through traditional and nontraditional methods, including social media and multisector coalitions." (Wakefield et al., 2021, p. 369)

ANSWERING THE CALL

New and well-established nurse leaders at all levels within practice and education settings are needed to lead change that results in achieving equity in health and healthcare. A strong response needs to come from nurses and the time is now. Each one of the over 4 million RNs in the United States has the opportunity to get involved. We must all share our expertise and competencies at board tables in our communities and nationally to improve the equity of healthcare for all. *The Future of Nursing 2020–2030: Charting a Path to Achieve Health Equity* (Wakefield et al., 2021) report provides a compelling case for the importance and impact of nursing leadership, giving every nurse the opportunity to be a part of the collective engagement of the profession to bring about profound and lasting change for the benefit of all those we serve.

WHY YOU?

Every nurse is a leader. Regardless of where you fall on the spectrum of nursing roles, education, and practice, there is a place for you to serve on a board that aligns with your skills, qualifications, experience, and passion. Each nurse is responsible for discovering and pursuing a leadership path that meets with personal and professional goals, interests, abilities, and career timeline.

NURSES ON BOARDS COALITION

The Nurses on Boards Coalition (NOBC) is a national endeavor with the overarching goal of improving the health of communities and the entire nation through engaging nurses as active board members. NOBC was created in direct response to the 2011 *The Future of Nursing: Leading Change, Advancing Health* recommendation of increasing the number of nurse leaders in pivotal decision-making roles on boards and commissions that work to improve the health of everyone in America (IOM, 2011). *The Campaign for Action*, an initiative of the AARP Foundation, AARP, and the Robert Wood Johnson Foundation, initially assembled the group as part of their collaborative effort to implement the recommendations of the IOM report through the Future of Nursing: Campaign for Action. The NOBC first convened in 2014, and later that year publicly announced its strategic measure of ensuring that at least 10,000 board seats were filled by nurses in 2020. In its formative days, funded through a Robert Wood Johnson Foundation grant, NOBC was housed within the American Nurses Association (ANA), and the American Nurses Foundation (ANF) served as the fiducial agent for the organization until it became a 501(c)3 public charity in 2017.

NOBC represents national and state efforts by nurses and others to build healthier communities in America. With 24 national member organizations, their collective mission is to improve the health of communities and the nation through the service of nurses on boards and other bodies. NOBC has always been committed to increasing nurses' presence and influence on corporate, health-related, and other boards, panels, and commissions. Now that the NOBC's initial key strategy to ensure that at least 10,000 board seats are filled by nurses has been achieved, NOBC can leverage this collective accomplishment to measure the impact of nurses on boards and raise broader awareness that all boards would benefit from the unique perspective of nurses to achieve the goals of improved health and efficient and effective healthcare systems at the local, state, and national levels.

Nurses represent the largest segment of the healthcare workforce, are considered the most trustworthy of all professions, and play a huge role on the frontlines of care in our schools, hospitals, community health centers, long-term care facilities, and many other places. Their perspective and influence must be considered at decision-making tables (NOBC, 2021a). Without the voice of nursing, all too often, decisions are made in the absence of information regarding disease prevention, health equity, and SDOH. Such decisions can and do result in changes in the health of communities, but those changes sometimes go in the wrong direction, creating health disparities. NOBC proposes that nurses are uniquely qualified to provide the data and information needed to inform boards of the information needed to make the best decisions for the health and welfare of those they serve.

REVIEW OF RELEVANT LITERATURE IN NURSING, HEALTHCARE, AND OTHER DISCIPLINES

Prior to the release of the *Future of Nursing Report* in 2011 (IOM, 2011), very little had been written about the concept of nurses serving on boards. With the release of the IOM recommendation suggesting that nurses get involved in the boardroom, followed by the creation of the NOBC, nursing leaders began to expound on the concept and disseminate through publications and presentations.

Curran (2015) published the first book about nurses on boards entitled *Nurse on Board: Planning Your Path to the Boardroom*. In this book, Curran (2015) provides an excellent overview of board basics and trends as well as descriptions of several nurse leaders, as well as their paths to the boardroom and board service. Much of Curran's writing focuses on the need for more board positions to be held by nurses, stating, "Nurses represent the largest labor force in hospitals, are the largest human resource expense and, most importantly, are closest to the patients, their families, the physicians, and many other key stakeholders. Yet they have little to no input into the governance of healthcare organizations, regardless of their level in those organizations. Only a small fraction of healthcare board positions are held by nurses. The thousands of healthcare organizations, hundreds of disease-focused organizations, and innumerable nursing organizations will be greatly improved when informed nurses serve on their boards" (Curran, 2015, p. xxx). Much of Curran's work contributed to the creation and strength of NOBC.

Also in 2015, Patton et al. published the first edition of a nursing leadership textbook, *Nurses Making Policy: From Bedside to Boardroom* (2015), that provided "a hands-on approach designed to help graduate students and nurses across a variety of settings develop health policy skills in order to advocate for patients and work empowerment at the bedside, boardroom, or in state and national politics" (Patton et al., 2015, p. XV).

A widely distributed white paper sponsored by Capella University and NOBC entitled *Nurses on Board: The Time for Change Is Now* (2017) provided a detailed overview of why nurses bring a different and much-needed set of competencies to the table that would otherwise not be found in the absence of a nurse in the discussion. The paper proposed that all nurses should accept their leadership responsibility and become involved in their communities through service on boards, commissions, and appointments (Robinson et al., 2017).

Also, in 2016, McBride published "Serving on a Hospital Board: A Case Study." In this article, she outlined her personal service on a large academic medical center board of trustees and described how nurses are uniquely qualified to lead a board's quality and patient safety committees. Furthermore, McBride noted that nurse service on boards endorses recognition of the value of nurses, which also promotes an overall more diverse makeup of the board (McBride, 2016).

Sundean and colleagues (2018) published results of an explanatory, sequential, mixed-methods study which highlighted nurse-specific knowledge, skills, and perspectives that augment board governance. Sundean proposed that nurse board leadership is an influential factor needed in healthcare policy making to ultimately achieve healthcare transformation. The study also validated that preparation and self-promotion are important for nurse board appointments. Additionally, the researchers recommended that nurses should be appointed to boards of directors based on their knowledge, skills, and perspectives about healthcare. In doing so, the board leadership leverages the public's trust in nursing, advances the profession, and positions nurses to influence healthcare transformation (Sundean et al., 2018).

In 2019, the concept of nurses serving on boards gained international attention. The International Council of Nurses included a story in their International Nurses Day publication outlining a case study of NOBC in the United States. This article illustrated the collaboration of nursing organizations' efforts to achieve collective goals (Harper, 2019). This international spotlight resulted in numerous requests for assistance to create collaboration among nurses across the globe.

An article series showcased the value of nursing through the service of nurses on boards, commissions, and appointments. Each of the articles held a specific focus, including the importance and impact of nurses serving on boards (Harper & Benson, 2019); attaining a seat at the table through process, preparation, and potential (Harper & Wray, 2019); preparing and pursuing board opportunities by providing a practical guide for nurse leaders to serve on a board (Cleveland & Harper, 2020); and readying oneself for board service by identifying key competencies and discovering one's path to the boardroom (Harper & Benson, 2020a).

Harper and Benson (2020b) highlighted the importance of nurses on boards in the chapter "Taking Your Place at the Table: Board Appointments and Service." Harper and Benson outlined the unique position that nurses provide in helping boards identify the healthcare needs of those they serve and affirmed that nurses' insight brings value not only to the nurses themselves, but also to their employers and to the communities in which they live and work (Harper & Benson, 2020b).

Nurses in academia have unique knowledge, skills, resources, and networks that can be leveraged for effective board service. Seibert and Harper (2020) outlined how board service provides nurse faculty an opportunity to contribute to societal change. The authors described how board service may help nurse faculty meet academic institutional requirements for engagement within the community.

Another series of articles by Harper and colleagues provided information about the outcomes of nurses on boards and the preparation needed to serve on boards. The first article by Harper (2021) focused on the positive measurable outcomes of an action coalition; specifically, an increase in the number of nurses in the state who served on a board. This increase was due to an organized effort in the state to provide frequent, repetitive messaging to the state's nurses through networks established in state nursing organizations and through social media. The messaging reinforced the national NOBC that conveyed (a) encouragement to serve as a way to give back to their communities through board service, (b) information regarding educational sessions to prepare nurses to serve through a "Get on Board" training program provided free of charge to nurses across the state, and (c) personal assistance to nurses to identify the right board for them, create their one-page board bio, and apply for board membership (Harper, 2021). The second article by Brewington (2021) highlighted how nurses should be prepared for serving and supported to serve on boards. The NOBC Board Competencies Model and the NOBC Board Readiness Model were unveiled as tools for nurses to identify and edify their role as a board member (Brewington, 2021). The third article by Harper and Benson (2021) provided an overview of why nurses are uniquely qualified for board service and what competencies nurses bring to board service and included a helpful list of board types, board readiness questions, the process one would follow to select the right board, and the value of serving to the individual nurse as well as the benefits to the community (Harper & Benson, 2021).

Patton et al. continued their work in this arena and published a third edition of *Nurses Making Policy: From Bedside to Boardroom* (2022). This edition contains a number of references to the need for nurses to serve on boards, on commissions, and in appointments across their communities and the nation and noted the many benefits to our communities with a focus on improving the SDOH across the nation.

> Nursing has the numbers to be a powerful influence. The profession has a well-established, respected national association (ANA) with state and local affiliates. In addition to the ANA, many associations at the national, state, and local levels address the special interests of nurses. Working together, these groups can be leveraged to strengthen nursing's influence across healthcare at the organizational, local, state, national, and international levels. Considerable effort has been made through the Nursing Community, a coalition of more than 60 associations representing over one million nurses; the Campaign for Action at the Center to Champion Nursing in America [(CCNA)]; and the Nurses on Boards Coalition to expand nursing's influence through the placement of nurses in key positions. Nurses associations are working on key appointments at the state level. Often, these positions are perceived to be only hospital- or health-focused boards. However, relevant experience and/or influence can be garnered by serving on boards of community-based affiliates of nonprofit organizations, schools, libraries, food banks, and agencies related to environmental hazards, to name a few. These efforts can expand influence into all the communities where nurses live and work. (Patton et al., 2022, pp. 464–465)

KEY CONCEPTS OF BOARD SERVICE FOR THE NURSE MANAGER

DEFINITION OF BOARDS

The definition of "boards" presented here is intentionally broad to encompass the wide range of governance roles available for nurse leaders to consider, pursue, and serve. Boards are defined as governing bodies that have strategic influence to improve the health of communities and the nation. This includes any corporate, governmental, nonprofit, advisory, or governance boards or appointments that have fiduciary and/or strategic responsibilities (NOBC, 2021b).

TYPES OF BOARDS

Traditionally, nurses have served in governance roles within the nursing profession where nurses have already achieved dominant representation. The dedicated nurse leaders who have served and continue to serve on important nursing association boards and boards of nursing have laid the foundation that prepared nurses to gain significant, necessary skills and experience to expand their reach and impact by serving in much broader and unlimited board opportunities beyond the profession. The following examples depict the variety of opportunities.

PRIVATE AND PUBLIC CORPORATE BOARDS

Corporate industry board structures range from small start-up companies and entrepreneurs to large corporate enterprises. Corporate governing bodies may oversee operations within insurance, finance, manufacturing, agriculture, food and beverage, technology, medical devices, pharmaceutical, and transportation, as well as other product and service industries.

NONPROFIT, NON-NURSING BOARDS

This category includes all types of nonprofit organizations regardless of size that serve the needs of communities, states, our nation, and global missions. Examples include philanthropic boards and foundations such as United Way, American Red Cross, public health-board of directors, local food pantries, literacy councils, poverty advisory groups, and elder adult services, as well as many other human services. All hospital or health system boards (private, public, and nonprofit health provider organizations) are included in this category.

ADVISORY BOARDS

Advisory boards provide strategic advice to the organization, but advisory board members don't typically have a voting role. All types of organizations may offer advisory board roles. Many nurses begin their initial board service on advisory boards.

APPOINTED AND ELECTED POSITIONS

Appointments by the president, governor, mayor, or legislature are numerous and varied. Nurses may be appointed to commissions, task forces, or leadership positions. Citizen-elected boards such as school boards, county board of supervisors, and other local, municipality, and county boards also are included in this category (NOBC, 2021b).

CASE SCENARIO

UNITED WAY

SITUATION

One of the strategic focus areas of United Way is thriving families. Nurse MP recently served on a United Way Review Panel that decides allocation of grants to organizations that service families and people in need. While this isn't a formal board of directors, it is a critical volunteer panel that impacts decisions about the types of community services available to families in need.

A nurse's perspective is extremely helpful in identifying issues related to accessing healthcare. Nurses who work in the community/public health/home health/school nursing have a special nuanced understanding of the needs of their communities and the people they are serving.

OUTCOME

Nurse MP's experience in home health was valuable to the review panel's decision to allocate funding for nurses who work for a family agency in a low-income population. Within the family agency, the nurses' role was critical in motivating, supporting, and providing continuity of care that was otherwise lacking to these families. The other members on the panel had no idea that nurses working in public health tend to make less money and often have less support. Nurse MP's nursing perspective led to a favorable outcome for the health of the community.

Nurse MP highly encourages nurses to participate in their local United Way committees and considers it an honor to be part of this group, sharing that serving the community in this way was the most valuable volunteer work Nurse MP has done since retirement. Nurse MP stresses that service on governing bodies provides invaluable experience for nurses to learn about assessing an organization's functions, including financial operations. As nurses become part of a decision-making body, they witness how outcomes are measured and agency priorities are established. This perspective allows a better understanding of the needs in your community and generates ideas for how you might be able to help meet those needs.

DISCUSSION QUESTIONS

1. How is serving on a panel such as this different than serving on a board of directors?
2. How would you go about trying to convince a group of individuals that the SDOH must become a priority in the community?
3. Nurse MP served on a panel. What are other types of governing bodies within which nurses can serve?

VARIETY OF OPPORTUNITIES TO SERVE

Nursing leaders can raise their voices within an array of board types. Available governing roles offer a variety of options regarding scope, purpose, and venues. For example, nurses may serve on boards whose scope is a start-up, such as a digital health or biotech company, or range as large as a multisystem corporation. Board options also include a variety of purpose and venue such as boards that promote healthcare, education, or advocacy within large and small organizations at the local, state, national, or international level. There is most definitely a board that is a good fit for every nurse who is ready to answer the call.

⬣ **CASE SCENARIO**

NONPROFIT RESIDENTIAL HOME FOR TERMINALLY ILL PATIENTS

SITUATION

Nurse BK is a nursing director for a large hospital in the Midwest and serves on the board of directors for a not-for-profit community organization which funds and operates a residential home for terminally ill patients with no financial means to cover their outpatient care and no place to go for their final days. Nurse BK has recently been elected to serve as the president-elect of the board. During the pandemic of 2020, the organization struggled with the decision to allow visitors in the facility. Some staff believed that they must allow family members and close friends to visit the terminally ill patients who resided in the home.

OUTCOME

Based on Nurse BK's clinical background and experience in the hospital in which they were employed, coupled with their experience with the psychosocial needs of patients (especially dying patients), Nurse BK urged the other members of the board of directors to follow the guidelines of the Centers for Disease Control and Prevention (CDC) and the other hospitals and healthcare facilities in the city by keeping all visitors out of the facility until it was safe to allow them to return. Through the presentation of data-driven evidence, Nurse BK was able to convince the other members of the board that unless they could test and provide the personal protective equipment (PPE) needed to keep the visitors and the patients safe, the patients would be at great risk. Once it was safe, access was made available to again allow the patients to die with a loved one at their side rather than with a nurse or certified medical assistant. Though Nurse BK initially received some backlash for sharing their concerns, other board members (including a physician) all agreed that it was in the best interest of the patients, visitors, and staff. The outcome of the decision resulted in zero cases of COVID-19 in the facility for over a year.

DISCUSSION QUESTIONS

1. Why would a nurse be the best one to present the case for changes in the visitation policy?
2. In this case, who benefitted from the information that Nurse BK shared with the board?

⬣ **WHAT EVERY NURSE MANAGER NEEDS TO KNOW ABOUT BOARD SERVICE**

- Nurses make great board members! Nurses bring a unique set of skills and competencies to the boardroom. Gained through education and experience, these competencies closely match the competencies that most boards seek.
- Self-assessment of board readiness is key in identifying what type of board is right for you.
- Understand your own personal and broader barriers and facilitators of board success.
- Confidence is vital to your successful pursuit of board opportunities.
- Each board has its own dynamics and culture; understand the organization's culture, values, and guiding principles before agreeing to serve on a board.
- When deciding what board is right for you, start with an open mind, understand your personal mission, assess your readiness to serve, prepare a board-ready biography, and contact the organization.
- Supporting board service is an executive role for all nurse leaders.

BOARD COMPETENCIES

Nurses bring a unique set of skills and competencies to the boardroom. The nursing lens offers insights into health promotion, disease preventions, and patient-centered outcomes. Gained through education and experience, these competencies closely match the competencies that most boards seek.

In 2015, a group of nurse leaders involved with the NOBC Support Work Group set out to define the major competencies that nurses bring to the boardroom. The Work Group interviewed over 100 nurse leaders across the nation who were at various levels of involvement with their personal board service (Brewington, 2021). Through these interviews, the group extrapolated a list of five specific competencies that they felt were the most highly needed by boards: mission driven, financial knowledge, communication, cultural competence, and leadership.

MISSION DRIVEN

Nurses are motivated by and guided by the mission to provide quality care. We set goals for patient outcomes, for quality improvement, and for our career paths. In our practice, we measure success by achievement of quality outcomes and alignment with our personal values. This steadfast commitment to accomplishing what they believe is right for those they serve, likewise, would benefit an organization where they serve as board members and consequently could drive a high level of improvement in high-quality, equitable healthcare for all.

FINANCIAL KNOWLEDGE

Nurses often hesitate to commit to serving on boards because they underestimate their competence with analyzing financial reports. Whereas nurses who have worked in senior level positions in their employment settings have experience with managing large budgets, most nurses manage their own budgets and understand the concepts needed to analyze documents such as balance sheets, operating income versus loss statements, changes in assets/equity, and cash flow.

COMMUNICATION

All board members must be skilled communicators and have the ability to communicate effectively, professionally, calmly, confidently, and collegially in all settings. This competency is one which is developed early in the career of nurses and builds over time. Being able to foster the trust of others and build the bonds that result in the respect of other board members promotes an environment where others listen and ultimately consider nurse input to make better decisions for the organization.

CULTURAL AWARENESS

As outlined in one of the conclusions of the NASEM's *The Future of Nursing 2020–2030: Charting a Path to Achieve Health Equity* (Wakefield et al., 2021), nurses must play a primary role in assuring high-quality care to patients of all cultures and in all settings.

> Conclusion 9-1: Nurse leaders at every level and across all settings can strengthen the profession's long-standing focus on social determinants of health and health equity to meet the needs of underserved individuals, neighborhoods, and communities and to prioritize the elimination of health inequities. (Wakefield et al., 2021, p. 11)

In light of this important recommendation, all nurses and nurse board members must not only recognize, but also embrace differences in cultures, values, beliefs, and behaviors. Once differences are recognized, nurses can provide high-quality, equitable care to all. To achieve equity in healthcare, one must possess a high level of understanding of diversity, equity, and inclusion. Nurses possess a high level of cultural humility and are uniquely qualified to successfully and effectively conceptualize and put into action all the SDOH and provide the type of care that is equitable and desired by patients/clients and community members of underrepresented minorities. Nurses are well equipped for this role on any board.

LEADERSHIP

Through experiences within formal education and exposure to leadership roles, both formal and informal, nurses shape their own personal leadership styles early in their careers. Often, we think of leadership as the act of guiding and supporting others to achieve mutually agreed upon goals. In nursing, leadership is not dependent on role or title, but rather inherent in all who work with teams to improve the health of patients and communities.

NURSES ON BOARDS COALITION BOARD COMPETENCIES MODEL

Utilizing the competencies created through the survey, the NOBC Work Group amplified the list of competencies and divided them into three groups to create the NOBC Board Competencies Model (see Figure 20.1). In this model, competencies are divided by level of skill and experience into the categories of self-leadership, organizational management and leadership, and civic/professional leadership (NOBC, 2021e).

Nurses are encouraged to utilize the NOBC Board Competencies Model to identify which type of board is the right fit for them at a specific point in time in their career trajectory. As depicted by the domains in Figure 20.1, the model demonstrates how nurses move from one domain to the next. For example, after meeting the basic competency level, nurses may be ready to transition to the next level for a different type of board appointment. Over time, nurses gain new experiences and competencies that prepare them to move outside their personal self-leadership and into the next domain, organizational management and leadership. Here, they begin to reach outside their personal education and practice realm to strengthen the types of organizations on whose board they may wish to serve. Eventually, nurses gain the experience needed to enter the domain of civic/professional leadership. High-level boards seek nurses who can function at this level and are excited to appoint them to board positions within their organizations where they can demonstrate their political prowess, innovative thinking, and leadership in policy and governance within a community, region, or at the national level (Harper & Benson, 2020a).

BOARD READINESS

Utilizing the concepts developed in the NOBC Board Competencies Model, the Work Group members felt the need to take the next step, which included the development of a second model focused on the readiness of a nurse to serve. Based on the Novice to Expert Model developed by Benner (1982), the Work Group ranked the specific competencies and sub-competencies outlined in the first model by order of skill and then categorized them by areas of performance into levels of complexity of boards and appointments (see Figure 20.2). The authors of the model assumed that most nurses would begin with the skills and competencies found in the self-management domain and work their way up to the higher-level skills and competencies required for organizational management and leadership, ultimately arriving at the competencies needed to address civic and professional

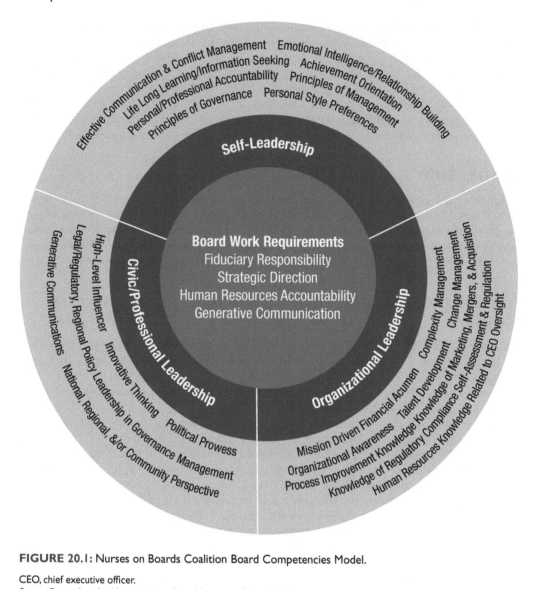

FIGURE 20.1: Nurses on Boards Coalition Board Competencies Model.

CEO, chief executive officer.
Source: Reproduced with permission from Nurses on Boards Coalition; www.nursesonboardscoalition.org.

leadership. The model also supports the belief that nurses often move fluidly between the domains as they encounter new skills and competencies needed by specific board placement. The arrows in this model demonstrate the reality that though a nurse may possess expertise in one area of a domain, further development may still be needed in another area due to a lack of experience or skill. This model provides an operational framework for nurses contemplating a specific board, allowing them to self-assess where they fall into the specific domains as well as to evaluate their need for further professional development in other areas (Harper & Benson, 2020a).

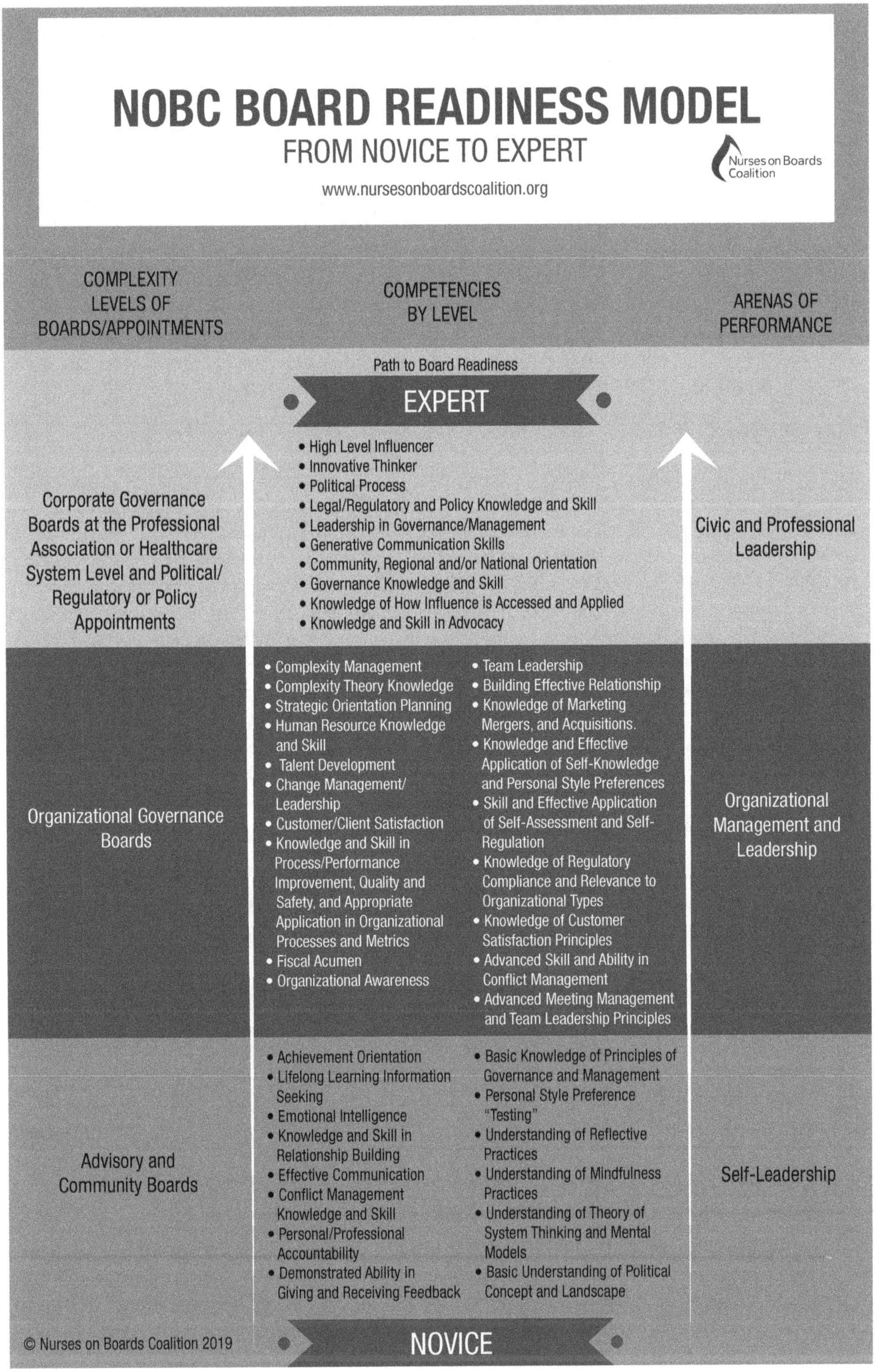

NOBC BOARD READINESS MODEL
FROM NOVICE TO EXPERT
www.nursesonboardscoalition.org

Nurses on Boards Coalition

COMPLEXITY LEVELS OF BOARDS/APPOINTMENTS	COMPETENCIES BY LEVEL	ARENAS OF PERFORMANCE

Path to Board Readiness

EXPERT

Corporate Governance Boards at the Professional Association or Healthcare System Level and Political/Regulatory or Policy Appointments	• High Level Influencer • Innovative Thinker • Political Process • Legal/Regulatory and Policy Knowledge and Skill • Leadership in Governance/Management • Generative Communication Skills • Community, Regional and/or National Orientation • Governance Knowledge and Skill • Knowledge of How Influence is Accessed and Applied • Knowledge and Skill in Advocacy	Civic and Professional Leadership

Organizational Governance Boards	• Complexity Management • Complexity Theory Knowledge • Strategic Orientation Planning • Human Resource Knowledge and Skill • Talent Development • Change Management/Leadership • Customer/Client Satisfaction • Knowledge and Skill in Process/Performance Improvement, Quality and Safety, and Appropriate Application in Organizational Processes and Metrics • Fiscal Acumen • Organizational Awareness	• Team Leadership • Building Effective Relationship • Knowledge of Marketing Mergers, and Acquisitions. • Knowledge and Effective Application of Self-Knowledge and Personal Style Preferences • Skill and Effective Application of Self-Assessment and Self-Regulation • Knowledge of Regulatory Compliance and Relevance to Organizational Types • Knowledge of Customer Satisfaction Principles • Advanced Skill and Ability in Conflict Management • Advanced Meeting Management and Team Leadership Principles	Organizational Management and Leadership

Advisory and Community Boards	• Achievement Orientation • Lifelong Learning Information Seeking • Emotional Intelligence • Knowledge and Skill in Relationship Building • Effective Communication • Conflict Management Knowledge and Skill • Personal/Professional Accountability • Demonstrated Ability in Giving and Receiving Feedback	• Basic Knowledge of Principles of Governance and Management • Personal Style Preference "Testing" • Understanding of Reflective Practices • Understanding of Mindfulness Practices • Understanding of Theory of System Thinking and Mental Models • Basic Understanding of Political Concept and Landscape	Self-Leadership

© Nurses on Boards Coalition 2019

NOVICE

FIGURE 20.2: Nurses on Boards Coalition Board Readiness Model.

Source: Reproduced with permission from Nurses on Boards Coalition; www.nursesonboardscoalition.org.

CASE SCENARIO

BANK BOARD OF DIRECTORS

SITUATION

Nurse KG is a nurse entrepreneur. They sold their company after serving as chief executive officer (CEO) for 15 years. The CEO of Nurse KG's local bank approached Nurse KG about submitting their nomination to be considered to serve on the largest area subsidiary bank board. The CEO of the bank had observed Nurse KG's leadership skills through founding their business, scaling and growing the business, engaging in the local community, and serving in national industry roles.

Nurse KG didn't know much about the banking business, but when asked to represent the voice of the client, Nurse KG agreed to submit their nomination for consideration. Nurse KG embraced the opportunity to be the voice of the client as important decisions were made in the boardroom that impacted services for clients and the client experience. Nurse KG spent significant time preparing for the interview and thinking about how to contribute as a board member.

OUTCOME

Eventually, the nominating committee selected Nurse KG as a board director. Nurse KG learned much about the banking business during their term as a board director and continues to contribute by applying specific and relevant nursing skills such as strategic planning, assessing the environment, critical thinking skills, risk management, and always considering the implications of decisions on clients. Several years later, Nurse KG was asked to serve as the chair of one of the board's committees and as a mentor to novice board members.

Nurse KG's advice to other nurses considering board service is to not let your own perceptions of your abilities limit you from getting outside of your comfort zone. Take a leap of faith and serve on a board when you are given the opportunity. The best place to start is on a local nonprofit board. Remember, no one board member must have all the skills. The board functions and contributes as one body, based on the collective skills, qualifications, and experience of all board members. Most importantly, keep in mind that the nursing perspective is relevant on all types of boards.

DISCUSSION QUESTIONS

1. Why did the bank CEO invite Nurse KG to serve on the board?
2. Do you think Nurse KG had reservations about serving on a board?
3. Nurse KG encouraged nurses to volunteer for board service. Identify strategies to find the best fit for you.
4. Nurse KG provided good advice about how the board functions as one body. Identify some other tips of how to be an effective board member.
5. Nurse KG serves as a mentor to novice board members. According to the NOBC Support Roles for Board Success Model, what are some other support roles for experienced nurse board members?

BARRIERS AND FACILITATORS OF SUCCESS

There are several barriers and facilitators that one might face while preparing for and pursuing board opportunities. While each nurse's experience is unique, a good place to start is by looking inside yourself. Nurses frequently share that they don't feel confident enough to pursue board opportunities. They express concern that they aren't prepared to contribute as a board member. Time is also often a real or perceived barrier. Nurses may hesitate to make a commitment to serve on a board, given their busy schedules. All board leaders are busy people, and most nurses who serve on boards have made it a priority to clear a space to have time to serve in these important roles. The time commitment varies with each board. Nurses should inquire about the expected time commitment before agreeing to serve. Most boards meet on a monthly or quarterly basis. While it takes time to prepare and participate in board meetings, there is usually a way to fit board service into one's busy schedule, especially when you serve on a board that aligns with your personal passion.

Facilitators of successful board membership include the fact that nurses make great board members. The skills, experience, and qualifications that are developed in nursing practice, both within clinical settings and in communities, are a natural fit to serve in governance roles. The increasing emphasis on board diversity, equity, and inclusion creates a sense of urgency for boards to identify candidates with diverse perspectives. However, boards often struggle identifying candidates beyond the circle of those known to them. Board leaders are frequently receptive to learning about potential candidates when approached, so it's a time of great opportunity for nurses to come forward and raise their hands to indicate their interest in serving.

The increased visibility of the nursing profession provides fertile ground for an abundance of new leadership roles for nurses. The COVID-19 pandemic of 2020 emphasized the value nurses bring to the healthcare setting and set up an extremely positive regard for the nursing profession. Due to this heightened awareness, there is increased interest, emphasis, and receptivity for including nurses as candidates for all types of board roles.

BOARD DYNAMICS AND CULTURE

Each board has its own unique dynamics and culture. Potential board candidates need to understand the organization's culture, values, and guiding principles, as adopted and abided by the organization and board's leadership, before agreeing to accept a board appointment. To assess the culture, talk to the organization's leadership and meet with other board members. Your reputation as a board member is tied to the organization and thus you must make sure your values align with the organization.

Diversity, inclusion, and equity are key elements that shape the culture in the boardroom. The following definitions will help you to explore these elements as you are considering the best fit for your board service as well as contemplating your role in creating an optimal board culture.

DIVERSE

All organizations can best realize their missions by drawing on the skills, talents, and perspectives of a broad, diverse range of leaders. Board leaders should embody their organization's values and beliefs and represent the population served to foster advocacy. "The diversity of viewpoints that comes from different life experiences and cultural backgrounds strengthens board deliberations and decision-making" (BoardSource, 2021, para. 5).

INCLUSIVE

A governing body must create and sustain a culture of inclusion to establish the trust, candor, and respect among the board members that is needed for efficient, effective board operation. An inclusive culture fosters sharing of perspectives, experiences, and wisdom within the boardroom that enhances dialogue and decision-making. "An inclusive board culture welcomes and celebrates differences and ensures that all board members are equally engaged and invested, sharing power and responsibility for the organization's mission and the board's work" (BoardSource, 2021, para. 6).

EQUITY-FOCUSED

A key function of a board is to identify the needs of the population served by the board in context and then prioritize the resources and strategies to best meet the needs. "An awareness of how systemic inequities have affected our society and those an organization serves enables boards to avoid blind spots that can lead to flawed strategies, and creates powerful opportunities to deepen the organization's impact, relevance, and advancement of the public good" (BoardSource, 2021, para. 7).

Nurses serving on boards play a key role in shaping a culture of inclusion. While having a diverse board is important, making sure all voices are heard is the only way to tap into the collective experience and perspectives of each board member. Consider the following questions as you think about your role in creating board culture.

- Why is inclusion an important aspect of board effectiveness and impact?
- When serving in your current or prior board roles, what have you observed or experienced about the role of board leadership in making all board members feel welcome and comfortable participating in board discussions?
- What are potential or real barriers to an inclusive board culture?
- What actions can you take as a board member to encourage inclusion, and that all voices are heard and valued?
- How does inclusion look and feel different in a virtual environment?

As nurses, we often talk about self-care and care for others. These concepts are also relevant in the boardroom. Key steps to promoting a culture of self-care and care for others in the boardroom include allowing space for reflections, giving others your full attention, recognizing and appreciating others, expressing empathy, sharing humanity, and being aware of biases. During challenging times, consider the impact of fatigue on board deliberations by ensuring focused agenda topics and scheduling shorter meetings. Nurse leaders can contribute to a positive board culture regardless of the type of board by making sure discussions are aligned with the mission and strategies of the organization, considering the implications of decisions on all stakeholders, and celebrating wins along the way.

CASE SCENARIO
RISE RECOVERY BOARD OF TRUSTEES
SITUATION

Nurse ST serves on the Rise Recovery Board of Trustees as their expert on addiction outcomes. Based on Nurse ST's expertise in the field and ability to share data regarding the mental health needs of the community, the board recently completed a retreat where addiction outcomes moved to the forefront of the board discussion. Through Nurse ST's influence, the board declared that the aggregation of outcomes is now a top priority. Nurse ST felt this was a big win for themselves and for the mental health of the community but shared that it took a while serving on the board before they were able to influence decisions in this way.

OUTCOME

Because nurses are among the most trusted professions, we need to leverage that trust to address the health-related issues within an organization. Nurse ST believes that once a nurse joins a board of interest, one must remain patient and quietly assess where one can best contribute. This takes time, so Nurse ST advises to stick with it and don't get discouraged. Once trust and respect are developed, the board may ask you to take a leadership role, so always be ready to step up and make an impact just like Nurse ST did with the mental health of their community.

DISCUSSION QUESTIONS

1. Do you think that the same decision would have been made regarding the closer focus on mental health if Nurse ST had not been involved in the discussion and able to bring their expertise to the conversation?
2. What are your personal thoughts on Nurse ST's suggestion that nurses serving on boards need to be patient and gain the respect and trust of other board members prior to suggesting strong changes in the direction of the discussion or board?

HOW TO DECIDE WHAT BOARD IS RIGHT FOR YOU

Identifying the board opportunity that is the right fit for the right nurse at the right time can be the most difficult part of the decision-making process. Many nurses have shared testimonials about their board service and how they arrived on the board that was right for them. Through those testimonials, a list of strategies was developed that may be helpful when making such a decision.

- Start with an open mind. There are many options out there and no one should jump into the first board opportunity that comes forward before careful consideration.
- Understand your personal mission. What areas, causes, or services make your heart eager to serve?
- Assess your personal readiness to serve on a board and assess the organization you are being asked to represent. Ask questions of yourself and the organization about time commitment, expectations for financial giving, financial status of the organization, how well the services and products of the organization match their mission, and so on.
- Prepare a personal board-ready biography. This document is not a resume or a curriculum vitae. It is a one-page overview of who you are, your experience as it relates to the organization, your previous or current board experience, and what you would bring to their board.
- Contact the organization. Call or email the CEO or executive director of the organization and ask to meet with them to discuss your interest. You could also contact a current board member (you can usually locate these contacts on the organization's website) and ask about the board duties and if there would be interest in adding a nurse to their board.
- Register your interest in serving on a board with the NOBC at www .nursesonboardscoaliton.org. Once registered, NOBC will assist you in identifying opportunities to serve that may be of interest to you.
- NEVER underestimate the value that you bring to a board. Boards are hungry for new board members who will commit to their mission. Undoubtedly, the competencies and skills that you can bring to their boardroom will benefit the decisions they make regarding the health of the community, state, or nation.

◆ CASE SCENARIO

MEALS ON WHEELS AND CHAMBER OF COMMERCE BOARDS

SITUATION

Nurse GN got involved with Meals on Wheels after being introduced to the idea through the NOBC website. Nurse GN works with clientele who rely on food pantries to get the food that they need because there are no grocery stores within walking distance. The board was impressed with Nurse GN's commitment to the cause and work ethic from their volunteer role delivering meals and helping at the food pantry, so they invited Nurse GN to serve on the board.

Nurse GN quickly became known in the community for their nursing leadership and commitment to contributing to a better community. Through this network of community connections, Nurse GN was invited to serve on the local Chamber of Commerce Board. Nurse GN accepted this role so they could have a greater impact in shaping the strategies and policies that would foster a stronger economy and better community services for all those in the community.

OUTCOME

Nurse GN advises nurses who are interested in board service to start by taking an inventory of the skills one already possesses. Nurse GN believes that nurses have skills in negotiation, organization, and crisis management that can benefit the community. They recommend that nurses get to know an organization before agreeing to serve on the board, because the reputation of the board in which a nurse serves has a direct reflection on the nurse. Nurse GN advocates for patients and believes that all nurses can and should advocate for consumers of the services of the organizations on whose boards they serve. Nurse GN strongly believes nurses have much to contribute, especially through bringing humanity into conversations in the boardroom and not focusing solely on the numbers.

DISCUSSION QUESTIONS

1. How did Nurse GN get started on their board journey?
2. What lessons from this case can be applied to all nurses considering board service?
3. Nurse GN recommends that a nurse should get to know an organization before agreeing to serve on the board. List some key questions that a nurse might ask to get to know an organization.

THE BOARD INTERVIEW

Most boards interview potential candidates for board seats prior to issuing an invitation to serve. During this interview, the nurse must come prepared just as they would for an interview for an employment setting. While awaiting the interview day, spend time on the website of the organization reading and learning about the organization, including its mission, values, and strategic plan.

On the day of the interview, dress professionally, show up early, introduce yourself, shake hands with everyone, and come with a list of well-thought-out questions. You will want to first answer all their questions about your experience on boards, your interest in their organization, how you learned about the opportunity, and so on. Then, it will be your turn to ask any questions you have that have not already been answered. Be sure to ask about time commitment, financial donation expectations, fundraising requirements and orientation to the board. Also, confirm that the organization carries directors and officers liability insurance coverage for their board members.

Before accepting a board seat, a best practice is to meet with the board chair to discuss expectations, to learn more about the role and impact of the board, and to gain a full understanding of why you were selected to serve as well as how you can best contribute. You will want to understand what the board feels it does very well, what aspects could be improved, and how the board evaluates their effectiveness and identifies strategic gaps. Be sure to review with the board chair the strategic plan and the top priorities for the board, what needs to happen for the board to have the greatest impact, and your role in this process. Before leaving the interview, be sure to confirm the next steps in the selection process. Often, the full board will need to vote to approve new members, so do not be surprised if the process takes a while, depending on the board meeting frequency and the timing of a specific and expected open board seat.

DOS AND DON'TS IN THE BOARDROOM

Just as in most settings, there are guidelines and protocols to follow when serving on a board. Consider the following tips to ensure that you contribute value and impact in the boardroom. First, be "all in" by learning everything you can about the organization and those they serve. Be prepared, review the agenda, plan strategic questions, and focus on what's most important. Ask questions of the organization's leadership and/or board chair prior to the board meeting if there is anything on the agenda that you don't fully understand. Second, establish rapport with board colleagues and aim to establish trust with everyone.

Third, engage fully while keeping the mission of the organization at the forefront. Keep an open mind on all topics until you hear the perspectives of your board colleagues. If you have something to say, speak up. That's why you are there. Make your points clearly and succinctly. Listen to what's being said and what's not being said and use questions to elevate or redirect discussion. Inform the board chair if you are unable to attend or participate for any reason and always ask how you can help. And most importantly, be YOU!

In contrast, there are some behaviors to avoid. To maintain perspective, try not to get too deep into operations. Also be careful to not dominate conversations or "over explain" your position or be inflexible. These behaviors don't reflect respect for the opinions of other board members and can cause the board to disengage from listening to a particular board member or not seriously consider the member's point. Acknowledge that unanimous agreement on every topic is not realistic; however, consensus once a decision has been made is essential for fluent operations. Remember, in the end, the board speaks with one voice, regardless of anyone's personal views.

◼ WHAT EVERY NURSE EXECUTIVE NEEDS TO KNOW ABOUT BOARD SERVICE

PREPARING FOR SUCCESSFUL BOARD SERVICE

Board service is an extension of leadership and all nurses are leaders. Nurse executives must remember to model behaviors that one wants to create in the team. By serving on community and national boards and sharing those experiences with the members of the team, nurse executives help build a culture of caring for the community in which they serve. When leaders see their leaders giving of their time, talents, and treasure to causes in the community, they may begin to recognize the importance of giving back. By sharing the knowledge gained through board service, leaders can encourage and mentor others to follow.

It is important that every nurse know that support structures and resources are available to prepare and support them through their board service. NOBC created a third model, the NOBC Support Roles for Board Success Model, in 2021 to provide a visual depiction of support roles for nurses as they build their board service experience (see Figure 20.3). The support roles outlined include those of preceptor, coach, mentor, and sponsor. Though they can sometimes overlap and at any given time a nurse board member may engage in more than one role, the four roles are truly unique from each other. The nurses who serve in these roles provide much-needed support to prepare and empower less experienced nurses to thrive on boards (NOBC, 2021d).

Most new nurse board members pair with a seasoned board member assigned to serve as a preceptor. Like preceptorships within the clinical setting, the board preceptor is a content expert skilled in assessing needs, teaching specific tasks, and developing the competencies of the new board member on a short-term basis. This support role provides one-to-one, time-specific assistance to orient the new person to the role of board member.

Nurse board members may also seek a mentor as a more lasting resource. A mentor is a voluntary role created through a personal request of the nurse to someone whom they believe possesses the skills and competencies they would like to emulate. The mentor is usually perceived as a trusted advisor to the mentee. Mentorships are usually long-term relationships that deepen over time.

Occasionally, a nurse board member needs skill development in a specific area. In this case, the board member may seek out the counsel of a coach. The coach–trainee relationship employs goal oriented, personal/professional development for a specific skill or competency. The coach, as often seen in sports, serves as a skilled observer who can advise on how to improve specific skills, point out areas of concern, and guide the trainee to maintain personal accountability.

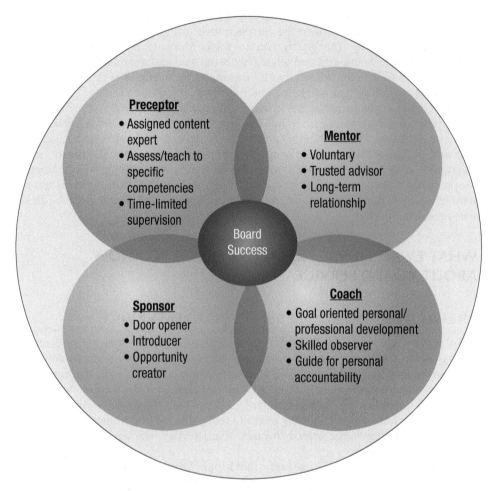

FIGURE 20.3: Nurses on Boards Coalition support roles for Board Success Model.

Source: Reproduced with permission from Nurses on Boards Coalition; www.nursesonboardscoalition.org.

Once a nurse has reached a high level of competency and skill serving on boards, they are often "noticed" by a colleague who is well connected and respected. In this case, the role of sponsor may be applied. The sponsor serves as a door opener who can introduce and vouch for the less experienced nurse creating opportunities that could not be achieved without the sponsor's connections and reference.

Each of these four roles are important to the development of up-and-coming nurse board members and are often fulfilled by experienced nurse executives. These roles provide another way for nurse leaders to demonstrate their commitment to teaching and supporting the next generation of nurses.

◆ | CASE SCENARIO

SENIOR LIVING BOARD AND CORPORATE INSURANCE BOARD

SITUATION

Nurse PM has served on many boards since the age of 30. Their parents were both community leaders and believed that giving back is an essential part of one's life journey. Nurse PM followed their guidance and wisdom.

Nurse PM frequently told their friends in business that nurses are talented contributors to society and that nurses often have skills not typically represented on boards. Nurse PM promotes nurses as good listeners, good problem-solvers, and compassionate humanitarians with diverse educational backgrounds and holistic approaches to societal challenges. While serving on the nursing faculty of the local university, a globally recognized gerontologist faculty colleague approached Nurse PM about taking their place on the board of a local senior living community. This colleague was just too busy to continue to serve in the role. They approached Nurse PM based on observation of Nurse PM's knowledge, experience, and passion for serving older adults and being a role model for students. When asked, Nurse PM jumped at the chance to serve! Nurse PM viewed it as an opportunity to engage their students in the senior living experience and perhaps spark an interest in them to consider a nursing career in gerontology. A few years later, Nurse PM was asked to join the board of a corporate insurance company. One of the corporate board members had learned about Nurse PM's service on the senior living board.

OUTCOME

Nurse PM reflects that they learned many things through serving in board roles. Nurse PM learned to listen more, to reach out to those with less "voice," and to be patient and respectful; all lessons that made them a better contributor and leader.

DISCUSSION QUESTIONS

1. What was Nurse PM's motivation for serving on boards?
2. Why do you think Nurse PM was selected to serve on the senior living board?
3. Why was Nurse PM selected for the corporate insurance company board?
4. Based on Nurse PM's service on a corporate board, use the NOBC Board Readiness Model (see Figure 20.2) to identify the competency level and list specific competencies required at this level.

BOARD SERVICE: A PRIVILEGE AND A RESPONSIBILITY

As nurse leaders, we must all recognize that serving in board roles includes a privilege that comes with great responsibility. We must not lose sight of the expectations that come with the title of board member. Board members must accept the following list of nurse board member expectations.

- Attend all meetings, actively engage.
- Be prepared for all meetings.
- Serve on a board committee.
- Understand the organization's business.
- Get to know the leadership and staff.
- Ask strategic questions.
- Comply with rules and regulations.
- Declare any potential conflicts of interest.
- Focus on the mission.
- Listen more, talk less.

Likewise, the board member must also recognize and accept the collective expectations of the board and its members as denoted in the following list.

- Act in the best interests of the organization and all who are served.
- Ensure all voices are heard.
- Once a vote is taken, support the board's decision publicly.
- Provide feedback and evaluate performance to raise the level of efficiency, effectiveness, and impact.

- All boards benefit from the unique perspective of nursing to achieve the goals of improved health and efficient, effective healthcare systems at the local, state, and national level. Nurses are well versed in many of the critical skills essential to board effectiveness, which enable them to optimally contribute to boardroom discussions and decision-making.

- Five specific competencies that contribute to highly effective board service are mission driven, financial knowledge, communication, cultural competence, and leadership.

- After meeting the basic competency level, nurses can access resources and mentors to master new competencies that enable them to serve on more complex boards where they can demonstrate their political prowess, innovative thinking, and leadership in policy and governance within a community, region, or the national level.

- Consider different types of boards, commissions, or appointments that you may be interested in pursuing, including corporate, governmental, nonprofit, advisory, or governance boards that have fiduciary or strategic responsibilities that align with your skills, qualifications, experience, and passion.

- One of the greatest rewards of board service comes from working alongside other dedicated board members to advance the mission and impact for each organization. In almost every case, the value we receive is far greater than what we give.

- Look around where you live and work. Pursue a board seat for an organization where you care deeply about their mission, and claim your place to make a difference right now. There is no better time than today to begin your journey to the boardroom.

- Never underestimate the value you bring to a board.

SUMMARY

"The time is always right to do right."

Dr. Martin Luther King, Jr. (1965)

REWARDS OF BOARD SERVICE

Through our own experience, the authors of this chapter have found board service to be professionally and personally rewarding. We know first-hand the privilege and responsibility of board service and have experienced both extrinsic and intrinsic rewards. The greatest rewards come from knowing we have made and are continuing to make a difference, working alongside other dedicated board colleagues to advance the mission and impact for each organization. We have found that in almost every case, the value we receive is far greater than what we give.

As nurses serve on more community boards outside their work environment, they gain fresh perspectives that can be applied in their own organization. These fresh perspectives often positively affect job satisfaction. Nurses may find inspiration in sharing their nursing knowledge to improve the health of those served by the board's organization and find a renewed fulfillment of purpose; in other words, a reminder of why we became nurses in the first place.

Board service can be rewarding to nurses both personally and professionally. It not only requires them to exercise leadership; it expands those skills and advances their capabilities and knowledge. It gives nurses the chance to meet people and enhance their professional networks. And it can be inspirational and empowering. (Sue Hassmiller, PhD, RN, FAAN, as cited in NOBC, 2021c)

SENSE OF URGENCY—THE TIME IS NOW!

There has never been a more opportune or crucial time for nurses to raise their voices in boardrooms across our country. *The Future of Nursing 2020–2030: Charting a Path to Achieve Health Equity* report (Wakefield et al., 2021) provides a strategic roadmap to guide our endeavors to become the nursing voice in the boardroom. As each nurse is unique, we can determine a path that aligns with our skills, qualifications, and passion (Wakefield et al., 2021).

Everybody wins when nurse leaders at all levels serve on the boards of nonprofit and community health organizations. Communities experience improved health. Nurses increase their job satisfaction and grow professionally. And healthcare organizations who support the volunteer efforts of their nurse executives reap the benefit of new insights, best practices, and enhanced reputation (Benson & Harper, 2017).

To shape strategies and policies that create health equity for all, it is imperative for nurses to serve in diverse governance roles. This is a time of unprecedented opportunity for nurse leaders and the profession to make a significant and lasting impact. Look around where you live and work, pursue a board seat for an organization where you care deeply about their mission, and claim your place to make a difference right now. There is no better time than today to begin your journey to the boardroom.

END-OF-CHAPTER RESOURCES

◻ DISCUSSION QUESTIONS

1. Why is it important for nurses to serve in governance roles?
2. How can nurses identify, prepare for, and pursue opportunities to serve on boards?
3. What are the benefits to communities and the nation when nurses serve in governance roles on boards, commissions, and appointments?
4. What competencies make nurses uniquely qualified to serve as successful board members?
5. What is your personal plan to bring your nursing expertise to the boardroom, commission, or appointment?

◻ ADDITIONAL RESOURCES

- Nurses on Boards Coalition: https://www.nursesonboardscoalition.org/
- Nurses on Boards Coalition. (2019). *NOBC board competencies, readiness, and support roles for board success models.* https://documentcloud.adobe.com/link/track?uri=urn:aaid:scds:US:3459e0e9-3a0e-4900-9cb8-2af7f036dd39#pageNum=1
- Healthcare Trustees of New York State. (2008). *Boardroom basics: What every trustee needs to know.* https://htnys.org/governance/docs/boardroom_basics.pdf
- North Carolina Nurses Association. (n.d.). *Readiness assessment for board service.* https://www.nursesonboardscoalition.org/wp-content/uploads/Readiness-Assessment-4-17-19.pdf
- American Nurses Foundation & Nurses on Boards Coalition. (n.d.). *Introducing nurses on boards: getting on board.* https://www.nursesonboardscoalition.org/wp-content/uploads/Getting-on-Board-Final.pdf
- Ohio Action Coalition. (2017, November 22). *Board meeting simulation.* https://www.youtube.com/watch?v=QiMpg-S59is

◉ LEARNING EXERCISES FOR STUDENTS

Mock Board Meeting

A small group of learners can learn the value of the nurse perspective in the boardroom through participating in a mock board meeting. To begin this activity, the facilitator creates an agenda topic which would provide the nurse board member with an opportunity to share their clinical expertise and judgment regarding health promotion, disease prevention, or SDOH. This agenda item could be funding a health fair, policies for reporting COVID-19 exposure, resources for minority residents, or any other hot topic. Next, one learner takes the role of the nurse board member, while the others assume the role of board members from the business sector, community citizens, philanthropists, and so on. Then, the learners proceed to address the agenda item. To wrap up the mock board meeting exercise, participants should reflect upon how the discussion and the decisions made would be different without the nursing voice.

Mock Board Interview

A good strategy to help a nurse gain confidence with their board readiness competencies, appreciate the value of a nurse perspective, and enhance interview skills is to engage in a mock board interview. This activity involves pairing learners with a partner with one playing the nurse and the other playing the CEO of the organization or the chairman of the board of the organization. The organizational leader begins by asking the nurse what competencies and expertise they bring to the board and why they would make a good board member for the organization. Once complete, the students could switch roles and repeat the exercise. A debrief discussion should focus on the learner's reflections of their own board readiness, value to a board, and interview skills.

◉ GLOSSARY OF KEY TERMS

- **Board:** A governing body that represents all stakeholders, meets at regular intervals to set strategy and policy, and provides oversight of organizational management, outcomes, and risk management.
- **Board service:** Serving in a governance role as a volunteer or paid director.
- **Governance:** An extension of leadership applied in the boardroom that encompasses the scope of the board's (profit and nonprofit) responsibilities to provide oversight to an organization's fiduciary and operational effectiveness.
- **Nurses on Boards Coalition (NOBC):** An independent 501(c)(3) public charity representing national nursing organizations, whose mission is to improve health in communities across the nation through the service of nurses on all types of boards.

SPRINGER PUBLISHING CONNECT™ | A robust set of instructor resources designed to supplement this text is located at http://connect.springerpub.com/content/book/978-0-8261-7795-7. Qualifying instructors may request access by emailing textbook@springerpub.com.

REFERENCES

Benner, P. (1982). From novice to expert. *The American Journal of Nursing, 82*(3), 402–407. https://doi.org/10.2307/3462828

Benson, L. (2018). *NOBC survey "Why should nurses serve on boards?"* [Unpublished work].

Benson, L., & Harper, K. J. (2017). Why your nurses should serve on community health boards. *BoardRoom Press, Governance Institute, 28*(1), 1–2. https://www.nursesonboardscoalition.org/wp-content/uploads/BRP_2017_02_V28N1_Why-Your-Nurses-Should-Serve-on-Community-Health-Boards_Benson_Harper.pdf

BoardSource. (2021). *Diversity, inclusion, and equity.* https://boardsource.org/research-critical-issues/diversity-equity-inclusion

Brewington, J. G. (2021). The journey Nurses on Boards Coalition preparation and support work group. *Nursing Administration Quarterly, 45*(1), 18–25. https://doi.org/10.1097/NAQ.0000000000000446

Cleveland, K. A., & Harper, K. J. (2020). Prepare and pursue board opportunities: A practical guide for nurse leaders to serve on a board. *Nursing Economic$, 38*(2), 94–97.

Curran, C. (2015). *Nurse on board: Planning your path to the boardroom.* Sigma.

Harper, K. J. (2019, May). Nurses on boards: A case study. Health for all: Nursing, global health, and universal health coverage. *International Council of Nurses International Nurses Day 2019 Resources and Evidence, 55.*

Harper, K. J. (2021). The *Future of Nursing* report set the stage for healthier Hoosiers. *Nursing Administration Quarterly, 45*(1), 46–51. https://doi.org/10.1097/NAQ.0000000000000450

Harper, K. J., & Benson, L. S. (2019). The importance and impact of nurses serving on boards. *Nursing Economic$, 37*(4), 209–212. https://www.nursesonboardscoalition.org/wp-content/uploads/The-Importance-and-Impact-of-Nurses-Serving-on-Boards.pdf

Harper, K. J., & Benson, L. S. (2020a). Are you ready for board service? Identifying key competencies and discovering your path to the boardroom. *Nursing Economic$, 38*(6), 316–319, 323.

Harper, K. J., & Benson, L. S. (2020b). Taking your place at the table: Board appointments and service. In D. J. Mason, E. Dickson, M. R. McLemore, & G. A. Perez (Eds.), *Policy & politics in nursing and health care* (8th ed., pp. 400–405). Elsevier.

Harper, K. J., & Benson, L. S. (2021). The value of including the nursing perspective in the boardroom. *Nursing Administration Quarterly, 45*(3), 192–196. https://doi.org/10.1097/NAQ.0000000000000470

Harper, K. J., & Wray, R. (2019). Attaining a seat at the table: Process, preparation, and potential. *Nursing Economic$, 37*(6), 324–327.

Institute of Medicine. (2011). *The future of nursing: Leading change, advancing health.* National Academies Press.

King, M. L. (1965). *Remaining awake through a great revolution.* https://www2.oberlin.edu/external/EOG/BlackHistoryMonth/MLK/CommAddress.html

McBride, A. B. (2016). Serving on a hospital board: A case study. *Nursing Outlook, 65*(4), 372–379. https://doi.org/10.1016/j.outlook.2016.12.006

Moore Foundation. (2015, June 2). *Lessons in leadership: The Betty Irene Moore speaker series* [Video]. YouTube. https://youtu.be/eTZ6FbSXBkQ

Nurses on Boards Coalition. (2021a). *About our story.* https://www.nursesonboardscoalition.org/about

Nurses on Boards Coalition. (2021b). *Frequently asked questions: What is your definition of a board?* https://www.nursesonboardscoalition.org/resources/faqs

Nurses on Boards Coalition. (2021c). *Home page.* https://www.nursesonboardscoalition.org

Nurses on Boards Coalition. (2021d). *NOBC Support Roles for Board Success Model.* https://www.nursesonboardscoalition.org/resources/for-nurses

Nurses on Boards Coalition. (2021e). *Resources: For nurses: Helpful documents.* https://www.nursesonboardscoalition.org/resources/for-nurses

Patton, R., Zalon, M., & Ludwick, R. (Eds.). (2015). *Nurses making policy: From bedside to boardroom.* Springer Publishing Company.

Patton, R., Zalon, M., & Ludwick, R. (Eds.). (2022). *Nurses making policy: From bedside to boardroom* (3rd ed.). Springer Publishing Company.

Robinson, F. P., Harper, K. J., & Benson, L. S. (2017). *Nurses on board: The time for change is now* (White paper). Nurses on Boards Coalition & Capella University. https://www.nursesonboardscoalition.org/wp-content/uploads/2017/06/NursesOnBoard-TimeforChange.pdf

Sanford, K. (2021). Improving engagement, operations: Including nurses on governing boards has multiple benefits. *Healthcare Executive, 36*(1), 32–33. https://healthcareexecutive.org/archives/january-february-2021/improving-engagement-operations

Seibert, S. A., & Harper, K. J. (2020). The scholarship of application: Opportunities within the NOBC. *Teaching and Learning in Nursing, 15*(2), 152–154. https://doi.org/10.1016/j.teln.2020.01.005

Sundean, L. J., Polifroni, E. C., Libal, K., & McGrath, J. M. (2018). The rationale for nurses on boards in the voices of nurses who serve. *Nursing Outlook, 66*(3), 222–232. https://doi.org/10.1016/j.outlook.2017.11.005

Wakefield, M. K., Williams, D. R., Le Menestrel, S., & Flaubert, J. L. (Eds.). (2021). *The future of nursing 2020–2030: Charting a path to achieve health equity.* National Academies Press. https://doi.org/10.17226/25982

CHAPTER 21

RELATIONSHIPS BETWEEN BOARD AND MANAGEMENT

Pamela Austin Thompson[1]

"Governance is not about the budget lines [and] personnel issues. . . . It is about values and vision and strategic leadership."

John Carver (as cited in Annie E. Casey Foundation, n.d., p. 2)

LEARNING OBJECTIVES

- Identify how staff can operationalize the strategic plan for an organization.
- Demonstrate understanding of the major components of the board of directors/trustees for healthcare organizations.
- Evaluate how nurse leaders can contribute to the strategic focus of a board.
- Create a model situation to demonstrate key components of relationships among boards, management, and operations.

INTRODUCTION

The environment for healthcare has become more and more complex. The patient care delivery system is changing rapidly, especially because of the COVID-19 crisis. Although hospitals remain central to the delivery system, patient care continues to move into the community, expanding the focus of hospital and health system strategic plans. Multihospital systems are emerging, and healthcare organizations are increasingly partnering with the community to meet community needs (Lúanaigh & Hughes, 2016). Boards are also adapting their function and becoming more attuned to this changing environment. This chapter explores how boards govern and how nurse leaders can influence the governance and operations of the organization.

Healthcare organizations are governed by a board of directors/trustees and are responsible for the strategic direction of the organization. High-performing boards partner with the organization's senior management to align operations with the strategic direction. This partnership can be well known within the organization, or it can be somewhat removed from the day-to-day experiences of the staff. Nurse leaders should know the functions of governance and how they might inform and impact governance to further the provision of high-quality patient care (Meynell & Sedel, 2012).

The federal tax status of healthcare organizations provides an initial categorization of their focus. For-profit status or investor-owned status means that profits are directed to the shareholders of the company or corporation. Not-for-profit means that profits are directed back

---

[1] *The author wishes to acknowledge the work of Hannah Holmes, who provided outstanding assistance in the completion of this chapter.*

into the organization for the benefit of the community served and for charitable purposes. These distinctions guide the work of the boards and their operations. Nurse leaders should be familiar with this designation to understand the implications it has on operations and the provision of patient care. Healthcare institutions in both for-profit and not-for-profit categories want to be financially successful but their focus on the use of profit margins will differ.

Duties of board members, however, should be the same for both for-profit and not-for-profit boards. These duties, referred to as fiduciary responsibilities, include duty of care, duty of loyalty, and duty of obedience (Curran, 2016). In addition, each organization has a mission and vision to guide the work and values that describe "how" they will accomplish the mission and vision. Using these statements, the boards develop strategic plans to guide the organization. The management teams oversee the operations to achieve the mission, as laid out by the board. This partnership between board and management is critical to achieving success. Nurse leaders can understand both strategic direction and operations to achieve that plan and determine how best to impact the delivery of high-quality patient care.

Boards provide strategy, policy, fiscal oversight, and quality and safety goals. Much of this work is delegated to board committees. These committees offer opportunities for nurse executives and nurse managers to become involved with governance. It is critical that nurse leaders understand how to relate at the board level, rather than wait for direction to trickle down through the organization's hierarchy.

In this chapter the author proposes that both nurse managers and nurse executives have a role to play in their organization's governance.

HEALTHCARE TRENDS FOR BOARD AND MANAGEMENT

Hospitals have faced significant challenges over the past 5 years. Consolidations of independent hospitals are resulting in hospital systems and smaller hospitals are finding it increasingly difficult to remain independent. Reimbursement methodologies are changing, making financial success more challenging. Beginning in 2020, COVID-19 dramatically changed the way care is delivered. The complexity of the COVID-19 patients crippled some health systems and resulted in more deaths than hospitals could manage. COVID-19 created the greatest crisis the healthcare community has faced since the devastating Spanish Flu one hundred years ago.

These challenges have also caused healthcare organizations to look closely at their boards. The competencies of board members are under greater scrutiny. Boards are seeking to increase board diversity, so the board reflects the community served. New models of care, such as telemedicine/telehealth, are expanding at a rapid rate. Communities are asking for more accountability from their healthcare providers. Workforce shortages are present in all roles in healthcare. Physician relationships are gaining more importance for hospitals and board leadership (Price, 2019; Totten, 2018).

How are boards responding to these challenges? How are boards adapting to maintain high performance? How is this affecting the board and management relationship? These are questions that are being addressed by boards today.

MAJOR ATTRIBUTES AND FUNCTIONS OF BOARDS

While there are many attributes and characteristics of high performance in board governance, the following are most relevant to nurse leaders. These are detailed in Curran's resource *Nurse on Board: Planning Your Path to the Boardroom,* which is a frequent reference for the subject matter (Curran, 2016).

1. Maintaining a governance structure that brings value to the organization

2. Safeguarding both the value and reputation of the organization

3. Clarity of role and focus of the board

4. Effective leadership of the board coupled with an open relationship with the CEO and management that creates a board–management partnership

5. A board team that is balanced with respect to expertise and temperament

6. A culture of respect and trust that permits the board to function as a team

7. Clarity around mission and key organizational strategies

8. Willingness to challenge the status quo

It is important for nurse leaders to understand what a board does so that they can provide targeted input and be more effective. There are three core responsibilities that all board members must accept as part of their role (Box 21.1). These duties are referred to as the fiduciary responsibilities which are legal duties that they will be held accountable for meeting. They are:

Duty of care: In making decisions, the board must use the same diligence that a reasonable person would use given a similar set of facts. This requires board members to explore the facts before making decisions to ensure that their actions are in the best interests of the organization (Curran, 2016). In practice, it requires the board to be informed and willing to debate issues to ensure that "how" they make decisions is thorough.

Duty of loyalty: The board member agrees to always put the good of the organization first, ahead of personal or other considerations. The allegiance requires that they respect the confidentiality of board meetings and avoid conflicts of interest for themselves, especially those that result in personal gain (Curran, 2016). To document this, many boards require members to submit a conflict-of-interest statement that outlines potential conflicts that may arise. This allows the board to take necessary precautions if conflicts do arise. The goal is to ensure that all board members act as independent agents, serving the organization needs first and foremost.

Duty of obedience: The board member agrees to comply with all laws, rules, and regulations that apply to the organization. This also requires members to support the organization's mission, bylaws, policies, and procedures (Curran, 2016). For not-for-profit hospitals, it means that board members must ensure that the charitable purpose is protected. This duty is important because failing to abide by laws and regulations could result in significant harm and disruption to the organization. Some may assume that the board's fiduciary role only applies to oversight of finances. However, it extends beyond finances and addresses how boards make decisions, the alignment of board member intentions with the best interests of the organization, and the mandate to be law-abiding in their actions.

It is also helpful to understand the Internal Revenue Service (IRS) tax status of the organization. There are two major types of assignments for healthcare facilities. The easiest way to understand the distinction is knowing how the organizations' profits are managed.

BOX 21.1: FIDUCIARY ROLES AND DUTIES

- **Duty of care:** In making decisions, the board must use the same diligence a reasonable person would use with a similar set of facts.

- **Duty of loyalty:** The board member agrees to put the organization first, ahead of personal gain, thus avoiding conflicts of interest.

- **Duty of obedience:** The board member agrees to comply with all laws, rules, and regulations that apply to the organization.

Source: Data from Curran, C. (2016). *Nurse on board: Planning your path to the boardroom.* Sigma Theta Tau International, Center for Nursing Press.

For-profit healthcare organizations are governed as corporate businesses. Profits are provided back to the shareholders or owners of the corporation. Examples include Tenet Heathcare Corporation and Healthcare Corporation of America (HCA). These corporations pay federal, state, and local taxes.

Not-for-profit healthcare organizations invest profits back to the organization for the benefit of stakeholders. Profits can be used to fund capital expenditures or long-term financial reserves. These organizations do not pay federal, state, or local taxes. In exchange for no taxes, they focus on their work to meet their community's needs and meet a charitable mission. Examples include academic medical centers (AMCs), community hospitals, faith-based organizations, and some hospital systems.

These two distinctions provide the foundation for the board's governance perspective and strategic planning. Both for-profit and not-for-profit healthcare institutions must meet federal, state, and local requirements for healthcare facilities. This includes regulatory agencies like The Joint Commission (TJC), Medicare, Medicaid, and state licensing agencies. Both for-profit and not-for-profit agencies are also interested in providing quality to their patients and clientele. The differences lie in their goals for their financial profits. The key difference is that for-profit organizations are accountable to their shareholders who usually expect to receive the profits. Not-for-profit organizations use profits to invest in the facility and meet the needs of the communities they serve.

As stated in the previously listed attribute 5, a high-performing board requires a balance and breadth of expertise; one organization that is devoted to broadening the expertise of boards is the Nurses on Boards Coalition (NOBC). The NOBC works to identify nurses interested in serving on a board and matches this interest with boards who want to have a nurse on their board. As of 2021, NOBC has documented 10,000 nurses who occupy a seat on a board. NOBC focuses on healthcare boards, community boards, non-nursing associations, and corporate and business boards. They have developed a comprehensive model for the competencies of board members. Their focus on developing the expertise of nurses serving on boards is critical to the success of the NOBC goals. Securing board seats for nurses is important, but equally as important is the competency of nurses who occupy a seat on a board. NOBC serves as a resource, advocate, and promoter of the voice and expertise of nurses in governance roles (www.nursesonboardscoalition.org).

THE RELATIONSHIP OF BOARD AND MANAGEMENT

One of the key roles of the board is to create and adhere to a strategic direction that moves the organization toward achieving its mission. This calls upon the board to envision the future for the organization, considering the environmental, political, and social factors that will be encountered. The point where the board and management create one of their strongest bonds is the division of the strategic priorities into its two components—the future path and the details for how to get there (Meynell & Sedel, 2012). The governance strategic plan and the management's focus on operations can make this happen. Management usually refers to senior management, those individuals who report to the chief executive officer (CEO) or chief operating officer (COO), and the other management staff who direct and manage the facility/system departments. Senior management is the usual group that works most closely with the board (Murphy, 2018).

For the nurse executive of the organization, this is where they can have the greatest impact. The board conceptualizes the strategic direction and priorities for the organization, but it is the management team that usually takes that and creates the actual plan and tactics to achieve those priorities. As the leader of patient care, the nurse leader can play a significant role in how the plan is operationalized.

This is also true for the nurse manager. Nurse leaders can address the priorities related to patient care, quality, safety, and ambulatory care. They understand how to create measurable outcomes and incorporate a systems perspective to achieving the goals.

Management develops the implementation plan for the strategies and establishes the metrics for evaluating achievement of goals. Usually, there are progress reports provided to the board. The nurse executive can attend the board meetings and participate in the dialogue addressing the priorities. If the metrics are reported by another member of the executive team, the nurse executive can still enhance the dialogue about the reports. It provides the opportunity for the nurse executive to establish a presence at the board meeting by giving voice to the contributions of nursing.

Key to the strategic plan is a well-articulated mission, vision, and values statement (Price, 2018). Fundamental attributes of these statements are as follows:

- **Mission:** What the organization does to meet the needs of shareholders (for-profit) or stakeholders (not-for-profit)
- **Vision:** The aspirational statement of what the organization wants to be in the future
- **Values:** Statements of key behaviors that members of the organization demonstrate in their pursuit of the mission and strategic plan

These statements become a lens for the organization to judge the strategic and operational actions. Are their initiatives aligned with achieving the mission and ultimately the vision? Do they exemplify the values in their internal and external interactions? These elements should form the foundation for actions of the organization (Price, 2018).

A perfect example of how important initiatives come to the board and organizations occurred in May of 2021. The National Academies of Sciences, Engineering, and Medicine (NASEM) released the first draft of the consensus study report of the *Future of Nursing 2020–2030: Charting a Path to Achieve Health Equity* (Wakefield et al., 2021). This report is a call to action for nurses to advance health equity in the United States. It outlines a path for the nursing profession to reduce inequities that prevent all people from achieving their full health potential. The report identified nine recommendations to achieve this goal that focus on social determinants of health (SDOH), environmental health, health equity, and nurses' health and well-being. It also calls for involvement of healthcare organizations, foundations, government agencies, payors, and education programs to work with nurses to achieve these all-encompassing goals (Wakefield et al., 2021).

Nurse leaders can take responsibility for sharing the report and its recommendations with governing boards. Not-for-profit boards focus on the health of their communities, and this report can augment strategic plans to address community benefit and improve the health of their communities.

The report highlights that nurses can be advocates and leaders in achieving health equity (Wakefield et al., 2021). They connect with people, patients, and communities to promote health and well-being. Boards can support and strengthen this work if they are aware of its goals. Nurses who occupy a board seat can also bring the report to the board and share the recommendations and highlight how they align with the organization's strategic plan. The report outlines work for the next decade to improve health. It will be important for nurse leaders to advocate for health equity for all. The management and board relationship can be a productive venue for these recommendations to be nurtured.

THE BOARD AND MANAGEMENT PARTNERSHIP

In high-performing organizations, there is a strong partnership between the board and the management team. The board focuses on the strategic direction and priorities, and the management team creates the operational plan to achieve those strategies. The partnership demonstrates how each brings forward their insights and creates constructive dialogue and action.

For the nurse leader, it is critical to understand what makes this partnership successful. Knowledge of how the board functions and communicates facilitates effective participation in the partnership. Basic structural elements like the meeting schedule, meeting agendas, communication between meetings, committees, and the role of the chair and the executive committee are elements the nurse executive should understand. The main committees that nurses serve on include the quality and safety committee, talent development and workforce committees, and strategic planning committees. If a nurse chairs a committee, they may also serve on the governance committee (Lúanaigh & Hughes, 2016). They can, in turn, educate other nurse leaders in how the board functions. Many nurses did not learn about board governance in their initial nursing education. Preparing nurse leaders to bring a voice to governance is a role that nurse executives can play in their own organizations (Sundean et al., 2019).

Questions that the senior nurse leader can utilize to assess the board include:

1. Who writes the reports for the board? This is usually someone on staff and not the board members themselves. Knowing this offers the opportunity to advocate for inclusion of specific points or data related to patient care, nursing, or quality that might otherwise be omitted.

2. How do the nurse leaders officially provide input? Asking targeted questions of the person writing the reports can demonstrate a willingness to help and an interest in staying involved in the future.

3. Who attends board meetings? Are there other nursing colleagues? This is important as this provides another opportunity to participate in board dialogue and bring the nurse perspective and expertise.

4. Who presents reports at the board meetings? Do individuals who do not understand issues related to patient care report on patient care? In that case, the nurse leader can aid the person reporting. The goal would be for the board members to experience the expertise that a nurse can bring. This can also pertain to non-patient care issues, as the nurse executives' areas of expertise are not limited to patient care and nursing. Nurses are system thinkers and can see how one issue may impact other issues. They also interact with a multitude of departments and understand how the organization functions. They can be strategic in their approach to problems or issues. Most importantly, they understand the value of relationships in a complex organization (McBride, 2017).

5. Who staffs board committees? Staffing the committees can provide access to the development of committee agendas, what topics will be discussed, and the inclusion of different voices in the committee discussions. Nurses can staff committees if it isn't possible to be named a member of the committee. The quality and safety committee is a critical placement for the expertise of a nurse leader.

Each organization will have unique answers to these questions. Board discussions can range from closed to open processes. For example, some boards may only meet with the CEO and the CEO relates all information to the board. Others may have the entire management team present, and reports are provided by select management staff. Nurse leaders should assess their own organization's approach and know when there are opportunities to have the voice of nursing and patient care included in board deliberations or when it is appropriate to advocate for inclusion.

● CASE SCENARIO

ADDRESSING COMPENSATION VARIANCES

SITUATION

COVID-19 caused an extreme increase in the census of the ICU. Medical–surgical bed occupancy decreased because no elective surgery was being done. Because of the overcapacity in the ICU, medical–surgical beds were being used for COVID-19 patients.

The nurse executive attends board meetings as a guest. The chief financial officer (CFO) is new to the organization and has only been at the hospital for 6 months. Prior to coming, the CFO was working in the private sector at an investment firm. The CFO has been asked to provide a report to the board explaining why there has been such an increase in compensation for nursing when beds in the medical–surgical unit have been closed. The nurse executive approached the CFO to ask if they would like to review the variances together. The CFO declined the offer and presented at the next board meeting. The board asked numerous questions about the variances, but the CFO was not able to answer their questions. The CFO was asked to come back to the board meeting with the answers.

DISCUSSION QUESTIONS

1. What can the nurse executive do now? What could the CFO do now?
2. If you were the nurse executive, how would you answer these questions? If you were the nurse executive, what would you look at to explain the variances? What advice would you give the CFO about what else they could explore to explain the variances?

THE ROLE OF STRATEGY, POLICIES, AND COMMITTEES

How does the board develop its strategy, policies, fiscal oversight, quality and safety goals, and other governance functions? Keep in mind that the board's role is not to engage in operations, but rather to provide the higher-level strategic guidance to those responsible for operations.

The strategic plan usually addresses a 3- to 5-year period and is updated annually. The current healthcare environment makes it difficult to plan for 5 to 10 years, as organizations may have done in the past. The plan can be developed by a special task force, the full board, or a combination of groups.

The policies of the board include nominations for board members and officers, election of officers, and term limits of officers. A code of conduct for board members may be developed by the board. Most boards have policies for confidentiality, support for decisions of the majority, respect for differing perspectives of other board members, and how members contribute and participate in board discussions. All of these are aimed at encouraging high-quality dynamics.

High-performing boards are efficient with their time together in official board meetings. Discussions about strategic directions and growth are reserved for full board participation. The more detailed work of the board is delegated to committees or task forces. Usually, committees have formal charges or charters, can be chaired by a member of the board, and present summary reports to the board.

Committees also provide the opportunity for non-board individuals to participate in specific conversations offering the input of select stakeholders (Box 21.2). The most common board committees include an executive committee, a governance and nominating committee, a finance committee, audit and compliance, a compensation committee, a talent development/workforce development committee, a strategic planning committee, a quality and safety committee, a research and education committee, and task forces.

BOX 21.2: BOARD COMMITTEES

- Audit and compliance
- Compensation
- Executive
- Finance
- Governance/nominating
- Quality and safety
- Research and education
- Strategic planning
- Talent development
- Task forces

EXECUTIVE COMMITTEE

This committee is chaired by the board chairperson. Members usually include the officers of the board such as vice chair, secretary, treasurer, and the chairs of the major committees. This committee can convene between official board meetings to discuss or decide on issues requiring immediate action. Any actions taken by the executive committee are reported to the whole board.

GOVERNANCE AND NOMINATING COMMITTEE

This committee oversees the board effectiveness. It may be the same membership as the executive committee or an expanded membership. One of its chief responsibilities is the recruitment of new board members. This committee ensures that the make-up of the board encompasses the competencies and expertise necessary to govern well. Unfortunately, there are few nurses on healthcare governance boards. Only 2% to 6% of boards have nurses serving. The NOBC is working hard to increase nursing representation. Chapter 20, "Board Leadership and Responsibilities," provides excellent insight into what a nurse can bring to board deliberations (Rudisill & Benson, 2021).

FINANCE COMMITTEE

This committee is charged with the financial oversight of the organization. It ensures there are adequate financial resources to achieve the strategic plan and the core business of the organization. The finance committee covers revenue, expenditures, capital budgets, investment strategies and performance, and long-term financial planning to accommodate growth. The goal is to ensure adequate resources exist to achieve the organization's mission.

AUDIT AND COMPLIANCE

This committee focuses on the internal financial controls and processes. It ensures that these controls function to create healthy and legal financial practices. Federal rules require audit committee members to be independent with no personal relationship with governance. To achieve this, many organizations contract with independent audit companies to perform the audit reviews.

Compliance is the organization's ability to meet requirements of regulatory bodies such as TJC and federal payment programs such as Medicare and Medicaid. There are numerous regulatory agencies from local, state, and federal bodies that require compliance. This committee also reviews internal financial functions to ensure they are sound financial practices. Reports from independent evaluators come to this committee and then on to the board.

Sometimes the finance and audit and compliance committees are combined. This is especially true in smaller organizations. As organizations become larger and more complex, better oversight of these functions is achieved when they are split between two separate bodies.

COMPENSATION COMMITTEE

This committee is responsible for establishing the compensation package of the CEO. The CEO is the only management role that the board hires, evaluates, determines the compensation package, and can terminate. All other employees ultimately are accountable to the CEO. This committee may use outside firms to benchmark compensation, but the committee recommends the final package to the board for approval. On occasion, the committee may also have a role in the compensation of select senior executives or major changes in pay for large workforce groups.

TALENT DEVELOPMENT/WORKFORCE DEVELOPMENT COMMITTEE

This committee works with human resources to approve programs that ensure a well-trained and well-educated workforce for the organization, especially related to succession planning. This has become even more important as sections of the workforce experience shortages. Because nursing is such a large percentage of the organization's workforce, boards are especially attuned to quality patient care being tied to a well-educated and skilled nursing cadre.

Sometimes the compensation and talent development/workforce development committees are combined. This is especially true when leadership development initiatives and succession planning are included in both committees.

STRATEGIC PLANNING COMMITTEE

The development of the strategic plan can be accomplished in a variety of ways. It can be a separate committee, it can be a function of the full board, or it can be part of another committee's charge. Many organizations hire consultants to lead the planning work. Whatever the structure, it is a critical job to accomplish. Most organizations have 3- to 5-year plans with priorities and major tactics. Operating plans are completed yearly, follow the budget calendar, and guide day-to-day operations. Organizations with robust and nimble plans are better able to flex to the complex changes in today's healthcare environment. Mission is the driving force, but the appearance of sudden challenges like COVID-19 can cause plans to be adjusted.

QUALITY AND SAFETY COMMITTEE

This committee is charged with setting standards and monitoring achievement for overall quality and safety provided by the organization. Most organizations use quality scorecards that set targets and then measure achievement or lack of achievement on a quarterly basis. Scorecards can track improvements, standard adherence, serious safety events, and select screening efforts. For performance that is not on target, indicators can be further analyzed for cause of not meeting targets, actions to remedy, and timelines to re-evaluation. Hospital-acquired conditions (HACs), like pressure ulcers, falls, and adverse drug events, can affect reimbursement from Medicare, so these are closely monitored. Publicly reported quality data lends itself to benchmarking with other organizations. This can provide information about where other improvements can be made. Some quality and safety committees also monitor patient experience data. This makes it possible to correlate the quality data with patient experience and look for trends. Although staff engagement usually is not part of the quality committee, it can also be included to see if there are any relationships between these three measurements. Quality committees can also be assigned to manage the community benefit surveys completed by local communities. Not-for-profit hospitals use this data to develop their charitable benefit plans for the communities they serve.

Nurse leaders should be involved with the quality work of the organization and this committee would be an excellent place to be members. The nurse executive should also consider attending this committee's meetings, if not as a member, then in an *exofficio* status. Angela McBride, PhD, RN, FAAN, FNAP, ANEF, provides an excellent case study of what a nurse can do to elevate quality and safety as the chair of a board's quality and patient safety committee. She believes that nurses' orientation to systems is an asset to the board's institutional support of quality and safety (McBride, 2017).

Safety is also a focus of the quality committee. It includes both patient safety and staff safety. There are monitoring actions that dictate education programing and process improvement.

Healthcare organizations want to be safe for patients and families. Incidents like patient injury from falls, pressure ulcers, and medication errors should not happen. Safety issues for staff include prevention of needle sticks, illness from blood-borne pathogens, and back injuries from inappropriate lifting. Safety science provides insights into why these events might happen and how to mitigate them. Human factors science guides the work to keep hospitals safe. Nurse leaders are critical players in safety work because they understand what actions make systems safer for patients and staff. They can bring diverse topics of quality and safety to the quality committee and eventually to the board. They can lead conversations about quality metrics and other measurements such as patient experience and staff engagement. They can create relationships between metrics and variables, where others might not have experienced or observed the relationships. Nurse leaders understand what the board dialogue could cover, what quality care entails, and what to do with the measurements (Janes et al., 2021; McNally, 2018; Willard-Grace et al., 2021).

RESEARCH AND EDUCATION COMMITTEE

This committee is usually present in AMCs and focuses on the academic mission of AMCs. It addresses research completed at the organization. Historically, this is physician-led research that is funded by outside resources such as the National Institutes of Health. Nurse leaders can bring forth nurse-led research to be included in the committee's work. There are also other professions that may have research, such as pharmacists and physical therapists. Education focuses on professional academic programs like medical schools, nursing schools, and pharmacy schools associated with the organization. This committee can also review the grants and costs of providing education resources for the organization. The board learns of the contributions of research and education in the reports of this committee.

TASK FORCES

The board creates task forces when there is work to be done that does not fit into standing committees. The work is time limited and narrowly focused. A group is convened and charged with a specific task, completes that work, reports to the board, and is then disbanded. This is an excellent way to have short-term, focused work groups efficiently address an issue and then cease to meet. Examples of task forces could be planning a board event that will only happen once, developing a board response to a specific topic, or deciding on award nominations for a yearly recognition event.

These are the usual committees of boards. They remain the major working components of the board. Their work and outcomes are reported to the board. Nurse leaders can influence governance by being involved in the committee work. They can volunteer to serve on committees and become active members. This gives nurse leaders the opportunity to shape agendas and dialogue of important topics of the board. In her case study of being on a board, Dr. Angela McBride details how she was able to redirect the work of an AMC quality and safety committee to be more efficient and effective (McBride, 2017). She served on this board for 12 years, and notes that some changes take time, especially those that depend on establishing relationships of trust and credibility.

KEY CONCEPTS FOR NURSE EXECUTIVES

There are several topics that the nurse executive should know about the board and the relationship with management. Knowledge of what constitutes excellence in board governance is critical. It is difficult to judge the effectiveness of a board unless the nurse executive understands the structures of good governance. The most successful relationship between board and management is a respectful partnership. The nurse executive has much to offer to this partnership, especially related to quality patient care, workforce issues, community needs, and the business of healthcare. The nurse executive should be familiar with the board's strategic plan, the organization's strategic plan, and how nursing is integrated into those plans. Even though the nurse executive may only be an official member of a few committees, they should know the charges of all committees. This creates the ability to gauge possible input in quality, finance, workforce, strategic planning, or compliance with TJC and regulators. The nurse executive can assist other senior management colleagues with their assignments by offering input and collaborating on common areas of work. For example, the nurse executive may have details for the finance committee on why patient care is causing a rise in expenses. COVID-19 and the dramatic increase in the cost of PPE (personal protective equipment) would demonstrate this.

Nurse executives understand the context of how care is delivered and the impact on other organization departments. They use a systems approach and knowledge that is not limited to nursing or patient care. They can synthesize information that would be valuable for board discussions.

The nurse executive needs to know how to introduce and present information so that it is understood by the board. Most board members are not clinicians and may not be familiar with the jargon used in healthcare. Nurse executives should provide comprehensive information in a manner that all board members understand. It is also essential that nurse executives have a broad knowledge base to include challenges that their organization may be facing in the healthcare environment. This includes what is happening in their local and regional market, financial pressures, reimbursement issues, overall workforce status, and political issues that may impact the organization's ability to do business. Most hospitals follow legislative issues and are clear where advocacy is needed. Nurse executives who can discuss these issues as well as nursing and patient care can become valuable members to management and the board.

Members of the board and management should possess good communication skills, engage in respectful debate, and manage possible conflicts. Nurse executives have skills in navigating conflict and can role model effective interpersonal behaviors that benefit the board. Nurse executives are also strategic and systems thinkers, which can better shape the conversations. Nurse executives understand the importance of relationships and how they can impact the work of healthcare. It is the currency of how the work gets done. It is through relationships that trust and credibility are established. Nurse executives should be skilled in this area.

The key is for the nurse executive to feel comfortable offering perspectives and opinions. Being silent in board meetings or management meetings does not demonstrate the power of the voice of nursing or their value as a healthcare executive.

An important step for the nurse leader is to do their own assessment of the board and how it functions by exploring key questions (Box 21.3).

BOX 21.3: QUESTIONS A NURSE LEADER CAN ANSWER TO ASSESS A BOARD

- Who are the members of the board? What is their background?
- Who is the chair of the board? What is their background?
- What are the board committees? Who are the chairs?
- Who attends the board meetings?
- Who attends the committee meetings?
- How does a nurse leader provide input to the board meeting and to committee meetings?
- Who reports on what topics/agenda items at board meetings?
- How do people get appointed to the committees?
- Are there nurses on the board as voting members? On committees?
- What is the strategic plan for the board/organization? Where does nursing impact the strategic plan? How often is the board updated on progress of the plan?

INTERVIEW WITH A NURSE EXECUTIVE

Michelle Janney, PhD, RN, FAAN, was the chief nursing officer (CNO) at a major AMC and was then promoted to executive VP/COO of the healthcare system. She believes her role when working with the board is to focus on strategic issues and not operations. The board can be advisory to management by bringing their diverse perspectives and expertise to the work of the organization. It is management's responsibility to create a relatable context for discussions. In her organization, management provides a board packet for meetings that contains executive summaries and the important questions where the board can provide input and guidance.

She cautions nurse leaders to avoid focusing on the negative aspects of nursing and instead demonstrate competence in managing challenges. It is important to link nursing's work to the organization's mission, vision, values, and strategic plan. In this way, the board can appreciate the linkages to the board's work. She also advises nurse leaders to work with board chairs before finalizing presentations to ensure the chair has input. It is helpful for nurses to focus on patients and patient care and not always just nursing. Other members of management can be helpful role models for creating productive relationships with the board.

Dr. Janney encourages nurse executives to develop their roles as healthcare executives who can speak to all aspects of healthcare. She encourages nurse leaders to forge relationships across all disciplines. This strategy can establish a reputation of focusing on "us" as a healthcare team (M. Janney, personal communication, August 12, 2021).

KEY CONCEPTS FOR NURSE MANAGERS

Nurse managers can begin their education of board governance early in their careers. The nurse executive can mentor the nurse manager and educate them about the role of governance, how the board is structured, the work of committees, and how the nursing strategic plan is aligned with the organization's strategic plan that is developed to align with the organization's mission, vision, and values adopted by the board.

Nurse managers know how care is delivered on their unit(s). They are familiar with quality indicators and measurements. They should be aware of their unit(s)' engagement and patient experience scores. All this knowledge makes them perfect candidates for quality committees, talent development committees, and specific task forces. They can explain patient care and also gain an understanding of what is important to the board.

Nurse managers can also be a conduit for information that will assist the nurse executives during board dialogue. Creating a desire to influence governance is a critical development for early careerist leaders. They should be encouraged to bring forth questions related to board actions and plans as they seek understanding of governance. As nurse executives mentor nurse managers, they create a succession plan for the knowledge that nurse leaders should have to optimally participate in the governance of their organizations. Nurse managers may continue their career development and become nurse executives. Knowledge regarding boards and governance when they are nurse managers will serve them well as they progress in their leadership and management roles. This focus on what is needed as a nurse executive will make them stronger healthcare executives and can expand the voice of nursing.

 CASE SCENARIO

FILLING A BOARD VACANCY

SITUATION

You are a nurse manager or the senior nurse executive of the management team. The board expects three board members to reach their term limits in the upcoming year. The nominations committee has made it known that they would like the names of potential candidates to fill these positions. The current three members are vacating the following positions: member of the quality committee, member of the talent development committee, and chair of the audit and compliance committee. There are no nurses on the board, and that has been the case for the last 15 years. The last nurse was a CEO of a community hospital in the system. You see this as an opportunity to put forward a nurse as a candidate. You know several colleagues who you think might be interested and you approach them with information about the opportunity.

DISCUSSION QUESTIONS

1. What would you tell the candidates about the opportunity?
2. What questions would you ask the candidates?
3. How would you propose each nurse's candidacy?

WHAT EVERY NURSE MANAGER NEEDS TO KNOW

- What creates excellence in board governance
- How the board is structured and its usual operations/interactions with staff
- The charges for all committees
- How the nursing strategic plan is aligned with the organization/board's strategic plan
- How care is delivered in the patient care areas
- Manager's unit(s) scores for patient engagement and patient experience
- Quality metrics and outcomes for manager's unit(s) and how they relate to the overall hospital scores, metrics, or outcomes
- The board's agenda and what is discussed and decided that can be shared with staff
- How to present clinical information to nonclinicians on the board and in committees

THE LIVED EXPERIENCE OF THE AUTHOR, PAMELA AUSTIN THOMPSON, MS, RN, FAAN

During my career, I have been in a senior management role (CEO) reporting to a board, as well as on state and national boards, a hospital board, a healthcare system board, and association boards. I have chaired several of these boards. This has given me a perspective of functioning effectively as management and as a director/trustee. The most important thing that I have learned is the ability to establish effective relationships. I believe relationships are the currency of our work in management and governance.

It is also necessary to actively engage in self-reflection to learn from situations that are successful and especially from situations that don't meet our expectations. Because I have been elected/appointed to boards to represent nursing, I believe that it is important to also demonstrate my knowledge beyond nursing early in my tenure on a board. This allows me to be viewed as an expert or competent in other aspects such as finance, strategic planning, decision-making, governance, research, and education.

I have found it productive to do more listening than talking. I can synthesize what I hear in dialogue and move the conversations in constructive new paths. My most developed skill is asking questions. A well-placed question can clarify, redirect, and augment dialogue and debate.

In working with boards, it is critical to be truthful and establish trust and credibility. If trust is lost, it is almost impossible to regain it. Seek clarity to understand the board and the board members' perspectives.

Don't strive to be right—strive to be competent, confident, curious, and a good communicator.

Understanding how a board functions is to understand the foundation of a healthcare organization. Nurse leaders can influence how a board understands nursing, patient care, and quality and safety and why it is critical to organizational success. Nurse involvement can also promote better governance, especially related to the inclusion of different perspectives. Nurse leaders can include community perspectives and create stronger stakeholder relationships. Ultimately, the organization can achieve optimal governance.

> *"An effective group spirit on a board is one that attracts its members,*
> *makes them want to work with one another, and gives them a sense of pride and*
> *satisfaction in the program and the board itself."*
>
> *(Houle, 1989, p. 120)*

KEY POINTS

- Healthcare organizations are governed by a board of directors/trustees and are responsible for the strategic direction of the organization.

- The fiduciary responsibilities of the board members include the duty of care, the duty of loyalty, and the duty of obedience. These are the foundational responsibilities of all boards.

- The management staff are responsible for operationalizing the strategic plan to accomplish the mission, vision, and values. They also manage the business of the organization in caring for patients and the community.

- The mutual relationship between the board and management is critical to the success of the organization.

- Nurse leaders should understand board roles, board structure and function, and how nursing and patient care fit into the overall organization plan.

- Nurse executives can be advocates for nursing and high-quality care in their relationship with the board.
- Nurse managers should be exposed to board governance and functions to understand the importance of the management and board relationship.

END-OF-CHAPTER RESOURCES

DISCUSSION QUESTIONS

1. What are the key components of board governance that nurse leaders can influence?
2. Why is board governance and the management relationship rarely discussed in nursing leadership conversations?
3. Why should more nurse leaders be included on quality and safety committees?
4. What are the obstacles that nurse leaders must overcome to be considered for board-related work?
5. Name the contributions that nurse leaders can make to boards and their committees that would strengthen their governance oversight.

ADDITIONAL RESOURCES

- The American Hospital Association (AHA)—This association has a special interest group for trustees and multiple resources for hospitals and management: https://www.aha.org
- Nurses on Boards Coalition (NOBC): https://www.nursesonboardscoalition.org
- The Governance Institute: https://www.governanceinstitute.com
- Board Source: https://boardsource.org

 A robust set of instructor resources designed to supplement this text is located at http://connect.springerpub.com/content/book/978-0-8261-7795-7. Qualifying instructors may request access by emailing textbook@springerpub.com.

REFERENCES

Annie E. Casey Foundation. (n.d.). *Charter schools: Creating effective governing boards.* https://charterschoolcenter.ed.gov/sites/default/files/files/field_publication_attachment/Creating%20Effective%20Govering%20boards_0.pdf

Curran, C. (2016). *Nurse on board: Planning your path to the boardroom.* Sigma Theta Tau International, Center for Nursing Press.

Houle, C. (1989). *Governing boards: Their nature and nurture.* Jossey-Bass.

Janes, G., Mills, T., Budworth, L., Johnson, J., & Lawton, R. (2021). The association between health care staff engagement and patient safety outcomes: A systematic review and meta-analysis. *Journal of Patient Safety, 17*(3), 207–216. https://doi.org/10.1097/PTS.0000000000000807

Lúanaigh, P. Ó., & Hughes, F. (2016). The nurse executive role in quality and high performing health services. *Journal of Nursing Management, 24*(1), 132–136. https://doi.org/10.1111/jonm.12290

McBride, A. B. (2017). Serving on a hospital board: A case study. *Nursing Outlook, 65*(4), 372–379. https://doi.org/10.1016/j.outlook.2016.12.006

McNally, K. (2018). *Nurses in the boardroom.* American Hospital Association Trustee Services. https://trustees.aha.org/sites/default/files/trustees/nurses-boardroom.pdf

Meynell, L., & Sedel, R. (2012). *In touch with the board: What makes for a high-performing board?* Russell Reynolds Associates. https://resources.finalsite.net/images/v1583208379/isbeijing/gzngci70bzs1mcfgwsio/in-touch-what-makes-for-a-high-performing-board_1.pdf

Murphy, A. (2018, December 20). *5 essential qualities of an effective board member*. https://greatboards .org/5-essential-qualities-of-an-effective-board-member/

Price, N. (2018, July 23). *Defining the role of a hospital board of trustees*. BoardEffect, A Diligent Brand. https://www.boardeffect.com/blog/defining-role-hospital-board-trustees/

Price, N. (2019, March 11). *What are the qualities of an effective non-profit board of directors*. BoardEffect, A Diligent Brand. https://www.boardeffect.com/blog/what-are-qualities-effective-nonprofit-board -directors

Rudisill, P., & Benson, L. (2021). Achieving 10,000 board seats filled by nurses: Nurses improve health across communities. *Nursing Economic$, 39*(3), 6–10.

Sundean, L., White, K., Thompson, L., & Prybil, L. (2019). Governance education for nurses: Preparing nurses for the future. *Journal of Professional Nursing, 35*(5), 346–352. https://doi.org/10.1016/j .profnurs.2019.04.001

Totten, M. (2018, June 11). *Becoming a visionary board*. American Hospital Association. https://trustees .aha.org/articles/1381-becoming-a-visionary-board

Wakefield, M. K., Williams, D. R., Le Menestrel, S., & Flaubert, J. L. (2021). *The future of nursing 2020– 2030: Charting a path to achieve health equity*. National Academies Press. https://doi.org/10.17226/ 25982

Willard-Grace, R., Knox, M., Huang, B., Hammer, H., Kivlahan, C., & Grumbach, K. (2021). Primary care clinician burnout and engagement association with clinical quality and patient experience. *Journal of the American Board of Family Medicine, 34*(3), 542–552. https://doi.org/10.3122/ jabfm.2021.03.200515

SECTION VIII
SPECIAL TOPICS

CHAPTER 22

UNANTICIPATED TRANSITIONS

Theresa L. Champagne and Ashley M. Carlucci

"Times of transition are strenuous, but I love them. They are opportunity to purge, re-think priorities, and be intentional about new habits. We can make our new normal any way we want."

Kristin Armstrong

LEARNING OBJECTIVES

- Identify the knowledge gap for nurse managers and nurse executives by exploring examples of unanticipated transitions.
- Delineate leadership styles and skills that have demonstrated benefit in times of unanticipated transitions.
- Analyze skill sets to enhance professional growth during unexpected transitions in healthcare organizations.
- Create a scenario in which there is a positive outcome of an unexpected transition in an organization.

INTRODUCTION

The nurse manager and the nurse executive will experience many transitions over the course of their professional career. Some may be anticipated transitions, and some may be unanticipated. An anticipated transition by definition is one that is expected to occur and its timing is predictable and can therefore include robust planning. In contrast, an unanticipated transition is a change that is not expected and does not follow any predictable timeline or course of events. While there are similarities and differences between the two, the opportunity to learn and grow from both are tremendous.

Anticipated and unanticipated transitions may be internal or external in nature. Some examples of internal transitions include organizational chart changes, unanticipated financial challenges, or an organizational reduction in (work)force (RIF), which may include one's own position elimination. Examples of external transitions include organizational mergers or acquisitions, local or global competitive market changes, relationship changes, and environmental events including natural disasters, such as recent weather events and the COVID-19 global pandemic, which can cause unanticipated care delivery model changes.

The type of transition and the response will determine the impact of the anticipated and the unanticipated transition. Anticipated transitions often include the elements of planning, trialing, evaluating, and implementing, then revising as needed with clear timelines and goals in a controlled way. These same ideas need to be in the forefront during unanticipated transitions, despite the higher sense of uncertainty and chaos. Edmunson (2015) noted that unanticipated change brings tremendous learning opportunities, and it is most important to share these lessons learned not only within one's own organization but nationally and globally so other healthcare organizations can gain knowledge from challenging experiences.

The nurse manager will be better prepared to meet these anticipated and unanticipated transitions by developing and utilizing certain skills including open and honest communication, emotional intelligence, focusing on the core values of the organization, and engaging in trust-building behaviors during these times of transitions. Other leadership skills needed during times of transition and change include being present and visible for staff while rounding with purpose, showing staff compassion, and managing these stressful times with self-care activities.

Likewise, the nurse executive will need to develop and focus on some of these same skills while leading during times of transition. Additionally, the nurse executive may also need to fill in the knowledge gap for the nursing team in order to onboard the nursing team with the transition and extend team support. Other important skills besides open and honest communication include negotiating skills, relationship building, and data analysis. Aligning staff under the organizational mission, vision, and value system, as well as cultural considerations, are also key during times of transition, allowing staff to focus on a common goal.

The purpose of this chapter is to explore transitions, anticipated and unanticipated, that the nurse manager and nurse executive are likely to experience during their career. We begin with a brief review of relevant literature on some anticipated and unanticipated transitions and change. Different types of transitions are then discussed. Examples and scenarios are described in order to provide the nurse leader with ways to reshape their situation to a desired state and make them better prepared to face future challenges. Suggestions for developing specific skills and identifying tools that have proven to be useful during anticipated transitions and unanticipated transitions are presented so the nurse leader will be better prepared to lead when faced with the unexpected. These skills may help the nurse leader to turn unanticipated transitions that have the potential to be a crisis or turbulent in nature into opportunities to improve and grow.

REVIEW OF THE RELEVANT LITERATURE

The most recent literature written on leadership and transitions focused on the unexpected global pandemic, which has had many consequences and has driven sudden transitions. Many nurse leaders shared leadership experiences during the pandemic. Caroselli (2020) described the importance of role modeling with intention following her experience as a nurse leader in a healthcare system in New York City during the pandemic. The challenges of leading nursing during times of turbulence and uncertainty were described by Hertel (2020). Balluck et al. (2020) described how unanticipated increased patient volumes required staffing model changes to team nursing. The literature also describes the sudden technology shift to the use of telemedicine to deliver essential health services as a result of the pandemic (Centers for Disease Control and Prevention [CDC], 2020).

The increased number of mergers and acquisitions in healthcare across the country is also documented in the literature. In 2018, the *American Journal of Nursing* (AJN) reported mergers and acquisitions have risen dramatically in number over the past 10 years, increasing from 74 in 2010 to 115 in 2018 (Sofer, 2020). While there is an abundance of literature on the business effect on cost of mergers and acquisitions, there is not a lot of research on the effects on quality of patient care or leadership postmerger or acquisition. In 2018, Robinson and Knight published results of a qualitative study on the chief nurse executive (CNE) perspective of hospital acquisitions after 15 different acquisitions. An interesting finding was that similar themes were found whether the CNE was part of the acquiring organization or part of the organization being acquired. The four most common themes were communication, respect, staff turnover, and lack of a clear transition plan. The importance of effective communication during organizational transitions was a similar theme reported by Nelson and Pilon (2015). Beaulieu et al. (2020) found no evidence of improved quality of patient care, nor any improvement in patient experience, readmission rates, mortality, or clinical process measures after acquisitions. Chesley's (2020) research suggests that organizational culture and the ability of organizations to align culture postmerger is an important predictor of the success of a merger.

INTERNAL TRANSITIONS

ORGANIZATIONAL CHART CHANGES

The reporting structure of an organization, which defines who reports to whom, is often outlined on an organizational chart. Changes to the organizational chart are a common occurrence in healthcare. As one leader leaves an organization, reporting structures may change and nurse executives and nurse managers may be asked to change their scope of oversight or take on new responsibilities. Nurse leaders may even be assigned roles and responsibilities that are out of their areas of expertise. When these organizational chart changes occur, nurse leaders often find themselves in a role that becomes very different than the role and responsibilities that they accepted when hired. It is important to ensure, when these changes occur, that their job description is updated to reflect the new roles and responsibilities. Nurse leaders also may find themselves reporting to a person with different values or a leadership style different from their previous leader. These are times when a nurse leader must self-reflect and determine if the new reporting structure is a good fit; if not, it may be time to explore other opportunities.

Another challenge during organizational change is that the nurse leader be required to implement organizational decisions that are sometimes in conflict with the needs of the frontline staff or with their own internal values. This conflict or managerial dissonance, as described by Galura (2020), may have either a positive or negative outcome depending on whether the manager can externalize responsibility of the transition. A nurse manager is much more likely to embrace an organizational decision that seems in conflict with staffing needs if able to understand factors that caused the need to act and how this action will help the organization meet its goals. Nurse executive responsibilities include helping their frontline managers understand the organizational goals and decisions through open communication so they can externalize responsibility of difficult transitions or change. The ability to externalize the rationale for change will more often allow the nurse manager to support even difficult transitions.

Self-advocacy is important during these unanticipated organizational chart transitions. With a new reporting structure, the nurse leader should be sure to talk about their accomplishments and goals with their new supervisor. With added responsibility, compensation, if appropriate, should be discussed. This may be difficult to do during uncertain times and times of financial strain. Yet if a nurse leader is accepting a greater scope of responsibility, it is not unreasonable to request additional compensation if none is offered. Nurse leaders often feel that they will put their jobs in jeopardy if they request additional compensation. Fear of negatively impacting a new relationship may deter the nurse leader from having a compensation discussion. Seeking out coaching on having a conversation around compensation is recommended if this is an area of discomfort for the nurse leader. A well prepared, thoughtful conversation may relieve the anxiety these conversations can create, thus making it easier to self-advocate and request to be compensated for additional responsibilities and broader spans of control.

UNANTICIPATED EVENTS CAUSE FINANCIAL CHALLENGES

There are many causes for unanticipated financial challenges for healthcare organizations. Some of these include unforeseen revenue gaps. Others include an unanticipated loss of a key physician in small health systems, loss of volume due to competition in an organization's patient catchment area, staffing shortages where the organization must resort to using expensive locum or agency to staff key areas, and shrinking reimbursement, to name a few. The size of the healthcare system or organization will depend on the impact that an unanticipated revenue loss will have. For example, a larger health system may be better able to withstand the loss of a physician if there are multiple physicians providing the same subspecialty care. However, a healthcare system or program that is small may be devastated by the same loss.

Consider this scenario: A mid-sized not-for-profit health system had started a cardiac surgical program, hiring one full-time and one part-time cardiac physician at the start of the program. The program was profitable and growing in volume for its first 3 years. Just as they were considering opening a second operating room (OR) and recruiting an additional physician, the full-time cardiac surgeon died unexpectedly, bringing the program to a near standstill. The lost revenue impacted not only the cardiac OR but also projected ICU volumes and other inpatient volumes, as well as outpatient volumes in the cardiac rehabilitation program. Some specially trained staff left the organization as the process of recruiting a new physician took several months.

While it is important to evaluate risk, some cases like this one could not be predicted, and the revenue loss was substantial to this organization. A larger cardiac program that employed multiple full-time cardiac surgeons may not have felt the loss of one surgeon as deeply as this small program did. What are some of the other consequences of the sudden closure of a program one might expect? What would be the role of nurse managers and nurse executives in addressing those consequences?

It is important to recognize that decisions one makes during unanticipated financial challenges may have a different impact depending on the size of the organization. Large organizations with capital reserve and a healthy positive margin may be able to withstand a financial strain of a program failure much easier than that of a small rural health system with a weak margin and no reserve. Risky decisions that may involve financial loss if a program implementation fails to yield a projected return on investments (ROI) must be carefully considered among smaller organizations that are experiencing financial instability. An unanticipated revenue loss in these situations may even lead to a closure or bankruptcy situation. For this reason, often institutions bring in consultants who have expertise in certain areas to advise them on program development prior to implementation to mitigate risk.

WORKING WITH CONSULTANTS

An unfortunate reality is that when an organization is undergoing deep financial troubles, it may turn to consulting firms that have expertise in cost savings. These consultants analyze the organization's current state, often by department, and make recommendations for efficiencies and improved revenue. Some senior leaders put more credibility to highly paid consultant work than their own leadership team recommendations. Typically, the nurse leader is asked to provide large amounts of data that describe operations including full-time equivalents (FTEs), supply spend, staffing schedules, patient volumes, and scopes of service. They will then take the data presented, analyze it, and compare it to national trends and benchmarks. Frequently, the data is presented with visual charts and grafts with recommendations for improved efficiencies. The group may or may not be consulted to then stay and work with the various teams to implement these recommended changes, or the organization may leave it up to their leadership team to implement changes. The nurse leader's responsibility is to validate that the data presented is an accurate depiction of what is actually being described in their area of expertise. Data presented should not be taken for its face values. For example, when FTE data is presented, it is important to understand if orientation hours are included, what job codes are included or excluded in the data, shifts, and if patient acuity is considered.

Consider this scenario: One financially challenged organization hired a consulting firm to evaluate ED volumes and FTE requirements. After the data gathering and analysis was final, the consultants presented a picture of an overstaffed ED based on volumes and presented this data to the senior team. The nurse manager reported being understaffed on a daily basis and was shocked when the recommendation was to cut staff. On further investigation as to what was included in the FTE numbers presented, it was discovered that the roll up of numbers included the 1:1 sitters required for the behavioral health patients. The average daily census for behavioral health patients was 5 to 6 patients per day. The consultants had used payroll data to determine staffing numbers, not understanding the ratio requirements for certain patient populations, and in turn misrepresented staffing needs. When this error was corrected, their analysis did demonstrate a staffing need, not an opportunity for cost saving through staffing cuts. Had the nurse manager not validated the data, unrealistic expectations could have been part of the implementation plan for cost savings in the ED.

Developing skills for data analysis is critical for nurse managers and nurse executives, especially when consultants are presenting data and making recommendations for improvement. The nurse leader does not always have control over what data is presented to the consultants for analysis. The importance of understanding one's own data and asking questions about what is being presented is important. There are many programs available to develop data analysis skills. Being able to present data about one's area of oversight in a clear, understandable way is an important skill to develop credibility. Validated, well-presented data is a powerful tool and necessary to support business plans and change initiatives that abound during many transitions, but it is especially important when cost-cutting recommendations come from outside consultants. One of the most common recommendations that come from consulting firms that have been hired to help the organization identify cost savings is a reduction in the workforce.

REDUCTION IN WORKFORCE AND POSITION ELIMINATION

Organizations under financial strain, depending on severity and the ability to withstand the strain, may turn to an RIF and position eliminations as a cost savings tactic to close the budget gap. One of the most common unanticipated transitions that a nurse leader will face in her career is an RIF. As staff or FTEs are usually the most expensive part of any nursing budget, this is the area that is usually targeted, before service elimination is considered by an organization. The nurse leader may be asked for input as far as position elimination or simply be told what positions will be eliminated. Today, staff reductions are such a challenge because cost-cutting initiatives have been going on in healthcare systems for decades now with shrinking reimbursements and rising cost of supplies and equipment. It may seem like a daunting task at first when asked to develop plans requiring staff to do more with less, when leaders and staff are already feeling they are overworked and as lean as possible.

Reductions in workforces often require the nurse leader to be involved in employee terminations. This is one of the most difficult tasks that any nurse leader must perform in a professional career. Even when terminating an employee for a performance issue, these conversations are emotionally charged and anxiety provoking, at best. It is often recommended that these conversations are witnessed, and many organizations will have a member of the human resource staff present for the conversation. While there are varying strategies, it is recommended to keep the conversation short, stick to the facts of the matter, and show the employee compassion. When there is suspicion that the employee may be highly emotional or hostile, it may be recommended to have hospital security either present or at least be notified of the termination, so that they may be immediately available if needed. These are difficult conversations at best and often do not go as planned. However, it is always prudent to plan for the worst-case scenario. Human resource staff may be available to explain the separation package if there is one and answer questions about health insurance coverage and unemployment benefit eligibility.

Nurse managers and executives are not immune to position elimination during workforce reductions. Depending on the organization, there may or may not be notice given that the nurse leader's job will be eliminated. It is important to recognize that job eliminations are business decisions and not a reflection of a leader's personal contributions to the organization. Middle and upper management positions are frequent targets in workforce reductions because higher salary positions that do not directly impact patient care are generally viewed as a more cost-effective cut than frontline staff cuts. This is especially true in a union environment, as non-union position elimination is generally much less complicated than positions protected by a collective bargaining agreement. While these unanticipated transitions are usually emotionally charged moments and one of the most stressful events in one's career, it is important to remain professional and focus on the positive experiences a former position and employer provided. By embracing the event as a time to seek new opportunities, the nurse leader is likely to experience new possibilities and professional growth.

 CASE SCENARIO

WORKFORCE REDUCTION

SITUATION

A nurse manager had oversight of several units in the surgical service line. The nurse manager's areas were meeting goals, including financial targets set by the organization. Their FTE budget was at the low end of recommended staffing levels based on Association of periOperative Nurses (AORN) standards, the organization that sets standards for perioperative areas. The nurse manager was aware that other service lines were not meeting targets and were operating over budgets set for their areas. The health system suddenly found itself in a revenue shortfall due to sudden state budget cuts to hospitals and lower reimbursements than anticipated when the hospital budget was set. Senior leadership of the organization chose to address this revenue shortfall with an RIF. Each service line was given target numbers to meet the collective reduction needed for the organization to meet budget.

APPROACH

Initially this nurse manager faced internal conflict and was angry with the mandate, the organization, and the person the nurse manager reported to as these numbers seemed arbitrary—it had not been explained how these target numbers were assigned. The nurse manager had high anxiety as they were faced with implementing a plan that they felt would not meet the needs of the frontline staff that reported to them. The nurse manager did not know how to get the rest of their leadership team to accept the plan when they themself were struggling. To add to the stress, the nurse manager had a short timeline to present the plan for the surgical service line. The nurse manager finally met one-on-one with their senior leader to discuss their concerns. Together, they were able to determine that by not filling several open positions and by eliminating just one of the low-performing clinical leads on the team, the nurse manager could meet the targeted reduction numbers. After gaining a better understanding of the cause of the financial shortfalls, the nurse manager was able to externalize responsibility (state budget cuts in this case) and accept the plan for the good of the organization.

OUTCOME

While able to get the team on board with the reduction plan, it soon became evident that this RIF was not accepted by the team without consequence. Uncertainty and lack of trust caused by this RIF resulted in other staff on the leadership team stepping down for staff positions, which they felt were more secure. It was over a year before these clinical lead positions would be filled. Additionally, there was a palpable lack of trust between the leadership team and the frontline staff that also took many months to rebuild. Rebuilding trust included continual open and honest communication with the nursing leadership team, staff engagement in planning new workflows, and the nurse leaders being present for the frontline staff with frequent rounding and recognition. Over time, relationships improved and slowly trust was rebuilt.

DISCUSSION QUESTIONS

1. Why was the nurse manager's ability to externalize the conflict important in this case scenario?

2. What are some other tactics that this nurse manager could have used after the reduction in the workforce to rebuild trust with the frontline staff?

EXTERNAL TRANSITIONS

MERGERS AND ACQUISITIONS

Hospital and health system mergers and acquisitions have been dramatically increasing in numbers over the past 10 years. Rising cost, shrinking reimbursement, increasing nontraditional competition (e.g., CVS and Walmart), and the value-based reimbursement model of the Affordable Care Act (ACA) have all contributed to shrinking hospital margins. Mergers and acquisitions often occur to contain cost, increase buying power, and give institutions more leverage when negotiating contracts with health insurers (Chesley, 2020). A merger occurs when two hospitals or health systems combine to form a new joint organization. In contrast, an acquisition is a takeover of one organization by another. Both mergers and acquisitions can cause uncertainty, low morale, nurse burnout, and less job satisfaction (Sofer, 2020). Leading staff through these transitions is both a challenge and a tremendous learning opportunity for nurse managers and nurse executives.

Acquisitions can be sudden or take months to complete. Robinson and Knight (2018) reported the experience of one CNE who walked in to find that the hospital was closing that day. In contrast, consider this scenario:

One financially stressed health system had been seeking partnership for several months. A request for purchase (RFP) process was held, and 50 health systems were invited to consider a merger or acquisition; however, this process failed to lead to a merger or acquisition. The health system finally negotiated an acquisition, but the conditions included that the health system go through a debt consolidation process, or bankruptcy, first so that the acquiring facility would not have to absorb the financially stressed health system's debt load. A nondisclosure agreement was signed between the two health systems so there could be no formal announcement or discussion about the intended acquisition. The negotiating process for setting a purchase price prior to the Chapter 11 bankruptcy filing took over 9 months. The senior leadership team was not able to be completely transparent in their communication about what was happening and the rumor mill at every level created uncertainty. Staff resignations increased, morale sank, and open positions had few applicants as the months dragged on with no clear communication of the path forward while uncertainty continued. Some nursing units closed due to staff shortages.

Effective communication has been identified as one of the most important elements of a successful transition during acquisition (Robinson & Knight, 2018), yet as this scenario demonstrates, transparency and communication is not always possible, and sometimes legally restricted. The unfortunate reality is that communication during these times is often lacking, disorganized, or conflicting. This leaves the nurse manager and nurse executive in a difficult situation. During these uncertain times, it is even more important to be present with the staff. It is also important to admit when you do not know the answer to questions or that you are not allowed to talk about certain topics. Admitting that you have no answer is better received than being absent as staff then focus on misinformation that abounds.

It is important to have a brief high-level discussion on bankruptcy, a situation mentioned in the previous scenario. There are generally two major types of bankruptcy that a healthcare organization may fall into: Chapter 7 bankruptcy or Chapter 11 bankruptcy. A Chapter 7 bankruptcy is when the organization closes its doors, and the assets are sold off in order to cover the debt owed by the organization. This usually occurs when the organization cannot raise enough cash on hand to cover payroll. In a Chapter 11 bankruptcy, an auction is held after a Chapter 11 bankruptcy is declared and another organization agrees to buy the organization's assets once debt is restructured. If there is an asset purchase agreement signed with another organization prior to the declaration of the bankruptcy, the organization enters the bankruptcy process with a "stalking horse," which gives the prospective buying organization certain privileges during the auction process. The bankruptcy process is a very complex, time-consuming process which is highly regulated by the legal system and can take many months before an acquisition meets all final approvals. During a bankruptcy, the courts oversee all spending. At times, an ombudsman may be assigned to oversee clinical practice if it is determined that because of lacking resources, the quality of patient care is in jeopardy. While this is a very difficult time for any organization, emerging from bankruptcy with a hospital and services intact and able to continue to provide care locally is key for the community served and is a tremendous learning experience at any leadership level.

Integrating the culture of the acquiring and the acquired organization is another important consideration during mergers and acquisitions. Organizational culture can be defined as a system of shared values, beliefs, and assumptions that employees have. There is abundant evidence in the literature that supports the idea that integrating organizational culture is one of the most important predictors of the success or failure of any merger or acquisition (Chesley, 2020). Cultures of the two organizations should be considered before an acquisition and continually monitored after the merger or acquisition. Aligning the new organization under one shared mission, vision, and values can assist the cultures of the two organizations to become one. It has been reported that there was not always a formal plan on integration. In fact, Robinson and Knight (2018) reported in their research that of the 15 acquisitions they reviewed, very few reported a transition plan in place on day one once the acquisition/merger was finalized. More commonly, a plan is developed over the course of the first 6 months to a year when full assessments of strengths and weaknesses of each organization can be determined. That is the time of evaluations on what services should be consolidated and which services should expand. Frequently, moving to one electronic medical record, billing system, and payroll system is usually prioritized as the first step in the integration process for operations.

While mergers and acquisitions are certainly challenging and stressful, CNEs have reported positive experiences and new opportunities. Important to note is that it may take up to 2 to 5 years before organizations are fully integrated after an acquisition or merger. CNEs reported committee work between the two organizations presented learning and relationship building opportunities. Advice from CNEs who had experienced the stress of an acquisition included to remain professional, stay patient and focused, and continue to do what is right at all times (Robinson & Knight, 2018). Respect in all interactions has also been reported as one of the most important values as new relationships are being formed during integration.

Other advice from CNEs from an acquired organization included to not assume that the acquiring leadership team knows you or your accomplishments. It was recommended that the nurse leader should be sure to tell members of the new organization about current roles, goals, outcomes, and accomplishments of their past and current work. Frequent meetings within the new reporting structure are helpful to accomplish this if possible (Robinson & Knight, 2018).

 CASE SCENARIO

ACQUISITION OF ONE CRITICAL ACCESS HOSPITAL BY A LARGER COMMUNITY HOSPITAL

SITUATION

A mid-sized community health system acquired a financially stressed 35-bed critical access hospital (CAH) located about 20 minutes to the north. This hospital had always been viewed by the acquiring organization as a competitor, and many patients from that area already used the specialty services provided by the health system. Acquisition seemed like a logical move. There was not a lot of communication about future plans and the impact of the acquisition on the leadership team before the announcement that the acquisition was finalized. Prior to the acquisition and after the announcement, there was a perception on the staff's part that the acquisition would put a financial strain on the parent organization. With little communication about the goals or benefits that the organization would achieve, staff was less than enthused when integration goals and teams were assigned.

APPROACH

Soon after the announcement of the acquisition, integration teams were set up to address immediate needs including finance and human resources. Of note, both nursing staffs were under different collective bargaining agreements with different unions, which did complicate alignment of pay practices for the nursing staff. Some departments merged immediately, including environmental services, facilities, and food services. Others, including nursing, began integration meetings about 3 months into the acquisition. Nursing was given the task to align policies and practices in both the outpatient (OR, ED, and gastrointestinal [GI]) and inpatient (ICU and medical–surgical) units. At the nursing leadership meetings, it soon became clear that these two organizations had very different cultures and there was a reported lack of respect during some of the interactions between managers from the two organizations. The two teams were still treating each other as competition rather than one organization. Nursing leadership had just come under one chief nursing officer (CNO) from the parent company, which also had not been well received by the CAH.

OUTCOMES

To address behaviors, the CNO brought both groups of nurse leaders together, set expectations of mutual respect, and aligned the team all under the same goal of policy and practice alignment for the different service areas. Relationship building was key in finding common ground so the teams could work together. Frequent meetings and being present on both campuses each week helped build trust between the teams. Over a 1- to 2-year period, the teams were able to achieve policy and practice alignment in most areas. They were also able to shift some volumes between campuses that were mutually beneficial. There were many lessons learned along the way. For example, when some patients who were receiving chemotherapy were shifted to the CAH for treatment, it was found that pricing was much higher at the CAH, which was a patient dissatisfier. However, since both organizations still had separate insurance contracts and licensure, that situation took time to rectify. After that incident, insurance contracts were renegotiated prior to volume shifts. Several services were consolidated, an RIF happened to the parent company, and, after a 3-year period, a much smaller CAH with many consolidated services remained but did realize financial stability.

DISCUSSION QUESTIONS

1. What could the parent organization have done prior to the acquisition of the CAH to ensure a smoother integration?
2. What other big challenge might you expect the CNO to face during nursing integration?

COMPETITIVE MARKET CHALLENGES

Most healthcare organizations face competitive market challenges. While these challenges may be more pronounced in larger cities with multiple health systems or urban settings, they can still occur in small community and rural settings. Competition in a rural healthcare setting can even be more devastating financially than in a bigger city where there are plenty of patients to support two healthcare centers. Ambulatory surgical centers, walk-in clinics, and the pharmaceutical companies and big box stores getting into the walk-in clinic business for urgent care are a few examples of external factors that have created competitive market challenges for many health systems, big and small. These pop-up care companies have been siphoning volume and revenue out of healthcare systems for many years. Additionally, they may also compete for a shrinking workforce, which creates additional challenges. While these challenges are difficult to predict, the nurse executive and nurse manager must be ready to address the staffing challenges and volume adjustments these events create. Market competition can also create relationship challenges between organizations and private providers and provider groups. A common example of this is when a private orthopedic group opens its own surgical center, which then becomes a direct competitor to the health system where these providers still practice. Maintaining relationships during these times in an attempt to continue to capture some of the orthopedic volume has been a challenge that many organizations have faced.

RELATIONSHIP CHALLENGES

One of the key competencies for nurse managers and executives is relationship building (American Organization of Nurse Executives [AONE] & American Organization for Nursing Leadership [AONL], 2015). Strong relationships that are built on trust inspire leaders, engage staff, and build loyalty. Today more than ever, positive relationships are needed for healthcare systems to face these commonplace financial challenges of growth, downsizing, or restructuring. The challenge occurs because there are continual internal and external forces during times of transition that strain relationships, break trust, and cause betrayal. These incidents of betrayal, the opposite of trust, may occur within or between departments, or outside organizations and are sometimes beyond the nurse leader's control. The truth of the matter is that trusting relationships are continually changing as small or large events of betrayal occur. Nurse managers and executives must continually work on building trusting relationships to counteract all the things that happen during these times of change that are negatively impacting relationships.

All the transitions discussed have the potential to strain relationships. Reductions in the workforce events can certainly strain even the best relationships, as discussed in the first case scenario. Lack of clear communication during mergers and acquisitions and uncertainty lead to gossip and false stories. As the rumor mill grows, often ill intent is assumed. Uncertainty during times of financial strain can lead to competition for scarce resources and backstabbing among staff and departments to acquire them.

As all these transitions have the potential to break trust and strain relationships, practicing strategies that build trust are important during times of transition. The most important element in building trust and relationships is to first trust in one's own self and capabilities. Building trust begins first with the nurse leader's positive attitude, positive intention, and role modeling positive behaviors. Active listening, following through on requests, and closed loop communication are some strategies to help build trust and regain staff confidence. These are important behaviors all the time, but they are even more important during times of transition. The challenge is that times of transition require lots of energy, dedication, and self-awareness at a time when every moment and interaction can be energy draining. A positive attitude and positive affirmations bring increasing energy, build strong relationships, and can even repair strained relationships and broken trust.

Reina and Reina (2015) described a seven-step process for rebuilding trust after times of betrayal which frequently happen during transition. By actively choosing to respond to a betrayal, trust can be rebuilt, allowing damaged relationships to heal and grow stronger (Box 22.1). This

---

BOX 22.1 THE SEVEN-STEP PROCESS FOR REBUILDING TRUST

1. Observe and acknowledge what has happened
2. Allow feelings to surface
3. Give and get support
4. Reframe the experience
5. Take or acknowledge responsibility
6. Forgive
7. Let go and move on

Source: Reproduced with permission from Reina, D., & Reina, M. (2015). *Trust and betrayal in the workplace* (3rd ed., pp. 143–163). Berrett-Koehler.

process may take some time during transitions. However, following these steps will allow for a better understanding of the events that occurred and will create an environment that allows the nurse leader and the staff to heal and to begin to trust once again (Reina & Reina, 2015).

ENVIRONMENTAL CHALLENGES

The COVID-19 pandemic is a good example of an unexpected environmental transition that has occurred in recent times. This global pandemic brought several changes to the healthcare system that had not been experienced previously. While the pandemic affected health systems for an extended period, other environmental challenges—for example, weather events such as the recent tornadoes and hurricanes experienced over the past few years—have also had lasting impacts on many health systems' abilities to deliver care. Emergency preparedness drills, which are a regulatory requirement for many organizations, give health systems and nursing teams' opportunities to prepare for these environmental challenges. These events can occur at any time. Developing surge plan policies and team nursing delivery care models, and ensuring that all staff are familiar and understand expectations should such an event occur, is paramount. Too often, such emergency preparedness drills lack full participation from leadership and frontline staff and lessons learned are not fully shared, leaving the staff and organizations unprepared when these events occur.

Participating in an emergency preparedness drill that requires opening the Incident Command Center, a universal way to run an emergent event, is a great experience for every nurse leader. It is an important exercise to test communication systems, determine how quickly staff and supplies can be mobilized, and determine gaps or areas that need improvement. Such drills give an organization the ability to identify weaknesses and correct them before an actual event occurs. Full participation from all departments and units is a requirement for a successful drill. Additionally, participation in debriefing or hot-wash at the end of these drills gives an opportunity to plan improvements when gaps are identified and the ability to celebrate what went well. Again, like in many other situations encountered, communications before, during, and after these drills are key to ensuring nurse leaders and staff are prepared to handle sudden environmental events when they occur.

◘ WHAT EVERY NURSE MANAGER NEEDS TO KNOW ABOUT UNEXPECTED TRANSITIONS

One of the most important leadership skills for unanticipated transitions is open and honest communication. The importance of communication is addressed in previous chapters but cannot be overstated. This is probably the most common theme discussed when considering all examples of transition. The unknowns are scary and when communication is lacking, the team starts to draw their own conclusions of what they think is happening. At times, nurse managers will not be able to share fully the changes that are coming with frontline staff, but as much as possible communicating with their employees that they will share information when they are able is important to build and maintain trust. Effective leadership is understanding the needs of others and not reflecting personal emotions or judgment onto others. Communicating well and being able to deal with conflict in a way that motivates a team to work together and fosters collaboration will be a huge success factor for a leader.

Emotional intelligence (EI) is a skill needed during times of transition. As discussed in Chapter 5, "Emotional Intelligence," EI is the ability to know, understand, and control one's own emotions while also being able to identify, understand, and empathize with others in a social situation. EI helps nurse leaders and nurses to understand not only what the patient needs emotionally but also what the frontline staff need in order to provide excellence in their daily caring of others; this is also important during times of uncertainty that transitions bring. Nurse leaders with high EI communicate based upon the needs of the individual they are directing the communication to at the time. They tailor the style to what they observe in communications to have a positive interaction and work to accomplish a common goal. They are able to be the speaker and also listen and empathize with their audience. High EI leaders are able to understand the perceptions of others and change communication as needed. Perceptions are the truth to the person who believes them and high EI leaders can recognize and understand perceptions that both negatively and positively influence behaviors. This in turn allows them to communicate in a way that motivates others to understand the high EI leader's meaning.

Codier (2014) describes that nurses with high EI attributes are able to show positive conflict resolution and work better in teams, which leads to higher job satisfaction. Employee retention occurs when the nurses are satisfied with their work environment created by their nurse leader. With leaders who have high EI, the work environment is collaborative and positive, which lessens the likelihood of staff turnover. Coladonato and Manning (2017) also describe positive consequences of high EI as the ability of the nurse leader to manage emotions in their work environment and develop positive relationships with their staff. This leads to significantly higher job satisfaction and retention of staff.

Trust among the team, as discussed, is important yet fragile during times of unanticipated change. Visibility with frequent rounding with the team helps maintain trust during uncertain times. Questions will arise through the unknown, and while leaders are not expected to know all the answers, open feedback and follow-up to questions is imperative. Not having all the answers opens the manager up to vulnerability that can be uncomfortable. Be open to suggestions and also criticism from others that can be used for professional growth to improve and strengthen relationships and trust. The manager needs to remain flexible and role model the set tone that is expected on the unit. The response of the leader can have a ripple effect on the team; if the manager is calm, collected, and hopeful during a crisis, it will help to reduce anxiety. Open communication and active listening allow for questions and prevent false information from being spread around the unit.

Many nurse leaders have a very large span of control with multiple units, and being available and visible to everyone can be quite the challenge. During times of transitions, rounding on the team every day multiple times a day should be a top priority. Purposeful leadership rounding, when done effectively, can have a large positive impact on the trust of the team. Times of transition are usually also very time consuming for many different aspects, so rounding can be pushed aside when there does not seem to be enough hours in the day. Nurse managers should be cautious not to fall into this trap and view the rounding time as a time to assess the work environment.

Core values are what drive the thoughts and actions of an individual. The leader should recognize and understand their personal core values and how these fit into the organization. It is imperative that an individual's core values match those of the organization they are entrusted to lead. Yoder-Wise et al. (2021) describe that agile leaders' core strengths are their own internal values that guide their decision-making and refer to this as the leader's true north or purpose in life. A lack of alignment causes mistrust and anguish for not only the leader but also the employees, especially during times of transition or uncertainty. Being able to rely back to personal core values will allow the leader to make decisive decisions quickly when needed that support the organization's values.

Trust and collaboration may also need to be rebuilt after a period of unforeseen transitions as discussed. Supporting a culture of openness and learning is important to ensure human error mistakes are discussed and allowable while processes are addressed to prevent future error. Human error is inevitable, and leaders make mistakes or bad judgment calls as well. Being transparent and supporting a culture of learning and process improvement toward a common goal will help to gain and maintain trust. Admitting when a process is broken or an error in judgment occurred along with having a plan to mitigate or correct the issue can be difficult but presents the leader as human and trustworthy. An environment that is punitive or not compassionate will negatively affect the entire department.

Empathy and compassion are hugely beneficial to individuals and organizations, especially during times of transition and uncertainty. A leader who is able to listen and understand another's emotions and reactions can choose different approaches based upon the employee's need at that moment. Understanding what employees need and how to help them succeed is a core piece to compassionate leadership. A compassionate and empathetic environment spreads from individuals to other individuals in the department and starts with the leader's role modeling and engagement.

Empathy may be difficult to achieve if one is feeling stressed or burned out, so self-care of the leader is also an important factor that needs to be a priority. Setting boundaries and specifically calling out self-care activities can be hugely beneficial to an individual. Many leaders believe that self-care is nonsense or they do not have time; recognizing this resistance can help to change the leader's focus. Self-care is individualized and can take many different forms, but it begins with the leader consciously recognizing what works for them and utilizing these tools to decrease stress and invest in themselves. It can be as simple as taking a deep breath or a short walk around the room, or creating positive moments for others that in turn make the leader happier and more satisfied. Leadership is hard and sets the tone for others through either negative emotions or positive, self-resilient emotions.

WHAT EVERY NURSE MANAGER NEEDS TO KNOW

- Frequent, transparent communication is paramount during times of transition.
- Focus should be on developing EI and empathetic communication skills.
- Being present with staff helps maintain trust that can be broken during times of transition.

WHAT EVERY NURSE EXECUTIVE NEEDS TO KNOW ABOUT UNEXPECTED TRANSITIONS

Nursing leadership has inevitably been a learn-on-the-job, trial-by-fire type of experience. Nurse manager leaders are typically chosen to "move up the ladder" based on excellent clinical skills and motivation. Nurse executives also typically have a motivational factor, but how does one fill the knowledge gap of experiences that are unknown while also focusing on developing and retaining the nurse manager level talent? The AONL has identified five core competencies that nurse executives must develop: communication and relationship management, knowledge of healthcare and environment, leadership, professionalism, and business and principles. Gaining knowledge in each of these categories is important for success. Developing a network of fellow leaders is also a significant element of effective executive leadership to fill the knowledge gap and share experiences. Grow a mentorship circle of professionals that have similar roles, or meet in an environment that is inspirational to the nurse executive role and organizational values. Learn the resources that are out there to ask questions and gain knowledge of unexpected challenges.

One of the core competencies from AONL is communication and relationship management. Nurse executives are responsible for communicating to multiple stakeholders at different levels of the organization as well as the community stakeholders. They will facilitate conflict resolution among team members of various backgrounds to work toward a common goal. Creating a trusting environment for not only those that report to the executive but also those that report to operational manager/director levels below the executive is imperative.

Communication at the executive level becomes more complex with greater responsibilities to establish and maintain relationships. Daily rounding to different areas becomes more of a priority to understand what is taking place at the frontline level and how the executive can remove barriers. The relationships at this level become less individualized than the nurse manager has with direct staff. The executive must develop strategies to follow through with communication to a large team and engage staff in decision-making that may affect multiple areas of the organization. Presenting the larger picture and negotiating with multiple groups for a common outcome based upon strategy is important to achieve organizational goals. Maintaining credibility and respect when not working as closely with a group is a balance that can become overwhelming and stressful to be in multiple locations at the same time. Much like the nurse manager level, purposeful leadership rounding can be easy to set aside for competing priorities and is even more important to maintain/establish good rapport with the frontline caregivers. Staff must be able to relate and trust the nurse executive to be engaged in the team outcome. A study of various nurses completed by Easler (2021) found that leaders were more interesting and pleasing in person than through written communication, which supports the importance of personal relationships. Knowing the staff's name, listening, and demonstrating caring behaviors were the key skills that were recognized during this study. Visible leadership shows the priority and value the nurse executive has in the frontline staff.

Nurse executives are also expected to understand and anticipate market needs and what is or is not being met in order to help the organization grow and improve. Recruiting and retaining talent in key areas to maintain or grow services is crucial and requires leaders to look toward the future needs and adjust based upon the organizational workforce needs. This may mean trying something outside the norm in innovative ways that other leaders may push back upon or not fully support. Having a vision that inspires others to think differently and support ideas that can and will fail at some point sets the tone for the organization to grow. Failure is inevitable and necessary to make the leader stronger and more resilient in times of uncertainty. Yoder-Wise et al. (2021) encourage leaders to embrace ignorance for growth; although not having the answers can feel counterintuitive to managing the team, it allows for different perspectives to be heard and innovation to occur. Executives need to be comfortable with failure and look for the learning opportunities and knowledge gained during the experience.

A nurse leader will need to understand more than just clinical needs of their departments at the manager level and the entire nursing workforce for the nurse executive; a strong business acumen is also required. There are many different angles of data that will come across the nurse executive's desk, and the ability to digest, understand, explain, and take action on this data will be vital. During times of unexpected transition, a nurse executive will need to be able to review and analyze research data in order to make quick decisions. Understanding statistics and ways data is collected and presented will help the nurse executive know new trends or support initiatives with evidence-based practices. Nurse executives must know if the data is credible or not and how to translate the data into action and vision when needed. Credibility of the leader to analyze data and provide direction during times of unanticipated challenges will help caregivers navigate throughout the unknown if the trust is established.

High EI is also important for the nurse executive, especially when establishing and retaining trust of the caregivers in which we serve. Credibility is built through consistent words and actions. A nurse executive does not have as much direct connection as a nurse manager who has more interactions with frontline caregivers on a daily basis, so the interactions one has must be meaningful and impactful. Easler's (2021) study also found that nurses viewed their senior leader's actions and behavior as more important than their words. Not all actions were recognized, but those that were surprising or abnormal were remembered more during times of transition, and being present in person so the nurse can feel and sense the leader's intentions was imperative. Highly emotionally intelligent leaders are able to build relationships by showing control over emotional situations and not acting impulsively. They decrease the anxiety of others around them and analyze the tone of environment to provide direction that instills confidence and motivation. Emotionally intelligent leaders are real and experience both the positives and the negatives of the team. They take responsibility when things do not go right and give credit to the team when things go well, but they also create a balance through self-reflection for improvements.

Part of the core responsibility of the nurse executive is developing a nurse management leadership team through inclusive leadership. Nurse managers and future nurse leaders seek mentors, not just preceptors, so it is important to have ongoing conversations about strengths and opportunities (Armstrong et al., 2021). As a nurse executive, one must assess and leverage the strengths of the team and develop and coach the weaknesses. Different personalities do better with different situations, and knowing what each individual contributes while working to improve and strengthen organizational goals through stretch assignments and opportunities is important. Understanding the team and having frequent conversations toward goal setting will assist with coaching and redirecting when needed in order to achieve outcomes. Trust is also gained with the team by allowing them to think of their own process ideas and providing direction instead of commanding. Just as frequent self-assessment is important for the nurse executive, coaching the team to take self-assessments and share strengths will help them develop further as well.

A good onboarding plan should be developed to ensure that the new nurse manager is welcomed into the team and supported along the way. More frequent time spent up front to develop the leader will be a benefit to the entire leadership team. Assigning a fellow manager mentor for the new leader to connect with and talk through situations that arise will also assist the team. During times of unanticipated changes, a newer leader may not have all the skills developed to think quickly when decisions are needed to affect the unit; trial and error with support of the executive in front of the team is necessary. Course corrections can take place after the situations through guidance and direction in a private setting. Roussel et al. (2020) describe the differences between a routine manager and a leader as the ability to accept or challenge the structures and processes as they are. Changes are required, and leadership experiences help to navigate reality versus current processes that need to be improved. New nurse leaders will need to be encouraged to challenge the status quo without fear of punishment or negative reflection. A nurse executive must encourage and positively influence the team to improve themselves by trying new things and not fearing failure.

As nurses, one of our principal values is taking care of others and promoting healing through compassion and well-being. It is typical to place others' well-being above the nurses' own self, and this includes nurse leaders. The impact of COVID-19 has tested resilience and strength of all leaders and requires us to take action to place self-care and well-being as an essential value going forward (Armstrong et al., 2021). A nurse executive is looked at as a model, and others from frontline to leadership positions will take notice of what is promoted by the executive. Yoder-Wise et al. (2021) describe a healthy work environment as one that starts at the top with role models from leaders who make healthy decisions and show behaviors to reduce stress, improve resilience, and enhance decision-making. Self-care must be a priority and encouraged for not only the leadership team but also the nurse executive. Taking a few moments to self-reflect on the day or send along an appreciative note will help center the leader for the good things in the day and help move past the negative things. Leadership is difficult at times, and mistakes or wrong decisions will be made. How the leader reflects and moves past this to course correct reflects the integrity and values of the individual.

- Communication, while still paramount, becomes more difficult when all information is not able to be shared.
- Leadership presence with frontline staff is even more important at the executive level, although often more difficult to achieve.
- Relationship management is critical to success during transitions.
- The shift from clinical competence to business skills and competencies becomes most important during times of transition.

KEY POINTS

- Nurse executives need to assist their team in externalizing difficult organizational decisions.
- Developing competencies in statistical analysis is an important skill to acquire.
- Compassion and exercising EI are important during position elimination.
- Self-care and promoting one's own well-being is as important as ensuring the well-being of one's team.

SUMMARY

As healthcare appears to be in a state of constant change, nurse managers and nurse executives will continually be faced with navigating through change, sometimes in the form of anticipated or unanticipated transitions. Some of the common internal transitions that the nurse leader will experience during their career include a change in role and responsibilities and in the organizational chart, managing unanticipated financial challenges and dealing with the consultants these challenges bring, reductions in workforce, and even one's own position elimination. Other more complex transitions include mergers and acquisitions and even bankruptcy. A change in the competitive market may cause external transitions beyond the control of the organization, including relationship challenges. And finally, unanticipated environmental events, including weather events and health epidemics such as the COVID-19 pandemic, will continue to trigger unanticipated transitions, and new care delivery models will evolve as leaders pivot to be able to address the healthcare needs of the communities that are served. The response to each of these challenges and the ability to successfully lead staff during these times will determine the outcomes.

Nurse managers and nurse executives can prepare for these transitions by developing their competencies and skills, many described by AONL, that they depend on during times of relative calm. Communication and being present with staff, similar to skills needed for good leadership in times of status quo, are identified as key components to navigating transitional times successfully. Open and honest communication helps fill in the knowledge gap during times of rapid change and uncertainty. But even with the constant communication, trust can be broken and relationships damaged during these stressful times and transitions. Rebuilding trust and mending relationships takes time and effort, and the nurse leader must have the EI to recognize the needs of the staff as well as their own needs as a leader. An inclusive leadership style has demonstrated success in leading teams through transitions. Showing compassion and empathy and offering and participating in self-care and other needed interventions and therapies will help staff decompress and heal to regain confidence and demonstrate the resiliency needed to face the next challenge on the horizon.

END-OF-CHAPTER RESOURCES

● DISCUSSION QUESTIONS

1. The importance of communication is a common theme when discussing management of both anticipated transitions and unanticipated transitions. Describe some different communication skills that would be useful to a nurse leader to develop and utilize when managing transitions.
2. Discuss some of the challenges that a nurse leader may experience during an organizational merger or an acquisition.
3. There were other anticipated and unanticipated transitions discussed in this chapter. Discuss these and name others that you may have experienced.

● ADDITIONAL RESOURCES

- Reina, D., & Reina, M. (2015). *Trust and betrayal in the workplace* (3rd ed.). Berrett-Koehler.
- *Mergers and acquisitions: Strategies, execution and postmerger management.* Harvard Business School. https://www.exed.hbs.edu/programs-organizations/mergers-acquisitions
- 2021 podcast: *Merger and acquisition science: Preserving value:* https://coachingforleaders.com

● LEARNING EXERCISES FOR STUDENTS

We have all experienced some transitions as nurse leaders. Sharing experiences in group discussion becomes a learning opportunity for all.

1. Discuss one anticipated transition that you have been faced with in your nursing career to date. What went well? Looking back today, what would you have done differently? How would that have changed the outcome for you?
2. Discuss one unanticipated transition that you have experienced in your nursing career. Would you have changed anything in the response to that event?
3. What are some of the similarities between the two events and what are some of the differences?

● GLOSSARY OF KEY TERMS

- **Acquisition:** A takeover of one organization by another where the parent organization purchases the assets of another organization and the two become one system.
- **Anticipated transition:** A change that is expected to occur; the timing is predictable in nature and can therefore include robust planning.
- **Merger:** When two organizations agree to combine their organizations to become one larger organization.
- **Organizational chart:** A leadership chart that outlines the reporting structure, defining who reports to who for the entity that the chart represents.
- **Unanticipated transition:** Change that is not expected and does not follow any predictable timeline or course of events.

REFERENCES

American Organization of Nurse Executives & American Organization for Nursing Leadership. (2015). *Nurse executive competencies*. https://www.aonl.org/system/files/media/file/2019/06/nec.pdf

Armstrong, L., Spivey, P., & Doran, M. (2021). Contemporary engagement strategies for nurse leaders. *Nurse Leader*, *19*(4), 360–365. https://doi.org/10.1016/j.mnl.2021.03.011

Balluck, J., Asturi, E., & Brockman, V. (2020). Use of the ADKAR® and CLARC® change models to navigate staffing model changes during the COVID-19 pandemic. *Nurse Leader*, *18*(6), 539–546. https://doi.org/10.1016/j.mnl.2020.08.006

Beaulieu, N. D., Dafny, L. S., Landon, B. E., Dalton, J. B., Kuye, I., & Michael McWilliams, J. (2020). Changes in quality of care after hospital mergers and acquisitions. *New England Journal of Medicine*, *382*(1), 51–59. https://doi.org/10.1056/NEJMsa1901383

Caroselli, C. (2020). A journey through unchartered territory: A nurse executive's frontline pandemic response. *Nursing Economic$*, *38*(3), 164–171.

Centers for Disease Control and Prevention. (2020, June 10). *Using telehealth to expand access to essential health services during the COVID-19 pandemic*. U.S. Department of Health and Human Services. https://www.cdc.gov/coronavirus/2019-ncov/hcp/telehealth.html

Chesley, C. G. (2020, March/April). Merging cultures: Organizational culture and leadership in a health system merger. *Foundation of the American College of Healthcare Executives*, *65*(2), 135–150. https://doi.org/10.1097/jhm-d-18-00213

Codier, E. (2014). Making the case for emotionally intelligent leaders. *Nursing Management*, *45*(1), 44–48. https://doi.org/10.1097/01.numa.0000440634.64013.11

Coladonato, A. R., & Manning, M. L. (2017). Nurse leader emotional intelligence. *Nursing Management*, *48*(9), 26–32. https://doi.org/10.1097/01.numa.0000522174.00393.f2

Easler, L. (2021). Nurses' aesthetic responses and emotional judgments to senior leaders' use of language, action, and behavior. *Nurse Leader*, *19*(4), 366–370. https://doi.org/10.1016/j.mnl.2021.03.008

Edmunson, C. (2015). Moving forward: Lessons from unplanned change. *The Journal of Nursing Administration*, *45*(2), 61–62. https://doi.org/10.1097/NNA.0000000000000158

Galura, S. (2020). On the frontlines of nursing leadership: Managerial dissonance and the implications for nurse managers and health care organizations. *Nurse Leader*, *18*(5), 476–480. https://doi.org/10.1016/j.mnl.2020.05.012

Hertel, R. A. (2020). Navigating turbulence as a leader. *MedSurg Nursing*, *29*(3), 141–142.

Nelson, K. E., & Pilon, B. (2015). Managing organizational transitions: The chief nurse perspective. *Nurse Leader*, *13*(3), 71–76. https://doi.org/10.1016/j.mnl.2014.09.011

Reina, D., & Reina, M. (2015). *Trust and betrayal in the workplace* (3rd ed.). Berrett-Koehler.

Robinson, R., & Knight, S. (2018). Hospital acquisitions. The chief nurse executive perspective. *Nursing Management*, 34–40. https://doi.org/10.1097/01.numa.0000533767.28005.d2

Roussel, L., Harris, J. L., & Thomas, P. L. (2020). *Management and leadership for nurse administrators*. Jones & Bartlett Learning.

Sofer, D. (2020, May). The cult of the Colossus: A dramatic rise in hospital mergers and acquisitions. *American Journal of Nursing*, *120*(5), 19–20. https://doi.org/10.1097/01.NAJ.0000662772.53382.ce

Yoder-Wise, P. S., Crenshaw, J. T., & Wilson, R. C. (2021). Leading with agility and grace when the path is unclear. *Nurse Leader*, *19*(3), 259–263. https://doi.org/10.1016/j.mnl.2021.02.008

CHAPTER 23

THE NURSE LEADER'S ROLE IN PHILANTHROPY

Kate Judge

> *"Philanthropy is about solving problems."*
>
> *Naveen Jain (as cited in Boyle, 2018, para. 21)*

LEARNING OBJECTIVES

- Describe how philanthropy can have an impact on nurses and nursing practice.
- Identify competencies that nurses bring to philanthropy and resource generation.
- Analyze ways in which you can engage colleagues in philanthropic activities and goal setting.
- Create a model scenario that demonstrates benefits of engaging in fundraising.

INTRODUCTION

Philanthropy directed at nursing is a relatively new phenomenon. When achieved, there is the potential for significant improvements in patient care and nursing practice and education (Bolton et al., 2014). Nursing today does not command a leading share of the financial resources contributed to nonprofits as through philanthropy. Nursing and nurses' patients are poorer—literally—for this inequity. But that is changing as nurse leaders engage in more intentional philanthropic conversations and identify the resources they need to deliver the best care possible. Engaging in fundraising can both generate greater resources for nursing practice and patients and be foundational to personal and professional growth and advancement for the nurse leader involved.

WHAT IS PHILANTHROPY?

Philanthropy is literally the love of humankind. The desire to aid in the common good is a part of virtually all communities and traditions. Providing assistance, whether a meal to a new or hungry neighbor, or providing clothing or housing to a victim of a disaster, is a value built into communities world-wide.

The current concept of philanthropy is based upon definitions of "charity" defined as "something done or given for the benefit of our fellows or the public" (*Knight's Estate*, 1894, as cited in Zunz, 2012, p. 16). In the United States, formal philanthropy emerged after the Civil War, when the wealthy and powerful used financial contributions to shape community affairs with modern and more universal strategies for human progress, although not all communities or "humans" benefited equally from those contributions. In community life, philanthropy led to creation of libraries, hospitals, museums, universities, and medical research.

In addition to financial resources, philanthropy also relates to the giving of time and talent as a volunteer. However, for the purposes of this chapter, we focus on philanthropy that is monetary.

Philanthropy in healthcare primarily covers two areas. The first is meeting basic needs and addressing temporary relief such as providing a meal, shelter, or basic care. For example, a community health center seeks contributions to augment services not covered by insurance, or it raises funds to provide transport or food vouchers. Assistance in meeting basic core needs is an important safety net for individuals globally.

The second area is the extra investment of dollars that enable an organization to reach a new state or provide a long-term solution to a significant problem. An example of this may be a donor creating a fund to provide scholarships for students from communities that are underrepresented in nursing, such as students of color or students from rural communities.

Nursing's connection with philanthropy has roots dating back to the 19th century and the formal organization of nursing with the creation of the American Nurses Association (ANA) in 1896 (Bazzy, 2018). To date, there have been few studies or articles on nursing and philanthropy, but given nurses' central role in care—acute, ambulatory, and home—and the unprecedented visibility of nurses during the COVID-19 pandemic, increased giving to nursing and documenting and studying that giving are all contributing to new interest in the impact of philanthropy in nursing practice.

WHO PROVIDES PHILANTHROPIC SUPPORT?

There are five primary sources of philanthropic giving: individuals (living and posthumously), estates, foundations, corporations, and government agencies. While government agencies are not calculated in the annual philanthropic giving reports, they do support needed programs, especially nursing education.

In 2020, a total of $471 billion was given as part of formal philanthropy (Giving USA, 2021). Of that, $42.12 billion was contributed to health overall, which included giving to large health systems and hospitals, organizations focused on specific health issues and diseases, as well as special events.

The vast majority of the funding (69%) was provided by individuals (e.g., grateful patients, caring community members, and interested parties). Individuals—those that nurses care for every day—make small contributions such as "rounding up" at a convenience store, make annual contributions and organize the collections of funds and materials, and donate large gifts. It is not only the Rockefellers or Gateses who give, and it is not just large gifts such as Ezra Cornell's gift to create Cornell University or the Chan Family's naming of the School of Public Health at Harvard. Most large contributors began with modest gifts as they started a long-term relationship with an organization or cause. Helping to build these relationships over time is a perfect way for nurse leaders to play a critical role in philanthropy.

Often, the donors who leave money in their wills and/or estates are modest annual donors who have a long history of giving. Appreciation for every gift—regardless of size—is important, just as every patient is important regardless of their ability to pay for care. Gifts through individual's estates provided an additional 9% of overall giving in 2020.

Sometimes significant donors have no history of active giving to an organization and then make a large gift at the time of their death. Often referred to as the millionaire donor next door giving, anecdotes abound. One example: Phyllis A. Stone, who lived in a modest house and drove an old car. She bequeathed nearly all of her estate to charity, leaving more than $6 million to local Albany, New York, charities when she died at the age of 91 in 2013.

Often nurses feel they cannot relate to fundraising because it is perceived as being associated only with mega rich individuals. That is not true. The honest and heartfelt relationship that is established when a potential donor admires nursing and asks, "How can I help?" is related to authenticity and appreciation—something nurses have in spades.

Foundations, the next largest type of donors, provided 19% of total giving in 2020. These organizations range widely in size and purpose. They run the gamut from small family-based foundations focused on community issues to large, established organizations with national or international priorities. There are different types of foundations with different legal requirements for distributing funds. There are public resources, guides, and documents such as an organization's tax filings that may provide insight into a foundation's priorities, in addition to any public-facing information provided by the foundation itself.

Corporations provided the final 4% of giving in 2020. Corporations often align giving with company interests or mission or the communities where their employees live and work. Often, companies generate and receive a disproportionate share of public recognition for their giving in contrast to individuals who provide the largest percentage of philanthropic dollars.

TYPES OF DONATIONS

There are two principal categories of donations, specifically designed to control how the contributions may be used by the recipient. The first category is "unrestricted," which leaves the determination of how funds will be used to the receiving organization. Annual fundraising efforts that cover operational costs are the greatest source of unrestricted funds.

A second category is "restricted," which indicates use of a gift by the recipient is restricted to a certain purpose as identified by the donor. Restrictions can be for specific projects or for a type of activity. The other type of common restricted contribution is one that is held permanently in reserve and only the interest earned on the gift is spent. This is called an endowment.

Most organizations have annual giving campaigns, which are time-limited efforts to raise donations. These typically follow the organization's budget cycle. The other common type of fundraising effort is for a "capital campaign." This is a longer, usually multiyear, time-limited fundraising effort that seeks to raise a substantial amount of money—significantly more than an annual campaign.

FUNDRAISING ROLES

Successful fundraising is a collective endeavor. It involves professional fundraising staff and expertise, often located in an organization's "development" or "advancement" office. This staff has specific expertise in identifying, cultivating, soliciting, and thanking donors so that they are informed, engaged, and inclined to make additional gifts. Administrative leadership is also engaged in setting priorities and goals for fundraising and in maintaining communication with prospective and current donors. Every successful solicitation or fundraising campaign requires a champion who ensures that the needs of the institution and project are prioritized (Paul et al., 2017).

One of the most important roles in fundraising is in telling the story of the need or problem to be solved and who will benefit. This is a role where nurse leaders and frontline nurses can excel. No one knows better what patients experience and need than nurses do. Providing the narrative and descriptions of real people and their real needs is the most compelling element in any fundraising effort. It is essential in "making the case."

◆ CASE SCENARIO
THE INVITATION TO MEET A POTENTIAL DONOR

The new chief nurse executive (CNE) receives a call from the fundraising department to help arrange a tour for a board member of the facility's new memory center. The CNE hasn't met any of the fundraising staff yet and sees this as a two-fold opportunity to make new connections in the organization and community.

The CNE is strategic in thinking this is an opportunity to make connections and build their reputation as a resource to be counted on now and in the future. Engaging in a visit with a board member can accomplish multiple goals.

DISCUSSION QUESTIONS

1. What are two quick things the CNE can do to prepare?
2. How can the CNE involve nurses on the unit?
3. What should the CNE do after the visit?

MAKING THE CASE

All too often, what nurses do and what resources nurses need to thrive are invisible. They are invisible to patients, to leaders, and to prospective donors. When nurses downplay their contributions to care delivery, assessment, and intervention when talking with patients, the expertise of nursing care is invisible. This is especially detrimental if it is done when a patient or family member is expressing gratitude and asks what they can do to help or recognize the outstanding care they received.

A case for support can make nursing's critical role in care visible. A case can range from a fundraising letter to a donor or group of donors to a comprehensive multiyear, multimillion dollar written and visual documentation of an organizational transformation funded through philanthropy. A good example of this is a university or hospital capital campaign brochure. The goal is to make the case compelling with persuasive content that shares an exciting future state and inspires a donor to give.

A case for support needs to answer several key questions: What is the problem needing to be solved? How does that problem translate to everyday people? Why is it important to solve this NOW? How will the problem be solved? How much will it cost and how long will it take?

Answering the latter two questions requires solid and conservative planning. The gift or giving experience could be derailed if solutions are overpromised (e.g., "All of a patient's life issues will be solved with one type of intervention"). If the cost of the project is greater than the case identifies, a project can stall, and the donor could lose respect for the business acumen of the organization and leaders involved.

Ultimately, a case for support is a story about people and needs. It needs to include emotion and color. It is not simply a request filled with statistics or general statements. For a nurse, this means gathering the facts and the personal stories around a particular need; in other words, identifying the costs involved in addressing the problem as well as the consequences of *not* addressing the problem. Each is part of the compelling story.

The case is a combination of business case and brief compelling story that will appeal to a donor's interests. It is helpful to imagine yourself as the donor: Is the story compelling enough for you to make a gift? An essential part of making a case is getting input and feedback.

Get feedback and buy in from nurses, leadership, and the professional development staff. This accomplishes several key things. First, the ability to engage and advise expands the network of people that know and care about an issue. It provides an opportunity for shared governance and professional development for nursing staff. It also connects the fundraising staff directly to nursing. That has two benefits. The first is that fundraisers feel like a valued part of the care team. Second, when a prospective donor asks an organization's fundraising staff what the needs are, they will know much more and have a ready answer.

Since nurses provide the majority of patient care and interaction—especially in acute care settings—they can be essential to healthcare philanthropy priority setting if they are active and ready participants in fundraising.

CASE SCENARIO

BUILDING A CASE FOR SUPPORT

An organization is beginning its strategic planning process. The chief nursing officer (CNO) wants to identify several investments that could support the nurses working at the facility and translate into improved care. The CNO anticipates having 3 months to build a case for support.

The CNO cannot guarantee that the investments needed will make their way into the strategic plan, but developing the case for support can increase appreciation by staff nurses of their importance of crafting communication about resource needs to both organizational leadership and donors. It can also serve as a ready document when a donor asks what is needed. Finally, it helps build a broader culture of philanthropy where everyone is involved.

DISCUSSION QUESTIONS

1. How can the CNO engage frontline nurses in preparing the case for support?
2. What are key elements needed in the case?

 CASE SCENARIO

ANSWERING THE QUESTION "HOW CAN WE HELP"?

In discussing a patient case with their manager, the primary care nurse at a hospice facility shares that a patient's family has requested a way to help the nurses or facility in recognition for the exemplary care they have provided. The nurse shares that they assured the family that all patients receive equal care and that knowing they've made a difference is all the thanks necessary. The family asks on several subsequent visits about finding some way to help. The nurse asks their manager how they should answer. Should the nurse suggest a gift or something for the patients to enjoy, such as decorations for a common area? A basket of food?

DISCUSSION QUESTIONS

1. What organizational resources could the nurse manager turn to for advice and partnership?
2. What resources would be helpful so the nurse could respond to the family's request the first time?
3. In what nonfinancial ways could the family recognize the nurses?

HOW TO APPLY EXISTING NURSING COMPETENCIES TO PHILANTHROPY

COMMUNICATION

Effective communication is central to nursing leadership and plays an essential role in fundraising and philanthropy. Clear, sincere, and compelling communication about organizational needs in human terms engages donors and helps them decide if this is the right cause to support. Strong and appreciative communication helps build relationships with donors and key organizational staff such as the development staff. Engaging donors in philanthropic projects could include presentations, small meetings, and written communications including notes of thanks.

INTERPERSONAL RELATIONSHIPS

Strong communication helps build the relationships that provide the foundation of philanthropy. Equal with donor's interests in a cause is their belief and connection to those asking for the donation. Nurses can draw upon their skills in listening, being empathetic, and valuing the individual in their relationships with donors and with the fundraising team.

Engaging with donors is a natural extension of nursing's engagement with patients (Hitchings et al., 2012). Nurses' ability to understand people and situations is both fundamental to providing care and raising money. This includes their ability to listen deeply to aspirations and needs, their skill in building supportive interpersonal relationships that exhibit empathy for a person's needs and dreams, and their commitment to communicate clearly and authentically.

TEAM ENGAGEMENT

Nurses' reliance on colleagues with complementary expertise is a natural bridge to creating a successful fundraising effort. Engaging with nurses who provide direct care helps nurse leaders understand and better communicate the needs of nurses and patients to the administration and donors.

LEADERSHIP

One of the most important leadership skills that nurses bring to philanthropy is setting the tone and communicating the message that philanthropy is everyone's business. Nurse leaders do this by demonstrating their own philanthropy and giving a gift. They demonstrate leadership and build a broad culture of philanthropy each time they engage publicly with donors and connect those donors to those at the bedside who make care possible.

BUSINESS

Philanthropy, which is emotional and personal, is built on financial needs and the investment, dissemination, and use of funds. Nurse leaders can use their business experience to build a case for support and provide input and feedback on organizational priorities that may require philanthropic support. The nurse leader also demonstrates a knowledge of the full variety of financial streams that provide resources to an institution.

MYTHS ABOUT FUNDRAISING

In her article "Fundraising Tips for Nurse Leaders and Nurse Executives" (2014), Joyce Fitzpatrick drew upon her years of fundraising experience as an academic leader and dean of the Frances Payne Bolton School of Nursing at Case Western University to address the illusionary barriers to nurse leaders in fundraising. Her message was clear: Nurses are essential to better healthcare enabled by philanthropic giving (Fitzpatrick, 2014).

One of the common myths about philanthropy and nursing is that the only purpose of fundraising is to secure financial contributions. Fundamentally, fundraising and philanthropy are about building relationships around important work that needs to be done. Joining a need with a means to address it is a positive experience for both sides: the donor and the recipient.

Successful solicitations of donors provide new financial resources to meet the organization's mission and support nurses. It also helps the donors' feel they are making a difference. Volunteerism has even been shown to translate into physical health and well-being (Oman, 1999). Acts of gratitude are valuable to both sides of the equation. It is important to remember that while philanthropy is based on relationships, the person asking for money is not asking for their personal benefit. In that way, it is not personal; it is all about a problem needing to be solved.

Other myths include that successful fundraising is just about knowing the right wealthy people who have to give away their money. With 1.54 million charities in the United States, fundraising is competitive and donors, especially donors making significant gifts, expect that there is rigor in the fundraising experience (The Urban Institute, 2019). This ranges from their expectation that they will receive a strong case for support to being able to weigh the need against their own priorities and passions. Nurses' ability to listen, understand, and empathize with peoples' needs and goals is a strong foundation for fundraising.

These foundational skills apply to engaging with all types of donors, including individuals, corporations, and foundations. The need to do one's homework and understand what the potential donor is interested in is essential. What have they funded in the past? If they are a corporation or foundation, what are their stated goals, priorities, and limitations? Do they expect anything in return for their contribution? This is especially important to understand when working with companies who have responsibilities to shareholders and often use philanthropy for corporate gain.

The idea of self-interest in giving should be factored into any solicitation. All of us have interests that drive our decisions. Sometimes they are purely altruistic, but often they are influenced by a more complex array of personal desires and priorities. Successful fundraising can incorporate them all if conversations are open and comprehensive. If ethical issues are identified by the potential recipient, it is important to raise them with the fundraising team and with the potential donor. Successful fundraising requires planning, strong communication, attention to detail, personal affinity and a combination of skills and relationships.

WHAT EVERY NURSE MANAGER NEEDS TO KNOW ABOUT PHILANTHROPY

Given that it is in your and the donor's interest to connect, you can be ready when someone—a patient, a family of a patient, your friends and family—asks how they can help. Having an answer ready makes it easier for you and the asker. If you can quickly provide a website or a brochure, you increase the likelihood that they will follow through with their offer. In a busy world, and with competition among nonprofits in the United States, readiness and ease of giving stand out.

Nurse managers play a critical role in the philanthropy team. It is not all on their shoulders to fundraise, but their leadership sets the overall appreciation for the power of philanthropy in the department and demonstrates a key competency in nursing of valuing teamwork and being a team player. Like a care team, a philanthropy team is made up of people with different expertise who join together to address a clear goal and outcome. Like healthcare, it is complicated, it is personal, and it takes time and practice.

Part of working as a team in philanthropy is helping your executive leader build a case for support. You have the intimate knowledge of what is needed and why and how that translates into better outcomes for nurses and patients. You possess something that is essential to effective fundraising—the personal stories of need and impact. Donations are rarely made because of statistics; instead, they are made because of stories of real people—often one specific person. You bring a great value to your leadership and the development professionals when you can communicate about real patients and concrete needs. There is not a patient encounter that does not engage nursing; listening to when donors are grateful for "care" is a value you bring to the conversation.

WHAT EVERY NURSE MANAGER NEEDS TO KNOW

- Expressing gratitude for care helps the giver.
- You need to have a ready answer to "How can I help?"
- This is a team endeavor—your nurse leader and development professionals are resources.
- You can build your own case.

◼ WHAT EVERY NURSE EXECUTIVE NEEDS TO KNOW ABOUT PHILANTHROPY

Successful fundraising draws upon the mantra of the right person asking the right person at the right time for the right thing (cause and amount). It starts with identifying the need and making the case and involves setting your sights high enough for the gift to matter. Having not enjoyed a large share of the healthcare philanthropic giving pot in the past, nurse leaders can sometimes underestimate how much is needed to accomplish a goal and how likely donors are to generously support nursing. Setting sights and expectations high demonstrates the importance of nursing practice and nursing's essential role in care delivery. Successful philanthropy helps illuminate nursing overall and brings its importance out in the open.

Philanthropic priority setting, planning, and execution often involve top leadership—professional and volunteer. Those are important relationships for any nurse in the c-suite. They lead to further opportunities, like invitations to sit on community boards or engage in new projects and teams.

In every interaction, there is the opportunity to make what nursing is more explicit and central to the organization's public presentation. In this way, a nurse executive plays a vital incremental role in changing nursing's landscape in their organization. Each time a significant gift is made to nursing—from naming a school to establishing a scholarship fund—it becomes a more visible option for other donors. For example, when Barbara and Donald Jonas decided to focus their philanthropy on nursing because it was an "uncrowded field," they provided visibility to the profession and its social value (National Center for Family Philanthropy, 2007).

The relationships that are created in the process of philanthropy provide a richness that extends far beyond an exchange of financial resources. Donors can make connections with others they know who can provide advice, funding, and expertise that can enhance a project or healthcare institution. Donors have stories about why they care about a cause, and they often have business acumen which can help a nurse executive with making a future case. Their kindness and generosity of spirit can be uplifting for the leader and can be shared with frontline nurses. There can never be enough people expressing gratitude to nurses. Building a relationship between a donor and a leader's team pays in both directions.

One of the great benefits of philanthropy is the ability for a gift to have a lasting impact on a cause. A gift that is restricted by the donor for endowment means that the original gift—say a gift of $100,000—cannot be used, but the interest earned off that gift can and must be used. Preserving the original principal of the gift ensures that in the future there will be funding available. A common example is a scholarship endowment that generates dollars for financial assistance for a nurse's education or professional development every year. The principal typically grows as well so that over time the annual interest available increases to provide more financial assistance.

Working with your organization's administrative, fundraising, and volunteer leadership provides unique opportunities to grow communication skills and executive presence, and expand a nurse leader's network. This can lead to new professional and volunteer experiences. Given the importance of philanthropy to healthcare institutions, developing experience in philanthropy is an asset for any aspiring chief executive officer (CEO) or dean. It also can provide a connection that could lead to a volunteer leadership opportunity—like an invitation to board service in a non- or for-profit institution.

WHAT EVERY NURSE EXECUTIVE NEEDS TO KNOW

- Set your sights high.
- Philanthropic discussion puts you at a critical table.
- It's about more than money.
- It can provide a lasting resource: endowment.
- Engaging in philanthropy prepares you for other leadership opportunities—like CEO or board service.

KEY POINTS

- Developing relationships with donors and organizational professional fundraisers is key to creating allies in connecting the power of philanthropy to nursing.
- Engaging in the pursuit of philanthropy puts nurses together with key organizational and volunteer leaders and positions nurses as ambassadors of the organization.
- Nurses are vital to successful fundraising by bringing to donors their real patient experiences and stories and employing their skills of empathy, listening, and interpersonal dynamics.
- Philanthropy and its required skills are aligned with those skills and expertise of frontline nurses, nurse managers, and nurse leaders.

SUMMARY

Drawing upon some of the basic tenets of nursing practice, nurses, regardless of position, can engage in philanthropy and the pursuit of financial resources for the betterment of patient care. An overview of the history and current state of philanthropy reveals a landscape rich with potential for nurses. By engaging with donors, nurses can access resources that extend beyond dollars. These include connections to other influencers, ideas and knowledge, kindred spirits and volunteers, and new leadership opportunities. Nurses' ability to develop deep and lasting relationships has, in many institutions, led to transformative gifts, and serves as a blueprint for other nurses' leadership step into philanthropy.

END-OF-CHAPTER RESOURCES

◆ DISCUSSION QUESTIONS

1. How important are relationships to raising money?
2. What other value do key donors and volunteers have?
3. How would you go about creating your own case for support?

◆ ADDITIONAL RESOURCES

- Bolton, L. B., Swanson, J., & Zamora, E. (2014). Ensuring the availability of the nursing workforce through philanthropy: A case study. *Nursing Administration Quarterly, 38*(4), 327–331. https://doi.org/10.1097/NAQ.0000000000000053
- Association for Healthcare Philanthropy: https://www.ahp.org
- Association of Fundraising Professionals: https://afpglobal.org

⬤ GLOSSARY OF KEY TERMS

- **Case for support:** An outline or written narrative that uses clear and compelling language to describe what financial resources are needed and what they will accomplish if given.

- **Charity:** Giving help, usually in the form of money.

- **Donor:** A person or organization that has contributed financially to a nonprofit organization.

- **Philanthropy:** Love of humankind which inspires acts of donation of time and money.

- **Prospect:** A prospective donor. Often this is a donor who is considering a second or different additional contribution.

 A robust set of instructor resources designed to supplement this text is located at http://connect.springerpub.com/content/book/978-0-8261-7795-7. Qualifying instructors may request access by emailing textbook@springerpub.com.

REFERENCES

Bazzy, N. (2018). The nurse philanthropist: Where care and cause meet. *Creative Nursing, 24*(1), 82–87. https://doi.org/10.1891/1078-4535.22.2.82

Bolton, L. B., Swanson, J., & Zamora, E. (2014). Ensuring the availability of the nursing workforce through philanthropy: A case study. *Nursing Administration Quarterly, 38*(4), 327–331. https://doi .org/10.1097/NAQ.0000000000000053

Boyle, A. (2018, October 23). *Naveen Jain explores the entrepreneurial frontier in 'Moonshots' book and business.* GeekWire. https://www.geekwire.com/2018/naveen-jain-explores-entrepreneurial-frontier -moonshots-book-business

Fitzpatrick, J. J. (2014). Fund-raising tips for nurse leaders and nurse executives. *Nursing Administration Quarterly, 38*(4), 294–298. https://doi.org/10.1097/NAQ.0000000000000053

Giving USA. (2021). *Giving USA annual report.* Giving USA Foundation. https://store.givingusa.org/ products/2021-annual-report?variant=39329211613263

Hitchings, K. S., Capuano, T. A., & Herzog, M. E. (2012). Friends of nursing: A community of caring to promote excellence in nursing practice, education, and research. *Journal of Continuing Education in Nursing, 43*(5), 211–217. https://doi.org/10.3928/00220124-20120201-27

National Center for Family Philanthropy. (2007). *Painting a family philanthropy canvas.* https://www .ncfp.org/2007/01/15/the-barbara-and-donald-jonas-family-fund-painting-a-family -philanthropy-canvas/

Oman, D. (1999). Volunteerism and mortality among the community-dwelling elderly. *Journal of Health Psychology, 4*(3), 301–316. https://doi.org/10.1177/135910539900400301

Paul, R., Hollenberg, E., & Hodges, B. D. (2017). Philanthropy in health professions education research: Determinants of success. *Medical Education, 51*(5), 511–520. https://doi.org/10.1111/medu.13231

The Urban Institute. (2019). *National Center for Charitable Statistics.* https://nccs.urban.org/publication/ nonprofit-sector-brief-2019

Zunz, O. (2012). *Philanthropy in America: A history.* Princeton University Press.

SECTION IX

CASE STUDIES FOR NURSE MANAGERS AND EXECUTIVES

CHAPTER 24

COMPREHENSIVE CASE STUDIES

■ **Comprehensive Case Study 1:** Human-Centered Leadership
Kay Kennedy, Lucy Leclerc, and Susan Campis

■ **Comprehensive Case Study 2:** Effective Mentoring Through Relational Leadership
K. David Bailey and Joseph P. De Santis

■ **Comprehensive Case Study 3:** Telehealth
Mary Joy Garcia-Dia

■ **Comprehensive Case Study 4:** Nurse-Led Innovation to Reduce Occupational Heat Stress of Operating Room Personnel
Jill Byrne

■ **Comprehensive Case Study 5:** Leadership to Drive Quality Through Direct-Care Nurse Feedback Using an Electronic Health Record Dashboard
Anne Pohnert and Mary A. Dolansky

■ **Comprehensive Case Study 6:** Resiliency
Deirdre O'Flaherty and Mary Joy Garcia-Dia

■ **Comprehensive Case Study 7:** Main Hospital: Perioperative Transition Unit
Garry Brydges

■ **Comprehensive Case Study 8:** Competition Within Healthcare Industry
Nathanial Schreiner and Stuart D. Downs

HUMAN-CENTERED LEADERSHIP

Kay Kennedy, Lucy Leclerc, and Susan Campis

HUMAN ERROR: AN UNCONSCIOUS DRIFT FROM SAFE BEHAVIOR

A new nurse with only 6 months' experience was caring for a cohort of three patients on the COVID-19 unit. After donning personal protective equipment (PPE) and administering the subcutaneous insulin dose for the brittle diabetic patient, the nurse realized that a tuberculin syringe, instead of an insulin syringe, had been used. This resulted in the patient receiving a significantly higher dose of insulin than was ordered. The novice nurse immediately notified the preceptor who, in turn, called the physician. The patient was carefully monitored, and no harm ensued.

In this scenario, the nurse clearly made an error. It could be described as a "human error," just like the many errors each of us make during a normal day. The obvious difference here is that this error could have led to dire consequences for the patient. If the error had gone unreported, and the patient unmonitored, the result could have been insulin shock, coma, or even death. In this case, the nurse immediately reported the error upon realizing the wrong dose had been given, and appropriate monitoring to prevent harm followed. This was an unintentional error.

The human-centered leader harnesses the dimensions of the upholder, the awakener, and the connector to approach the situation holistically (Figure CCS1.1). As an upholder, the human-centered leader aims to recognize the humanity in the novice nurse through a culture of caring. The leader avoids rushing to judgment and instead assesses the situation in an effort to get a complete picture of the situation and all the variables. The human-centered leader, as connector, creates a safe environment for the novice nurse, minimizing feelings of shame and embarrassment by recognizing the nurse is new to the profession and may be unfamiliar with specific unit policies and safety checks (i.e., second RN verification). The human-centered leader also consoles the novice nurse and accepts accountability for system improvements to prevent or mitigate the possibility of this happening to someone else. The leader recognizes the nurse's humanness and any unrealistic expectation for perfection, taking this opportunity to let the nurse know that errors are an essential teacher. Through these efforts, a culture of trust is fostered (Figure CCS1.1). The human-centered leader recognizes the complexity of caring for COVID patients who require rigorous attention to disease management, as well as adherence to use of PPE, may have contributed to the novice nurse's distraction while preparing the insulin. The leader as awakener involves the novice nurse in determining why and how the error occurred. The leader understands the limits of knowledge and recognizes blind spots by actively engaging the novice nurse in investigating opportunities to improve individually and at the unit level. The human-centered leader explains the goal is to make it difficult for another nurse to make a similar mistake in the future. The novice nurse is honored for the quick response to the known error and is involved in the process to make system improvements to promote patient safety, resulting in a strengthened culture of excellence (Figure CCS1.1). Lastly, the leader recognizes the

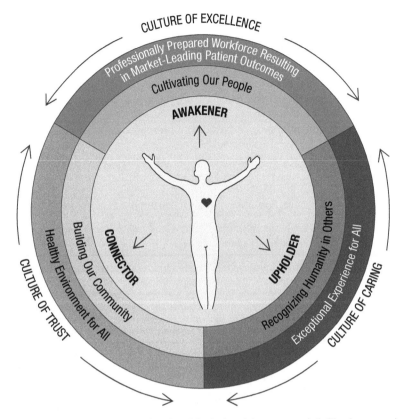

FIGURE CCS1.1: Human-centered leadership in healthcare model. The framework reflects an innovative approach to leadership in healthcare that starts with the leader's mind, body, and spirit as the locus of influence within local and larger complex systems. The human-centered leader realizes success in nurturing cultures of excellence, trust, and caring by being an awakener, a connector, and an upholder.

Source: Reproduced with permission from Leclerc, L., Kennedy, K., & Campis, S. (2021). Human-centred leadership in health care: A contemporary nursing leadership theory generated via constructivist grounded theory. *Journal of Nursing Management, 29,* 294–306. https://doi.org/10.1111/jonm.13154.

pandemic has disrupted nursing academia with varied and often limited clinical experiences. Some new nursing graduates may not have had the opportunity to enhance clinical skills and to strengthen clinical judgment. The human-centered leader uses this perspective to offer additional support for the novice nurse through educational opportunities designed to enhance clinical reasoning.

END-OF-CASE RESOURCES

◆ DISCUSSION QUESTIONS

1. If you were this novice nurse's manager, describe at least two ways you would harness the attributes of the upholder to ensure a culture of caring. Refer to Table CCS1.1 for definitions of each attribute and identify two attributes in your discussion and how you would apply them to this situation: mindful, others-oriented, emotionally aware, socially and organizationally aware, personally well and healthy.

2. How does the human-centered leader also effectively use their awakener skills to ensure that the same mistake doesn't happen again with another nurse? Using the

attributes of the awakener, describe at least two actions you, as the nurse manager, would take. Refer to Table CCS1.1 for definitions of each attribute (motivator, coach, mentor, architect, advocate).

3. Lastly, how does the human-centered leader, acting as a connector, focus on developing and maintaining a culture of trust? Describe two ways in which you, as the nurse manager, would use the attributes of the connector to ensure staff members continue to speak up when mistakes happen. Refer to Table CCS1.1 for definitions of each attribute (collaborator, supporter, edgewalker, engineer, and authentic communicator).

TABLE CCS1.1: Human-Centered Leadership in Healthcare: Dimensions, Attributes, and Definitions

Awakener	Cultivates our people → Culture of excellence
Motivator	Establishes a learning culture with high expectations for ongoing learning for self and others
Coach	Provides honest feedback, addresses behaviors inconsistent with learning culture
Mentor	Advises on member accountability for individual growth plans
Architect	Designs structures/processes so innovation can emerge
Advocate	Ensures resources are available for best practice and professional growth
Connector	**Builds our community → Culture of trust**
Collaborator	Unifies others around shared mission and vision
Supporter	Supports, recognizes, and appreciates independent problem-solving and individual contributions at the point of service
Edgewalker	Embraces change/chaos by endorsing experimentation of ideas to generate innovation
Engineer	Ensures people are plugged into processes/structures for emergence of new ideas
Authentic communicator	Builds mutual respect and trust through nurturing intentional connections with others
Upholder	**Recognizes humanity in others → Culture of caring**
Mindful	Focuses attention, awareness, and energy on present
Others-oriented	Supports with respect, kindness, empathy, and empowerment
Emotionally aware	Recognizes and embraces humanity at all levels, self-reflective
Socially and organizationally aware	Leads with an open mind
Personally well and healthy	Practices self-care, self-compassion, self-awareness

Source: Reproduced with permission from Kennedy, K., Leclerc, L., & Campis, S. (2021). *Human-centered leadership in healthcare: Evolution of a revolution.* Morgan James Publishing.

EFFECTIVE MENTORING THROUGH RELATIONAL LEADERSHIP

K. David Bailey and Joseph P. De Santis

INTRODUCTION

Many leadership styles exist, but those with elements that centralize around relationships remain the preferred style by many nurses and healthcare teams. More specifically, evidence suggests that nurses prefer relationship-oriented leaders who practice consistently from the positive leadership perspective (Alilyyani et al., 2018). Nurses also want to have relationships with their leaders and feel valued (Armstrong et al., 2021). Evidence from multiple international studies suggests that leaders who practice from a positive leadership style favorably influence the patient's experience, patient outcomes, and workforce indicators, including RN retention, reduced turnover, and nurse satisfaction (Alilyyani et al., 2018; Northouse, 2019; Oberleitner, 2019; Porter-O'Grady & Malloch, 2018; Saleh et al., 2018; Wong & Cummings, 2009).

The American Organization for Nursing Leadership (2015) established core competencies for nurse executives and leaders, including relational proficiency, creating a trusting environment, and mentorship. These three competencies serve as some of the essential elements for relational leadership practice. Relational leadership implies that a leader's effectiveness is based on the leader's ability to create and maintain productive working relationships with others within an organization. In relational leadership, the context of leadership is wholly encompassed by these relationships developed and maintained between the leader and the leader's followers (Wheatley, 2006). Although relationships between the leader and followers are highly valued (Clarke, 2018), little attention is given to the role of effective mentoring as an essential component of relational leadership. Because the leader–follower relationship is based on the need for the leader to formally or informally mentor followers at some point in the professional relationship, it is essential for leaders who practice relational leadership to understand and appreciate the need for effective mentorship (Goodyear & Goodyear, 2018). Therefore, the purpose of this section of the case study is to describe how effective mentoring in nursing is congruent with relational leadership.

BACKGROUND AND CONTEXT

Mentoring can be defined as "a seasoned (although not always older) mentor and a mentee with specific development goals. They engage in a long-term professional relationship that focuses on the development of the mentee in certain areas" (Disch, 2018, p. 437). Several other terms are also used to describe mentoring in nursing. These include coaching, leading, developing, guiding (Fitzpatrick, 2021), advising, advocating, counseling, role modeling, sponsoring, teaching, and tutoring (Disch, 2018).

It is well-known that effective mentoring in nursing benefits the mentor, the mentee (also referred to in some sources as the protégé [Disch, 2018; Goodyear & Goodyear, 2018]), and the organization. These benefits included higher levels of career satisfaction, increased workplace productivity, a better work–life balance, better clinical outcomes for clients (Disch, 2018), opportunities for growth and professional development, development of trust, and the opportunity to learn how to give and receive constructive feedback (Goodyear & Goodyear, 2018).

The importance of effective mentoring in nursing has been documented in the theoretical and empirical literature. An integrative review by Lin et al. (2018) analyzed commentaries, editorials, and perspective papers from published articles in nursing journals to identify common themes in nursing mentorship. The authors reported 35 themes that included common features of mentoring, characteristics of mentoring relationships, mentor-related factors, organization-related factors, and mentee-related factors. The authors concluded that both the long-term positive and negative effects of mentoring require further investigation.

THE RELATIONSHIP OF RELATIONAL LEADERSHIP AND EFFECTIVE MENTORING

Despite the volume of research and theoretical work on effective mentoring in nursing, little attention has been given to the relationship between relational leadership and effective mentorship in nursing. Despite this lack of theoretical and empirical work on this topic, some components of relational leadership are congruent with effective mentoring. Relational leadership requires inclusion, empowerment, purposefulness, and ethical practices, as well as being process-oriented (Komives et al., 2013). All these components are necessary to ensure that effective mentoring occurs.

To promote effective mentoring, nurse leaders need to consider the components of relational leadership as described by Komives and colleagues (2013). Many followers would welcome the opportunity to be mentored, and all followers who want mentoring should receive it, which makes the process more inclusive (Carter, 2020; Disch, 2018). However, to be effective, the mentoring relationship must have a common purpose and goals (Disch, 2018) to ensure that purposefulness occurs. The mentoring relationship must address logistical planning to structure the mentoring experience in a process-oriented manner (Vitale, 2018). The aforementioned components are included within an ethical framework so that the needs of both the mentor and mentee are handled with respect, acknowledgement, commitment to the mentoring process, and commitment to one another in the mentoring relationship (Milton, 2021). Building purposeful, process-oriented relationships with mentees that promote inclusivity, encourage empowerment, and are ethical would allow nurse leaders to mentor others effectively by using relational leadership approaches.

Consistent with relational leadership, Tjan (2017) developed a unique approach to mentorship. This author focused on how relationships can help mentors perform more effectively. Four components of the effective mentor emerged from this work:

1. The mentor needs to prioritize the relationship with the mentee over the mentoring relationship.

2. The mentor needs to focus more on the mentee's character and less on the mentee's competency.

3. Mentors should use more optimism and less cynicism.

4. Effective mentors value the importance of their relationship with their mentees more than the relationship with the organization.

These components, congruent with relational leadership, could assist the nurse leader and mentor with some easy, basic principles to guide the mentoring relationship.

IDENTIFIED OPPORTUNITY

Nurse leaders manage many responsibilities, including organizational outcomes and performance, patient safety and experience, regulatory requirements, workforce management and stabilization, cultivating healthy and safe work environments, and succession planning. Leadership development and succession planning require a lasting commitment to dedication for others' success through effective mentoring (Disch, 2018). Although the names have been anonymized, this case study illustrates how a relationship-based leader (MP) used effective mentoring strategies to support the growth of a rising leader (JM).

MENTORSHIP OPPORTUNITY

MP, who served as the chief nursing officer (CNO) for a medium-sized tertiary medical center, hired a clinical nurse, JM, as the Magnet® coordinator for the hospital. Although JM held a baccalaureate in nursing and professional clinical certification, JM had no formal leadership experience. JM embraced the coordinator position and exuded an energy that others easily welcomed. Within the first 3 years, JM excelled; however, JM wanted additional job-related challenges. JM completed a master's degree focusing on nursing leadership and earned a second professional certification in nursing leadership. Because of MP and JM's open and trusting mentoring relationship, JM shared that they wanted to pursue a formal nursing leadership position after the organization achieved its subsequent Magnet designation.

IDENTIFYING SOLUTIONS

Knowing the 2-year timeline ahead, MP used the opportunity to explore what type of nursing leadership position JM wanted to pursue. JM shared that they missed the clinical focus where they started as a new graduate 8 years prior; MP asked numerous questions to help broaden JM's thinking and to help establish an acceptable approach. Furthermore, because they worked in an academic health setting, MP provided JM with a list of course offerings available at the business school throughout the 2-year window to prepare JM for a role they hoped to achieve. MP also approved for the nursing administration budget to cover the cost of the courses JM took. Stunned, JM asked why MP would approve the organization to pay for the classes if JM planned to leave the Magnet coordinator role. MP explained that this was an opportunity to invest in JM because they wanted JM to be successful and have the skills needed to obtain the leadership position JM wanted. Without placing expectations on JM, MP added that they hoped JM remained within the organization in a leadership position, but if not, some other organization would gain a great leader.

Over the next 2 years, following the initial conversation, the focus of MP and JM's monthly mentoring meetings shifted to prepare JM for a leadership position. MP offered to help JM refine their resume, and they looked for additional opportunities that would help JM gain different skills internal and external to the organization. MP encouraged JM to become more involved in a professional nursing organization to demonstrate commitment to nursing leadership and shared their own personal experiences of the benefits of professional organization involvement. Already a member of several national and international professional nursing organizations, JM decided to join a committee of one of the organizations. Membership on this committee allowed JM to interface with other colleagues external to the system, where JM learned additional skills. MP identified several leadership conferences and supported JM's registration fees through the nursing administration cost center.

While preparing the organization for the virtual Magnet site visit, JM gained considerable skills at the system level as they worked with several departments that were outside of their home department, which included working with marketing, information technology, and the communications team. JM created an organized plan for a successful virtual site visit by collaborating with colleagues at the system nursing education department and the Magnet program director. The hospital achieved its second Magnet designation. Shortly after the virtual site visit, MP recognized three upcoming leadership changes that may create opportunities for JM, so MP shifted their conversations to additional preparatory work. While the organizational leadership changes were underway, MP wanted to maintain JM's high level of engagement through other learning opportunities.

Along with the system Magnet program director, MP encouraged JM and the Magnet coordinator of the other acute care hospital within the system to collaborate on a manuscript about preparing both hospitals for virtual site visits scheduled to take place several weeks apart to share lessons learned and strategies employed. The system Magnet program director and MP offered to mentor them through the manuscript development process and agreed to coauthor with them. Both of them jumped at the chance for this additional mentoring and learning opportunity. JM took the lead, created the project timeline, corresponded with the editor, and served as the first author of the article that is now in print.

BENEFITS OF MENTORING

Shortly after the article was published, JM requested to work a few clinical days per month to refamiliarize themself with the clinical setting. MP enthusiastically supported JM's request. This experience allowed JM to form new relationships and recognize what additional skills JM may need to develop before applying for a manager position. This experience also allowed JM to identify opportunities and form questions for the clinical team as they prepared for the interview process. MP met with JM frequently to ensure JM knew of the upcoming opportunities and steps they needed to prepare for the interviews. Through a multilevel interview process with the staff, the director, and other organizational leaders, the oncology department selected JM for the clinical nurse manager position. After accepting the leadership position, JM quickly asked if they could continue the mentorship discussions with MP. They continue to meet monthly as MP monitors JM's progress and supports JM in this new role.

KEY POINTS

- Relational leadership focuses on the quality of the relationship between the leader and followers.
- The quality of the mentor–mentee relationship influences effective mentorship.
- Relational leadership strategies provide the framework for leaders to be effective mentors through trusting relationships.
- Effective mentors invest in their mentee and provide experiential learning opportunities for individuals and professional growth.
- Opportunities for further conceptual and empirical work on relationship leadership and mentoring are available.

SUMMARY

Relational leaders can influence positive outcomes across multiple spheres, including patient care and staff retention (Avolio & Gardner, 2005). As illustrated in the presented case study, relational leadership practices combined with effective mentoring strategies can produce enhanced benefits for the mentee and the organization. MP, who served as JM's mentor, mentored JM through multiple growth opportunities during JM's tenure as the Magnet coordinator and helped JM achieve the goal of becoming a clinical nurse manager. However, extant literature specific to relational leadership practice with effective mentoring remains limited.

In order to advance the study of relational leadership and effective mentoring in nursing, a few opportunities for further development are evident. Nurse leaders and researchers can collaborate to develop a consensus definition of effective mentoring in nursing (Disch, 2018; Lin et al., 2018). This definition will help identify the essential components of effective mentoring in nursing and help with incorporating effective mentoring into relational leadership theories and practices.

This collaboration between nurse leaders and researchers to advance the study of effective mentoring in nursing is needed. This includes a rigorous evaluation of existing mentoring programs to identify essential components of effective mentoring (Disch, 2018) that will include larger samples and more complex methodologies to determine the effectiveness of mentoring (Lin et al., 2018). This research can be further extended by examining the relationship between relational leadership and effective mentoring.

Clinical practice (and perhaps academia) needs to re-examine and adjust the prevailing mentoring paradigm of mentoring in nursing. Although relational leadership was not specifically mentioned, McBride et al. (2017) suggested abandoning the 20th-century mentoring paradigm to adopt the 21st-century paradigm that changes how mentoring is viewed and valued by the mentor, mentee, and the professional organization. The use of this 21st-century mentoring paradigm may be the first step in incorporating relational leadership as an essential component of effective mentorship in nursing.

END-OF-CASE RESOURCES

◼ DISCUSSION QUESTIONS

1. Think about a time during your nursing career when you were mentored by another nurse. What were some positive aspects that promoted effective mentoring? What were some negative aspects that inhibited effective mentoring?

2. Think about a time during your nursing career when you mentored another nurse. What strategies did you use to ensure effective mentoring? What were some strategies that could have been used to make the mentoring more effective?

3. As a nurse leader who is responsible for mentoring others, how could you use principles of relational leadership to effectively mentor others?

4. Describe how the 21st century leadership paradigm (McBride et al., 2017) could be incorporated into relational leadership practices.

5. In the case study, identify the individual benefits for JM.

6. From the case study, identify the organizational benefits for investing in JM.

REFERENCES

Alilyyani, B., Wong, C. A., & Cummings, G. (2018). Antecedents, mediators, and outcomes of authentic leadership in healthcare: A systematic review. *International Journal of Nursing Studies, 83,* 34–64. https://doi.org/10.1016/j.ijnurstu.2018.04.001

American Organization for Nursing Leadership. (2015). *Nurse executive competencies.* https://www.aonl.org/sites/default/files/AONL/nec.pdf

Armstrong, L., Spivey, P., & Doran, M. (2021). Contemporary engagement strategies for nurse leaders. *Nurse Leader, 19*(4), 360–365. https://doi.org/10.1016/j.mnl.2021.03.011

Avolio, B. J., & Gardner, W. L. (2005). Authentic leadership development: Getting to the root of positive forms of leadership. *Leadership Quarterly, 16,* 315–338. https://doi.org/10.1016/j.leaqua.2005.03.001

Carter, B. (2020). Achieving diversity, inclusion and equity in the nursing workforce. *Revista Latino-Americana de Enfermagem (RLAE), 28*(2), 1–3. https://doi.org/10.1590/1518-8345.0000-3254

Clarke, N. (2018). *Relational leadership: Theory, practice and development.* Taylor & Francis Group.

Disch, J. (2018). Rethinking mentoring. *Critical Care Medicine, 46*(3), 437–441. https://doi.org/10.1097/CCM.0000000000002914

Fitzpatrick, J. (2021). Narrative nursing: Empowering nurse leaders. *Nursing Administration Quarterly, 45*(4), 324–329. https://doi.org/10.1097/NAQ.0000000000000-486

Goodyear, C., & Goodyear, M. (2018). Supporting successful mentoring. *Nursing Management, 49*(4), 49–53. https://doi.org/10.1097/01.NUMA.0000531173.00718.06

Komives, S. R., Lucas, N., & McMahon, T. R. (2013). *Exploring leadership for college students who want to make a difference* (3rd ed.). John Wiley & Sons.

Lin, J., Chew, Y. R., Toh, Y. P., & Krishna, L. K. R. (2018). Mentoring in nursing: An integrative review of commentaries, editorials, and perspectives papers. *Nurse Educator, 43*(1), E1–E5. https://doi.org/10.1097/NNE.0000000000000389

McBride, A. B., Campbell, J., Woods, N. F., & Manson, S. M. (2017). Building a mentoring network. *Nursing Outlook, 64*(3), 305–314. https://doi.org/10.1016/j.outlook.2016.12.001

Milton, C. L. (2021). Ethical implications for mentoring and the discipline of nursing. *Nursing Science Quarterly, 34*(4), 356–358. https://doi.org/10.1177/08943184211031589

Northouse, P. G. (2019). *Leadership* (8th ed.). Sage.

Oberleitner, M. G. (2019). Theories, models, and frameworks from leadership and management. In M. McEwen & E. M. Wills (Eds.), *Theoretical basis for nursing* (5th ed., pp. 376–408). Wolters Kluwer.

Porter-O'Grady, T., & Malloch, K. (2018). *Quantum leadership: Creating sustainable value in health care* (5th ed.). Jones & Bartlett Learning.

Saleh, U., O'Connor, T., Al-Subhi, H., Alkattan, R., Al-Harbi, S., & Patton, D. (2018). The impact of nurse managers' leadership styles on ward staff. *British Journal of Nursing, 27*(4), 197–203. https://doi.org/10.12968/bjon.2018.27.4.197

Tjan, A. (2017). *Good people: The only leadership decision that really matters.* Penguin Random House.

Vitale, T. R. (2018). Nurse leader mentorship. *Nursing Management, 49*(2), 8–10. https://doi.org/10.1097/01.NUMA.0000529932.9246.ab

Wheatley, M. J. (2006). *Leadership and the new science: Discovering order in a chaotic world* (3rd ed.). Berrett-Koehler Publishing.

Wong, C. A., & Cummings, G. G. (2009). The influence of authentic leadership behaviors on trust and work outcomes of health care staff. *Journal of Leadership Studies, 3*(2), 6–23. https://doi.org/10.1002/jls.20104

TELEHEALTH

Mary Joy Garcia-Dia

INTRODUCTION

For years, healthcare organizations have relied on analytics for syndromic surveillance which enables clinicians to respond in a timely manner and provide information for public health action, especially during an epidemic. Hughes et al. (2020) described syndromic surveillance as a public health intelligence tool that aids in early warning and monitoring of public health impacts. The surveillance process uses symptoms, preliminary diagnosis information, and rapid data collection methods where data sources can vary such as calls from the community of ill individuals, telehealth advice phone lines, primary care clinics, or the EDs. During the Ebola virus outbreak, organizations invested in infection control measures, supplies, education, and training of employees to promote the safety of patients, staff, and the public (Cianelli et al., 2016). The COVID-19 pandemic showcased the integration of syndromic surveillance and telehealth care to triage and address the surge of emergency and inpatient admissions. Healthcare providers and patients who worry about safety and avoid in-person contact due to the veracity and rapid spread of the virus adapted quickly in using virtual visit applications, text messaging, and video calls to communicate with each other. According to Chang et al. (2021), telehealth visits increased by 350% over pre-pandemic figures, accounting for more than nine million Medicare beneficiaries using the service from mid-March to mid-June 2020.

Telehealth refers to the practice of caring for patients remotely when the provider and patient are not physically present with each other. Telehealth uses electronic information and telecommunications technologies to support long distance clinical healthcare and has been in existence for decades (Groom et al., 2021). This expanded value of telehealth increased access to care, especially in rural and remote areas; improved the quality of care for people who may not have the opportunity to see a specialist using advanced technology; and reduced cost by providing the right care at the right time and in the right place (Yesenofski et al., 2015).

The American Telemedicine Association (ATA) provides guidance to clinicians around best practices and approaches for telehealth encounters. Nursing has been a key stakeholder in the research, development, and implementation of telehealth care models that include telephone calls to video visits. According to the American Academy of Ambulatory Care Nursing (AAACN; 2018), "telehealth is an umbrella term used to describe a wide range of services delivered in nontraditional modalities, across distances, by a variety of health-related disciplines" (p. 10). Based on the scope and standards of practice for professional telehealth nursing, RNs play a critical role and are accountable for providing care that follows the relevant federal requirements, state laws and nurse practice acts, regulatory standards, standards of professional ambulatory care nursing practice, other relevant professional standards, and organizational policies. The AAACN describes nurses as those who practice telehealth, promote the patient's optimal well-being, partner with providers and patients in managing acute and chronic disease and disability, coordinate care transitions, and provide end-of-life care and support.

BACKGROUND AND CONTEXT

According to an audit conducted by the United States Government Accountability Office (2017), telehealth and remote monitoring provide alternatives to healthcare that is commonly conducted at a physician's office, particularly for patients who cannot travel easily due to their remote location or disease condition (i.e., disability). The United States Government Accountability Office report defines "telehealth" as clinical services that are provided remotely via telecommunication technologies, whereas remote patient monitoring is a technology to enable monitoring of patients outside conventional clinical settings such as in the home. This may include monitoring patients who are diabetic, congestive heart patients, or cardiac patients' devices (pacemaker or internal defibrillator). The report noted that there are differences between state-to-state federal programs on statutes, regulations, licensing/privilege requirements, and reimbursement for telehealth services. The Centers for Medicare & Medicaid Services (CMS) have waived restrictions on where the telehealth visit needs to transpire (rural health clinic versus home-base or urban areas) to support the merit-based incentive payment system that pays clinicians based on quality and resource use. For example, providers can coordinate care through telehealth or use remote patient monitoring to gather information to determine a patient's proper dose of medication or combine a virtual consult with a near-site visit to a workplace clinic for laboratory testing. The report described how the Veterans Administration (VA) has used asynchronous telehealth (or store-and-forward) and offers telehealth services for mental health, primary care, rehabilitation, chronic care for diabetes, congestive heart failure, chronic obstructive pulmonary disease (COPD), hypertension, and depression, to name a few conditions.

The CMS issued temporary measures for Medicare, Medicaid, and the Children's Health Insurance Program (CHIP) to receive medical care through telehealth services during the COVID-19 public health emergency by expanding the list of covered services such as ED visits, initial nursing facility and discharge visits, home visits, and therapy services. During the pandemic, providers were empowered in good faith to use remote communication technologies such as FaceTime, Facebook, Messenger, Google Hangouts, Zoom, or Skype and avoid using public-facing apps like Facebook Live, Twitch, and TikTok (Health and Human Services, 2021). Patients and consumers utilized the approved social media apps to communicate with their providers and helped in their decision to access emergency care or simply shelter-at-home through virtual consult follow-ups. Anecdotal stories in the media highlighted how nurses in the hospital setting used iPads or their own personal phones to connect patients who are on isolation with their immediate family who are not able to visit, due to restricted guidelines. This minimized the feelings of isolation experienced by many patients and provided reassurance to their family members who worry about the patient's overall condition.

CHALLENGE AND OPPORTUNITY

Prior to the pandemic, healthcare organizations have integrated virtual visits as part of the urgent healthcare model to minimize unnecessary ED visits and reduce costs. Some of the goals and motivation to implement virtual visits identified in the literature are to improve efficiency; utilize resources effectively; reduce waiting times, particularly in emergency and urgent settings; and improve patient satisfaction (Hughes et al., 2020).

The increased number of patients who need isolation rooms and the unprecedented surge of COVID-19 cases compounded the daily operational issues encountered by administrators in dealing with patient throughput and care coordination. Healthcare enterprise systems encountered challenges in facilitating the bed management process (admission, discharges, and transfers) due to the surge of inpatient admissions and the volume of patients requiring ventilators and critical care. Healthcare administrators made quick decisions in expanding infrastructure and converting spaces into patient care areas while setting up flexible spaces (even hallways) for triage and holding areas due to the lack of inpatient beds, as well as to minimize the spread of infection.

The integration of telehealth concepts within the hospital care setting provides a viable solution where clinicians can continue to provide traditional care (assessment, providing treatments, nursing care) and combine virtual approaches to treat and refer patients through video calls with offsite physicians. An audio/video-capable portable monitor on wheels can be set up easily to start remote surveillance for a pod of patients (between 6 and 10 patients) on isolation and monitor them centrally to reduce unnecessary exposure and conserve personal protective equipment (PPE). Within the nurse's station or designated remote location, two to three remote nurses can monitor and telesit 20 to 30 patients, which can alleviate some of the clinical burden on clinical nurses at the telemetry or regular floors. By thinking out of the box, nurse leaders can incorporate virtual care while addressing staffing, bed shortages, and lack of PPE through telehealth.

CASE STUDY: VIRTUAL CARE

ROLE AND SCOPE OF RESPONSIBILITY

As the chief nurse executive (CNE) of a not-for-profit health system in the Midwest, MS oversees six sites that are geographically located in various boroughs.

- Site A: 500-bed Level I trauma center academic and research facility comprised of:
  - university medical school
  - dental school
  - school of allied health with nursing
- Site B: 420-bed Level III trauma regional hospital
- Site C: 150-bed Level III specialty hospital for:
  - cancer treatment
  - research center that also serves as a teaching facility for two universities
- Site D: 250-bed community hospital Level IV trauma center:
  - undergoing extensive renovation to expand to 180 inpatient beds
  - cardiac surgical specialty area
  - cardiac rehab with plans to expand emergency and trauma services
- Site E1: 10 walk-in clinics
- Site E2: Ambulatory surgery center (ASC) with plans to expand to 10 ASC within next 4 years

Over the past 5 years of a 10-year information technology (IT) strategy, the academic medical center and hospitals are undergoing renovation and the six sites have moved either from a hybrid or legacy system to an integrated enterprise platform with the following:

- inpatient and outpatient computerized provider order entry
- pharmacy and laboratory systems
- nursing and allied health electronic clinical documentation
- telehealth and remote monitoring of patients as part of the population health program for cardiovascular and diabetic care

In February of 2020, Sites A, B, and E1 implemented telehealth connecting patients with specialists in the university hospital. When COVID-19 cases started increasing in March 2020, an emergency meeting was called with all key stakeholders across the healthcare system in expanding the telehealth platform. The senior executive team and board of trustees requested to aggressively expand virtual care and remote monitoring to meet the unprecedented number of patients requiring acute and urgent care due to COVID-19. MS needs to reimagine care delivery and be innovative in using technology to support nursing, supplement staffing, and meet the demands of patient care. At the daily operations huddle with senior leadership and IT, the top priority for the hospitals is to maintain safety and prevent the spread of infection. The expansion of telehealth as a temporary option by the CMS to provide access to a vulnerable and underserved community created an opportunity to bring the practice of virtual care within the hospital walls and promote communication between providers and patients across the enterprise system. Senior leadership approved to scale-up telehealth visits and reduce face-to-face visits in the outpatient and urgent care centers (Sites A, B, D, E1/E2) to minimize risks of exposures of employees and non-COVID-19 patients. To provide a high-level guidance and direction, the clinical informatics team drafted a project plan to implement and deploy tele-sitting and remote monitoring in collaboration with IT across the different sites using a big-bang approach.

PROJECT SCOPE

The project scope identifies the sites that have existing telehealth capability (Table CCS3.1). An assessment was performed to determine the amount of hardware (monitor with audio/video capability) that needs to be deployed and the software license that will be added to the existing enterprise license. Additional support services need to be coordinated with the vendor to ensure that additional sites who do not have ports to connect virtually can be hooked to the internet with the necessary security protocols in place. Staff will be trained on how to set-up and use the remote surveillance function and a designated pool of IT volunteers with clinical experience are assigned to facilitate the central monitoring and manage a pod of patients. Go-live support will be provided by the vendor remotely as there are travel restrictions. To fast track the project, an additional resource was included to provide project management oversight. Post-implementation, this resource will transition to connect with patients, family, and the community in setting up access or providing training on how to use the virtual visit application.

TABLE CCS3.1: Project Scope

Description	Site A	Site B	Site C	Site D	Site E 1 & 2
Bed capacity	500	420	150	250	75–100 patients/day
Telehealth-ready	Yes	Yes	No	No	Yes
Hardware to be deployed	75	60	15	25	10
Telehealth software (enterprise license)	Add-on (50 users)	Add-on (50 users)	New	New	Add-on (20 users)
Software maintenance and support services (premiere with telephony)	N/A	N/A	Add port	Add port	N/A
Training/go-live	150	150	75	75	50
Professional services and extended warranty	N/A	N/A	New	New	N/A

PROJECT IMPLEMENTATION

The emergent need to deploy and implement a turn-on key telehealth solution is the guiding principle that will drive the project implementation of the telehealth project. There are risks associated with scope, resources, and timeline that require support from the IT department, technical team, subject matter experts from the clinical team, and the telehealth vendor. Resources are short with the ongoing pandemic and some staff may not be able to go onsite for design sessions and training. A majority of the work design and build will need to be facilitated remotely to keep staff safe. Remote learning and support will be considered depending on the clinical staff's availability to attend a classroom training. Table CCS3.2 outlines the high-level plan and activities that nurse leaders have to take into consideration in implementing the telesitting and remote monitoring project.

TABLE CCS3.2: Project Implementation

Telehealth Service Module	Description
Project management	A project manager (PM) will be assigned to this project once the contract is signed with the vendor. Activities will include workflow design, installation and implementation, end-user training, and go-live services.
Performance assessment services	The telehealth software application performance assessment will be conducted by internal IT to ensure that the network infrastructure can support the software's communications system.
Design workshop	A hands-on demonstration of the telehealth software app will be facilitated to train clinical and IT staff and set expectations for the fast-track implementation.
Workflow design services	A series of workflow design sessions to identify use case scenarios and document each site's clinical call flow. Nursing/providers will identify the clinical roles, groups, communication, escalation, and naming conventions that will be built for the telehealth solution.
System admin training	The vendor will provide system administration knowledge transfer services for up to three staff who will assume the system administrator role. A hands-on review will be provided to help desk staff to support end-users as they resolve connection, communication, and telehealth app issues.
Database development services	The implementation architect/engineer will develop and document the database according to agreed-upon workflow design requirements.
System installation, configuration, and testing services	System configuration of the telehealth app solution will be completed by the IT/clinical informatics team with vendor oversight.
Technical knowledge transfer services	The vendor will conduct 2 days of technical knowledge transfer services for up to 3 "customer" staff to prepare staff to support the technical architecture and configurations of the telehealth solution.
Third-party system alarm and event notification integration services	The PM will coordinate with third-party vendors to design and implement escalation and event notifications for delivery and presentation on the telehealth communication device for caregivers and other hospital staff.

(continued)

TABLE CCS3.2: Project Implementation *(continued)*

Telehealth Service Module	Description
Telehealth training and go-live support services	The vendor will train clinical trainers, designated super users, and end-users—use the train-the-trainer model if applicable; a scenario training will be coordinated with professional staff/clinical educators for simulation and development of policy and procedure.
Post-deployment assessment services	The post-deployment evaluation includes remote review of reports, on-site clinical walk-throughs, and clinical interviews to ensure end-user satisfaction with the solution. This will be conducted between 3 and 6 months post-go-live.

CLINICAL CONSIDERATIONS—REMOTE MONITORING

The care of COVID-19 negative patients with comorbidities and chronic conditions will need to be prioritized in Sites A, B, and D. Similar to the emergency triage process, the telehealth team will require a triage and escalation procedure to quickly assess patients, refer them to the appropriate specialty, provide treatment and education, or escalate patients with an urgent/emergent condition to a higher level of treatment. Depending on the severity of illness, aside from COVID-19, patients with arrhythmias or stroke and labor patients who are admitted in the ED are a priority. Due to limited beds in the telemetry and critical care units, the nursing informatics director proposed adopting the use of remote monitoring technology and utilizing this within the inpatient environment. The monitor screens with telehealth app that has video/audio capability can be distributed to patients who are in isolation or those who require close monitoring. This allowed clinical staff or IT clinical resources to monitor 10 patients in a centralized pod and helped alleviate the staffing shortage. By generating a dashboard report, COVID-19 patients who meet the criteria for discharge will be fast-tracked. Once discharged, a report is generated to add these patients to the list of remote COVID-19 follow-ups. These patients, based on COVID-19 discharge protocol, are monitored on the first, third, and fifth day post-discharge for any respiratory deterioration or abnormal vital signs. If the patient's condition worsens, the patient is referred remotely to a provider who will perform a virtual visit and determine if the escalation meets the criteria for emergency re-admission.

Sites E1 and E2 (clinic and ambulatory setting) stretched their capacity in providing COVID-19 testing and doing telephone call triage for individuals with symptoms who may not necessarily require hospitalization but still merit close monitoring. By deploying the telehealth monitors, staff connected virtually with emergency physicians and pulmonary specialists who then performed rapid assessment, treatment, and referral. For Site C (cancer and research center), offsite referrals and follow-up via virtual visits minimized the risk of immunocompromised patients for unnecessary exposure to the SARS CoV-2 virus. This also allowed oncology providers and other specialty providers to lessen their travel between sites and continue to provide care via telecommuting.

KEY POINTS

- Healthcare systems recognized the benefits of implementing virtual healthcare to improve patient engagement and lower cost.
- There was an urgent need to expand telehealth and remote monitoring to mitigate risks in spreading infection, promote safety, and deploy telehealth services effectively during the pandemic crisis.
- The lack of PPEs, nursing shortage, and mental exhaustion reported by clinicians create a challenge and an opportunity for healthcare systems to consider different models of staffing and care delivery.

SUMMARY

Overseeing an enterprise-wide healthcare system created tremendous responsibility and pressure on nurse leaders during the height of the COVID-19 pandemic and provided an opportunity to adopt telehealth technologies in providing care and treatment (Varma et al., 2020). The telehealth team shared that around 59% of all U.S. adults (including the older adult population) owns a portable device and there has been an increase in how patients use their health portal or go to the internet to look for medical information. By using existing algorithms to monitor and track patients daily, patients who can be remotely monitored at home alleviated the congestion in critical care and telemetry units and minimized the spread of infection to vulnerable patients.

There is an increased urgency to implement virtual care to minimize the barriers in accessing healthcare as a result of the impact of the pandemic, specifically restricted travel and quarantines. CMS regulations expanded the use and reimbursement of telehealth benefitting underserved populations, especially the older adult population. Telehealth methods have shown potential promise in improving healthcare delivery services, but their uptake has not been widespread as research studies continue to explore barriers and challenges associated with individual, organizational, cultural, ethical, and legal implications (Collier et al., 2016).

The implementation of a telehealth project requires interprofessional collaboration with diverse stakeholders, including clinical partners, electronic medical record (EMR) vendors, software programmers, network engineers, database administrators, and telecommunication specialists. These stakeholders need to look at complex and meaningful workflow processes that consider the patient and caregiver needs, usability and functionality of the application, systems and regulatory requirements, and organizational policy. Nurse leaders must be agile and flexible in crisis situations. Telehealth holds promise in reimagining how nursing can adopt its concepts and incorporate virtual care within the healthcare delivery and community settings.

END-OF-CASE RESOURCES

◼ DISCUSSION QUESTION

1. Analyze the telehealth project implementation scenario provided and form a team with various roles on Sites A to E. As the chief nursing informatics officer, (1) discuss with the team risks with the telehealth project, (2) highlight pros and cons, and (3) describe resources (financial and human) that are needed to meet the overarching goal to implement the project at the height of the pandemic.

◼ ADDITIONAL RESOURCES

The North American Nursing Diagnosis Association/International (NANDA; https:// nanda.org), the AAACN (www.aaacn.org), and the Nursing Special Interest Group of the American Telemedicine Association (ATA; www.americantelemed.org) are leaders of telehealth efforts in the United States. The International Council of Nurses (ICN; www.icn.ch) and the Nursing Special Interest Group of the International Society for Telemedicine and eHealth (ISfTeH; www.isfteh.org) lead worldwide efforts in standardizing nursing practice and supporting eHealth programs. Some articles and presentations on telehealth and remote monitoring are provided:

- ◼ Broderick, A. (2011). *Remote patient monitoring* [PowerPoint slides]. http://www .ehcca.com/presentations/readsummit3/broderick_ms1.pdf
- ◼ Philips. (n.d.). *Enterprise telehealth.* https://www.usa.philips.com/healthcare/ solutions/enterprise-telehealth

- Robert Wood Johnson Foundation. (n.d.). *Project Echo: Moving knowledge not people.* https://www.rwjf.org/en/how-we-work/grants-explorer/featured-programs/project-echo.html
- National Institutes of Health Office of Disease Prevention. (2021, November 15). *Pathways to Prevention Workshop: Improving rural health through telehealth-guided provider-to-provider communication* [Video]. YouTube. https://www.youtube.com/watch?v=BCic2p6y3aw

---

 A robust set of instructor resources designed to supplement this text is located at http://connect.springerpub.com/content/book/978-0-8261-7795-7. Qualifying instructors may request access by emailing textbook@springerpub.com.

REFERENCES

American Academy of Ambulatory Care Nursing. (2018). *Scope and standards of practice for professional telehealth nursing.* Author.

Chang, J. E., Lai, A. Y., Gupta, A., Nguyen, A. M., Berry, C. A., & Shelley, D. R. (2021). Rapid transition to telehealth and the digital divide: Implications for primary care access and equity in a post-COVID era. *The Milbank Quarterly, 99*(2), 340–368. https://doi.org/10.1111/1468-0009.12509

Cianelli, R., Clipper, B., Freeman, R., Goldstein, J., & Wyatt, T. H. (2016). *The innovation road map: A guide for nurse leaders.* https://www.nursingworld.org/globalassets/ana/innovations-roadmap-english.pdf

Collier, A., Morgan, D. D., Swetenham, K., To, T., Currow, D. C., & Tieman, J. J. (2016). Implementation of a pilot telehealth programme in community palliative care: A qualitative study of clinicians' perspectives. *Palliative Medicine, 30*(4), 409–417. https://doi.org/10.1177/0269216315600113

Groom, L. L., Brody, A. A., & Squires, A. P. (2021). Defining telepresence as experienced in telehealth encounters: A dimensional analysis. *Journal of Nursing Scholarship: An Official Publication of Sigma Theta Tau International Honor Society of Nursing, 53*(6), 709–717. https://doi.org/10.1111/jnu.12684

Health and Human Services. (2021). *Notification of enforcement discretion for telehealth remote communications during the COVID-19 nationwide public health emergency.* https://www.hhs.gov/hipaa/for-professionals/special-topics/emergency-preparedness/notification-enforcement-discretion-telehealth/index.html

Hughes, H. E., Edeghere, O., O'Brien, S. J., Vivancos, R., & Elliot, A. J. (2020). Emergency department syndromic surveillance systems: A systematic review. *BMC Public Health, 20*(1), 1891. https://doi.org/10.1186/s12889-020-09949-y

United States Government Accountability Office. (2017). *Report to congressional committees: Telehealth and remotes patient monitoring use in Medicare and selected federal programs.* GAO-17-365. https://www.gao.gov/assets/gao-17-365.pdf

Varma, N., Marrouche, N. F., Aguinaga, L., Albert, C. M., Arbelo, E., Choi, J., Chung, M. K., Conte, G., Dagher, L., Epstein, L. M., Ghanbari, H., Han, J. K., Heidbuchel, H., Huang, H., Lakkireddy, D. R., Ngarmukos, T., Russo, A. M., Saad, E. B., Saenz Morales, L. C., . . . Varosy, P. D. (2020). HRS/EHRA/APHRS/LAHRS/ACC/AHA worldwide practice update for telehealth and arrhythmia monitoring during and after a pandemic. *Journal of the American College of Cardiology, 76*(11), 1363–1374. https://doi.org/10.1016/j.jacc.2020.06.019

World Health Organization. (1998). *A health telematics policy in support of WHO's Health-For-All strategy for global health development: Report of the WHO Group Consultation on Health Telematics, 11–16 December, Geneva, 1997.* Author.

Yesenofski, L., Kromer, S., & Hitchings, K. (2015). Nurses leading the transformation of patient care through telehealth. *Journal of Nursing Administration, 45*(12), 650–656. https://doi.org/10.1097/NNA.0000000000000279

NURSE-LED INNOVATION TO REDUCE OCCUPATIONAL HEAT STRESS OF OPERATING ROOM PERSONNEL

Jill Byrne

INTRODUCTION

Nurses provide care, support, and interventions when advocating for individuals who suffer from pain and discomfort. Nurses are well-known for being creative and innovative throughout the advocating process to mitigate disparities, promote equality, and preserve human dignity. For example, a nurse (the author) advocated for surgical personnel who wear layers of personal protective equipment (PPE) by creating a cooling vest intervention to reduce thermal discomfort, fatigue, and dehydration the staff experienced. Advocating for patients is a gold standard in nursing; however, advocating for the occupational health and well-being of healthcare personnel takes courage, dedication, and internal and external support from institutional leaders.

Equally important to advocating and implementing a healthcare innovation is its adoption and sustainability in practice. Rogers's Diffusion of Innovation Theory is a widely used theoretical framework that recommends an innovation must be communicated over time among members of a social system (public, professional, and organizational) and adopted by stakeholders to be sustainable (Rogers, 2003). According to Rogers, there are five components (relative advantage, compatibility, complexity, trialability, and observability) necessary to determine if diffusion and adoption of an innovation will occur (Rogers, 2003). Rogers's Diffusion of Innovation Theory is used to describe the progression of nurse-led innovation in this case scenario.

BACKGROUND AND CONTEXT

RELATIVE ADVANTAGE

Initially, there was no strategic plan to implement the cooling vest; it was spontaneously developed to address an urgent issue of discomfort and incivility affecting surgical personnel experiencing heat stress under layers of PPE while performing surgery. Rogers defines the "relative advantage" of an innovation as the degree to which an innovation is perceived as better than the idea it supersedes (Rogers, 2003). Clinicians' satisfaction with the disposable cooling vest offers freedom of movement over the expensive tethered electric cooling units that are seldom used or available. The disposable cooling vest is a simple solution to thermal discomfort that is available for the entire surgical team, unlike the expensive reusable electric tethered units that are available for physician use only. The tubing in electric cooling units leak, leave puddles of cold water on the floor, and require regular safety cultures for bacterial growth from water remaining in the unit.

COMPATIBILITY

Rogers defines "compatibility" as the degree to which an innovation is perceived as being compatible with the needs of those adopting the innovation.

Increased body temperatures and sweating lead to discomfort, a lack of concentration, and an increased potential to develop heat-related illnesses from fatigue and dehydration. Once the cooling vest was introduced to the surgical staff, complacency to accept thermal discomfort as part of the job expectations was no longer necessary. On occasion, some surgical personnel sweat enough to drip onto the sterile surgical field or actually into the surgical incision. Surgical personnel that sweat excessively wrap their foreheads in gauze rolls to absorb the sweat while operating; however, the weight of the wet gauze often shifts downward, blocking vision. The cooling vest is effective to reduce sweat production and gauze-wrapped foreheads are no longer necessary.

COMPLEXITY

Complexity is a measure of the degree to which an innovation is perceived as difficult to understand and use. An innovation is more likely to be adopted if it is simple and well defined (Rogers, 2003).

For any person bothered by heat stress while wearing PPE, the cooling vest is lightweight, simple to use, and has a simple design with strategically positioned ice packs. Surgical staff members readily adopted the simplicity of the cooling vest; however, as simple as the innovation is, there are individuals who don't understand the need for a cooling vest in the operating room (OR). The president of the hospital, who was also a surgeon, stopped me in the hall and said, "I heard about the cooling vest you created. When do you put it on the patient?" I explained, "The cooling vest is worn by the staff over scrubs and under the sterile gown; after all, we are humans too!"

TRIALABILITY

Trialability is defined as the degree to which the innovation may be trialed and modified (Rogers, 2003).

During the first 5 years, iterations made to the cooling vest were based on feedback from the OR personnel who readily wore the cooling vest. Additionally, several reusable ice-pack products were trialed over the years to find a lightweight and flexible pack that added to the wearability and adoption of the cooling vest.

A surgical cooling vest product trial was conducted to measure the stakeholder's positive and negative preferences for use. Participants included surgeons, physician assistants, nurses, and surgical techs who operate in adult, pediatric, and newborn surgeries. The participants had a significantly positive response to the use, design, and perceived comfort of the cooling vest. The results of the product trial provided evidence for the manufacturing company to adopt the innovation and eventually establish a license agreement with the hospital system for use and production of the cooling vest.

OBSERVABILITY

Observability is ironically the degree to which the results of the innovation are visible to others (Rogers, 2003). As intuitive as the benefit of comfort was to OR staff, it was often difficult for individuals who weren't familiar with wearing PPE to understand. However, the visibility of a new innovation stimulates peer discussions among potential stakeholders. Resident rotations and visitors to the OR were able to observe the benefits the cooling vest provided for the staff, which increased requests for the cooling vests. Nonetheless, I was a one-person manufacturing system; sewing the cooling vests became time consuming, and managing the workload was extremely stressful. My dedicated efforts to sustain the availability of the cooling vest were fueled by seeing the improved comfort and well-being of individuals who were physically and mentally suffering from heat stress.

CHALLENGE AND OPPORTUNITY

ADOPTION AND SUSTAINABILITY

The early adoption of the cooling vest by OR personnel led to its sustainability during the first 5 years. In fact, staff members refused to operate if cooling vests were not available. Rogers explains that early majority adopters of an innovation make up about half of the social system's stakeholders (Rogers, 2003). I knew it was my ethical responsibility as a nurse leader to educate the remaining half of stakeholders, late adopters of the social system, to sustain the continued use and future manufacturing of the cooling vest.

Organizational barriers (lack of knowledge and cost issues) hindered the adoption of the cooling vest innovation for hospital administrators unfamiliar with the benefits the cooling vest provided for staff who were impacted by heat stress. Without previous evidence-based research of surgical personnel exposed to occupational heat stress while performing real-time surgical procedures, I had little chance of gaining adoption of the cooling system by these stakeholders, simply based on my observations. Instead, I utilized Selye's stress theory to describe the basic physiological and psychological reaction pattern associated with occupational heat stress based on the General Adaptation Syndrome (GAS; Selye, 1950). I educated administrators from the hospital system and corporate executives from a major healthcare manufacturing company about the GAS, a three-phase reaction pattern to heat stress. The "alarm reaction" describes the initial response to wearing PPE: increased vasoconstriction, which triggers peripheral blood flow to produce sweat to naturally cool the body. However, evaporation of sweat is blocked under the impervious layers of PPE, preventing any cooling from occurring. As the surgical personnel attempt to adapt to the thermally stressful event, the body's physiological responses are triggered to protect major organ function. Glucose is routed to the brain to improve cognitive functioning during the "stage of resistance." Eventually, prolonged exposure to stressful situations, like surgical procedures lasting several hours, causes individuals' heart rate, skin, and core body temperature to increase, which Selye describes as the "stage of exhaustion." Given the predictability of the GAS, the reaction pattern supports the hypothesis that heat stress may lead to fatigue and exhaustion of surgical personnel and secondarily may impact the safe care of patients. The theoretical perspective provided a clear explanation of the impact heat stress may have on surgical personnel. The late adopters, administrators, and manufacturing executives agreed to conduct a product trial to measure the surgical personnel's receptiveness to the cooling intervention.

Dedicated to advocating for OR personnel, I became accustomed to challenging events and conversations to close the knowledge gaps with administrators regarding the use of the cooling system. On one occasion, I met with a hospital system's materials management team, thinking, "Instead of feeling defeated by the usual statements of rejection from individuals who have never stepped foot into an OR, I developed an alternative plan." The members of the materials management team make important budget decisions about supplies that surgical teams use in the OR. "I learned from previous meetings that I must bring the business and corporate leaders into my world through imagery, provide a sensory experience, so I packed a duffle bag with the necessary supplies."

As the materials management team began the meeting with opening remarks, I targeted my volunteer opportunity: the woman who remarked, "I just don't understand why a cooling intervention is necessary because ORs are known for being cold." The woman agreed to participate in the sensory experience, and I dressed her in a 7-pound lead apron and full PPE (bouffant hat, mask, goggles, face shield, surgical gown, shoe covers, gloves). Fortunately for her, the ambient temperature of the meeting room was comfortable at 68°F. Standing next to the woman, I intentionally took my time describing the OR environment. Utilizing pantomimed actions, I depicted the size and average 35-pound weight of cumbersome instrument trays that are repetitively lifted on and off the instrument tables. I explained that I, as a circulating nurse, wore the lead apron and similar layers of PPE the day prior for an extensive emergency trauma surgery that lasted over 8 hours and the COVID status of the patient was unknown, so full PPE was required. Throughout the trauma case, I walked—and, when necessary, ran—to gather supplies and equipment. I showed the meeting attendees the app on my phone that records my digital wrist pedometer, and at the end of the shift I had 16,000+ steps recorded. I described the feeling of dehydration due to sweat, fatigue, and exertion. I explained the sense of embarrassment that surgical personnel experience in the OR suit to maintain their personal dignity while doffing the PPE without exposing their body-revealing drenched scrub clothing. Additionally, surgical personnel are often in a pinch for time between surgeries, and changing scrubs and freshening up is difficult.

Throughout my presentation, I occasionally glanced at the woman volunteer who was awkwardly fidgeting with the weight of the PPE, and I could see the glow of sweat developing on her brow as I spoke. I eventually turned my attention to her and asked, "Would you wear this ensemble and walk 8 miles without stopping or taking a drink of water?" She casually uttered, "It's great for weight loss." I answered, "I go to the gym for exercise, and I wear PPE to save lives." By the end of the meeting, the materials management team acknowledged that they would try to budget funds for OR personnel who would benefit from a cooling intervention. I ended the meeting with, "Now, let's talk about an endless supply of juice boxes!"

THE ROLE OF THE NURSE–INTRAPRENEUR

Nurse leaders are positioned in their roles to translate and support the vision and mission of an organization to the teams they oversee. However, they may not be the individuals equipped to create an innovation and/or the strategies to bring the idea forward, or even visualize the benefits of a particular innovation that is brought to their attention; that is what intrapreneurs are known for. Intrapreneurs create the innovation, strategies, and process to move the vision forward within the organization, which requires support from organizational leaders. Foley (2016) identified three types of intrapreneurs that fuel innovation. Behavioral assessment tools can identify the "creators" who establish the innovative idea, the "doers" who are task-oriented, and the "implementers" who are known to bring the ideas to closure. Although rare, it is possible for one person to possess all three intrapreneurial characteristics. Individuals who have the complete set of intrapreneurial behaviors and competencies are among the most effective and successful intrapreneurs (Foley, 2016).

Intrapreneurs are typically described as not having financial risks within a company; however, I was only paid for the hours I worked as a staff nurse in the OR. I was not paid by the company for the countless hours to develop the cooling system. The financial sacrifices spread over a decade and included travel and hotel expenses; out-of-pocket expenses for equipment and supplies to sew approximately 500 cooling vests over 7 years; hours preparing presentations; using vacation time to cover time away from work to attend meetings, presentations, and conferences that provided opportunities to network and bridge the gaps between academic, healthcare system, and corporate partnerships; and school loans which will last through the next decade.

PERSEVERANCE AND TENACITY

What does the perseverance and tenacity of a nurse–intrapreneur look like over a decade?

The descriptions of the concepts began with literature reviews and conversations with nurse leaders in academia to confirm my observations and substantiate the need for occupational heat stress research; enrolling in a doctoral nursing program; endless discussion with institutional leaders, academic leaders, and executives from a corporate healthcare services company; participating in interviews (video, virtual, and print), podcasts and webinars, and presentations at local, national, and international conferences; securing a U.S. patent and an Investigator-Initiated Research Study grant to fund the heat stress research to support the efficacy of the cooling system; all performed without losing sight of my personal mission and goal—"to improve the health and well-being of individuals exposed to occupational heat stress, fatigue, and exertion."

LEADERSHIP CHARACTERISTICS

Leadership issues that interrupt the progression of innovation: Are leaders able to lead with humility? Can they identify leaders with effective empathetic characteristics who are comfortable supporting a staff member's idea without formally or informally presenting the idea, product, or process as their own innovation? Transparent and empathetic characteristics of nurse leaders are imperative to keep intrapreneurs engaged to move ideas, processes, or products forward. Perhaps, if leaders represent the mission and vision of the healthcare system and sign agreements to remove themselves from the temptations of unlawful authorship and potential innovation royalties, effective empathetic leaders may prevail. Several nurse–intrapreneurs have shared stories with me over the years regarding how they stepped back from or were eliminated from developing an idea when the nurse leaders presented the idea as their own and failed to give credit to the nurse–intrapreneurs.

As a nurse–intrapreneur, I was able to connect resources to establish relationships, improve communication, and build trust between academic, corporate, and healthcare organizations. In order to bridge the gaps, interconnectivity was necessary. I became familiar with nondisclosure agreements (NDAs), conflict of interest (COI) requirements, internal review board (IRB) processes, and data use agreements (DUA), as well as met with legal and business teams to provide clinical insight as contractual agreements were being drafted.

KEY POINTS

- Utilization of theoretical frameworks builds new knowledge to support the adoption and sustainability of an innovation.
- Consider the importance and benefits of interconnected partnerships to develop new innovations and advance healthcare.
- Transparent and empathetic characteristics of nurse leaders are imperative to keep intrapreneurs engaged to move ideas, processes, or products forward.

SUMMARY

The use and adoption of the cooling vest intervention by OR personnel provides important information about mitigating occupational heat stress, a well-known problem occurring around the world in ORs and healthcare units where PPE is required. Advocating for change to improve the comfort and well-being of surgical personnel embodies where the real innovation exists. Nurse leaders in healthcare can cultivate and support intrapreneurs to bridge the organizational gaps to maximize nurse-led innovation.

END-OF-CASE RESOURCES

⬡ DISCUSSION QUESTIONS

1. Consider a nurse-led innovation that appeared to be adequately intuitive or optimal to improve a process or patient care, although it lacked sustainability. Which of the tenets from Rogers's Diffusion of Innovation Theory could be considered to address the issue of sustainability?

2. When assessing characteristics of successful nurse leaders, what characteristics are imperative to cultivate and engage intrapreneurs?

3. Knowing that interconnected partnerships lend themselves to successful innovation, who should nurse leaders include on the innovation team and what benefits would the collaboration offer to the success of the innovation?

 SPRINGER PUBLISHING **CONNECT™** A robust set of instructor resources designed to supplement this text is located at http://connect.springerpub.com/content/book/978-0-8261-7795-7. Qualifying instructors may request access by emailing textbook@springerpub.com.

REFERENCES

Foley, S. (2016). *3 types of intrapreneurs*. Corporate Entrepreneurs. https://corporate-entrepreneurs.com/2016/3-types-of-intrapreneurs

Rogers, E. M. (2003). *Diffusion of innovations* (5th ed.). The Free Press: A Division of Simon & Schuster.

Selye, H. (1950). Stress and the General Adaptation Syndrome. *British Medical Journal, 1*(4667), 1383–1392. https://doi.org/10.1136/bmj.1.4667.1383

LEADERSHIP TO DRIVE QUALITY THROUGH DIRECT-CARE NURSE FEEDBACK USING AN ELECTRONIC HEALTH RECORD DASHBOARD

Anne Pohnert and Mary A. Dolansky

INTRODUCTION

Improving quality by implementing evidence-based practice (EBP) into direct-care nursing practice, at face value, seems relatively straightforward. As Nike says in their ads "Just do it!" It seems simple to describe the innovation, communicate it, train the staff, and implement it; however, effectively implementing, scaling, and sustaining EBP or any quality or safety initiative over the long term is not so easy. It takes leadership and governance—influencing staff, vision, strategic planning of structures, and process accountability.

BACKGROUND AND CONTEXT

In 2018, the Institute for Healthcare Improvement (IHI) introduced "Age-Friendly Health Systems" and the "4Ms Framework" with an aim to spread this evidence-based approach to caring for older adults to over 1,000 hospitals and ambulatory care practices by the end of 2020. IHI brought together an expert panel of geriatric specialists, physicians, nurses, social workers, pharmacists, and others from various healthcare settings who identified over 90 EBP approaches to caring for older adults. Over a series of workshops, these care approaches were distilled into the 4Ms: What Matters Most (referencing patient priorities of care), Medication (minimizing risks of medications for older adults in line with the American Geriatric Society [AGS] Beer's Criteria List), Mentation (assessing and treating depression, dementia, and delirium), and Mobility (helping older adults stay active as long as they are able). All of the 4Ms are meant to "do no harm" and to work together synergistically as each of the "Ms" interact with the others to produce overall improvements in care.

The leadership team valued the Age-Friendly 4Ms as it provided a patient-centered approach and enhanced safety and dimensions of quality. The value of age-friendly care was consistent with other quality initiatives in the organization including enhanced services related to chronic disease management. The strategic vision and plan unfolded to have all APRNs and RNs who were caring for patients 65 and older in the organization implement assessing and acting on the 4Ms into each clinic visit to improve patient outcomes. To address the opportunity of implementing the EBP and improving quality and ensuring safety, the director of clinical quality and a leadership team planned the implementation of the 4Ms in a large ambulatory care practice.

From a leadership standpoint, designing an approach to implement the 4Ms required a quality culture that embraced principles of a learning organization and a growth mindset.

One key strategy proposed was to implement a long-term feedback mechanism, which would give direct-care nurses a report of how well they are doing in implementing the 4Ms. It was decided that a dashboard of 4Ms quality indicators within an electronic health record (EHR) would be developed. The dashboard would provide each nurse with their performance data that would allow them to innovate and improve their performance.

CHALLENGE AND OPPORTUNITY

In order to develop a dashboard, the quality director and leadership team created a plan that answered the following questions: How will the 4Ms be defined within the clinical workflow at a particular healthcare setting? Once defined, how will the 4Ms be documented in the record? How can the 4Ms Framework EHR elements be made reportable (as reportable elements in an EHR are required in order to build an electronic report or dashboard)? What exactly does the leadership team want to drive in terms of performance?

The nurse leadership team sought input from the nurses who were documenting the care in order to determine how to best integrate the 4Ms into care for patients 65 and older in the ambulatory setting and what approaches to the documentation of the 4Ms would be best. Conducting several early observations of visits where they had the nurse implement the 4Ms and multiple tests of small changes was a critical process to design an effective approach to adding the EBP into the clinical workflow and to documenting it effectively.

After working with the nurses and determining the definitions, the clinical workflow, and the documentation approach, the leadership team set up several meetings to design and build the documentation system. This was a complex project to integrate the documentation into an existing EHR in an appropriate place, to make each element of the documentation reportable, to test the assumptions about how it would work, and to test the final product before introducing it to the nurses.

The process involved an official request to the department of data analytics to engage an EHR designer to support the build of the documentation workflow. Each step of the way, the nurse leadership team requested feedback from the frontline nurses, challenged the approach to ensure it would work as desired, and considered the implications of the design in terms of impact to the visit time, the clinical workflow, the nurse–patient interaction, and the functionality of the future reports.

At the same time the documentation workflow was developed, the nurse leader was thinking ahead to the quality dashboard implications and the need to produce reportable elements and configure them in a way so that all staff would clearly understand the dashboard elements related to the 4Ms. This included how the data would appear and which elements would be included, such as how many or what percentage of eligible visits with patients 65 and older included one or more of the 4Ms or all 4Ms together each month. Small pilot tests were done with nurses with considerable feedback that led to the need to change some critical components. Once developed and prior to launch, the nurse leaders took the time to share the documentation workflow and dashboards with a small group of nurse managers and direct-care nurses to complete a user test and get feedback on final changes to be completed.

After launching the entire 4Ms EBP framework, with the aim of implementing the 4Ms into eligible visits, part of the communication strategy was for nurse managers to cascade the use of the dashboard to each direct-care nurse so they would understand how each month they could monitor their progress and test improvements of their EBP implementation. In addition to the dashboard, a performance metric was put in place as a structural strategy to drive the change.

KEY POINTS

- Leaders establish the vision for quality improvement and drive the quality culture within an organization.

- Transformational leaders understand how to communicate data in a way that inspires performance and engages the nursing team to improve their own practice.

- Leaders who understand principles of complexity leadership, such as repetitive cycles of testing and experimentation, effectively enable and inspire staff to engage in rapid and continuous change.

- Quality improvement requires measurement of data points for analysis of progress toward the goals of a quality improvement implementation project. A dashboard that demonstrates how a direct-care nurse is improving their own practice can be an effective tool to drive performance.

SUMMARY

A large APRN convenient care practice was seeing an increase in the older adult population in various clinics. Senior leadership identified a gap in EBP frameworks for quality and safe care of older adults. The leaders had cultivated a vision for quality by recognizing nurses for quality patient care, being committed to professional development and training, measuring quality performance, and by structuring quality into practice through the use of clinical guidelines embedded in clinical workflows and in EHR documentation. The leaders launched a new evidence-based care framework for the care of older adults, the IHI 4Ms Framework of assessing and acting on What Matters Most, Medication, Mentation, and Mobility. This framework required an understanding of implementation science and complexity leadership. An important step of the implementation process was to define how to provide 4Ms care and then how to document the care. The leaders used rapid cycle tests of change and "Plan-Do-Study-Act" (PDSA) experiments with direct-care nurses in real patient visits. These tests of change in definition and documentation laid the groundwork for measuring quality care and quality improvement. Identifying data points that measured progress toward improvement eventually led to the development of national level reports and individual provider dashboards. These reports and dashboards were a key process step for driving quality improvement and implementation. Using principles of transformational leadership, the leaders understood how to effectively communicate data to inspire performance in a learning culture which is dedicated to quality care. This created a cycle of feedback and improvement that drove quality care of the individual older patient.

END-OF-CASE RESOURCES

◼ DISCUSSION QUESTIONS

1. High reliability is not just important for safety initiatives. It also has a role in quality initiatives as well. What components of high reliability are evident in the case study?

2. How did psychological safety principles support the quality initiative that targeted the implementation of evidence into practice?

3. Pick one of the methods to foster continuous learning suggested in Chapter 15, "Quality and Safety" (e.g., growth mindset, design principles, and agile approach) and describe what the method consists of and how this method could be integrated into the case study.

4. Transformational leadership is an essential leadership style to foster quality and safety. What transformational leadership characteristics can be added to improve performance?

5. Complexity leadership strategies have emerged with the challenges of the COVID-19 pandemic. What have we learned about these leadership strategies that can assist leaders in quality initiatives to enhance the implementation of EBP?

6. Reflecting back to the innovation of the EHR and the use of design-thinking, what are the steps to take as a leader and who are the stakeholders to engage in the process?

 A robust set of instructor resources designed to supplement this text is located at http://connect.springerpub.com/content/book/978-0-8261-7795-7. Qualifying instructors may request access by emailing textbook@springerpub.com.

RESILIENCY

Deirdre O'Flaherty and Mary Joy Garcia-Dia

INTRODUCTION

Nurses and other healthcare clinicians have suffered from alarming rates of burnout, depression, stress, and compassion fatigue, which have been the focus of studies by researchers for many years (Aliem & Hashish, 2021). Nurses bear witness to the best and worst situations and do their best to ease the burden on a daily basis. The accumulation of life experience, personality traits, and protective factors precipitate resilience to surface from within. The cumulative effect of responding to tragic and often untimely events could vary depending on one's exposure to clinical experiences. The dynamic nature of nurses' response to life and death situations, the possession of hope characterized by self-efficacy and coping, is often described as resilience (Garcia-Dia et al., 2013). It is known as the ability to bounce back after adversity, to be able to cope and strive. Yet, the process of bouncing back and constant exposure to stresses can put a strain on one's emotional, physical, and mental capacity over time (Foster, Cuzzillo, et al., 2018; Foster, Roche, et al., 2018). The unprecedented emotional toll, extreme workloads, and moral distress suffered by healthcare workers during the COVID-19 pandemic amplified worker burnout, making this a public health concern. It is critical for nurse leaders to promote resiliency measures that can support nurses' psychological safety in mitigating risks impacting patient safety and staff retention.

Research on the concept of resilience has evaluated that it is a dynamic process where heredity and environmental factors are mediated by mindfulness and coping; in other words, controlled exposure to risk rather than avoidance (Bonanno, 2004; Rutter, 2006). Although the phenomenon has been studied by many disciplines, it is only within recent years that resilience in nursing has been studied. Gillespie et al. (2007) and Reyes et al. (2015) advocate that resilience theory should be included in the curriculum for nursing education and orientation programs. According to Masten (2014), resilience is a dynamic, positive adaptation process toward adversity, and it involves the capacity of an individual or system to adapt successfully to disturbances that threaten system function, viability, and development. Nurse leaders have a major influence and responsibility in providing a workplace environment that promotes individual nurses' organizational resilience and engagement.

According to Rangachari and Woods (2020), organizational resilience has three essential elements: foresight, coping, and recovery. It is also known to have three interconnected levels: individual, team, and organizational levels. A resilient organization supports these essential elements across the three levels, using them to promote safety, anticipate failures, and adapt to circumstances of failure through lessons learned. At the same time, the organization restores safe conditions after failure ensues. Organizational resilience arises from systems in the form of communication structures developed by leaders that allow learning from foresight, coping, and recovery strategies of individual workers.

A review of literature shows the critical importance of a workplace environment that implements resilience training strategies to reduce burnout, increase staff retention, and improve patient safety (Rangachari & Woods, 2020). The success of this resilience training program requires supporting both nurse leaders and their clinical staff in providing the essential tools to utilize in increasing one's resiliency.

Cleary et al. (2014) stated that managers and organizations are accountable for developing and maintaining staff resilience through providing professional development opportunities and a flexible work environment. Nurse leaders and managers who strive to create a workplace environment rooted in mutual trust and psychological safety are more engaged with clinical staff in collectively creating a full-level resilient organization.

BACKGROUND AND CONTEXT

In the American Nurses Association (ANA) Enterprise Healthy Nurse, Healthy Nation survey, the results showed that out of 18,000 respondents, 79% of nurses rated themselves at high risk for workplace stress (Pabico & Carpenter, 2020). With the arrival of the pandemic, the nurses faced an unprecedented crisis that had a significant impact on the nursing workforce. The majority of healthcare organizations faced a major problem regarding how to sustain an adequate healthcare workforce. Many nurses were quitting their jobs while others opted for early retirement. A literature review showed that healthcare workers experienced physical and psychological impacts including anxiety, sleeping difficulties, fear, and burnout (Jo et al., 2021). This turnover is on the rise, which leaves nurse leaders not only dealing with staffing shortages but also addressing the emotional toll caused by moral injury because of the pandemic. Nurse leaders and nurse managers are challenged on how to maximize each clinician's individual resilience while maintaining a safe workplace environment.

CHALLENGE AND OPPORTUNITY

THE STAFFING CRISIS

It is essential for healthcare leaders, institutions, and government agencies to provide both tangible (adequate personal protective equipment [PPE]) and intangible support (social and emotional) to sustain nurses' capacity to provide care and remain resilient. Leaders need to be acutely aware of the pulse of the unit and foster an environment of optimism through strategies that create work–life balance, assist in critical reflection to problem-solve, offer mentorship, build resolutions, facilitate professional governance, and empower their teams to nurture caring environments (O'Flaherty et al., 2018). Nurse leaders like SL are on a leadership succession planning pathway that has been supported by their institution and championed by their director. As the nurse manager of a surgical specialty unit, SL has received several resignation letters from the nursing team. SL feels upset and frustrated after a fifth nurse chose to leave in the past 2 months. The ongoing resignations seem like a revolving door and make SL feel powerless. In their reflections, SL has invested so much time and effort in developing the unit and an A-team. Yet no matter what SL has done over the past few months, this rapid turnover is getting out of control, and SL cannot prevent it or stop it from happening.

This scenario is not unique in SL's organization or any other healthcare organization. The turnover statistics are consistent with the latest report released by the International Center on Nurse Migration (ICNM). According to the 2021 survey results of 5,000 nurses and nurse managers in the United States, the "pandemic impact on intention to leave was rated high overall and was highest in nurses with 25+ years of experience and in managers/directors. 11% of the total sample indicated they intended to leave their position, and 20% were undecided" (Buchan et al., 2022, p. 24). The report noted these two combined scenarios can potentially cause instability in the workforce if not reversed or rectified. Exit interviews glean that staff are leaving for work–life balance, travel assignments, and transitioning to other clinical areas such as critical care within the organization. The capacity to cope and function in stressful workplace environments may vary based on one's culture, educational background experience, and upbringing (Garcia-Dia & O'Flaherty, 2016). It is important to recognize that the value of unit-based and organizational leadership is central to supporting nurses' health and wellness, which, in turn, impacts the delivery of quality care and nurses' resilience.

AG, the nursing director who oversees SL's unit, is concerned not only with the turnover but how the current shortage can impact SL. Prior to the pandemic, SL was on a leadership succession planning pathway that has been supported by their institution and championed by their director. SL exceeds unit benchmarks and goals but might be at a point where they could be at risk of also resigning. AG schedules a strategy planning meeting to review the turnover data and recruitment plans.

During the meeting with AG, SL mentions a recent study where it was noted that there have been positive outcomes when staff have participated in education programs that developed their leadership, communication, and delegation skills and nurtured resiliency to sustain a healthy work environment. This open communication and transparency sparked their energy to create resilience boosting strategies for the unit. SL would like to collaborate with the professional development and human resources departments to participate in the design and planning of a program for the team with a similar focus and emphasis on building resilience skills. As a nurse manager, SL has learned the value of infusing leadership and delegation skills as a support to expanding staff's roles as charge nurses. AG strongly supports this and suggests gathering the stakeholders and advises that this idea be added to the next professional governance council agenda to involve the clinical nurses in the design. The literature on resilience among nurses reveals that resilience builds resources and increases the capacity to cope with workplace burnout and stress (Delgado et al., 2017).

BUILDING RESILIENT LEADERS

Recognizing the competing priorities and the need to maintain a stable clinical team that has been impacted by turnover and hiring newer graduates, AG believes in fostering interprofessional collaboration and developing resilient leaders like SL. Workplace programs that have concentrated on resilience building strategies such as focusing on emotional responses to stress and cultivating empathy and reflective practice to foster resilience have been known to be effective (Foster, Cuzzillo, et al., 2018; Foster, Roche, et al., 2018). It has also been noted that environments where staff report feeling valued and supported by leadership, and the utilization of stress-reducing interventions that infuse joy at work (Carter & Hawkins, 2019), can increase staff resiliency (Andersen et al., 2021). Other studies on resilience among nurses reveal that resilience builds resources and increases the capacity to cope with workplace burnout and stress (Delgado et al., 2017).

The promotion of initiatives to reduce stress in the workplace such as practices that can be incorporated into the daily routine can serve to strengthen the team and staff well-being. Currently SL's team has a gratitude jar where team members, patients, and visitors can write a comment of gratitude for the staff. These positive comments are shared weekly during a morning brief between shifts, and this has been a positive experience. The practice is well received and is a contributing factor that has impacted staff engagement; the unit consistently is rated top tier for engagement, and this is one of several practices that have been supported by the organization to promote well-being, recognition, and a healthy workplace. Promoting self-care and optimism by such gestures as grateful moments and building hardiness foster an organizational response to support well-being.

After the staff's meeting and with the guidance of the human resources department, the team came up with a resilience toolkit program to build resilience. The key elements of the program were to make connections with each other and team members, avoid seeing crises as unsurmountable, utilize the concepts of mindfulness debriefing, and accept that change is part of the work routine and living our lives. Each team member utilized an icon to symbolize the practical steps to carry out the hardiness tool gaming app. This tool will be accessible via a QR code where they can take a pause throughout the day to practice resilience and apply easy-to-use exercises that focus on self-care that is often overlooked by the majority of the nurses. The group collated the top five exercises that can be integrated in their daily practice either at the workplace or at their own home environment.

- C—have compassion for yourself and others, strive to nurture yourself
- A—ask for help and/or assist others who may need help with intention
- R—means to reflect and remain true to yourself
- E—exercise and eat healthy
- S—sleep adequately (8 hours/day) and smile, laugh, and be cheerful

The major focus of the resilience toolkit is to emphasize self-care through building nurses' interpersonal strengths. It encourages individuals to draw strength from hardship, support positive relationships, and build on the resilience skills that they already have internally as a trait (Foster, Cuzzillo, et al., 2018; Foster, Roche, et al., 2018).

LOOKING AHEAD FOR THE LONG HAUL: ORGANIZATIONAL RESILIENCE

Recent literature available post-pandemic cites the value of organizational support and including nurses in the development of policy and procedures as resilience sustaining factors (Jo et al., 2021). The central theme in resilience studies is the need for the work environment to support nurses as they handle emotionally challenging situations to strengthen their emotional bank and in turn their resilience. The value of interprofessional collaboration, teamwork, and nurses' psychological ability to contend with daily stressors is of the utmost importance. Another recommendation from the literature review identified the importance of team building. According to Baik and Zeirler (2019), team supports the relevance and correlation to positive outcomes including enhanced patient safety, cultural change, efficient workflow, better quality of care, and job satisfaction. Harnessing the value of teamwork, a shared mental model, trust, and respect allows for a positive work environment.

Organizations are recognizing and supporting the value of programs that focus on employee well-being. In collaboration with chaplaincy, human resources and holistic nurses in several institutions have established initiatives to serve as an adjunct to fostering empathy and recognition of challenging patient and/or staff tragic events. Programs such as Schwartz Rounds focus on the interprofessional response to care, moral distress, and caregiver and staff feelings. Additionally, organizations like Northwell have instituted a Team Lavender, which is an interdisciplinary group of professionals dedicated to supporting colleagues during times of crisis, stress, and/or trauma (Barden & Giammarinaro, 2021). This peer support model has been positively correlated with a culture of safety and employee engagement. The philosophy of caring for ourselves so we can care for others aligns with the resilience toolkit in creating a culture of care personally and professionally.

KEY POINTS

- Burnout, nursing shortages, and nursing recruitment and retention are ongoing challenges for the nurse manager, nurse leader, and the overall organizational structure.

- Applying resilience concepts that leverage an individual's internal resilience as a trait and a process are strategies that nurse leaders can adopt in promoting a culture of safety and support.

- Organizations have a moral obligation to keep the passion and joy for nursing burning to keep the workforce and workplace in a stable, healthy, and positive state.

SUMMARY

Promoting joy and meaning in work are integral to the value of the nurses' role and supporting an environment where staff are engaged and satisfied. With emphasis on the Quadruple Aim, efforts to improve quality, patient experience, cost containment, and team performance are essential organizational goals that are in accordance with national health system priorities endorsed by the Institute for Healthcare Improvement (IHI; Feeley, 2017). Resilience as a theoretical framework can be used by nurse leaders in creating professional development programs and initiatives that address nurses' engagement, correct adverse workplace environments, reduce turnover, and foster joy and meaning, helping staff know that what we do matters in nurses' work. Additionally, this is supported by Haizlip et al.'s (2020) research where it was noted that a sense of mattering was affirmed in nurses by feeling appreciated by their organization, patients, and colleagues, as well as through interactions between team members. It correlates to lower levels of burnout and relates to nurses' understanding of their commitment to nursing. Value and meaning in work, as well as the relationships that allow us to have and appreciate humor and be brave enough to laugh at ourselves and the situation, are some strategies that nurses can apply in their daily work and home environment.

END-OF-CASE RESOURCES

◼ DISCUSSION QUESTIONS

1. As a nurse leader, certain situations can impact your moral compass. What interventions would you recommend that organizations can utilize to address moral distress or compassion fatigue?
2. With the increased turnover in your unit, what initiatives can be in place to support staffing?
3. Should nursing look at predictive models that can provide an on-demand balanced staffing?

SPRINGER PUBLISHING
C**O**NNECT™

A robust set of instructor resources designed to supplement this text is located at http://connect.springerpub.com/content/book/978-0-8261-7795-7. Qualifying instructors may request access by emailing textbook@springerpub.com.

REFERENCES

Aliem, S., & Hashish, E. (2021). The relationship between transformational leadership practices of first-line nurse managers and nurses' organizational resilience and job involvement: A structural equation model. *Worldviews on Evidence-Based Nursing, 18*(5), 273–282. https://doi.org/10.1111/wvn.12535

Andersen, S., Mintz-Binder, R., Sweatt, L., & Song, H. (2021). Building nurse resilience in the workplace. *Applied Nursing Research, 59*, Article No. 151433. https://doi.org/10.1016/j.apnr.2021.151433

Barden, A., & Giammarinaro, N. (2021). Team Lavender: Supporting employee well-being during the COVID-19 pandemic. *Nursing, 51*(4), 16–19. https://doi.org/10.1097/01.NURSE.0000734020.32604.fe

Baik D., & Zierler B. (2019). Clinical nurses' experiences and perceptions after the implementation of an interprofessional team intervention: A qualitative study. *Journal of Clinical Nurse, 28*, 430–443. https://doi.org/10.1111/jocn.14605

Bonanno, G. A. (2004). Loss, trauma, and human resilience: Have we underestimated the capacity to thrive after extremely aversive events? *American Psychologist, 59*(1), 20–28. https://doi.org/10.1037/0003-066X.59.1.20

Buchan, J., Catton, H., & Schaffer, F. A. (2022, January). *Sustain and retain in 2022 and beyond: The global nursing workforce and the COVID-19 pandemic*. International Council of Nurses, CGFNS International, & International Centre on Nurse Migration. https://www.icn.ch/system/files/2022-01/Sustain%20and%20Retain%20in%202022%20and%20Beyond-%20The%20global%20nursing%20workforce%20and%20the%20COVID-19%20pandemic.pdf

Carter, K., & Hawkins, A. (2019). Joy at work: Creating a culture of resilience. *Nursing Management, 50*(12), 34–42. https://doi.org/10.1097/01.NUMA.0000605156.88187.77

Cleary, M., Jackson, D., & Hungerford, C. (2014). Mental health nursing in Australia: Resilience as a means of sustaining the specialty. *Issues in Mental Health Nursing, 35*, 33–40. https://doi.org/10.3109/01612840.2013.836261

Delgado, C., Upton, D., Ranse, K., Furness, T., & Foster, K. (2017). Nurses resilience and the emotional labor of nursing work: An integrative review of empirical literature. *International Journal of Nursing Studies, 70*, 71–88. https://doi.org/10.1016/jijnurstu2017.02.008

Feeley, D. (2017, November 28). *The Triple Aim or the Quadruple Aim? Four points to help set your strategy*. Institute for Healthcare Improvement. https://www.ihi.org/communities/blogs/the-triple-aim-or-the-quadruple-aim-four-points-to-help-set-your-strategy

Foster, K., Cuzzillo, C., & Furness, T. (2018). Strengthening mental health nurses' resilience through a workplace resilience programme: A qualitative inquiry. *Journal of Psychiatric and Mental Health Nursing, 25*(5–6), 338–348. https://doi.org/10.1111/jpm.12467

Foster, K., Roche, M., Delgando, C., Cuzzilo, C., Giandinoto, J., & Furness, T. (2018). Resilience and mental health nursing: An integrative review of international literature. *International Journal of Mental Health Nursing, 28*, 71–75. https://doi.org/10.1111/inm.12548

Garcia-Dia, M. J., DiNapoli, J. M., Garcia-Ona, L., Jakubowski, R., & O'Flaherty, D. (2013). Concept analysis: resilience. *Archives of Psychiatric Nursing, 27*(6), 264–270. https://doi.org/10.1016/j.apnu.2013.07.003

Garcia-Dia, M. J., & O'Flaherty, D. (2016). Resilience. In J. J. Fitzpatrick & G. McCarthy (Eds.), *Nursing Concept Analysis: Applications to Research and Practice* (pp. 237–248). Springer Publishing Company.

Gillespie, B. M., Chaboyer, W., & Wallis, M. (2007). Development of a theoretically derived model of resilience through concept analysis. *Contemporary Nurse, 25*(1–2), 124–135. https://doi.org/10.5172/conu.2007.25.1-2.124

Haizlip, J., McCluney, C., Hernandez, M., Quatrara, B., & Brashers, V. (2020). Mattering: How organizations, patients, and peers can affect nurse burnout and engagement. *The Journal of Nursing Administration, 50*(5), 267–273. https://doi.org/10.1097/NNA.0000000000000882

Jo, S., Kurt, S., Bennett, J. A., Mayer, K., Pituch, K. A., Simpson, V., Skibiski, J., Takagi, E., Karaaslan, M. M., Ozluk, B., & Reifsnider, E. (2021). Nurses' resilience in the face of coronavirus (COVID-19): An international view. *Nursing & Health Sciences, 23*(3), 646–657. https://doi.org/10.1111/nhs.12863

Masten, A. (2014). Global perspectives on resilience in children and youth. *Child Development, 85*, 6–20. https://doi.org/10.1111/cdev.12205

O'Flaherty, D., Fitzpatrick, J. J., Garcia-Dia, M. J., Arreglado, T., & Dinapoli, J. (2018, March 19). *Cultivating a culture of resilience: A nursing leadership initiative*. Poster presented at the Sigma Nursing Education Research Conference 2018: Generating and Translating Evidence for Teaching Practice, Washington, DC. http://hdl.handle.net/10755/623908

Pabico, C., & Carpenter, H. (2020, September 7). Coping with emotional stress. *American Nurse Today*. https://www.myamericannurse.com/coping-with-emotional-stress

Rangachari, P., & Woods, J. L. (2020). Preserving organizational resilience, patient safety, and staff retention during COVID_19 requires a holistic consideration of the psychological safety of healthcare workers. *International Journal of Environmental Research and Public Health, 17*(12), Article 4267. https://doi.org/10.3390/ijerph17124267

Reyes, A. T., Andrusyszyn, M.-A., Iwasiw, C., Forchuk, C., & Babenko-Mould, Y. (2015). Resilience in nursing education: An integrative review. *Journal of Nursing Education, 54*(8). 438–444. https://doi.org/10.3928/01484834-20150717-03

Rutter, M. (2006). The promotion of resilience in the face of adversity. In A. Clarke-Stewart & J. Dunn (Eds.), *Families count: Effects on child and adolescent development* (pp. 26–52). https://doi.org/10.1017/CBO9780511616259.003

MAIN HOSPITAL: PERIOPERATIVE TRANSITION UNIT

Garry Brydges

INTRODUCTION

Main Hospital is a for-profit hospital with a 585-bed capacity. The hospital chief executive officer (CEO) Bill McInroy has plans to expand hospital operations in the perioperative setting. A new 30-bed perioperative transition unit is being developed to care for patients in the postoperative setting and short-term stay. The perioperative transition unit is a redesigned approach to patient care innovations focusing on value-based healthcare delivery targeting high-quality care, cost effectiveness, and healthcare economics. The hospital CEO and chief nursing officer (CNO), Margaret Werrington, PhD, MBA, RN, collaborated with subspecialty surgeons performing a range of oncological surgeries. The perioperative transition unit is focused on incorporating techniques in enhanced recovery after surgery. Since enhanced recovery after surgery programs demonstrate significant quality enhancements, increase patient satisfaction, and reduce cost of care delivery, Mr. McInroy transitioned the hospital to a shared risk approach under the Centers for Medicare & Medicaid Services (CMS) value-based programs. Under the Medicare and Children's Health Insurance Program (CHIP) Reauthorization (MACRA) Act, the hospital decided to follow the alternative payment model of bundled payment systems for each episode of care per oncological service line.

BACKGROUND AND CONTEXT

In partnership with the oncological surgeons, several outcome metrics were identified to benchmark against similar services nationally (Table CCS7.1). The hospital-acquired conditions identified with the oncological surgeons included hospital-acquired pressure injuries (HAPI), catheter-associated urinary tract infections (CAUTI), falls, postoperative nausea and vomiting (PONV), pain, postoperative ileus (POI), respiratory depression, surgical site infections (SSI), postoperative cognitive disorder (POCD), length of stay (LOS), and 30-day readmission rates.

Mr. McInroy tasked chief nursing officer (CNO) Werrington, PhD, MBA, RN, and her leadership team to develop a personnel salary budget with a staffing matrix, capital budget, and operating budget. The forecasting for the 30-bed unit includes 9,000 patient days, average daily census (ADC) at 25 cases, 82% occupancy rate, average acuity 3.3, and average workload indexed at 81.4. The staffing make-up includes a nurse manager, APRNs, RNs, LPNs, and patient care assistants (PCAs). The forecasted patient volume for the fiscal year is 6,395 patients. The perioperative transition unit operates 7 days per week due to each patient requiring a LOS beyond 1 day. The RNs, LPNs, and PCAs work 8-hour shifts. The provider-to-patient ratio is 1:3. The hours per patient day are 9.73. All staff, except APRNs and manager, receive shift differentials such as 10% for the 3 p.m. to 11 p.m., 20% for the 11 p.m. to 7 a.m., an additional 5% for weekends (any shift), and 50% for overtime. The nonproductive hours for each employee are based on 40 hours per week or 2,080 hours per year.

TABLE CCS7.1: National Benchmark Outcomes and ERAS Economic Impact

Outcome	Cost	Incidence (non-ERAS)	Target (ERAS)
Length of stay	$2,064.00/day	6–10 days	<1–3.3 days
30-Day readmission rate	$11,200.00	5.40%	<2.10%
Postoperative ileus	$10,247.00	15.60%	<7.80%
Urinary retention/infection	$1,357.00	2.00%	<0.50%
Thromboembolic event	$4,159.00	2.20%	<1.30%
Postoperative nausea and vomiting	$87.12	15.00%	<7.00%
Respiratory depression	$568.00	3.30%	<1.10%
Surgical site infection	$34,407.00	5.60%	<2.00%

ERAS, enhanced recovery after surgery.

Source: Data from Bartels, K., Mayes, L. M., Dingmann, C., Bullard, K. J., Hopfer, C. J., & Binswanger, I. A. (2016). Opioid use and storage patterns by patients after hospital discharge following surgery. *PLoS One, 11*(1), e0147972. https://doi .org/10.1371/journal.pone.0147972; Hilton, W. M., Lotan, Y., Parekh, D. J., Basler, J. W., & Svatek, R. S. (2013). Alvimopan for prevention of postoperative paralytic ileus in radical cystectomy patients: A cost-effectiveness analysis. *BJU International, 111*(7), 1054–1060. https://doi.org/10.1111/j.1464-410X.2012.11499.x; Jenks, P. J., Laurent, M., McQuarry, S., & Watkins, R. (2014). Clinical and economic burden of surgical site infection (SSI) and predicted financial consequences of elimina-tion of SSI from an English hospital. *Journal of Hospital Infection, 86*(1), 24–33. https://doi.org/10.1016/j.jhin.2013.09.012; Laloto, T. L., Gemeda, D. H., & Abdella, S. H. (2017). Incidence and predictors of surgical site infection in Ethiopia: Pro-spective cohort. *BMC Infectious Diseases, 17*(1), 119. https://doi.org/10.1186/s12879-016-2167-x; Oderda, G. M., Gan, T. J., Johnson, B. H., & Robinson, S. B. (2013). Effect of opioid-related adverse events on outcomes in selected surgical patients. *Journal of Pain and Palliative Care Pharmacotherapy, 27*(1), 62–70. https://doi.org/10.3109/15360288.2012.751956; Parra-Sanchez, I., Abdallah, R., You, J., Fu, A. Z., Grady, M., Cummings III, K., Apfel, C., & Sessler, D. I. (2012). A time-motion economic analysis of postoperative nausea and vomiting in ambulatory surgery. *Canadian Journal of Anesthesia/Journal canadien d'anesthésie, 59*(4), 366–375. https://doi.org/10.1007/s12630-011-9660-x; Shepard, J., Ward, W., Milstone, A., Carlson, T., Frederick, J., Hadhazy, E., & Perl, T. (2013). Financial impact of surgical site infections on hospitals: The hos-pital management perspective. *JAMA Surgery, 148*(10), 907–914. https://doi.org/10.1001/jamasurg.2013.2246; Touchette, D. R., Yang, Y., Tiryaki, F., & Galanter, W. L. (2012). Economic analysis of alvimopan for prevention and management of postoperative ileus. *Pharmacotherapy, 32*(2), 120–128. https://doi.org/10.1002/PHAR.1047; Wu, A. K., Auerbach, A. D., & Aaronson, D. S. (2012). National incidence and outcomes of postoperative urinary retention in the Surgical Care Im-provement Project. *American Journal of Surgery, 204*(2), 167–171. https://doi.org/10.1016/j.amjsurg.2011.11.012.

TABLE CCS7.2: Staffing Patterns: Daily Staffing

Workload				Total
Nurse manager				1
APRN				4
	7 a.m.–3 p.m.	3 p.m.–11 p.m.	11 p.m.–7 a.m.	
Staff RN	7	4	2	13
LPN	3	2	2	7
PCA	2	2	1	5
Total	12	8	5	30

PCA, patient care assistant.

Other nonproductive hours include 3 weeks' vacation, 6 days sick leave, 8 holidays, and 3 personal days. Other benefits received from the hospital include 6.25% Federal Insurance Contributions Act (FICA), 1.25% Medicare, 6.7% health insurance, 1.5% life insurance, and 4.33% other. The hourly rate per employee is $62 per hour for the nurse manager, $65 per hour for the APRN, $36.50 for each staff RN, $23 per hour for each LPN, and $15 per hour for each PCA (Table CCS7.2).

CNO Werrington collaborated with CEO McInroy and the chief financial officer (CFO) to review the overall projected financials for the perioperative transition unit. Although the hospital is reimbursed under bundle payment systems, the team utilized Medicare Part A fee-for-service rates to determine the initial projected revenues for the unit. The average third-party payor reimbursement was projected at $2,080 per patient and Medicare was projected at $1,025 per patient. The payor mix is approximately 40% Medicare and 60% private insurers. The budgeted variable costs for medications and lab tests are projected at $351,725 and $30,000 for other variable costs. In addition to salaries and benefits, other fixed costs include building expenses at $416,244, office supplies at $2,400, transportation and travel at $67,236, advertising and branding the units to the community at $30,000, consultants such as legal and accounting at $25,200, liability insurance premiums at $104,400, and capital equipment depreciation at $373,428. The tax rate for the hospital is 15%. Also, hospital-acquired complications such as POI result in prolonged hospital LOS. In this case, a POI results in an additional 4-day LOS.

CHALLENGE AND OPPORTUNITY

A challenge confronting nurse leaders is understanding how to define and implement quality measures from a financial perspective. Also, an appreciation for reimbursement methodologies is essential for nurse leaders in generating personnel budgets, operational budgets, forecasting, and program innovations. Collaborative partnerships with the CEO, CFO, physicians, and other team members are opportunities that must be explored by every nurse leader.

KEY POINTS

- Developing local financial benchmarks for patient care based on the evidence is crucial.
- The importance of translating quality care and patient outcomes into financial outcomes enhances a nurse leader's ability to better justify resources.
- The nurse leader should be able to develop a staffing matrix outlining the full-time equivalent (FTE) requirements and related costs, as well as the operational benchmark drivers impacting FTE requirements.
- The importance of understanding revenue sources, variable costs, fixed costs, and methods for controlling cost of care through enhanced patient care remain essential nurse leader competencies as healthcare increases in complexity.

SUMMARY

The Main Hospital perioperative transition unit demonstrates a range of important tasks in developing financial literacy in leadership. Collaboration with a range of stakeholders is an imperative for project success. With hospital stakeholders, a range of operational projections based on volume and cost is the initial step. Next, a staffing model and associated personnel costs to implement the service require a few basic financial principles specific to staffing models. The other important financial aspect of project development is revenue. Value-based healthcare delivery is a concept focused on quality of care. The professional and technical aspects of revenue generating are optimized through strict control of variable costs, fixed costs, and high-quality care. Finally, operational and clinical care benchmarks act as a gauge to the level of quality care with associated cost reduction and revenue optimization. Some examples discussed include skin breakdown, perioperative ileus, and POI. The nursing leader with strong financial acumen can assimilate and master each of these financial elements, resulting in a high-quality, value-based care delivery model.

END-OF-CASE RESOURCES

DISCUSSION QUESTIONS

1. In a table, calculate the ADC and hours per patient day (HPPD) for the perioperative transition unit.
2. In a table, calculate the coverage factor for the perioperative transition unit.
3. Determine the total FTE requirements and skill mix to staff the perioperative transition unit.
4. Using bundle payment systems as the form of hospital reimbursement, explain the importance of benchmarking against national hospital-acquired conditions. (Hint: Use Table CCS7.2 to answer the question.)
5. Based on the projected patient volume and perioperative transition unit outcome targets, calculate the projected financial impact. Why is the focus on hospital-acquired conditions important for nurse leaders?
6. Calculate the total income, total variable costs, total fixed costs, contribution to margin, and net earnings for the perioperative transition unit.

A robust set of instructor resources designed to supplement this text is located at http://connect.springerpub.com/content/book/978-0-8261-7795-7. Qualifying instructors may request access by emailing textbook@springerpub.com.

COMPETITION WITHIN HEALTHCARE INDUSTRY

Nathanial Schreiner and Stuart D. Downs

INTRODUCTION

The healthcare system is a rapidly changing, complex environment in which we encounter constantly shifting dynamics ranging from patient care to government regulations. Within this contextual healthcare paradigm, administrative decisions, especially those related to finances, affect every variable and component of health-related operations and, most importantly, determine the future fiscal and operational viability of the entity. Given the complexities of healthcare, the variables and potential outcomes of these administrative decisions are not readily evident. These decisions are often comprised of known and unknown variables, which increase the inherent risks within the decision-making process. While financial decisions are not always made within the context of an opportunity related to financial gain, many administrative healthcare decisions are made to mitigate unexpected challenges, including loss stemming from decisions made by outside entities and competing healthcare systems. Within this case study, we present a situation that mimics the challenges related to the increased competition for market share of a geographic area consisting of a well-insured patient population.

This case study will explore two key financial terms/methods: *strength, weakness, opportunity, threat (SWOT) analysis* and *opportunity cost*. A SWOT analysis is a method that examines internal strengths and weaknesses of an entity, such as a hospital, in relation to external opportunities and threats within the context of a specific situation, such as an opportunity to expand a service line to meet population demand. Opportunity cost, which was briefly introduced in Chapter 18, "Macro Components of Healthcare Financing," is the loss of potential gains from alternative decisions when a specific decision is made. Mathematically, opportunity cost is expressed as the gains from the option not chosen divided by the gains from the option that is selected; thus, what is lost/what is gained. As aforementioned, opportunity cost is not easily determined; however, decisions are informed by factoring in as many variables as possible when determining the best option, including those within the context of healthcare. A SWOT analysis provides a methodological approach for identifying and incorporating these variables into the process of making an informed decision via the principles of opportunity cost. Within this case study, we present a relevant situation demonstrating how a SWOT analysis can inform healthcare decision-making framed within the context of opportunity cost.

BACKGROUND AND CONTEXT

You are the chief nursing officer (CNO) of a 150-bed, suburban hospital that is part of a larger healthcare network located within a metropolitan city where the flagship hospital, a large tertiary medical center, is located downtown. Your hospital, along with two other smaller hospitals, are "feeder" hospitals that transfer, or funnel, patients of higher acuity or who need specialized care to the flagship facility. Despite the smaller size of your hospital as compared to the flagship, your location within a middle to upper-class suburban area has provided the strongest profits per patient for the health system. Recognizing your hospital has the strongest net profits within the system, it is often referred to as the "jewel" of the health system. Additionally, the wealth of privately insured patients from your geographic area has brought increased net profits to the flagship hospital since all patients requiring specialized/higher acuity care (i.e., trauma, heart, stroke, transplant, obstetrics) are referred to or transported downtown.

Since your hospital was built 30 years ago, it has been the only provider of acute care for the population of the western suburbs. Unfortunately, the aging population within your geographic area has over time started to erode your payor mix. The once well-employed, well-insured population your hospital served is now retiring, which has shifted your payor mix from a majority of private insurers to Medicare reimbursement. Furthermore, as the children of these individuals began to have families of their own, they moved to areas further west due to cheaper/available land, thus slowly shifting the market dynamics from which your hospital has benefited over the last three decades.

The areas west of the current suburbs in which your hospital is located, which were previously rural farmland, are now becoming the in-demand areas for new businesses and their employees to live. These sleepy towns and townships are now experiencing rapid growth. Recently, this rapid growth has been exacerbated by the confirmation of a global technology firm agreeing to build a new chip manufacturing company in one of the townships. The company has projected that over 7,000 employees will be needed to run this new facility, although the number of new jobs that will be initially created in this area has been estimated at three times this number. Five-year projections in population growth for the township is nearly 500%. The shift in a younger, well-insured population migrating to the western areas coupled with the announcement of this new global technology firm with plans for building a new chip manufacturing plant has prompted a renewed sense of urgency by your healthcare system to integrate into this area.

CHALLENGE AND OPPORTUNITY

At the most recent board meeting, you have been tasked to conduct a SWOT analysis of current clinical services provided by your hospital in relation to the anticipated healthcare needs of the population/area within the areas west of your location. Your SWOT analysis will provide critical information and serve as the foundation for identifying opportunities for the potential growth/expansion of clinical services into this area.

You and your team sit down to discuss how to go about conducting this SWOT analysis. Based on your team's prior experience and education, you decide the first step is to identify the current state of healthcare in this geographic region, including any relationships with major stakeholders. Understanding how these stakeholders drive patient preference/volume is essential to forecasting future clinical needs.

MAJOR STAKEHOLDERS

THE HEALTHCARE SYSTEM

Your hospital system is the dominant healthcare provider west of downtown, with all four hospitals located on the west side of the city. Additionally, your hospital provides the majority of inpatient care for the specific areas of interest west of the current suburbs. Access to your hospital is approximately 4 minutes from the highway, providing for reasonably quick access to the facility for patients, family, and staff. Currently, you have no trauma, stroke, or chest pain certification at your facility as these patients are stabilized in your ED and transferred to the downtown flagship for higher acuity care. Benefitting from your strong payor mix, your hospital facilities are top notch, and you enjoy low staff turnover. Associated with low turnover, your nursing staff is the best paid within the hospital system, has low patient-to-nurse staffing ratios, and has ample ancillary resources inclusive of a robust nursing education department, IV team, and a float pool. Additionally, your nursing staff is highly seasoned, averaging 8 years of experience. You have a strong primary care and internal medicine presence within your immediate suburban area, providing nearly 60% of your inpatient census. From a surgical services perspective, general surgery and orthopedic cases are your primary focus and source of inpatient surgical volume, although you also have a large outpatient surgery center that provides gastrointestinal (GI); ear, nose, and throat (ENT); and pain management services to your community. Your hospital provides inpatient care for adult and geriatric psychiatric patients as well as outpatient obstetrical services, although newborn deliveries are only performed at the flagship hospital, which is a distance of approximately 17 miles from your hospital.

INDEPENDENT FAMILY/PRIMARY CARE PROVIDERS

Two private practices have traditionally provided care for the population in this area. Both practices are owned and staffed by third-generation physicians who have deep roots in the community. Providers at both practices are credentialed at your hospitals and amiable relations are maintained between your system and these practices, although no contract exists between these providers and your system.

Ten years ago, prior to your arrival as CNO, your hospital system inquired about purchasing these practices. A cost/benefit analysis demonstrated that, at their current payor mix, patient volume, and billed relative value units (RVUs) in relation to the asking price for acquisition, the purchase would be cost prohibitive and result in a negative return of investment (ROI) of approximately 30%. In response to not acquiring either of these practices, your hospital system leased medical office space and fully staffed a family practice in order to establish a foothold in this area. Initial projects demonstrated a slim margin (3%) on the ROI associated with this venture, but after 2 years at this location, this practice incurred a substantial loss in ROI (–15%). This loss stemmed from two reasons: lower than forecasted volume and poor payor mix associated with the patients for whom care was provided at this practice. Instead of accruing additional losses associated with operating this practice, your system decided to lose the practice, and wrote off the remaining debt associated with this venture as sunk cost. Qualitative inquiry into why the practice performed poorer than initial projections revealed that the area's population was loyal to the family practice physicians from whom they had sought care for years, and also felt your system's family practice was "too corporate" and "didn't have a hometown feel to it."

EMERGENCY MEDICAL SERVICES

Emergency medical services (EMS) in the neighboring area west of you are comprised of smaller fire departments with some of the smallest townships sharing EMS operated by individuals holding only part-time and volunteer status positions. In total, there are seven different fire departments for which your facility serves as medical control within this area to your west. Interfacing with these departments can be difficult, as the lack of full-time employees makes scheduling taxing at best. This has also made continuing education and training for these various departments frustrating for your EMS coordinator and medical director as it is difficult to schedule and conduct given these circumstances. These issues coupled with fewer patient transports due to a sparse population within the community has led to a lukewarm relationship between these departments and your hospital, although the majority of EMS transported patients are treated in your ED based on proximity. A few of your nurses have family and friends who work for these fire departments and have conveyed that many of the firemen feel the departments in close proximity to your hospital that bring the majority of the EMS-transported patients to the ED receive preferential treatment by staff. Furthermore, due to having a much smaller financial budget related to their tax base, changes in policy and procedure do not take into account their limitations associated with equipment, staffing, and/or training.

MAJOR EMPLOYERS

Your hospital system provides the current health plan for many of the townships' employees, including the district school system. The local governments have been, up to this point, the largest employer in this area and your system is due to renew/renegotiate the contract for these district employees at the end of this year. Additionally, your system also has healthcare contracts with several small manufacturing companies within the area, although the largest of these contracts is for just over 100 employees.

To date, there has been no meeting to discuss a potential relationship/deal between your healthcare system and the new technology company moving into the area. Various physicians and C-suite individuals have informally met some of the representatives from the company at community events, thus suggesting the relationship, although no formal discussions have been entertained. Additionally, based on the economic impact and national exposure this electronic chip plant brings to the area, it is speculated that the rural areas to the west are primed for a massive expansion in population, infrastructure, and business/economic bases.

OPPORTUNITY COST

As defined in the introduction, opportunity cost is the cost of an alternative decision in relation to the choice chosen. It is important to understand that (a) not choosing to proceed with a course of action is considered an opportunity cost, and (b) not all opportunity costs are associated with a beneficial choice. Opportunity cost is also related to decisions made when faced with situations in which financial losses are unavoidable where the best decision might mitigate some of the potential losses; however, a financial loss will be incurred regardless of the option chosen.

LOSS MITIGATION

As stated in the introduction to this case study and this section, not all situations are cut and dry, nor do they always end with the best possible outcome, especially within the complexities of a dynamic, constantly changing healthcare environment. Thus, in any business-related context, there are always known and unknown entities that are looking for strategic and financial opportunities in relation to your own aspirations.

After you present your findings to others in the C-suite and the board, major initiatives are undertaken based on your suggestions in conjunction with another group's input (e.g., finance, marketing). Hospital administrators and the governing board of your healthcare system have been meeting with various city and township officials, as well as the management team of the tech company, in order to establish affiliations/connections. Initially, discussions between all parties appear to be positive, with discussions ranging from reestablishment of satellite healthcare facilities (i.e., primary care practices) in nearby towns to becoming the provider of care for the new tech company at a negotiated rate. Over the weekend, an emergency meeting convenes at your system's downtown campus, during which you are informed that your competitor has purchased land near the new chip plant and is moving forward with building a state-of-the-art hospital at this site. For the first time in 30 years, there will be direct competition for patients in your immediate primary service area.

Initial reports on details of your competitor's new hospital are alarming. This hospital is projected to have between 200- and 250-bed capacity and a full range of inpatient services, including those not offered at your hospital (i.e., obstetrics, cardiothoracic/interventional cardiology, neurosurgery). Additionally, a 24-bed ED that aims to have trauma, chest pain, and stroke accreditations, in conjunction with a 10-bed fast track for non-emergent ED patients, is also included in the plans.

KEY POINTS

- Nurse leaders play a crucial role in the planning and implementation phases of healthcare services to maximize market share and the provision of care within existing communities.

- Competitiveness within healthcare systems affect every variable of health-related operations, and financial decisions are not always made within the context of an opportunity related to financial gain.

- Many administrative healthcare decisions are based on mitigating unexpected challenges, including loss stemming from decisions made by outside entities, and including competing healthcare systems.

- A SWOT analysis is an effective methodological approach to assess internal areas in which a healthcare organization is performing well in order to maintain a strong competitive advantage, and utilized to illuminate external factors so that opportunities can be seized and solutions can be proposed to counteract and mitigate threats to the organization.

- Opportunity cost is a decision made based on the value of something you have to give up in order to make a decision about something else.

- An analysis of opportunities establishes organizational demand by studying external conditions that have the ability to inform strategy and vision for the organization.

SUMMARY

Within this case study, we presented a complex, multifaceted scenario in which a CNO is tasked with determining a response to a fluid, developing situation that will have a direct impact on the current and financial viability of the hospital as well as the healthcare system. Additionally, none of the potential responses that arise from this scenario are without substantial cost, financial and otherwise, demonstrating pervasive risk within healthcare decision-making, especially at a macro level. Furthermore, this case study was framed to demonstrate the importance of the nursing role within this decision-making process, especially focusing on the expertise nursing has in relation to the clinical operations of any healthcare system.

As part of this decision-making case study, we introduced SWOT methodology as a process to assist the nursing executive with identifying all possible options for decisions related to the scenario. Moreover, conducting the SWOT analysis allowed the CNO to identify key stakeholders who are "drivers" of patient volume to the healthcare system. Based on this information, the CNO could determine specific strengths, weaknesses, opportunities, and threats unique to each stakeholder, as well as the intersections of these dynamics among these parties in relation to responding to the needs of this patient population. Once the CNO had established the opportunities and threats within the current scenario, the CNO was able to examine the related opportunity costs of making one decision in comparison to the alternatives. Furthermore, this case study introduced the complexity of a known competing entity, who has similar goals to your healthcare system, and that changed the dynamic of opportunity cost of decisions made from those of gains relative to opportunities to minimizing losses relative to an imminent threat. Of most importance, this case study introduces the student to the difficulty presented in the inherent risk of healthcare decision-making, especially when faced with competition for limited resources constrained by the current and future financial health of an institution.

END-OF-CASE RESOURCES

◐ DISCUSSION QUESTIONS

1. Who are the major stakeholders that need to be considered within this analysis?

2. Based on the information provided in the previous sections, how is your hospital and hospital system positioned to adapt/succeed in accordance with these new developments/challenges? Based on your SWOT analysis, what are the strengths, weaknesses, opportunities, and threats associated with this unique situation?

3. Now, after completing your SWOT analysis, what are the opportunity costs, specifically related to the strategies identified in taking advantage of the strengths and opportunities or minimizing weakness and mitigating threats in relation to the provision of healthcare services needed to meet the needs of a rapidly expanding population to the west?

4. Based on the threat of a new competitor hospital being built in this rapidly emerging region to your west, what actions need to be taken? How does this new information alter your SWOT analysis? What is the opportunity cost associated with potentially taking new action/change in decision-making? Additionally, what do you need to spend to mitigate potential losses in relation to patient volume in the areas west of you and in the suburban area that has made you the "crown jewel" of your healthcare system?

INDEX

AACN. *See* American Association of Colleges of Nursing

AAFP. *See* American Academy of Family Physicians

ACA. *See* Affordable Care Act

academic medical centers (AMCs), 506, 512, 514

accountable care organizations (ACOs), 176–177, 181, 184–188
   performance-based risks, 186–187

ACHE. *See* American College of Healthcare Executives

ACNE. *See* associate chief nurse executive

ACOs. *See* accountable care organizations

ACPE. *See* American College of Physician Executives

ADC. *See* average daily census

Admission/Discharge/Transfer (ADT), 388–389, 391

ADT. *See* Admission/Discharge/Transfer

adverse events (AEs), 419, 426

AEs. *See* adverse events

Affordable Care Act (ACA), 173–174, 184, 191, 193, 200, 223, 307, 440, 451, 527

Agency for Healthcare Research and Quality (AHRQ), 222, 224, 228

Agency for Toxic Substances and Disease Registry (ATSDR), 41

agile methodology, 367–368

AHRQ. *See* Agency for Healthcare Research and Quality

AI. *See* artificial intelligence

AL. *See* authentic leadership

ALQ. *See* Authentic Leadership Questionnaire

ALSN. *See* Association for Leadership Science in Nursing

alternative sites of care, benefit designs, 194–195

AMA. *See* American Medical Association

ambulatory surgery center (ASC), 563

AMCs. *See* academic medical centers

American Academy of Family Physicians (AAFP), 229

American Association of Colleges of Nursing (AACN), 57–59, 415, 421–422

American College of Healthcare Executives (ACHE), 56, 62

American College of Physician Executives (ACPE), 56

American Medical Association (AMA), 172

American Nurses Association (ANA), 31–35, 37–38, 41, 49, 51, 56, 76, 88, 114, 248, 250, 480, 482, 540, 580

American Nurses Credentialing Center (ANCC), 40, 123, 125, 333, 335, 340

American Nurses Foundation (ANF), 480

American Organization for Nurse Executives (AONE), 33, 35, 63, 108, 135, 138, 302

American Organization for Nursing Leadership (AONL), 8, 32–33, 35, 40, 42–43, 45, 47, 56–59, 61–62, 64–65, 119, 138, 147, 159, 250, 267, 332–333, 412

American Recovery and Reinvestment Act (ARRA), 288

American Telemedicine Association (ATA), 561

ANA. *See* American Nurses Association

ANCC. *See* American Nurses Credentialing Center

ANCC Magnet Recognition Program, 335

ANF. *See* American Nurses Foundation

ANL. *See* authentic nursing leadership

ANLQ. *See* Authentic Nurse Leadership Questionnaire

AONE. *See* American Organization for Nurse Executives

AONL. *See* American Organization for Nursing Leadership

AORN. *See* Association of periOperative Registered Nurses

API. *See* application program interface
application program interface (API), 385–386
APs. *See* assistive personnel
ARRA. *See* American Recovery and Reinvestment Act
artificial intelligence (AI), 198
ASC. *See* ambulatory surgery center
assistive personnel (APs), 458, 461–463, 471
associate chief nurse executive (ACNE), 64
Association for Leadership Science in Nursing (ALSN), 147
Association of periOperative Registered Nurses (AORN), 16, 526
ATA. *See* American Telemedicine Association
ATSDR. *See* Agency for Toxic Substances and Disease Registry
authentic leadership (AL), 127–130
   nursing and, 127–129
   transformational leadership vs, 129–130
Authentic Leadership Questionnaire (ALQ), 127
Authentic Nurse Leadership Questionnaire (ANLQ), 129
authentic nursing leadership (ANL), 128
authentically present leadership
   act/speak and look, 6–7
   impactful messaging, 6
average daily census (ADC), 413, 424, 456–458, 461, 470, 585

Bar-On model, 100–101
belonging
   relationships, 74–75
   sense of, 77
benefit relief factor (BRF), 458
big data
   predictive analytics, 396–397
   7 Vs of, 397
blood pressure (BP), 175, 177
board governance
   attributes and characteristics, 504–506
   audit and compliance, 510
   committees, 509–512
   compensation committee, 510
   executive committee, 510
   fiduciary roles and duties, 505
   finance committee, 510
   governance and nominating committee, 510
   healthcare trends, 504
   policies, 509
   quality and safety committee, 511–512
   relationship/partnership with management, 506–508
   research and education committee, 512
   strategic direction, 503–504

   strategic planning committee, 511
   talent development/workforce development committee, 511
board leadership/service
   appointed and elected positions, 483
   barriers and facilitators, 490–491
   collective engagement, 479
   communication skills, 486
   competencies, 486
   concept of nurses serving on boards, 480–482
   cultural awareness, 486–487
   decision-making roles, 478–479
   diversity, 491
   dynamic culture, 491
   equity-focused, 491–492
   financial knowledge, 486
   formal education and exposure, 487
   governing roles, 477, 484
   identification of opportunity, 493
   inclusion, 491
   interviews, 493–494
   mission driven, 486
   nurse responsibilities, 478, 497
   Nurses on Boards Coalition (NOBC), 480, 487–489
   service guidelines and protocols, 494–495
boards
   advisory, 483
   definition, 483
   nonprofit, non-nursing boards, 483
   private and public corporate, 483
   types, 483
BP. *See* blood pressure
BPCI. *See* Bundle Payments for Care Improvement
BRF. *See* benefit relief factor
budget
   balanced schedule, 466–467
   capital budget, 454
   coverage factor/benefit relief factor, 458–460
   definition, 452–453
   financial reports, 465–466
   hours per patient day, 460–461
   off cycle resources, 468–469
   operating budget, 454, 465
   position control, 467–468
   process, 454–455
   productivity and benchmarks, 457–458
   salary, 455–456, 465
   skill mix, 461
   staffing, 466
   supply, 455
   types, 453–454
   volume projection, 456–457, 461–465

budgeting strategy, 180–181
Bundle Payments for Care Improvement
    (BPCI), 182, 187–188
  success strategies, 188

CAH. *See* critical access hospital
CAHPS. *See* Consumers Assessment of
    Healthcare Providers and Systems
care coordination, 173–174, 179
care delivery system (CDS), 40
Case Mix Index (CMI), 435, 439, 442, 447
case scenarios
  academic partnerships, 422
  access to healthcare, 484
  accountable care organization, 185–186
  advocacy-based project, 39–40
  authentic nurse leadership, 130
  board service, 485, 490, 492, 493–494,
      496–497
  board vacancy, 515
  care delivery, quality, and safety, 370–371
  career aspirations of colleagues, 91–92
  clinical practice outcomes, 288–289
  compensation variances, 508–509
  competency evaluation, 64–65
  complexity leadership, 364–367
  conflict resolution, 60–61, 420–421
  culture of inquiry, 341–343
  data management, 393–394
  decentralization, 292–293
  disaster response during COVID-19,
      299–301
  early career coaching and mentoring
      (novice stage), 153–154, 159–160
  emergency visits, avoidance and reduction,
      229–230
  emotional intelligence (EI), 103
  ethical and legal consideration, 248–249
  exemplary practice, 40
  financial implications, 249
  head trauma evaluation, 227–229
  healthcare environment, 424–425
  healthcare ethics, 176
  honoring others' work, 90
  hospital acquisition, 528–529
  human resource support, 414–415
  information technology, 394
  influencing beyond your team, 370–371
  Innovation Studio (Ohio State University),
      271–273
  late career coaching and mentoring
      (expert stage), 155–156, 161–162
  leadership development, 136–137
  leadership skills, 416–417
  Magnet Recognition Program, 340

Medicare Advantage programs, consumer
    questions, 190–191
  metric falsification, 17
  mid-career coaching (competent proficient
      stage), 154–155, 160–161
  mindfulness, 46–49
  nurse credentials, 340
  palliative care, 323–324
  payor mix, 440–442
  personal and professional accountability,
      415–416
  philanthropy, 541–542, 543
  potential donors, 541–542
  professional citizenship, 93
  professional practice model, 340
  professionalism, 423–424
  relationship management, 104–105
  robotics and artificial intelligence, 274–277
  self-care, 46–47
  servant leadership (SL), 134
  shared purpose, values, 90–91
  skill mix, 461
  social competence, 104–105
  staff working hours, 460
  strategic development and planning,
      320–321
  strategic management, 418–419
  system approach
    culture of inquiry, 341–343
    patient safety, 337–339
  systems thinking, 425–426
  TEAMSTEPPS and emotional intelligence,
      107–108
  telehealth, 247, 251
  transformational leadership, 43–44, 124, 126
  United Way Review Panel, access to
      healthcare, 484
  unqualified candidates, 16–17
  value-based care, 446, 446–447
  volume assumptions, 457
  wearable devices, 248
  workforce reduction, 526
case studies
  competition within healthcare industry,
      589–594
  electronic health record, 575–577
  human-centered leadership, 552–554
  innovation, 569–573
  mentoring, 555–559
  perioperative transition, 585–588
  resiliency, 579–583
  telehealth, 561–566
catheter-associated urinary tract infections
    (CAUTIs), 452, 585
CAUTIs. *See* catheter-associated urinary tract
    infections

CBAs. *See* collective bargaining agreements
CCM. *See* chronic care management
CCNA. *See* Center to Champion Nursing in America
CCO. *See* chief clinical officer
CDI. *See* clinical documentation improvement
CDS. *See* care delivery system
Center to Champion Nursing in America (CCNA), 482
Centers of Excellence (COEs), 194
CEO. *See* chief executive officer
certified neuroscience registered nurse (CNRN), 92
CFO. *See* chief financial officer
CGEAN. *See* Council for Graduate Education for Administrative Nursing
checklists, 19–20
CHF. *See* congestive heart failure
chief clinical officer (CCO), 10
chief executive officer (CEO), 10–11, 16–17, 63, 88–91, 123, 126, 131, 133–134, 278, 286, 296, 361, 452, 505–506, 508, 510, 515, 546, 585, 587
chief financial officer (CFO), 23, 508–509, 587
chief human resources officer (CHRO), 16, 134
chief medical officer (CMO), 91
chief nurse executive (CNE), 63–64, 90–91, 130, 147, 154–156, 287–288, 295–299, 302, 316–317, 320, 412, 416, 426, 452, 469, 522, 527–528, 541–542, 563
chief nursing officer (CNO), 10, 12, 16–17, 56, 64–65, 125–126, 131, 134, 136, 138, 160–161, 185, 292, 323, 442, 452–454, 469, 514, 529, 543, 557, 585, 589, 591, 594
chief operating officer (COO), 63, 90, 296, 506
Children's Health Insurance Program (CHIP), 191–192, 437, 439, 562, 585
CHIP. *See* Children's Health Insurance Program
CHRO. *See* chief human resources officer
chronic care management (CCM), 189
chronic obstructive pulmonary disease (COPD), 176–177, 205, 210, 214–215, 217, 562
clinical documentation improvement (CDI), 177
CMI. *See* Case Mix Index
CMO. *See* chief medical officer
CNE. *See* chief nurse executive
CNO. *See* chief nursing officer
CNRN. *See* certified neuroscience registered nurse
coaching
  Benner's stage for the staff and nurse leader, 153
  career scenarios, 153
  definition, 149
  development and retention, 149
  key attributes, 153
  process, 150–151
  research review, 151–152
  standards, 152–153
  uses of, 151
COEs. *See* Centers of Excellence
collective bargaining agreements (CBAs), 466
Columbia University School of Nursing (CUSON), 342
community health
  definition, 200
  neighborhood and built environment, 204–205
competency
  AACN's The Essentials series, 58–59
  ALSN's perspectives, 58
  future implication, 65–67
  IOM competencies, 58
  lifelong learning, 55–56, 63
  nine categories, 56
  QSEN project, 58
  recent publications, 56
complexity leadership model
  adaptive space and process, 364
  enabling practices, 365
  quality and safety, 363–364
Comprehensive Primary Care Plus (CPC+), 188–189
condition of participation (CoP), 250
congestive heart failure (CHF), 188, 247
Consumers Assessment of Healthcare Providers and Systems (CAHPS), 293
COO. *See* chief operating officer
CoP. *See* condition of participation
COPD. *See* chronic obstructive pulmonary disease
cost centers, 454–456, 458–459, 462, 467
Council for Graduate Education for Administrative Nursing (CGEAN), 58
courageous caring leaders
  cache of resources, 8
  challenges, 7–12
  characteristics, 4–5
  clarity of communication, 13
  clinical compassion, 14
  collective intelligence, 14–15
  connecting with all stakeholders, 16
  crisis tackling, 13
  description, 4
  human and material resources, 10
  investing in self, 8
  morality, 5–6
  motivating self and team, 16
  optimistic realism, 13

paradigms shifting, 10
patience with slow adapters, 15
preparedness, 7–8
principle-guided decisions, 14
relationship skills, 10–11
sustenance during challenging time, 26
task delegations, 15
three elements, 6–7
timelines, 15
COVID-19, 25, 31, 67, 92, 203, 229, 253, 265,
        275, 288, 297, 307, 314, 453, 485, 491,
        503–504, 531, 535–536, 540, 552, 572
    courageous caring leaders, 4, 8, 10–11
    disaster response during, 299–301
    human resource management, 422, 424–426
    information technology, use in, 389, 402
    quality and safety, 353, 366
    professionalism, 38, 41, 47
    social determinants of health, 210, 216
    strategic planning, 324–325, 418–419
    telehealth, 243–244, 246, 562, 564, 566
    unanticipated transition, 508, 511, 513, 521
    vaccination program, 225–226
CPC+. See Comprehensive Primary Care Plus
CPS. See creative problem-solving
CPT. See Current Procedural Terminology
creative problem-solving (CPS), 367
critical access hospital (CAH), 528–529
Current Procedural Terminology (CPT),
        385, 392
CUSON. See Columbia University School of
        Nursing

data analytics
    key elements, 394–395
    missing data, 396
    preprocessing, 395–396
data management, information technology
    ability to access and use, 387–389
    clinical use, 382–383
    database structure, 390–392
    hospital use, 383
    life cycle, 385–386
    nonclinical data, 384
    quality, 389–390
    storing and transferring, 392–393
    structured, 385
    technological resources, 386–387
    types of data, 384
    unstructured, 384–385
    using new system, challenges, 402–403
data use agreement (DUA), 392–393, 406, 573
deep learning, 401–402
define-measure-analyze-improve-control
        (DMAIC), 20

DEI. See diversity, equity, and inclusion
Department of Health and Human Services
        (DHHS), 200–201, 205, 218, 220, 222,
        224, 230
design thinking, 367
Det Norske Veritas (DNV), 250
DHHS. See Department of Health and Human
        Services
diagnostic-related groups (DRGs), 172, 187
DICOM. See Digital Imaging and Communica-
        tions in Medicine
digital imaging, 385–386, 392, 402
Digital Imaging and Communications in
        Medicine (DICOM), 385–386
diversity, equity, and inclusion (DEI), 35, 66,
        77, 120, 487, 491–492
DMAIC. See define-measure-analyze-
        improve-control
DNV. See Det Norske Veritas
DRGs. See diagnostic-related groups
DUA. See data use agreement

EAP. See employee assistance program
EBP. See evidence-based practice
EEOC. See Equal Employment Opportunity
        Commission
EHR. See electronic health record
EI. See emotional intelligence
electronic health record (EHR), 178, 181, 299,
        339, 381–385, 387–389, 393, 395, 397,
        403, 567, 576
electronic medical record (EMR), 245–247,
        249, 253, 567
emergency medical services (EMS), 591–592
emotional intelligence (EI), 99–115, 126, 131,
        135–136, 151, 161, 522, 531, 536
    Bar-On model, 100–101
    benefits, 112
    communication, 110–111
    concept, 99
    definitions, 100
    Goleman–Boyatzis Model, 101
    health and well-being, 113
    intervention strategies, 111
    Mayer and Salovey's model, 100
    mindfulness meditation practice, 102–103
    positive thinking, 104
    self-management, 102
    social competence, 104
    synopsis, 111–112
    teams and organization effectiveness, 106
    turnover intention, examples, 110
    work environment, 109–110
employee assistance program (EAP), 24, 49
EMR. See electronic medical record

EMS. *See* emergency medical services
enhanced recovery protocols (ERPs), 288
Environmental Protection Agency (EPA), 206
EP. *See* executive presence
EPA. *See* Environmental Protection Agency
Equal Employment Opportunity Commission (EEOC), 211
ERPs. *See* enhanced recovery protocols
ethics and integrity, in nursing, 34–35
evidence-based practice (EBP), 20, 333, 338, 341–345, 575–576
    professional competencies, 65
    telehealth, 246
executive presence (EP), 325
external transitions, mergers, and acquisitions, 527–528

Fast Healthcare Interoperability Resources (FHIR), 385–386
Federal Emergency Management Agency (FEMA), 453
Federal Insurance Contributions Act (FICA), 587
Federal Medical Assistance Percentage (FMAP), 191
Federally Qualified Health Centers (FQHCs), 192
FEMA. *See* Federal Emergency Management Agency
FHIR. *See* Fast Healthcare Interoperability Resources
FICA. *See* Federal Insurance Contributions Act
financial reports, 465–466
financial resources, overview, 451–452. *See also* budget
financing
    bundled payments, 445
    Case Mix Index (CMI), 439
    clinical quality, 444–445
    economic principles, 435–436
    government payor sources, 438–439
    gross domestic product (GDP), 436–438
    healthcare reimbursement, 438
    key terminologies, 436
    macroeconomics, 435
    payor mix, 439–440
    private insurance reimbursement, 439
FMAP. *See* Federal Medical Assistance Percentage
FQHCs. *See* Federally Qualified Health Centers
Franklin Delano Roosevelt, 13, 171–172
FRLT. *See* Full Range Leadership Theory
FTEs. *See* full-time equivalents

Full Range Leadership Theory (FRLT), 123–124
full-time equivalents (FTEs), 411, 413, 455–465, 467–468, 471, 587
Future of Nursing 2020–2030, 9, 57, 63, 65–66, 479

GAO. *See* Government Accountability Office
GDP. *See* gross domestic product
Government Accountability Office (GAO), 223
government payor programs, 183–185
    accountable care organizations, 184–185
    Medicare, 183–184
gravitas, 43
gross domestic product (GDP), 173, 435–437, 442–443

HACs. *See* hospital-acquired conditions
HAPIs. *See* hospital-acquired pressure injuries
HCA. *See* Healthcare Corporation of America
HCAHPS. *See* Hospital Consumer Assessment of Healthcare Providers and Systems
HCL. *See* human-centered leadership
Healthcare Corporation of America (HCA), 506
Healthcare Financial Management Association (HFMA), 56, 62
Healthcare Information Management Systems Society (HIMSS), 10
Healthcare Leadership Alliance (HLA), 56, 58
healthcare, new delivery model, 424
healthcare organizations
    care delivery models, 62
    executive triad, 42
    inequity, 66
    national programs, 172–173, 177
    organizational impact, 177
    political agendas, 8
    transformational leadership, 44
health disparities, 66
health maintenance organizations (HMOs), 172
Health Professional Shortage Areas (HPSAs), 224
Healthy People 2020, 201
Healthy People 2030, 201, 218
healthy work environment (HWE), 122, 124–125, 127–129, 134, 137
HFMA. *See* Healthcare Financial Management Association
high-deductible health plans, 193
high reliability organizations (HROs), 293, 355–356, 360
    quality and safety, 355–356

HIMSS. *See* Healthcare Information Management Systems Society
historical milestones in nursing, 32–33
HLA. *See* Healthcare Leadership Alliance
HMOs. *See* health maintenance organizations
hospital-acquired conditions (HACs), 444, 452, 468, 511
hospital-acquired pressure injuries (HAPIs), 452, 468
Hospital Consumer Assessment of Healthcare Providers and Systems (HCAHPS), 6, 10, 134, 451
Hospital Readmission Reduction Program (HRRP), 444
Hospital Value-Based Purchasing (HVBP), 444
hours per patient day (HPPD), 413, 456–458, 460, 463, 466, 471, 585
HPPD. *See* hours per patient day
HPSAs. *See* Health Professional Shortage Areas
HRM. *See* human resource management
HROs. *See* high reliability organizations
HRRP. *See* Hospital Readmission Reduction Program
human-centered leadership (HCL), 119, 134–135
human resource management (HRM), 411–427, 469
    key components of, 411, 413, 427
    nurse leader's role, 411–412
    staffing needs, 412–414
    strategic direction, 412
HVBP. *See* Hospital Value-Based Purchasing
HWE. *See* healthy work environment

ICD codes. *See International Classification of Diseases* codes
ICN. *See* International Council of Nurses
ICNM. *See* International Center on Nurse Migration
ICU. *See* intensive care unit
IDP. *See* individual development plan
IHI. *See* Institute for Healthcare Improvement
individual development plan (IDP), 36–37, 51
innovation
    assessment, 263
    competencies, 262–263
    cultures, 265–266
    definition, 260
    diagnosing, 263–264
    educational programs, 268–269
    entrepreneurship vs, 261–262
    evaluation, 264
    ideation rate, 273–274
    impact in healthcare, 260–261
    implementation, 264
    incentivize clinicians, 267–268
    job description and responsibilities, 269–270
    leading, 266–267
    listening, 266
    mentoring and coaching, 270
    organizational policies, 269
    partnerships, 270
    physical or virtual epicenter, 270–271
    planning, 264
    resilience, 264–265
    sustainable structures, 259–260, 267, 277–278
Inpatient Quality Reporting (IQR), 444
Inside Scoop (Murthy), 85
Institute for Healthcare Improvement (IHI), 8, 22, 62, 133, 293, 310, 319, 354, 361, 444, 575, 577
Institute of Medicine (IOM), 114
Institutional Review Board (IRB), 341, 392–393, 406
intensive care unit (ICU), 90, 92, 366
Internal Revenue Service (IRS), 201, 505
internal review board, 573
internal transitions
    organizational chart changes, 523
International Center on Nurse Migration (ICNM), 580
International Classification of Diseases (ICD) codes, 385, 438
    ICD-10 codes, 392, 395, 438
International Council of Nurses (ICN), 32–33
internet of things (IoT), 10
intimate partner violence (IPV), 207
IOM. *See* Institute of Medicine
IoT. *See* internet of things
IPV. *See* intimate partner violence
IQR. *See* Inpatient Quality Reporting
IRB. *See* Institutional Review Board
IRS. *See* Internal Revenue Service

JCHS. *See* Joint Center for Housing Studies
Joint Center for Housing Studies (JCHS), 217

Kouzes and Posner, five leadership practices, 125

laissez-faire leadership, 122–123
leadership. *See also specific leadership styles*
    ANA Competency Model, 316–317
    authentic leadership (AL), 127–130
    authentic nursing leadership (ANL), 128
    authentically present leadership, 6–7

leadership (*continued*)
    complexity model, 363–364
    development, 136–137
    education, 60
    human-centered, 119, 134–135, 552–554
    Kouzes and Posner, five leadership
        practices, 125
    laissez-faire leadership, 122–123
    relational leadership (RL), 119–122, 124–138
    servant leadership (SL), 119, 130–134, 137
    skills, 416–417, 544
    systems thinking, 425–426
    transactional leadership, 122, 123
    transformational leadership (TL), 122–126,
        129, 136–137
Leadership Practices Inventory (LPI),
    123, 125
learning health system
    concept, 381–382
    five observable characteristics, 406
liberating structures (LSs), 340
lifelong learning, 55–56, 63
LPI. *See* Leadership Practices Inventory
LSs. *See* liberating structures

machine learning, 398–399
    supervised, 399–401
    unsupervised, 401
Magnet designation, 335
Magnet Recognition Model, 125
Managed Care Organizations (MCOs), 192
Maslow's hierarchy of needs, 5, 75–76
Mayer and Salovey's model, emotional
    intelligence (EI), 100
MCOs. *See* Managed Care Organizations
media message services (MMS), 37
Medicaid, 191–192
Medical Group Management Association
    (MGMA), 462
medical record number (MRN), 391–392
Medicare Advantage programs, 190
Medicare Shared Savings Program (MSSP), 184
mentoring
    definition, 156–157
    development and retention, 149
    executive presence, 149
    intentionality, 148
    key attributes, 158
    process, 157–158
    QSEN graduate-level competencies, 147
    research, 158–159
    resource support, 148
    uses, 158
MGMA. *See* Medical Group Management
    Association

mindfulness, 46–49
MLQ. *See* Multifactor Leadership
    Questionnaire
MMS. *See* media message services
MRN. *See* medical record number
MSSP. *See* Medicare Shared Savings Program
Multifactor Leadership Questionnaire (MLQ),
    123–124
multigenerational workforce, 76–77

NAHN. *See* National Association of Hispanic
    Nurses
narrow networks, 194
NASA. *See* National Aeronautics and Space
    Administration
NASEM. *See* National Academies of Sciences,
    Engineering, and Medicine
National Academies of Sciences, Engineering,
    and Medicine (NASEM), 57, 63, 65, 200,
    203, 227, 479, 486, 507
National Aeronautics and Space Administra-
    tion (NASA), 244
National Association of Hispanic Nurses
    (NAHN), 33
National Black Nurses Association
    (NBNA), 33
National Coalition of Ethnic Minority Nurse
    Associations (NCEMNA), 33
National Council of State Boards of Nursing
    (NCSBN), 33
National Database of Nursing Quality Indica-
    tors (NDNQI), 122, 457
National Institute of Nursing Research
    (NINR), 33
National Institutes of Health (NIH), 33
National Patient Safety Foundation
    (NPSF), 354
natural language processing (NLP), 384,
    396, 398
NBNA. *See* National Black Nurses Association
NCEMNA. *See* National Coalition of Ethnic
    Minority Nurse Associations
NCSBN. *See* National Council of State Boards
    of Nursing
NDNQI. *See* National Database of Nursing
    Quality Indicators
NECs. *See* Nurse Executive Competencies
NIH. *See* National Institutes of Health
NINR. *See* National Institute of Nursing
    Research
NLP. *See* natural language processing
NMCs. *See* Nurse Manager Competencies
NOBC. *See* Nurses on Boards Coalition
NPA. *See* nurse practice act
NPSF. *See* National Patient Safety Foundation

Nurse Executive Competencies (NECs), 56, 316
nurse executives
  additional roles and responsibilities, 63–64
  authentic presence, 7
  board and the relationship with management, 512–513
  board service, 495–496
  clinical quality, 446
  coaching and mentoring, 162
  competencies, 56–57
  continuous education, 61
  emotional intelligence (EI), 104–105, 114–115
  equitable healthcare policies, 90
  failed predictions, 11
  financial acumen, 469
  giving credit to team, 16
  healthcare reimbursement, 440
  human resource management, 426–427
  incentives, 268
  information management and big data, 405
  innovation, 278–279
  interprofessional collaborations, 62
  interview, board service, 514
  membership in professional associations, 61–62
  organization goal, 301–302
  philanthropy, 546–547
  population health, 227
  professionalism, 50
  quality and safety, 372
  relationship-based leadership, 138–139
  relationship-centered orientation, 89
  self-care, 12
  strategic development and planning, 320
  system level CNO, 63
  system perspectives for organizations, 344
  telehealth, 252–253
  unexpected transitions, 533–536
  use of Nursing Leadership Mission Critical Checklist, 25
  value-based contracting, 185
nurse leaders
  board assessment, 513–514
  diversity, equity, and inclusion, 66
  emotional intelligence development, 101–103, 108–109
  future implications, 60
  TEAMSTEPPS, 107–108
  telehealth competency, 250
Nurse Manager Competencies (NMCs), 56–57
nurse managers
  accountability for self and staff, 16
  best practices, 12

board governance, 514–515
board service, 485
clinical quality, 445–446
coaching and mentoring, 162
competencies, 57
conflict management, 420–421
emotional intelligence (EI), 113–114
financial acumen, 469
formal structure, clinical practice, 59–60
healthcare reimbursement, 440
human resource management, 427
incentives, 268
information management and big data, 403–404
innovation, 278
knowing organizational models, 293–294
leadership education, 60
mentorship and coaching, 63
patient–staff balancing, 7
philanthropy, 545
population health, 226
professionalism, 49
quality and safety, 371–372
relationship-based leadership, 137–138
self-care, 12
sense of community, 91
strategic development and planning, 321–323
system perspectives for organizations, 343–344
telehealth, 252
three domains of strategy implementation, 59
unexpected transitions, 531–533
use of Nursing Leadership Mission Critical Checklist, 25
nurse researcher, advocacy role, 40
Nurses on Boards Coalition (NOBC), 480–483, 487–489, 493, 495–496, 506, 510
  NOBC Board Competencies Model, 480, 487–489
Nursing Leadership Mission Critical Checklist, 18–19
  accepting setbacks, 25
  caring, 20
  committing to evidence, 20
  components, 20
  emotional support, 24
  five languages of appreciation in the workplace, 23
  improving the patient experience, 21
  networking, 24
  nurturing and self-care, 23
  patient individuality, 20–21
  practice of reflection, 24
  reducing healthcare costs, 23

Nursing Leadership Mission Critical
    Checklist (*continued*)
    staff individuality, 21
    truthful dialogue, 21–22
    well-cared for workforce, 22
nurturing behaviors, 88–89

OLA. *See* Organizational Leadership
    Assessment
optimizing strategy, professionalism, 42
OQR. *See* Outpatient Quality Reporting
Organizational Leadership Assessment
    (OLA), 131
organizational models
    authority, 291
    change management, 294–295, 297
    contextual and structural dimensions,
        295–296
    decision-making, 291–292
    departmentalization, 291
    division of labor, 291
    evolution of structures, 286–288
    five contingency factors, 295–296
    functional process, 290
    horizontal and vertical integration, 297
    practical considerations in structuring
        organizations, 299
    redesigning, 296–297
    role of technology, 297–299
    span of control, 291
    structure, process, and goals, 285–286
organization, system perspective
    communication and relationship building,
        333–335
    controlling, 337
    directing, 336
    essential components, 331–332
    goal achievement, 341
    key competencies for gaining, 332–333
    organizing, 336
    planning, 336
    staffing, 336
    structural empowerment, 335–336
    succession planning, 46
    team thinking, 337
    thinking skills, 336–337
Outpatient Quality Reporting (OQR), 444

PAC. *See* political action committee
paid time off (PTO), 459, 467
PAM. *See* Patient Activation Measure
Pathway to Excellence (PTE), 125
Patient Activation Measure (PAM), 175
patient care assistants (PCAs), 585–587

patient safety organizations (PSOs), 354
PCAs. *See* patient care assistants
PCPs. *See* primary care physicians
PDCA. *See* plan-do-check/study-act
Pediatric Intensive Care Unit (PICU), 90
per member per month (PMPM), 178, 189
personal protective equipment (PPE), 62, 38,
        225, 275, 417, 419, 422, 485, 552, 563,
        566, 569–573, 580
PHAB. *See* Public Health Accreditation Board
PHI. *See* protected health information
philanthropy
    business experience, 544
    definition, 539–540
    effective communication, 543
    fundraising roles, 541
    in nursing practice, 539
    interpersonal relationships, 543–544
    leadership skills, 544
    making a case, 542
    myths about fundraising, 544–545
    nursing competencies, 543–545
    primary support, 540–541
    team engagement, 544
    types of donations, 541
PICU. *See* Pediatric Intensive Care Unit
plan-do-check/study-act (PDCA), 20
PMHNs. *See* psychiatric-mental health nurses
PMPM. *See* per member per month
political action committee (PAC), 38
population health
    concept, 199–200
    health inequities, 200
PPE. *See* personal protective equipment
PPS. *See* prospective payment systems
PR. *See* public relations
primary care physicians (PCPs), 176–177, 179–
        180, 183–184, 188, 190, 221, 224, 229–230
professional citizenship, 77–78
professional organizations, president's role, 93
professionalism, 423
    advocacy, 38–39
    allyship, 45
    common core competencies, 31–32
    equity, social justice, and allyship, 40–41
    ethics and integrity, in nursing, 34–35
    executive presence, 43
    individual ethics, 36
    membership advocacy, 39
    mentorship, 45
    organization's ethical standards, 35–36
    social media presence, 36–38
    sponsorship, 45–46
    tenets of cultural humility, 41–42
prospective payment systems (PPS), 172
protected health information (PHI), 249

PSOs. *See* patient safety organizations
psychiatric-mental health nurses (PMHNs), 109
psychological safety, 355, 357, 359–360, 371–372
PTE. *See* Pathway to Excellence
PTO. *See* paid time off
Public Health Accreditation Board (PHAB), 201
public relations (PR), 318

QA. *See* quality assurance
QI. *See* quality improvement
QSEN. *See* Quality and Safety Education for Nurses
Quadruple Aim, 9, 444
qualified workforce, 421, 423
quality and safety
   adaptive space and process, 364
   affecting factors, 354–355
   agile methodology, 367–368
   complexity leadership model, 363–364
   design thinking, 367
   designing and driving culture, 362
   governance, 361
   growth mindset, 360–361
   high reliability organizations (HROs), 355–356
   leadership competencies, 353–354
   mindfulness culture, 357
   organizational coherence, 362–363
   psychological safety, 357–360
   situation awareness levels, 357
   spread, sustain, and scale attributes, 369–370
   through influence, 369
   use of tools, 368
Quality and Safety Education for Nurses (QSEN), 57–59, 147, 333
   QSEN project, 58
quality assurance (QA), 445
quality improvement (QI), 445

registered nurses (RNs), 179
relational leadership (RL), 119–122, 124–138
   authentic leadership (AL), 127–130
   best approach, 135–136
   five main components, 120–121
   followership and engagement, 120–121
   human-centered leadership (HCL), 119, 134–135
   nonrelational styles vs, 122–123
   nursing-specific engagement, 122
   overview of specific theories, 119–120
   resonant leadership, 135
   servant leadership (SL), 119, 130–134, 137

transformational leadership (TL), 122–126, 129, 136–137
relationship management
   acknowledgment of failure, 87–88
   apology, role in, 81–82, 89
   being physically and emotionally attentive, 88
   belonging, 74–75
   check-ins and settling practices, 82–84
   diversity, equity, and inclusion (DEI), 77
   empathic language, 79–81, 89
   expressing gratitude, 89
   feedforward, 81
   forgiveness, 89
   generational preferences, 76–77
   genuineness, 73
   giving gifts, 89
   If You Knew Me, statements, 86
   Inside Scoop (Murthy), 85
   interpersonal, 76
   language, use in, 78–81
   listening, 88
   managing conflicts, 419–420
   meaningful connection (break bread together), 89
   minute matrix, 85
   person-centered language, 79
   professional, 77–78
   rituals, 82
   role of communication, 421–422
   Stepping Stones (Progroff), 85
   strength-based language, 79
   team charters, 86–87
   warm-up activities, 84–85
relative value units (RVUs), 591
remote monitoring, 562–564, 567
remote patient monitoring (RPM), 245–246, 253, 297
resonant leadership, 135
RL. *See* relational leadership
RNs. *See* registered nurses
RPM. *See* remote patient monitoring
RVUs. *See* relative value units

SDOH. *See* social determinants of health
self-care, 7, 12, 46–49
servant leadership (SL), 119, 130–134, 137
   advantages and disadvantages, 133
   characteristics and behaviors, 131–133
   follower outcomes, 133
   nursing and, 133
SIRS. *See* systemic inflammatory response syndrome
skilled nursing facilities (SNFs), 182, 185, 192
SL. *See* servant leadership

SNAP. *See* Supplemental Nutrition Assistance Program
SNFs. *See* skilled nursing facilities
SNOMED CT, 395
social determinants of health (SDOH), 175–176
  access to foods, 207–208
  age and disability discrimination, 211
  civic participation, 212
  COVID-19 crisis and vaccination program, 225–226
  crime and violence, 207
  discrimination, 209–210
  early childhood education and development, 220
  economic stability, 213–214
  education, 218–219
  employment, 216
  enrollment in higher education, 221
  environmental elements, 205–206
  food insecurity, 216–217
  gender discrimination, 210
  health literacy, 224–225
  healthcare access, 221–224
  healthy eating patterns, 207–208
  high school graduation, 220–221
  housing stock and quality, 206–207, 215–216
  incarceration, 211–212
  key influencers, 202–204
  language and literacy, 219–220
  LGBTQ+ discrimination, 211
  neighborhood and built environment, 204–205
  poverty, 215
  primary care, access, 224
  role in community health, 201–202
  shelter adequacy (housing instability), 217–218
  social and community concerns, 208–209
  social cohesion, 212–213
social inequities, 66
Society of Nurse Scientists, Innovators, Entrepreneurs, and Leaders (SONSIEL), 268
SONSIEL. *See* Society of Nurse Scientists, Innovators, Entrepreneurs, and Leaders
SSIs. *See* surgical site infections
standards of nursing practice, 33–34
Stepping Stones (Progroff), 85
strategic development and planning
  ANA Leadership Competency Model, 316–317
  assessment and analysis phase, 310–311
  balanced scorecard tool, 314–315
  best practices, 310
  corporate level, 317
  evaluation phase, 316

  execution phase, 314–315
  formulation phase, 313–314
  historical perspective, 308–309
  IHI recommendations, 319
  key actions, 326
  key stakeholders, questions, 313
  mission statement, sample, 311
  new payment models, 307–308
  nurse leader competency, 316
  organizational levels, 310
  reasons for failure, 327
  SWOT and SOAR analysis, 312
  10-step process, 317–319
  values, sample, 312
  vision statement, sample, 311
strategic management, nursing plan, 417–418
STS. *See* Systems Thinking Scale
Supplemental Nutrition Assistance Program (SNAP), 207
surgical site infections (SSIs), 585–586
systemic inflammatory response syndrome (SIRS), 366
Systems Thinking Scale (STS), 337

TCM. *See* transitional care management
technological advances, 10
telehealth
  delivery models, 243
  evidence-based practice and application, 246
  future consideration, 250–251
  history, 244
  means of communication, 246–247
  nursing competency, 250
  regulatory standards, 249–250
  terminology, 244–245
  use of, 245
The Joint Commission (TJC), 172, 244 250, 506, 510, 513
Thompson, Pamela Austin, 516
tiered networks, 193–194
TJC. *See* The Joint Commission
TL. *See* transformational leadership
transactional leadership, 122, 123
transformational leadership (TL), 122–126, 129, 136–137
  authentic leadership vs, 129–130
  "Four I's," 123–124
  Kouzes and Posner, five leadership practices, 125
  potential disadvantages, 126
transitional care management (TCM), 179
Triple Aim, 444

Ubuntu, 78
unanticipated transitions
  challenging experiences, 521–522
  competitive market challenges, 529–530
  environmental challenges, 531
  external transition, 527–528
  financial challenges, 523–524
  organizational chart changes, 523
  position elimination, 525–526
  reduction in workforce, 525–526
  relationship challenges, 530–531
  relevant literature, 522–523
  working with consultants, 524–525
U.S. Department of Agriculture (USDA),
    207–208, 216
University of Texas Medical Branch
    (UTMB), 271
USDA. *See* U.S. Department of Agriculture
UTMB. *See* University of Texas Medical Branch

value-based care (VBC), 171, 173–174, 177,
    183, 189
  benefit design, 193
  budgeting strategy, 180–181
  Bundle Payments for Care Improvement
    (BPCI) initiative, 187–188
  care management structure, 179–180
  care redesign, 177–178
  Centers of Excellence (COEs), 194
  Children's Health Insurance Program
    (CHIP), 191–192
  chronic disease management, 189–190
  closed network of services, 174
  commercial payors, 193
  Comprehensive Primary Care Plus (CPC+),
    188–189
  contracting performance, 181–182
  data and analytics, 174–175

  data-driven operations, 183
  fee-for-service versus, 173–174
  government payor programs, 183–185
  high-deductible health plans, 193
  Medicaid, 191–192
  Medicare Advantage programs, 190
  narrow networks, 194
  new innovative strategies, 189
  organizational impact and operational
    decisions, 177
  patient activation, 175
  patient attribution, 174
  physician alignment outcomes, 189
  predictive analytics and outcomes, 182–183
  reference pricing, 194
  resource alignment, 178
  risk stratification, 175
  social determinants of health (SDOH),
    175–176
  strategies, 174
  tiered networks, 193–194
  transitional care management hub, 178–179
  value-based insurance design, 194
  wellness and prevention, 175
value-based healthcare, 442–444
  international performance ranking, 443
value-based programs, 177–178, 180, 183
Value-Based Purchasing (VBP), 451
VBC. *See* value-based care
VBP. *See* Value-Based Purchasing
Veterans Health Administration (VHA), 159
VHA. *See* Veterans Health Administration

WHO. *See* World Health Organization
workforce, 412, 415, 423–424, 426–427
World Health Organization (WHO), 4, 19,
    32–33, 47, 175, 199–200, 207, 412,
    438, 561